Amyotrophic Lateral Sclerosis: Current Research

Amyotrophic Lateral Sclerosis: Current Research

Editor: Finn Cooper

MURPHY & MOORE
www.murphy-moorepublishing.com

www.murphy-moorepublishing.com

MURPHY & MOORE

Cataloging-in-Publication Data

Amyotrophic lateral sclerosis : current research / edited by Finn Cooper.
p. cm.
Includes bibliographical references and index.
ISBN 978-1-63987-044-8
1. Amyotrophic lateral sclerosis. 2. Motor neurons--Diseases. 3. Neuromuscular diseases. I. Cooper, Finn.
RC406.A24 A49 2022
616.83--dc23

Murphy & Moore Publishing,
1 Rockefeller Plaza,
New York City, NY 10020, USA

ISBN 978-1-63987-044-8 (Hardback)

Contents

Preface

Amyotrophic lateral sclerosis is a neurodegenerative and neuromuscular disease. It affects the motor neurons which control the voluntary muscles. Some of the symptoms of this disease are muscle twitches, stiff muscles, difficulty in swallowing or speaking, and muscle wasting. The treatment of amyotrophic lateral sclerosis involves improving the symptoms. Non-invasive ventilation and mechanical ventilation can be used to prolong life. Genetic and environmental factors can affect the chances of being affected by amyotrophic lateral sclerosis. One of the characteristic features of this disease is the death of lower motor neurons and upper motor neurons. The genes which are considered to be behind amyotrophic lateral sclerosis are classified on the basis of their function into cytoskeleton, protein degradation and RNA processing. This book discusses the fundamentals as well as modern approaches of amytrophic lateral sclerosis. It will also provide interesting topics for research which interested readers can take up. This book will provide comprehensive knowledge to the readers.

This book unites the global concepts and researches in an organized manner for a comprehensive understanding of the subject. It is a ripe text for all researchers, students, scientists or anyone else who is interested in acquiring a better knowledge of this dynamic field.

I extend my sincere thanks to the contributors for such eloquent research chapters. Finally, I thank my family for being a source of support and help.

Editor

1

Differential autophagy power in the spinal cord and muscle of transgenic ALS mice

Valeria Crippa[1,2], Alessandra Boncoraglio[1,2,3], Mariarita Galbiati[1,2], Tanya Aggarwal[4], Paola Rusmini[1,2], Elisa Giorgetti[1,2], Riccardo Cristofani[1,2], Serena Carra[3,5], Maria Pennuto[4,6] and Angelo Poletti[1,2]*

[1] *Sezione di Biomedicina e Endocrinologia, Dipartimento di Scienze Farmacologiche e Biomolecolari, Centro di Eccellenza sulle Malattie Neurodegenerative, Università degli Studi di Milano, Milano, Italy*

[2] *Centro InterUniversitario sulle Malattie Neurodegenerative, Università degli Studi di Firenze, Milano, Genova e Roma Tor Vergata, Italy*

[3] *Department of Cell Biology, University Medical Center of Groningen, Groningen, Netherlands*

[4] *Department of Neuroscience and Brain Technologies, Istituto Italiano di Tecnologia, Genova, Italy*

[5] *Sezione di Fisiologia e Neuroscienze, Dipartimento di Scienze Biomediche, Metaboliche e Neuroscienze, Università degli Studi di Modena e Reggio Emilia, Modena, Italy*

[6] *Dulbecco Telethon Institute Laboratory of Neurodegenerative Diseases, Centre for Integrative Biology (CIBIO), University of Trento, Italy*

Edited by:
Ricardo Tapia, Universidad Nacional Autónoma de México, Mexico

Reviewed by:
Jie Zhang, University of Texas Health Science Center at San Antonio, USA
Lee J. Martin, Johns Hopkins University School of Medicine, USA

****Correspondence:***
Angelo Poletti, Sezione di Biomedicina e Endocrinologia, Dipartimento di Scienze Farmacologiche e Biomolecolari, Centro di Eccellenza sulle Malattie Neurodegenerative, Università degli Studi di Milano, Via Balzaretti 9, 20133 Milano, Italy
e-mail: angelo.poletti@unimi.it

Amyotrophic lateral sclerosis (ALS) is a motoneuron disease characterized by misfolded proteins aggregation in affected motoneurons. In mutant SOD1 (mutSOD1) ALS models, aggregation correlates to impaired functions of proteasome and/or autophagy, both essential for the intracellular chaperone-mediated protein quality control (PQC), and to a reduced mutSOD1 clearance from motoneurons. Skeletal muscle cells are also sensitive to mutSOD1 toxicity, but no mutSOD1 aggregates are formed in these cells, that might better manage mutSOD1 than motoneurons. Thus, we analyzed in spinal cord and in muscle of transgenic (tg) G93A-SOD1 mice at presymptomatic (PS, 8 weeks) and symptomatic (S, 16 weeks) stages, and in age-matched control mice, whether mutSOD1 differentially modulates relevant PQC players, such as HSPB8, BAG3, and BAG1. Possible sex differences were also considered. No changes of HSPB8, BAG3, and BAG1 at PS stage (8 weeks) were seen in all tissues examined in tg G93A-SOD1 and control mice. At S stage (16 weeks), HSPB8 dramatically increased in skeletal muscle of tg G93A-SOD1 mice, while a minor increase occurred in spinal cord of male, but not female tg G93A-SOD1 mice. BAG3 expression increased both in muscle and spinal cord of tg G93A-SOD1 mice at S stage, BAG1 expression increased only in muscle of the same mice. Since, HSPB8-BAG3 complex assists mutSOD1 autophagic removal, we analyzed two well-known autophagic markers, LC3 and p62. Both LC3 and p62 mRNAs were significantly up-regulated in skeletal muscle of tg G93A-SOD1 mice at S stage (16 weeks). This suggests that mutSOD1 expression induces a robust autophagic response specifically in muscle. Together these results demonstrate that, in muscle mutSOD1-induced autophagic response is much higher than in spinal cord. In addition, if mutSOD1 exerts toxicity in muscle, this may not be mediated by misfolded proteins accumulation. It remains unclear whether in muscle mutSOD1 toxicity is related to aberrant autophagy activation.

Keywords: amyotrophic lateral sclerosis, motoneurons, autophagy, HSPB8, BAG3, BAG1, protein quality control

INTRODUCTION

Autophagy is a fundamental intracellular degradative pathway activated to respond to the accumulation of aberrantly folded (misfolded) proteins (Mizushima and Komatsu, 2011). Autophagy is required for the cellular protein quality control (PQC) system, which also includes molecular chaperones and the ubiquitin-proteasome degradative system (UPS) (Carra et al., 2012). These systems work together protecting cells particularly sensitive to misfolded protein toxicity, such as motoneurons (Rusmini et al., 2010; Bendotti et al., 2012; Carra et al., 2013). Motoneurons are major targets of toxicity in diseases linked to mutant proteins prone to misfold, such as in amyotrophic lateral sclerosis (ALS) (Pasinelli and Brown, 2006; Rusmini et al., 2010; Sau et al., 2011; Strong and Yang, 2011; Carra et al., 2012, 2013; Robberecht and Philips, 2013). Most ALS cases appear in sporadic (sALS) forms; only about 10–15% have familial (fALS) history, and are clinically indistinguishable from sALS. fALSs have been associated with mutations in different genes, such as the superoxide dismutase 1 (SOD1), TAR DNA-binding protein 43 (TDP-43), fused in sarcoma/translocated in liposarcoma protein (FUS/TLS), optineurin (Robberecht and Philips, 2013), or the C9ORF72 gene (Dejesus-Hernandez et al., 2011; Renton et al., 2011; Ash et al., 2013; Lashley et al., 2013; Mori et al., 2013). Notably, also the wild type (wt) forms of the mutated fALS proteins may show aberrant behavior in sALS (e.g., oxydized wtSOD1, cleaved C-terminus of wtTDP-43, etc.) (Neumann et al., 2006; Daoud et al., 2009; Bosco and Landers, 2010; Bosco et al., 2010), suggesting the existence of a common pathological mechanism. An explanation for this is that these proteins (either the modified wt or the mutant forms) have the propensity to misfold and aggregate forming insoluble inclusions that are a key neuropathological hallmark of ALS. Inclusions may alter several cellular functions, such as axonal transport, mitochondrial, and/or degradative activities, thereby leading or contributing to motoneuron death (Pasinelli and Brown, 2006; Cozzolino et al., 2008; Seetharaman et al., 2009).

In recent years, emerging evidences support the idea that also non-neuronal cells (e.g., surrounding astrocytes or Schwann cells, chemotactically attracted microglial cells, and target muscle cells) might contribute to disease onset and progression (Boillée et al., 2006), by making motoneuronal cells more sensitive to protein toxicity. For example, selective expression of mutant SOD1 (mutSOD1) in skeletal muscle induced atrophy associated with the loss of motoneurons in the anterior horn of the spinal cord (Dobrowolny et al., 2008a; Corti et al., 2009; Wong and Martin, 2010). However, mutSOD1 largely accumulates in spinal cord of transgenic mice expressing human G93A-SOD1 (Tg G93A-SOD1) (Cheroni et al., 2005, 2009; Basso et al., 2006, 2009; Bendotti et al., 2012), but not in skeletal muscle of the same mice at any stage of disease (Galbiati et al., 2012; Wei et al., 2012); thus, muscle cells better cope with misfolded mutSOD1 species than motoneuronal cells. This may be due to an higher muscular degradative capabilities compared to motoneurons (Onesto et al., 2011). In fact, in both cells, mutSOD1 clearance involves both UPS and autophagy, but both the proteasome and autophagy activities are higher in muscle cells than in motoneuronal cells.

The interplay between UPS and autophagy is finely regulated through a mechanism that involves the co-chaperones BAG1 and BAG3, which act as a switch between the two pathways (Luders et al., 2000; Carra et al., 2008a; Gamerdinger et al., 2009; Arndt et al., 2010; Zhang and Qian, 2011). BAG1 is expressed at relatively higher levels in young tissues, paralleled by higher UPS activity, while BAG3 is expressed at higher levels in aged tissues, characterized by higher autophagic activity (Gamerdinger et al., 2009), and the BAG3:BAG1 ratio determines the fate of client proteins to be degraded through either UPS or autophagy. Indeed, BAG1 routes substrates to UPS by interacting with a complex formed by the chaperone HSC70 and the ubiquitinating enzyme CHIP. UPS overwhelming or impairment, due to misfolded proteins, results in upregulation of BAG3 and its partner, the chaperone HSPB8 (a small heat shock protein involved in misfolded proteins recognition) (Wang et al., 2008; Du et al., 2009; Crippa et al., 2010b; Gentilella and Khalili, 2011; Carra et al., 2013). The increased BAG3:BAG1 ratio favors a stoichiometric HSC70/CHIP complex association to BAG3/HSPB8 complex, allowing the p62-mediated autophagic removal of CHIP-ubiquitinated substrates (Crippa et al., 2010b; Gamerdinger et al., 2011; Zhang and Qian, 2011; Carra et al., 2012, 2013). Interestingly, we found that mutSOD1 blocks the autophagic flux in motoneurons, but not in muscle cells (Onesto et al., 2011). This autophagic flux blockage can be counteracted by HSPB8, which participates together with BAG3/HSC70/CHIP in the autophagic clearance of several different misfolded proteins (polyQ containing proteins, mutSOD1, a truncated form of TDP-43) (Carra et al., 2005, 2008a,b, 2013; Crippa et al., 2010b). In addition, HSPB8 induces translation attenuation via phosphorylation of eIF2alpha (Carra et al., 2009), thereby decreasing the amount of aggregation-prone proteins to levels manageable by PQC.

In this study, we analyzed whether spinal cord, which comprises the two main cell targets of SOD1 toxicity, namely motoneuronal and astroglial cells, and skeletal muscle, differentially activate the HSPB8 mediated PQC system in response to mutSOD1 in tg G93A-SOD1 mice. The results demonstrate that the autophagic response of muscle tissue to the mutSOD1 expression is much higher than that found in the spinal cord of the same mice, suggesting that if mutSOD1 exerts toxicity in muscle, this may not be mediated by misfolded protein accumulation.

MATERIALS AND METHODS

ANIMALS

All the procedures involving animals and their care were carried out following the institutional guidelines and in accordance with national (D.L. no. 116, G.U. suppl. 40, Feb. 18, 1992), and international laws and policies (EEC Council Directives 86/609, OJ L 358, 1 DEC.12, 1987), and were approved by the Italian Institute of Technology Animal Care Committee. All the animals were kept under controlled temperature and humidity conditions with standardized dark/light cycles of 12 h each. Food (standard pellets) and water were supplied *ad libitum*. BL6JL Tg(SOD1)2Gur/J (Stock number 002297, Charles River, Wilmington, MA, USA) male mice or BL6JL-Tg(SOD1*G93A)2Gur/J (Stock number 002726, Charles River) male mice were crossed with wt female mice purchased (Stock number 100012, Charles River) or obtained in house by crossing C57Bl/6J female and SJL male mice. All the experiments were performed in mice coming from the F1 generation of the cross described above. Non-transgenic littermates were used as controls (NTg). Mice were genotyped by PCR on tail DNA as previously described (Gurney et al., 1994), using REDExtract-N-Amp Tissue PCR kit (Sigma-Aldrich, St. Louis, MO, USA). To evaluate disease stages, starting from the 8th week of age and twice a week, mice were tested for deficit by rotarod, and hanging wire by the same operator as previously described (Palazzolo et al., 2009). Body weight loss was also monitored. Disease onset was set as the time at which the mouse permanently starts to lose body weight. Four mice per group were anesthetized with isoflurane and sacrificed at 8 or 16 weeks of age, corresponding to presymptomatic (PS) or symptomatic (S) stage of disease. Quadriceps muscles and spinal cord were rapidly collected after the sacrifice, snap frozen in liquid nitrogen, and conserved at −80°C until RNA and protein extraction.

RNA EXTRACTION

Total RNA from frozen spinal cords or muscles was extracted using the standard TRI Reagent protocol based on the method developed by Chomczynski and Sacchi (Chomczynski and Sacchi, 1987). RNA was subsequently extracted in accordance to manufacturer's protocol (Sigma-Aldrich). The precipitated RNA was dissolved in RNase-free water. Total RNA (1 μg) was treated for 15 min at room temperature with 1 U of DNaseI (Sigma-Aldrich). Samples were reverse-transcribed using the High-Capacity cDNA Reverse Transcription Kit (Life Technologies Corporation, Carlsbad, CA, USA) according to the manufacturer's instructions, in a 20 μL volume. Primers for selected genes were designed via the Primer Express software (Life Technologies Corporation) and purchased from MWG Biotech (Ebersberg, Germany). Primer sequences were as follows: mouse HSPB8: 5′- ATA CGT GGA AGT TTC AGG CA -3′ (forward), 5′- TCC TTT GAC CTA ACG CAA CC -3′ (reverse); mouse BAG3: 5′- ATG GAC CTG AGC GAT CTC A -3′ (forward), 5′- CAC GGG GAT GGG GAT GTA -3′ (reverse); mouse BAG1: 5′- GAA ACA CCG TTG TCA GCA CT -3′ (forward), 5′- GCT CCA CTG TGT CAC ACT C -3′ (reverse); mouse MAP-LC3b: 5′- CGT CCT GGA CAA GAC CA -3′ (forward), 5′- CCA TTC ACC AGG AGG AA - 3′ (reverse); mouse p62: 5′- AGG GAA CAC AGC AAG CT -3′ (forward), 5′- GCC AAA GTG TCC ATG TTT CA -3′ (reverse); mouse GAPDH: 5′-CCA GAA CAT CAT CCC TGC AT-3′ (forward), 5′-CAG TGA GCT TCC CGT TCA-3′ (reverse). The evaluated efficiency of each set of primers was close to 100% for both target and reference gene. Real-time PCR was performed using the CFX 96 Real Time System (Bio-Rad Laboratories, Hercules, CA, USA), in a 10 μL total volume, using the iTaq SYBR Green Supermix (BioRad), and with 500 nmol primers. PCR cycling conditions were as follows: 94°C for 10 min, 40 cycles at 94°C for 15 s, and 60°C for 1 min. Melting curve analysis was performed at the end of each PCR assay to control specificity. Data was expressed as Ct values and used for the relative quantification of targets with the ΔΔCt calculation to give N-fold changes in gene expression. Values were normalized to those of GAPDH. To exclude potential bias due to averaging data transformed through the equation $2^{-\Delta\Delta Ct}$, all statistics were performed with ΔCt values. Each experiment was carried out with four independent samples, and each sample was run in duplicate wells.

The BAG3:BAG1 relative ratio was obtained considering the group of 8 weeks-old NTg female mice as control for the basal physiological condition of the PQC system. In particular, for each sample a single BAG3:BAG1 ratio was determined [measuring the $(\text{BAG3 } 2^{-\Delta\Delta Ct}/\text{BAG1 } 2^{-\Delta\Delta Ct})_{sample}$] and the mean BAG3:BAG1 ratio of control was subtracted [$(\text{BAG3 } 2^{-\Delta\Delta Ct}/\text{BAG1 } 2^{-\Delta\Delta Ct})_{control}$]. Finally, the resulting values were normalized by the mean BAG3:BAG1 ratio of the control 8 weeks-old NTg female mice.

WESTERN BLOTTING AND FILTER RETARDATION ASSAY (WB AND FRA)

Total proteins from frozen spinal cord or muscles were extracted in 1% SDS using the standard TRI Reagent protocol, in accordance with the manufacturer's protocol (Sigma-Aldrich). Protein concentration was determined with the bicinchoninic acid method (BCA assay, EuroClone, Pero, Milan, Italy). WB analysis was performed on 12% sodium dodecyl sulfate (SDS)-polyacrylamide gel electrophoresis loading 15 μg of total proteins. Samples were then electrotransferred to Nitrocellulose membrane (Bio-Rad) using the Trans-Blot Turbo (Bio-Rad). The membranes were treated with a blocking solution containing 5% non-fat dried milk powder (EuroClone) in TBS-T for 1 h and then incubated with the primary antibodies: (1) home-made rabbit polyclonal anti-HSPB8 (kindly provided by Dr Jacques Landry, Quèbec, Canada, dilution 1:1000); (2) rabbit-polyclonal anti-BAG3 antibody (Abcam, Cambridge, UK; dilution 1:1000); (3) rabbit-polyclonal anti-BAG1 (Santa Cruz Biotechnology, Dallas, Texas, USA; dilution 1:1000); (4) rabbit polyclonal anti-LC3 (Sigma; dilution 1:1000); (5) rabbit polyclonal anti-SQSTM1/p62 (Abcam; dilution 1:1000); (6) rabbit-polyclonal anti-GAPDH (Santa Cruz Biotech; dilution 1:1000); (7) rabbit-polyclonal anti-SOD1 (SOD-100; StressMarq, Victoria, BC, Canada; dilution 1:1000). Immunoreactivity was detected using goat anti-rabbit (sc-2004, Santa Cruz Biotech, dilution 1:5000) secondary peroxidase-conjugated antibody. Immunoreactivity was then visualized using the enhanced chemiluminescence detection kit reagent (ECL prime Western Blotting Substrate, GE Healthcare, Maidstone, UK). The same membranes were subsequently processed with different antibodies to detect the levels of different proteins in the same samples loaded on the gel, after stripping for 10 min at room temperature (StripABlot, EuroClone). Each experiment was carried out twice, with four independent samples.

FRA was performed using a slot-blot apparatus (Bio-Rad). 3 μg of total proteins were loaded on a 0.2 μm cellulose acetate membrane (Whatman, GE Healthcare), pre-incubated with 20% methanol, washed with water and then incubated with 1% SDS solution. After slight vacuum filtration, slot-blot membranes were probed as described for WB.

A ChemiDoc XRS System (Bio-Rad) was used for the image acquisition of WB and FRA.

STATISTICAL ANALYSIS

Statistical analysis was performed through two-tailed Student *t-test* for comparisons between 8 and 16 weeks mice of the same group (NTg/Tg wtSOD1/Tg G93A-SOD1) and two-way analysis of variance (ANOVA) for group comparisons, using the PRISM software (GraphPad, San Diego, CA, USA). Specific group pair(s) statistical difference was determined by the Bonferroni *post-hoc* test. Data were expressed as mean ± SD of four independent samples.

RESULTS

Our study has been performed on 8 (presymptomatic stage, PS) and 16 weeks-old (symptomatic stage, S) Tg G93A-SOD1 mice, compared to age-matched non-transgenic (NTg) and transgenic human wild-type SOD1 (Tg wtSOD1) mice. In addition, since gender differences have been reported to affect the age of onset and disease progression both in ALS patients (Kurtzke, 1982; Giagheddu et al., 1983; Rudnicki, 1999; Manjaly et al., 2010; McCombe and Henderson, 2010; Lee et al., 2013a) and rodent models of ALS (Veldink et al., 2003; Suzuki et al., 2007), with male gender being more susceptible, we analyzed males and females separately. Based on our data on the protective role of HSPB8 in ALS, which is mediated by autophagy, we analyzed the expression of this small chaperone in the spinal cord and muscle of Tg G93A-SOD1 mice and control mice. We also analyzed the expression of the two co-chaperones BAG3 and BAG1, which may mediate the PQC activity by selecting the proper degradative system to be activated in cells in response to proteotoxicity. Finally, we analyzed two widely used autophagic markers, LC3 and p62. Using homogenates of spinal cord and skeletal muscle derived from Tg G93A-SOD1 mice and age-matched NTg or Tg wtSOD1 mice, we first compared the levels of wtSOD1 and mutSOD1 in both the soluble and insoluble fractions in 8 (corresponding to PS stage) and 16 weeks (corresponding to S stage) male and female mice. As shown in **Figure 1**, soluble monomeric wtSOD1 and mutSOD1 were analyzed by western blot (WB; **A**: spinal cord; **B**: muscle). In the spinal cord of Tg mice the levels of wtSOD1 and mutSOD1 proteins were similar, while in skeletal muscle mutSOD1 levels were apparently lower as compared to wtSOD1 and no gender differences were observed. Using motoneuronal and muscle ALS models as well as tg G93A-SOD1 mice, we recently demonstrated that mutSOD1 accumulated both in motoneuronal cells and in spinal cord of tg mice (already at PS, increasing at S stage), but did not accumulate in ALS muscle cells and ALS muscle tissues at any age tested (Onesto et al., 2011; Galbiati et al., 2012). These data were recently confirmed and extended by Wei and coll. (Wei et al., 2013) using a different strain of tg G93A-SOD1 mice. Thus, here we repeated these experiments to provide a general view of mutSOD1 behavior in our mice. A representative filter retardation assay (FRA; **C**: spinal cord; **D**: muscle) illustrating the corresponding insoluble fractions of mutSOD1 is reported. The FRA analysis confirmed the presence of relevant amounts of mutSOD1 insoluble species in samples of S stage tg G93A-SOD1 mice. In muscle tissue, no mutSOD1 insoluble species were present, with the exception of samples obtained from tg G93A-SOD1 male mice at S stage (16 weeks), suggesting that muscle tissue may better cope with the misfolded fraction of mutSOD1 as compared to cells in the spinal cord.

Since we already showed that overexpression of HSPB8 prevents mutSOD1 intracellular accumulation by facilitating its clearance through autophagy (Crippa et al., 2010a,b), we analyzed HSPB8 mRNA levels in the spinal cord and skeletal muscle in response to wt or mutSOD1 expression. In spinal cord, we observed a significant increase of HSPB8 mRNA transcript levels in response to mutSOD1 expression in S stage (16 weeks) Tg G93A-SOD1 male mice as compared to age-matched NTg or Tg wtSOD1 mice (**Figure 2A**) (Crippa et al., 2010b). Interestingly, Tg G93A-SOD1 female mice did not show any significant increase of HSPB8 transcript level in response to mutSOD1expression, suggesting the existence of gender differences in the PQC system activated by misfolded proteins in spinal cord. In male 16-week-old NTg mice, the expression level of HSPB8 tended to decrease, even if it did not become statistically significant. However, we already shown that HSPB8 expression significantly decreases when older NTg mice (age-matched with Tg G93A-SOD1 mice at end stage of disease) were analyzed (Crippa et al., 2010a,b). In contrast to what we found in spinal cord, in the skeletal muscles of S stage (16 weeks) Tg G93A-SOD1 mice we observed a dramatic increase of HSPB8 mRNA (up to 8-fold) (**Figure 2B**). Importantly, this HSPB8 mRNA upregulation occurred in both sexes. HSPB8 mRNA levels were unaffected in both sexes in NTg and Tg wtSOD1 mice at all ages considered.

The robust induction of HSPB8 expression in response to mutSOD1 in muscle might serve to initiate and/or facilitate the clearance of aberrant mutSOD1 species. This may avoid the aggregation of misfolded protein and the accumulation to levels that cannot be managed by the PQC system. Considering that mutSOD1 species are degraded by the saturable UPS, but it can be preferentially degraded by the highly efficient autophagic system in presence of high levels of HSPB8 (Crippa et al., 2010b) and that the pro-degradative activity of HSPB8 is mediated by its partner BAG3, we analyzed the expression levels of BAG3 in both spinal cord and muscle (Carra et al., 2008b; Carra, 2009). We found that in the spinal cord of both male and female mutSOD1 mice BAG3 expression remains unchanged at PS stage (8 weeks), but it was significantly increased by approximately 3-fold compared to NTg or Tg wtSOD1 mice at S stage (16 weeks, **Figure 3A**). Furthermore, the mutSOD1-induced appearance of symptoms correlated with a great response of the HSPB8-BAG3-mediated PQC system also in muscle (**Figure 3B**). Curiously, in female mice, BAG3 expression differed from that of HSPB8, since it was upregulated by mutSOD1 both in spinal cord and in muscle of tg G93A-SOD1 mice at S stage.

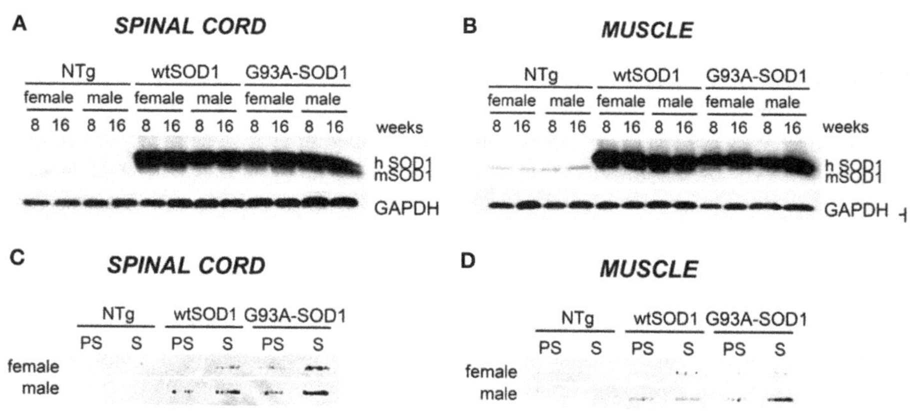

FIGURE 1 | Biochemical properties of wtSOD1 and mutSOD1 in spinal cord and muscle of ALS animal models. Western Blot (WB) analysis and Filter Retardation Assay (FRA) on proteins extracted from whole spinal cord (**A**, WB; **C**, FRA) or quadriceps muscles (**B**, WB; **D**, FRA) of female and male non-transgenic (NTg) mice, of mice expressing the wild type human SOD1 transgene (wtSOD1), and of mice expressing the G93A mutant form of human SOD1 (G93A-SOD1), at 8 (corresponding to presymptomatic stage, PS, in Tg G93A-SOD1 mice) or 16 weeks (corresponding to symptomatic stage, S, in Tg G93A-SOD1 mice). GAPDH was used to normalize protein loading. hSOD1, transgenic human SOD1; mSOD1, endogenous murine SOD1.

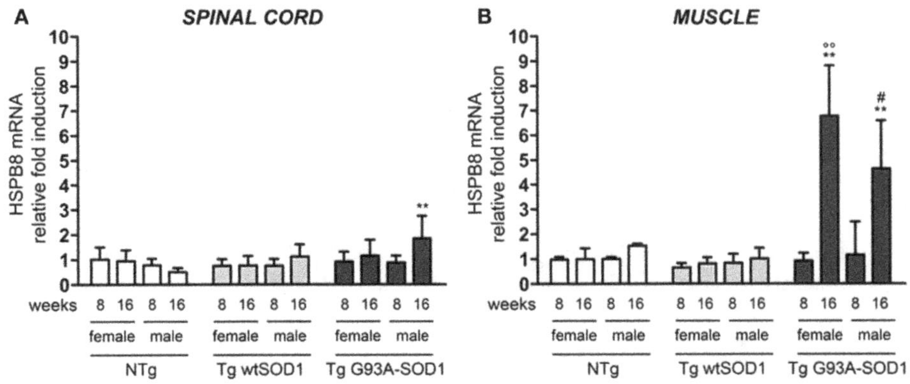

FIGURE 2 | Changes in HSPB8 levels in response to wt or mutSOD1 expression in spinal cord and muscle of ALS animal models. RT-qPCRs were performed on total RNA extracted from whole spinal cord **(A)** or quadriceps muscles **(B)** of female and male non-transgenic (NTg) mice, of mice expressing the wild type human SOD1 transgene (Tg wtSOD1), and of mice expressing the G93A mutant form of human SOD1 (Tg G93A-SOD1), at 8 (corresponding to presymptomatic stage, PS, in Tg G93A-SOD1 mice) or 16 weeks (corresponding to symptomatic stage, S, in Tg G93A-SOD1 mice). Data have been normalized to the amount of GAPDH mRNA, expressed relative to the levels determined in age-matched PS female NTg mice, taken as internal reference, and expressed as fold changes. Data are mean ± SD of four independent replicates. **(A)** $^{**}p < 0.01$ vs. age- and sex-matched NTg mice. **(B)** $^{**}p < 0.01$ vs. age- and sex-matched NTg mice and Tg wt SOD1 mice; $^{\circ\circ}p < 0.01$ vs. PS (8 weeks) female Tg G93A-SOD1; $^{\#}p < 0.05$ vs. PS (8 weeks) male Tg G93A-SOD1.

In light of our previous results showing that muscle cells possess a higher UPS activity with respect to motoneuronal cells (Onesto et al., 2011), we analyzed the expression of BAG1, which is involved in the re-routing of the misfolded proteins to proteasome-mediated substrates degradation. In spinal cord, BAG1 transcript levels were not affected by mutSOD1 expression (**Figure 3C**). On the contrary, BAG1 expression increased 2-folds in the skeletal muscle of S stage Tg G93A-SOD1 mice compared to all other groups analyzed (**Figure 3D**). This increase was similar in both sexes. These data suggest that proteasome-mediated substrate degradation is highly favored in muscle cells under proteotoxic conditions (e.g., misfolded mutSOD1 overexpression). We also estimated the ratio BAG3:BAG1 in each sample (**Figures 3E,F**) and found that this is always more elevated in muscle tissue, both in control and tg G93A-SOD1 mice, suggesting a predominance of the autophagic pathway, but it reaches higher levels at S stage of disease in response to mutSOD1. In the case of spinal cord, the BAG3:BAG1 ratio increases only at S stage (16 weeks) both in male and female tg G93A-SOD1 mice, suggesting that misfolded mutSOD1 could be re-routed to the autophagic system at this stage of disease (possibly not fully removed because of autophagic flux blockage).

Next, we asked whether the upregulation of the transcript levels of the genes described above results in an increase in protein expression. As shown in **Figure 4**, in the spinal cord **(A)**, HSPB8, BAG1, and BAG3 protein levels correlated with the data of gene transcription observed in the same mice. In skeletal muscle, we found that HSPB8, BAG3, and BAG1 were all up-regulated in Tg G93A-SOD1 mice at the S stage (16 weeks) of disease compared to Ntg and Tg wtSOD1 mice (**Figure 4B**). In the case of BAG3, the protein was up-regulated also at the PS stage (8 weeks). Little variation was observed in Tg G93A-SOD1 mice at S stage, while no major sex differences were noted. Also these data were perfectly in line and corroborate the mRNA expression analysis data reported above.

Since HSPB8 overexpression has beneficial effects in cell models of fALS, it is upregulated in human tissues from patients, and its mode of action requires the partner BAG3 and a functional autophagy system, we then analyzed the expression of two widely used markers of the autophagic flux: LC3 (which is overexpressed and associated with the autophagosome when autophagy is activated) and p62 (which is also upregulated during autophagy activation and is responsible for the insertion of ubiquitinated misfolded protein species into the autophagosomes). We found a moderate increase of LC3 mRNA selectively in the spinal cord of S stage (16 weeks) Tg G93A-SOD1 female mice (**Figure 5A**). In contrast, in skeletal muscle of Tg G93A-SOD1 mice (**Figure 5B**), LC3 expression was robustly increased at S stage both in male and female animals. p62 mRNA levels remained unchanged in spinal cord (**Figure 5C**), while they were increased in muscle of S stage female mice (**Figure 5D**). Notably, p62 levels increased also in Tg G93A-SOD1 male mice at S stage, even if this induction was not statistically significant.

Protein levels of LC3 and p62 as well as the conversion of free LC3-I to autophagosome-associated lipidated form of LC3-II were analyzed by WB (**Figure 6**). In spinal cord samples no major variations of p62 protein were observed, while the levels of LC3 protein were higher in Tg G93A-SOD1 mice (**Figure 6A**). Surprisingly, no conversion of LC3-I to LC3-II was observed, suggesting that the autophagic process is not massively activated in the spinal cord at these stages of disease. In skeletal muscle, p62 protein levels robustly increased in Tg G93A-SOD1 mice at both ages and in both sexes (**Figure 6B**). Moreover, at S stage (16 weeks), in skeletal muscle samples, the lipidated form of LC3 (LC3-II), which is the only one capable to associate with the newly formed autophagosomes, was increased in Tg G93A-SOD1 mice.

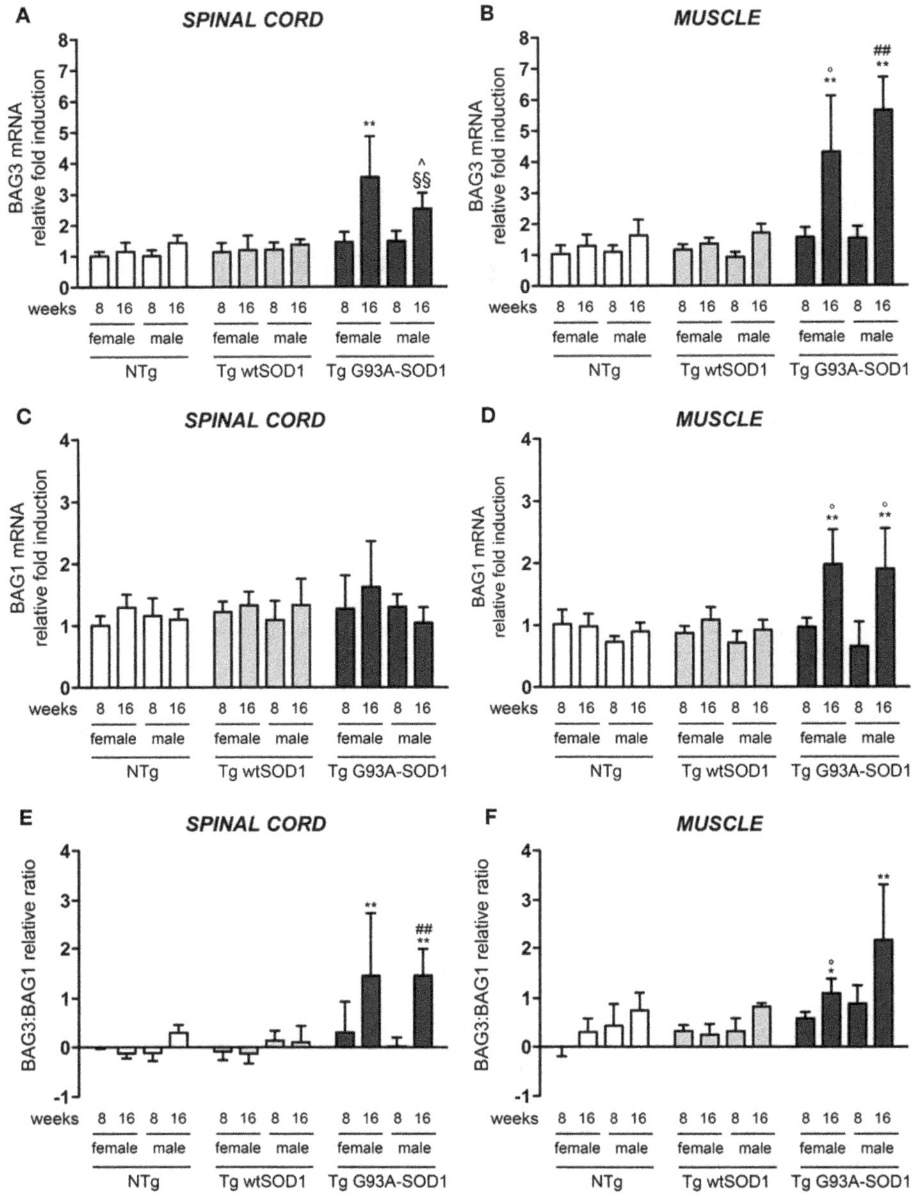

FIGURE 3 | BAG3 and BAG1 expression in spinal cord and muscle of ALS animal models. RT-qPCRs were performed on total RNA extracted from whole spinal cord **(A,C)** or quadriceps muscles **(B,D)** of female and male non-transgenic (NTg) mice, of mice expressing the wild type human SOD1 transgene (Tg wtSOD1), and of mice expressing the G93A mutant form of human SOD1 (Tg G93A-SOD1), at 8 (corresponding to presymptomatic stage, PS, in Tg G93A-SOD1 mice) or 16 weeks (corresponding to symptomatic stage, S, in Tg G93A-SOD1 mice). Data have been normalized to the amount of GAPDH mRNA, expressed relative to the levels determined in age-matched PS female NTg mice, taken as internal reference, and expressed as fold changes. Data are mean ± SD of four independent replicates. **(A)** RT-qPCR on BAG3 mRNA expression levels in whole spinal cord. $^{**}p < 0.01$ vs. age- and sex-matched NTg and Tg wtSOD1 mice; $^{\wedge}p < 0.05$ vs. age- and sex-matched NTg mice; $^{\S\S}p < 0.01$ vs. age- and sex-matched Tg wtSOD1 mice. **(B)** RT-qPCR on BAG3 mRNA expression levels in quadriceps muscles. $^{**}p < 0.01$ vs. age- and sex-matched NTg and Tg wtSOD1 mice; $^{\circ}p < 0.05$ vs. PS (8 weeks) female Tg G93A-SOD1; $^{\#\#}p < 0.01$ vs. PS (8 weeks) male Tg G93A-SOD1. **(C)** RT-qPCR on BAG1 mRNA expression levels in whole spinal cord. **(D)** RT-qPCR on BAG1 mRNA expression levels in quadriceps muscles. $^{**}p < 0.01$ vs. age- and sex-matched NTg and Tg wtSOD1 mice; $^{\circ}p < 0.05$ vs. sex-matched PS (8 weeks) Tg G93A-SOD1. **(E)** BAG3:BAG1 relative ratio of mRNA expression levels in whole spinal cord. Data represent variations of the relative levels of BAG3 and BAG1 normalized over the relative BAG3 and BAG1 levels of age-matched PS (8 weeks) female NTg mice (taken as internal reference, see Materials and Methods for details). $^{**}p < 0.01$ vs. age- and sex-matched NTg and Tg wtSOD1 mice; $^{\#\#}p < 0.01$ vs. PS (8 weeks) male Tg G93A-SOD1. **(F)** BAG3:BAG1 relative ratio of mRNA expression levels in quadriceps muscles. Data have been calculated as in **(E)**. $^{*}p < 0.05$ and $^{**}p < 0.01$ vs. age- and sex-matched NTg and Tg wtSOD1 mice; $^{\circ}p < 0.05$ vs. PS (8 weeks) male Tg G93A-SOD1.

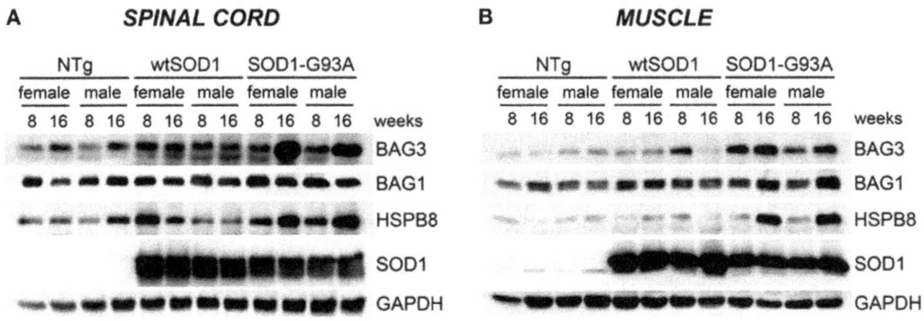

FIGURE 4 | HSPB8-BAG1-BAG3 protein levels in spinal cord and muscle of ALS animal models. Western Blot (WB) analysis on proteins extracted from whole spinal cord **(A)** or quadriceps muscles **(B)** of female and male non-transgenic (NTg) mice, of mice expressing the wild type human SOD1 transgene (Tg wtSOD1), and of mice expressing the G93A mutant form of human SOD1 (Tg G93A-SOD1), at 8 (corresponding to presymptomatic stage, PS, in Tg G93A-SOD1 mice) or 16 weeks (corresponding to symptomatic stage, S, in Tg G93A-SOD1 mice). GAPDH was used to normalize protein loading.

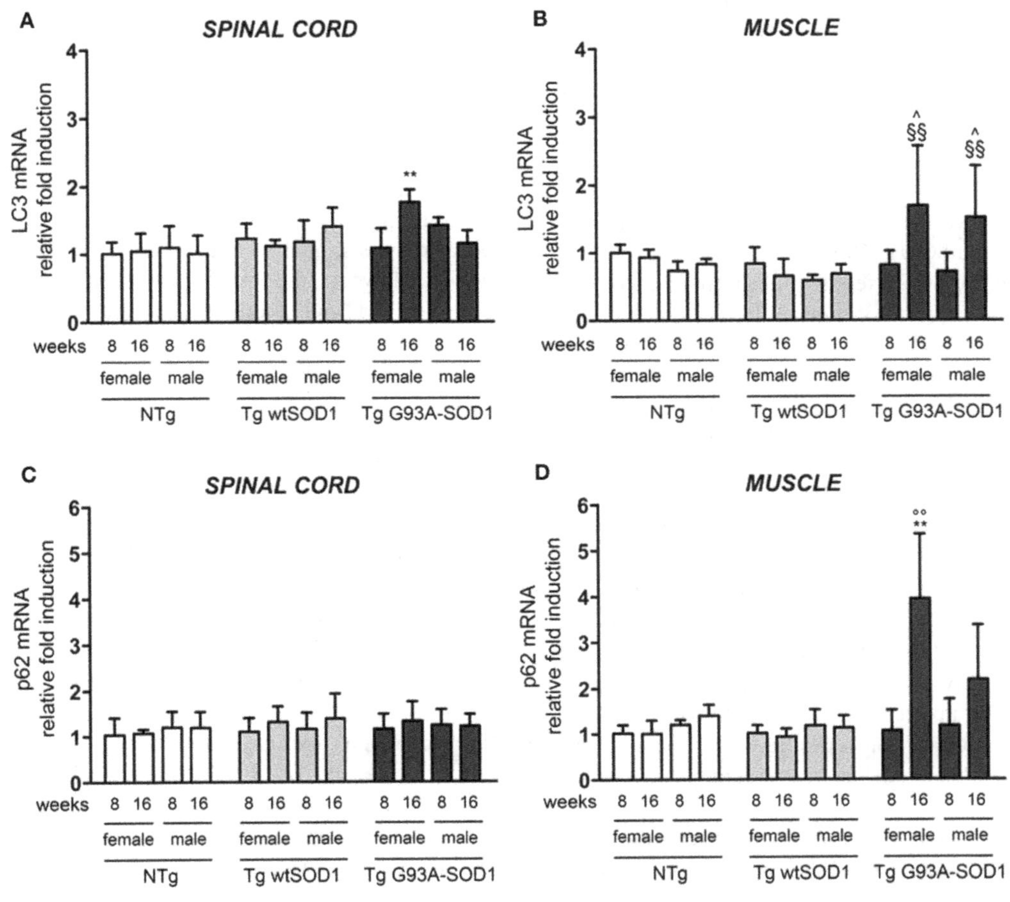

FIGURE 5 | LC3 and p62 expression in spinal cord and muscle of ALS animal models. RT-qPCRs were performed on total RNA extracted from whole spinal cord **(A,C)** or quadriceps muscles **(B,D)** of female and male non-transgenic (NTg) mice, of mice expressing the wild type human SOD1 transgene (Tg wtSOD1), and of mice expressing the G93A mutant form of human SOD1 (Tg G93A-SOD1), at 8 (corresponding to presymptomatic stage, PS, in Tg G93A-SOD1 mice) or 16 weeks (corresponding to symptomatic stage, S, in Tg G93A-SOD1 mice). Data have been normalized to the amount of GAPDH mRNA, expressed relative to the levels determined in age-matched PS female NTg mice, taken as internal reference, and expressed as fold changes. Data are mean ± SD of four independent replicates. **(A)** RT-qPCR on LC3 mRNA expression levels in whole spinal cord. $^{**}p < 0.01$ vs. age- and sex-matched NTg and Tg wtSOD1 mice. **(B)** RT-qPCR on LC3 mRNA expression levels in quadriceps muscles. $^{\wedge}p < 0.05$ vs. age- and sex-matched NTg mice; $^{\S\S}p < 0.01$ vs. age- and sex-matched Tg wtSOD1 mice. **(C)** RT-qPCR on p62 mRNA expression levels in whole spinal cord. **(D)** RT-qPCR on p62 mRNA expression levels in quadriceps muscles. $^{**}p < 0.01$ vs. age- and sex-matched NTg and Tg wtSOD1 mice; $^{\circ\circ}p < 0.01$ vs. PS female (8 weeks) Tg G93A-SOD1.

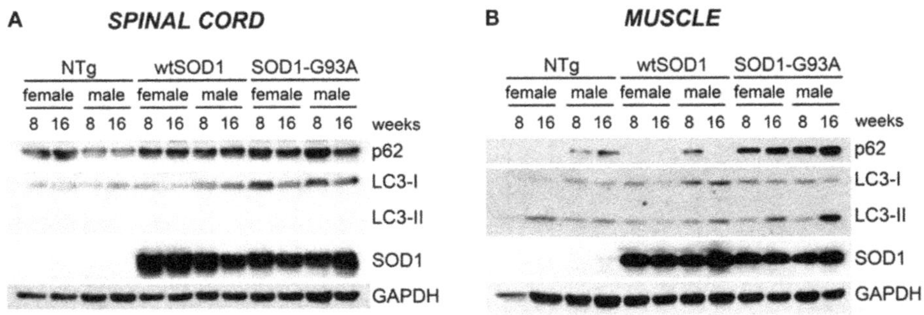

FIGURE 6 | Autophagic-markers (p62 and LC-3) protein levels in spinal cord and muscle of ALS animal models. Western Blot (WB) analysis on proteins extracted from whole spinal cord **(A)** or quadriceps muscles **(B)** of female and male non-transgenic (NTg) mice, of mice expressing the wild type human SOD1 transgene (Tg wtSOD1), and of mice expressing the G93A mutant form of human SOD1 (Tg G93A-SOD1), at 8 (corresponding to presymptomatic stage, PS, in Tg G93A-SOD1 mice) or 16 weeks (corresponding to symptomatic stage, S, in Tg G93A-SOD1 mice). GAPDH was used to normalize protein loading.

Collectively, these data strongly suggest that muscle, probably because of higher HSPB8, BAG1, and BAG3 expression, not only may better cope with misfolded mutant proteins, but also has a more intense autophagic response power compared to cells in the spinal cord.

DISCUSSION

In a previous study, we showed that spinal cord and muscle differently cope with mutSOD1 (Onesto et al., 2011). In fact, in Tg G93A-SOD1 mice mutSOD1 tends to accumulate in the spinal cord, while no accumulation of high molecular weight (HMW) species was found in muscles (Galbiati et al., 2012). Thus, the specific ability of spinal cord and skeletal muscle to handle misfolded protein aggregation and clearance (Cheroni et al., 2005, 2009; Basso et al., 2006, 2009; Bendotti et al., 2012; Galbiati et al., 2012; Wei et al., 2012) could be related to differences in their response to proteotoxicity, mediated by the PQC system. In this study we further investigated this aspect and found that mutSOD1 poorly accumulates in skeletal muscle, and only a mild increase of SDS-insoluble species of mutSOD1 is detectable in this tissue in Tg G93A-SOD1 male mice at the S stage (16 weeks), but not in female mice. This suggests that differences in the PQC system may also exist between the two sexes. Consequently, we then evaluated whether the expression pattern of specific factors of the PQC system shows a different expression profile in the spinal cord and muscle of a tg ALS mice model also considering possible gender differences.

To this purpose, here, we evaluated whether modifications occur at the initial stages of the PQC system, by focusing our attention on the HSPB8-BAG3 mediated pathway, involved in the autophagic process as well as on BAG1 pathway, involved in UPS mediated PQC. We then further investigated the autophagic process, since mutSOD1 induced alterations of UPS have already been analyzed by several investigators, reviewed in Bendotti et al. (2012), including us (Onesto et al., 2011). Autophagic response was analyzed using two well-known autophagic markers: LC3 and p62.

Our data clearly demonstrated that in both spinal cord and muscle HSPB8, BAG1, and BAG3 expression levels are not affected at early stage of disease (PS). The HSPB8-mediated PQC response was induced at the S stage of disease, and this activation was lower in spinal cord than muscle. Therefore, in spinal cord, the presence of misfolded mutSOD1 might not be sufficient to induce the activation of the PQC system *per se*, unless the disease is in an advanced phase, when motoneurons loss and/or alterations of muscle structures are present (Crippa et al., 2010b). Considering BAG3 and BAG1 expression, we found that their behavior was similar to that observed for HSPB8 at S stage (16 weeks). However, the BAG3 response appeared higher than that of BAG1, and BAG3 induction was also present in the spinal cord at S stage. Thus, cells in spinal cord have a lower capability than muscle cells to activate the HSPB8/BAG3- and BAG1-mediated PQC responses, and this might explain the larger accumulation of mutant misfolded proteins in this structure. It is of note that mutSOD1 expression results in the induction of both HSPB8 and BAG3 in the same structures, since HSPB8 activity is enhanced by BAG3 recruitment. Once the HSPB8-BAG3 interaction occurs, the complex recognizes the misfolded proteins and recruits the constitutively expressed chaperone HSC70 bound to the CHIP ubiquitinating enzyme (Arndt et al., 2010), allowing misfolded proteins removal by autophagy (Carra et al., 2008a,b, 2012, 2013; Arndt et al., 2010; Crippa et al., 2010b). In fact, CHIP ubiquitinates the target misfolded protein, which is then recognized by the protein p62 for its delivery to the nascent autophagosome (Arndt et al., 2010). Thus, HSPB8, BAG3, and the autophagy pathway may represent key players in the stress response elicited by mutSOD1 expression. Therefore, changes in their expression levels may correlate with the efficiency with which spinal cord and muscle cope with aggregate-prone mutSOD1.

On the other hand, the complex HSC70/CHIP can also associate to BAG1 to re-route substrates to UPS. When the proteasome component of UPS is overwhelmed or impaired by the misfolded proteins, HSPB8 and BAG3 are both highly induced. UPS inhibition is indeed a condition which occurs in motoneurons and muscle cells expressing mutSOD1 (Onesto et al., 2011), and the increase in the BAG3:BAG1 ratio allows BAG3 to more efficiently direct the HSC70/CHIP–associated substrates to autophagy for degradation (Zhang and Qian, 2011). Our data are in line with this working hypothesis, since in muscle we estimated that the BAG3:BAG1 ratio in tg G93A-SOD1 mice at S stage (16 weeks) is much higher than that observed in control mice. Conversely, in the spinal cord of tg G93A-SOD1 mice at S stage the BAG1 response is not detectable.

By following the auophagic response in muscle, our data here clearly show that at the S stage, muscle cells are still able to upregulate two essential players of the autophagic process, (a) p62, which recognizes the CHIP-ubiquitinated misfolded proteins in the HSPB8-BAG3-HSC70-CHIP complex, allowing their insertion into the autophagosome, and (b) LC3, which, after its activation to LC3, it is recognized by p62 and assists formation of autophagosomes. These steps are critical to initiate a correct autophagic flux required to clear the large excess of misfolded proteins from the cells during PQC response. This response does not efficiently take place in the spinal cord, since at S stage (16 weeks), misfolded mutSOD1 does not induce the overexpression of p62 and LC3, suggesting that the autophagic response in this structure is not as efficient as it is in muscle. In addition, in spinal cord very low basal levels of LC3-II form can be detected, suggesting that at these ages very few autophagosomes can be generated in response to mutSOD1. These data are consistent with previous reports obtained in the spinal cord of early symptomatic tg G93A-SOD1 mice, in which the LC3-I to LC3-II conversion, and thus, autophagy activation, occurs at very low levels, and it efficiently takes place only after the 17 week of age (Tian et al., 2011; Lee et al., 2013b). With disease progression, several autophagosomes appear in spinal cord motoneurons surviving at the end stage of disease (Li et al., 2008; Crippa et al., 2010b). This autophagic response can also be selectively activated in different cell types; for example LC3-I to LC3-II conversion can be visualized in cultured astrocytes in response to mutSOD1 (Kim et al., 2013).

With regards to the possible gender differences existing in the pathways here analyzed, we only found that, at S stage in tg G93A-SOD1 mice, the expression of p62 is significantly induced in skeletal muscle of female but not in that of male mice. These observations may help to explain why in skeletal muscle of tg G93A-SOD1 male mice mutSOD1 tends to accumulate in insoluble forms (see above). Interestingly, a mild increase of HSPB8 expression was present in spinal cord at S stage (16 weeks) of tg G93A-SOD1 male mice, but not in female mice. The molecular mechanism at the basis of this peculiar gender differences is unknown. Interestingly enough, there is a positive correlation between mutSOD1 accumulation and HSPB8 expression in the spinal cord of male tg G93A-SOD1 mice at S stage (16 weeks). This suggests that HSPB8 gene transcription increases in response to misfolded species accumulation. These data are in line with our previous results showing that an UPS impairment (which is know to result in a further mutSOD1 aggregation), lead to HSPB8 overexpression and stabilization (Crippa et al., 2010a,b; Bendotti et al., 2012; Carra et al., 2012, 2013). It remains to be determined why this HSPB8 overproduction fails to clear mutSOD1 insoluble species via autophagy (Crippa et al., 2010b; Rusmini et al., 2010).

By analysing the molecular and biochemical behavior of mutSOD1, we have previously elucidated several potential mechanisms of neurotoxicity associated with accumulation of misfolded proteins in motoneuronal cells (Sau et al., 2007, 2011; Crippa et al., 2010a,b; Onesto et al., 2011). For instance, the formation of HMW mutSOD1 species and aggregation correlated with an altered intracellular mutSOD1 distribution (Sau et al., 2007; Crippa et al., 2010b). In these conditions, mutSOD1 nuclear bioavailability was reduced in motoneuronal, but not in muscle cells (Sau et al., 2007; Crippa et al., 2010a,b; Onesto et al., 2011), an aberrant biochemical behavior that may result in a decreased nuclear protection from free radical species (Sau et al., 2007). In addition, by evaluating mitochondrial superoxide induced oxidation, using MitoSOX (a mitochondrial specific fluorogenic dye oxidized by superoxide) in motoneuronal NSC34 cell models of ALS, we found that mutSOD1 expressing motoneuronal cells are more sensitive to a superoxide-induced oxidative stress when compared to wtSOD1 expressing motoneuronal cells (Onesto et al., 2011). These mitochondrial alterations were not found in muscle C2C12 cells expressing either wt or mutSOD1 (Onesto et al., 2011). Therefore, mutSOD1 altered intracellular bioavailability, due to sequestration into aggregates, might result in a less efficient protection against free radical species damages in different subcellular compartments (Sau et al., 2007; Onesto et al., 2011).

Our results are in line with a recent report showing that protein misfolding, mitochondrial dysfunction and muscle loss are not directly dependent on soluble and aggregated mutSOD1 in skeletal muscle of ALS (Wei et al., 2012). Moreover, soluble mutSOD1 does not have direct effects on mitochondrial dysfunction as determined by quantifying the release of reactive oxygen species (ROS) in skeletal muscle mitochondria (Wei et al., 2012).

Interestingly, dysfunction of skeletal muscle and degeneration of neuromuscular junctions precede disease onset and motoneurons loss in tg ALS mice (Frey et al., 2000; Fischer et al., 2004). Notably, while the reduction of mutSOD1 expression in the skeletal muscle of tg ALS mice has no effect on disease progression (Miller et al., 2006), the selective expression of mutSOD1 in skeletal muscle induces atrophy and mitochondrial abnormalities in this tissue (Dobrowolny et al., 2008a; Corti et al., 2009; Wong and Martin, 2010). Moreover, mutSOD1-induced muscle damage leads to loss of mutSOD1-negative motoneurons in the anterior horn of the spinal cord, suggesting that mutSOD1 neurotoxicity can be exerted at different levels and its restricted expression in muscle can be sufficient to induce an ALS-like disease in mice (Dobrowolny et al., 2005, 2008a,b).

The data presented here clarify that mutSOD1 activates distinct pathogenetic pathways in muscle and motoneuron cells. In addition, the aggregation-independent mutSOD1 toxicity in muscle can be monitored at transcriptional levels. In fact, in our muscle cell models of ALS we observed specific alterations in the expression of typical genes controlling muscle pathways activated by nerve injury, or muscular atrophy [e.g., MyoD, myogenin (two myogenic regulatory factors), and TGFbeta1, which are markers for muscle fiber damage or atrophy] (Galbiati et al., 2012). Thus, muscle cells are able to better manage misfolded mutSOD1 species, even if misfolding is an intrinsic property of mutSOD1, and it does not depend on the cell environment (Dobson, 2003). It remains to be clarified whether the autophagic activation induced by mutSOD1 in muscle initially protective, when excessive, may become one of the toxic events mediating the deleterious activity associated with this mutant protein (Nassif and Hetz, 2011; Zhang et al., 2011). This hypothesis has already been proved in a ALS-related motoneuron disease, the Spinal and Bulbar Muscular Atrophy (SBMA) linked to an expansion of a polyQ stretch in the androgen receptor (ARpolyQ) (Poletti, 2004; Rusmini et al., 2013). Even in this motoneuron disease the mutant ARpolyQ affects both spinal cord and muscle, but it has been shown that an enhanced autophagy exacerbated skeletal muscle atrophy (Yu et al., 2011). Indeed, the genetic inhibition of autophagy in muscle, through haploinsufficiency for Beclin-1, a component of the autophagic initiation complex, mitigates skeletal muscle atrophy and prolongs survival of a tg SBMA mouse model (Yu et al., 2011).

Therefore, the toxicity exerted by mutant misfolded proteins in muscle cells is probably not related to the classical mechanism of intracellular protein aggregation, but other mechanisms of toxicity may be involved.

ACKNOWLEDGMENTS

AriSLA Foundation Italy (ALS_HSPB8 to Angelo Poletti and Serena Carra), Telethon—Italy (GGP06063 and GGP07063 to Angelo Poletti, GGP10037 to Maria Pennuto); Italian Ministry of Labour, Health and Social Affairs (Convenzione Fondazione Mondino/UNIMI to Angelo Poletti); Regione Lombardia (to Angelo Poletti and Valeria Crippa); Universita' degli Studi di Milano (to Angelo Poletti and Valeria Crippa); Fondazione CARIPLO (2008-2307 to Angelo Poletti); Fondation Thierry Latran, France (to Angelo Poletti and Maria Pennuto), Association Française contre les Myopathies (to Angelo Poletti), Muscular Dystrophy Association (196646 to Maria Pennuto), and Marie-Curie Reintegration Grant (FP7-256448 to Serena Carra).

REFERENCES

Arndt, V., Dick, N., Tawo, R., Dreiseidler, M., Wenzel, D., Hesse, M., et al. (2010). Chaperone-assisted selective autophagy is essential for muscle maintenance. *Curr. Biol.* 20, 143–148. doi: 10.1016/j.cub.2009.11.022

Ash, P. E., Bieniek, K. F., Gendron, T. F., Caulfield, T., Lin, W. L., Dejesus-Hernandez, M., et al. (2013). Unconventional translation of C9ORF72 GGGGCC expansion generates insoluble polypeptides specific to c9FTD/ALS. *Neuron* 77, 639–646. doi: 10.1016/j.neuron.2013.02.004

Basso, M., Massignan, T., Samengo, G., Cheroni, C., De Biasi, S., Salmona, M., et al. (2006). Insoluble mutant SOD1 is partly oligoubiquitinated in amyotrophic lateral sclerosis mice. *J. Biol. Chem.* 281, 33325–33335. doi: 10.1074/jbc.M603489200

Basso, M., Samengo, G., Nardo, G., Massignan, T., D'Alessandro, G., Tartari, S., et al. (2009). Characterization of detergent-insoluble proteins in ALS indicates a causal link between nitrative stress and aggregation in pathogenesis. *PLoS ONE* 4:e8130. doi: 10.1371/journal.pone.0008130

Bendotti, C., Marino, M., Cheroni, C., Fontana, E., Crippa, V., Poletti, A., et al. (2012). Dysfunction of constitutive and inducible ubiquitin-proteasome system in amyotrophic lateral sclerosis: implication for protein aggregation and immune response. *Prog. Neurobiol.* 97, 101–126. doi: 10.1016/j.pneurobio.2011.10.001

Boillée, S., Vande Velde, C., and Cleveland, D. W. (2006). ALS: a disease of motor neurons and their non-neuronal neighbors. *Neuron* 52, 39–59. doi: 10.1016/j.neuron.2006.09.018

Bosco, D. A., and Landers, J. E. (2010). Genetic determinants of amyotrophic lateral sclerosis as therapeutic targets. *CNS Neurol. Disord. Drug Targets* 9, 779–790. doi: 10.2174/187152710793237494

Bosco, D. A., Morfini, G., Karabacak, N. M., Song, Y., Gros-Louis, F., Pasinelli, P., et al. (2010). Wild-type and mutant SOD1 share an aberrant conformation and a common pathogenic pathway in ALS. *Nat. Neurosci.* 13, 1396–1403. doi: 10.1038/nn.2660

Carra, S. (2009). The stress-inducible HspB8-Bag3 complex induces the eIF2alpha kinase pathway: implications for protein quality control and viral factory degradation. *Autophagy* 5, 428–429. doi: 10.4161/auto.5.3.7894

Carra, S., Brunsting, J. F., Lambert, H., Landry, J., and Kampinga, H. H. (2009). HspB8 participates in protein quality control by a non-chaperone-like mechanism that requires eIF2{alpha} phosphorylation. *J. Biol. Chem.* 284, 5523–5532. doi: 10.1074/jbc.M807440200

Carra, S., Crippa, V., Rusmini, P., Boncoraglio, A., Minoia, M., Giorgetti, E., et al. (2012). Alteration of protein folding and degradation in motor neuron diseases: implications and protective functions of small heat shock proteins. *Prog. Neurobiol.* 97, 83–100. doi: 10.1016/j.pneurobio.2011.09.009

Carra, S., Rusmini, P., Crippa, V., Giorgetti, E., Boncoraglio, A., Naujock, N., et al. (2013). Different anti-aggregation and pro-degradative functions of the members of the mammalian sHSP family in neurological disorders. *Philos. Trans. R. Soc. Lond. B Biol. Sci.* 368, 20110409. doi: 10.1098/rstb.2011.0409

Carra, S., Seguin, S. J., Lambert, H., and Landry, J. (2008a). HspB8 chaperone activity toward poly(Q)-containing proteins depends on its association with Bag3, a stimulator of macroautophagy. *J. Biol. Chem.* 283, 1437–1444. doi: 10.1074/jbc.M706304200

Carra, S., Seguin, S. J., and Landry, J. (2008b). HspB8 and Bag3: a new chaperone complex targeting misfolded proteins to macroautophagy. *Autophagy* 4, 237–239.

Carra, S., Sivilotti, M., Chavez Zobel, A. T., Lambert, H., and Landry, J. (2005). HspB8, a small heat shock protein mutated in human neuromuscular disorders, has *in vivo* chaperone activity in cultured cells. *Hum. Mol. Genet.* 14, 1659–1669. doi: 10.1093/hmg/ddi174

Cheroni, C., Marino, M., Tortarolo, M., Veglianese, P., De Biasi, S., Fontana, E., et al. (2009). Functional alterations of the ubiquitin-proteasome system in motor neurons of a mouse model of familial amyotrophic lateral sclerosis. *Hum. Mol. Genet.* 18, 82–96. doi: 10.1093/hmg/ddn319

Cheroni, C., Peviani, M., Cascio, P., Debiasi, S., Monti, C., and Bendotti, C. (2005). Accumulation of human SOD1 and ubiquitinated deposits in the spinal cord of SOD1G93A mice during motor neuron disease progression correlates with a decrease of proteasome. *Neurobiol. Dis.* 18, 509–522. doi: 10.1016/j.nbd.2004.12.007

Chomczynski, P., and Sacchi, N. (1987). Single step method of RNA isolation by acid guanidinium thyocyanate-phenol chloroform extraction. *Anal. Biochem.* 162, 156–158. doi: 10.1016/0003-2697(87)90021-2

Corti, S., Donadoni, C., Ronchi, D., Bordoni, A., Fortunato, F., Santoro, D., et al. (2009). Amyotrophic lateral sclerosis linked to a novel SOD1 mutation with muscle mitochondrial dysfunction. *J. Neurol. Sci.* 276, 170–174. doi: 10.1016/j.jns.2008.09.030

Cozzolino, M., Ferri, A., and Carri, M. T. (2008). Amyotrophic lateral sclerosis: from current developments in the laboratory to clinical implications. *Antioxid. Redox Signal.* 10, 405–443. doi: 10.1089/ars.2007.1760

Crippa, V., Carra, S., Rusmini, P., Sau, D., Bolzoni, E., Bendotti, C., et al. (2010a). A role of small heat shock protein B8 (HspB8) in the autophagic removal of misfolded proteins responsible for neurodegenerative diseases. *Autophagy* 6, 958–960. doi: 10.4161/auto.6.7.13042

Crippa, V., Sau, D., Rusmini, P., Boncoraglio, A., Onesto, E., Bolzoni, E., et al. (2010b). The small heat shock protein B8 (HspB8) promotes autophagic removal of misfolded proteins involved in amyotrophic lateral sclerosis (ALS). *Hum. Mol. Genet.* 19, 3440–3456. doi: 10.1093/hmg/ddq257

Daoud, H., Valdmanis, P. N., Kabashi, E., Dion, P., Dupre, N., Camu, W., et al. (2009). Contribution of TARDBP mutations to sporadic amyotrophic lateral sclerosis. *J. Med. Genet.* 46, 112–114. doi: 10.1136/jmg.2008.062463

Dejesus-Hernandez, M., Mackenzie, I. R., Boeve, B. F., Boxer, A. L., Baker, M., Rutherford, N. J., et al. (2011). Expanded GGGGCC hexanucleotide repeat in non-coding region of C9ORF72 causes chromosome 9p-linked FTD and ALS. *Neuron* 72, 245–256. doi: 10.1016/j.neuron.2011.09.011

Dobrowolny, G., Aucello, M., Molinaro, M., and Musaro, A. (2008a). Local expression of mIgf-1 modulates ubiquitin, caspase and CDK5 expression in skeletal muscle of an ALS mouse model. *Neurol. Res.* 30, 131–136. doi: 10.1179/174313208X281235

Dobrowolny, G., Aucello, M., Rizzuto, E., Beccafico, S., Mammucari, C., Bonconpagni, S., et al. (2008b). Skeletal muscle is a primary target of SOD1G93A-mediated toxicity. *Cell Metab.* 8, 425–436. doi: 10.1016/j.cmet.2008.09.002

Dobrowolny, G., Giacinti, C., Pelosi, L., Nicoletti, C., Winn, N., Barberi, L., et al. (2005). Muscle expression of a local Igf-1 isoform protects motor neurons in an ALS mouse model. *J. Cell Biol.* 168, 193–199. doi: 10.1083/jcb.200407021

Dobson, C. M. (2003). Protein folding and misfolding. *Nature* 426, 884–890. doi: 10.1038/nature02261

Du, Z. X., Zhang, H. Y., Meng, X., Gao, Y. Y., Zou, R. L., Liu, B. Q., et al. (2009). Proteasome inhibitor MG132 induces BAG3 expression through activation of heat shock factor 1. *J. Cell. Physiol.* 218, 631–637. doi: 10.1002/jcp.21634

Fischer, L. R., Culver, D. G., Tennant, P., Davis, A. A., Wang, M., Castellano-Sanchez, A., et al. (2004). Amyotrophic lateral sclerosis is a distal axonopathy: evidence in mice and man. *Exp. Neurol.* 185, 232–240. doi: 10.1016/j.expneurol.2003.10.004

Frey, D., Schneider, C., Xu, L., Borg, J., Spooren, W., and Caroni, P. (2000). Early and selective loss of neuromuscular synapse subtypes with low sprouting competence in motoneuron diseases. *J. Neurosci.* 20, 2534–2542.

Galbiati, M., Onesto, E., Zito, A., Crippa, V., Rusmini, P., Mariotti, R., et al. (2012). The anabolic/androgenic steroid nandrolone exacerbates gene expression modifications induced by mutant SOD1 in muscles of mice models of amyotrophic lateral sclerosis. *Pharmacol. Res.* 65, 221–230. doi: 10.1016/j.phrs.2011.12.001

Gamerdinger, M., Hajieva, P., Kaya, A. M., Wolfrum, U., Hartl, F. U., and Behl, C. (2009). Protein quality control during aging involves recruitment of the macroautophagy pathway by BAG3. *EMBO J.* 28, 889–901. doi: 10.1038/emboj.2009.29

Gamerdinger, M., Kaya, A. M., Wolfrum, U., Clement, A. M., and Behl, C. (2011). BAG3 mediates chaperone-based aggresome-targeting and selective autophagy of misfolded proteins. *EMBO Rep.* 12, 149–156. doi: 10.1038/embor.2010.203

Gentilella, A., and Khalili, K. (2011). BAG3 expression in glioblastoma cells promotes accumulation of ubiquitinated clients in an Hsp70-dependent manner. *J. Biol. Chem.* 286, 9205–9215. doi: 10.1074/jbc.M110.175836

Giagheddu, M., Puggioni, G., Masala, C., Biancu, F., Pirari, G., Piras, M. R., et al. (1983). Epidemiologic study of amyotrophic lateral sclerosis in Sardinia, Italy. *Acta Neurol. Scand.* 68, 394–404. doi: 10.1111/j.1600-0404.1983.tb04849.x

Gurney, M. E., Pu, H., Chiu, A. Y., Dal Canto, M. C., Polchow, C. Y., Alexander, D. D., et al. (1994). Motor neuron degeneration in mice that express a human Cu, Zn superoxide dismutase mutation. *Science* 264, 1772–1775. doi: 10.1126/science.8209258

Kim, J., Kim, T. Y., Cho, K. S., Kim, H. N., and Koh, J. Y. (2013). Autophagy activation and neuroprotection by progesterone in the G93A-SOD1 transgenic mouse model of amyotrophic lateral sclerosis. *Neurobiol. Dis.* 59C, 80–85. doi: 10.1016/j.nbd.2013.07.011

Kurtzke, J. F. (1982). Epidemiology of amyotrophic lateral sclerosis. *Adv. Neurol.* 36, 281–302.

Lashley, T., Hardy, J., and Isaacs, A. M. (2013). RANTing about C9orf72. *Neuron* 77, 597–598. doi: 10.1016/j.neuron.2013.02.009

Lee, C. T., Chiu, Y. W., Wang, K. C., Hwang, C. S., Lin, K. H., Lee, I. T., et al. (2013a). Riluzole and prognostic factors in amyotrophic lateral sclerosis long-term and short-term survival: a population-based study of 1149 cases in Taiwan. *J. Epidemiol.* 23, 35–40. doi: 10.2188/jea.JE20120119

Lee, J. K., Shin, J. H., Hwang, S. G., Gwag, B. J., McKee, A. C., Lee, J., et al. (2013b). MST1 functions as a key modulator of neurodegeneration in a mouse model of ALS. *Proc. Natl. Acad. Sci. U.S.A.* 110, 12066–12071. doi: 10.1073/pnas.1300894110

Li, L., Zhang, X., and Le, W. (2008). Altered macroautophagy in the spinal cord of SOD1 mutant mice. *Autophagy* 4, 290–293.

Luders, J., Demand, J., and Hohfeld, J. (2000). The ubiquitin-related BAG-1 provides a link between the molecular chaperones Hsc70/Hsp70 and the proteasome. *J. Biol. Chem.* 275, 4613–4617. doi: 10.1074/jbc.275.7.4613

Manjaly, Z. R., Scott, K. M., Abhinav, K., Wijesekera, L., Ganesalingam, J., Goldstein, L. H., et al. (2010). The sex ratio in amyotrophic lateral sclerosis: a population based study. *Amyotroph. Lateral Scler.* 11, 439–442. doi: 10.3109/17482961003610853

McCombe, P. A., and Henderson, R. D. (2010). Effects of gender in amyotrophic lateral sclerosis. *Gend. Med.* 7, 557–570. doi: 10.1016/j.genm.2010.11.010

Miller, T. M., Kim, S. H., Yamanaka, K., Hester, M., Umapathi, P., Arnson, H., et al. (2006). Gene transfer demonstrates that muscle is not a primary target for non-cell-autonomous toxicity in familial amyotrophic lateral sclerosis. *Proc. Natl. Acad. Sci. U.S.A.* 103, 19546–19551. doi: 10.1073/pnas.0609411103

Mizushima, N., and Komatsu, M. (2011). Autophagy: renovation of cells and tissues. *Cell* 147, 728–741. doi: 10.1016/j.cell.2011.10.026

Mori, K., Lammich, S., Mackenzie, I. R., Forne, I., Zilow, S., Kretzschmar, H., et al. (2013). hnRNP A3 binds to GGGGCC repeats and is a constituent of p62-positive/TDP43-negative inclusions in the hippocampus of patients with C9orf72 mutations. *Acta Neuropathol.* 125, 413–423. doi: 10.1007/s00401-013-1088-7

Nassif, M., and Hetz, C. (2011). Targeting autophagy in ALS: a complex mission. *Autophagy* 7, 450–453. doi: 10.4161/auto.7.4.14700

Neumann, M., Sampathu, D. M., Kwong, L. K., Truax, A. C., Micsenyi, M. C., Chou, T. T., et al. (2006). Ubiquitinated TDP-43 in frontotemporal lobar degeneration and amyotrophic lateral sclerosis. *Science* 314, 130–133. doi: 10.1126/science.1134108

Onesto, E., Rusmini, P., Crippa, V., Ferri, N., Zito, A., Galbiati, M., et al. (2011). Muscle cells and motoneurons differentially remove mutant SOD1 causing familial amyotrophic lateral sclerosis. *J. Neurochem.* 118, 266–280. doi: 10.1111/j.1471-4159.2011.07298.x

Palazzolo, I., Stack, C., Kong, L., Musaro, A., Adachi, H., Katsuno, M., et al. (2009). Overexpression of IGF-1 in muscle attenuates disease in a mouse model of spinal and bulbar muscular atrophy. *Neuron* 63, 316–328. doi: 10.1016/j.neuron.2009.07.019

Pasinelli, P., and Brown, R. H. (2006). Molecular biology of amyotrophic lateral sclerosis: insights from genetics. *Nat. Rev. Neurosci.* 7, 710–723. doi: 10.1038/nrn1971

Poletti, A. (2004). The polyglutamine tract of androgen receptor: from functions to dysfunctions in motor neurons. *Front. Neuroendocrinol.* 25:1–26. doi: 10.1016/j.yfrne.2004.03.001

Renton, A. E., Majounie, E., Waite, A., Simon-Sanchez, J., Rollinson, S., Gibbs, J. R., et al. (2011). A hexanucleotide repeat expansion in C9ORF72 is the cause of chromosome 9p21-linked ALS-FTD. *Neuron* 72, 257–268. doi: 10.1016/j.neuron.2011.09.010

Robberecht, W., and Philips, T. (2013). The changing scene of amyotrophic lateral sclerosis. *Nat. Rev. Neurosci.* 14, 248–264. doi: 10.1038/nrn3430

Rudnicki, S. A. (1999). Estrogen replacement therapy in women with amyotrophic lateral sclerosis. *J. Neurol. Sci.* 169, 126–127. doi: 10.1016/S0022-510X(99)00234-8

Rusmini, P., Bolzoni, E., Crippa, V., Onesto, E., Sau, D., Galbiati, M., et al. (2010). Proteasomal and autophagic degradative activities in spinal and bulbar muscular atrophy. *Neurobiol. Dis.* 40, 361–369. doi: 10.1016/j.nbd.2010.06.016

Rusmini, P., Crippa, V., Giorgetti, E., Boncoraglio, A., Cristofani, R., Carra, S., et al. (2013). Clearance of the mutant androgen receptor in motoneuronal models of spinal and bulbar muscular atrophy. *Neurobiol. Aging* 34, 2585–2603. doi: 10.1016/j.neurobiolaging.2013.05.026

Sau, D., De Biasi, S., Vitellaro-Zuccarello, L., Riso, P., Guarnieri, S., Porrini, M., et al. (2007). Mutation of SOD1 in ALS: a gain of a loss of function. *Hum. Mol. Genet.* 16, 1604–1618. doi: 10.1093/hmg/ddm110

Sau, D., Rusmini, P., Crippa, V., Onesto, E., Bolzoni, E., Ratti, A., et al. (2011). Dysregulation of axonal transport and motorneuron diseases. *Biol. Cell* 103, 87–107. doi: 10.1042/BC20100093

Seetharaman, S. V., Prudencio, M., Karch, C., Holloway, S. P., Borchelt, D. R., and Hart, P. J. (2009). Immature copper-zinc superoxide dismutase and familial amyotrophic lateral sclerosis. *Exp. Biol. Med. (Maywood)* 234, 1140–1154. doi: 10.3181/0903-MR-104

Strong, M. J., and Yang, W. (2011). The frontotemporal syndromes of ALS. Clinicopathological correlates. *J. Mol. Neurosci.* 45, 648–655. doi: 10.1007/s12031-011-9609-0

Suzuki, M., Tork, C., Shelley, B., McHugh, J., Wallace, K., Klein, S. M., et al. (2007). Sexual dimorphism in disease onset and progression of a rat model of ALS. *Amyotroph. Lateral Scler.* 8, 20–25. doi: 10.1080/17482960600982447

Tian, F., Morimoto, N., Liu, W., Ohta, Y., Deguchi, K., Miyazaki, K., et al. (2011). *In vivo* optical imaging of motor neuron autophagy in a mouse model of amyotrophic lateral sclerosis. *Autophagy* 7, 985–992. doi: 10.4161/auto.7.9.16012

Veldink, J. H., Bar, P. R., Joosten, E. A., Otten, M., Wokke, J. H., and van Den Berg, L. H. (2003). Sexual differences in onset of disease and response to exercise in a transgenic model of ALS. *Neuromuscul. Disord.* 13, 737–743. doi: 10.1016/S0960-8966(03)00104-4

Wang, H. Q., Liu, H. M., Zhang, H. Y., Guan, Y., and Du, Z. X. (2008). Transcriptional upregulation of BAG3 upon proteasome inhibition. *Biochem. Biophys. Res. Commun.* 365, 381–385. doi: 10.1016/j.bbrc.2007.11.001

Wei, R., Bhattacharya, A., Chintalaramulu, N., Jernigan, A. L., Liu, Y., van Remmen, H., et al. (2012). Protein misfolding, mitochondrial dysfunction and muscle loss are not directly dependent on soluble and aggregation state of mSOD1 protein in skeletal muscle of ALS. *Biochem. Biophys. Res. Commun.* 417, 1275–1279. doi: 10.1016/j.bbrc.2011.12.126

Wei, R., Bhattacharya, A., Hamilton, R. T., Jernigan, A. L., and Chaudhuri, A. R. (2013). Differential effects of mutant SOD1 on protein structure of skeletal muscle and spinal cord of familial amyotrophic lateral sclerosis: role of chaperone network. *Biochem. Biophys. Res. Commun.* 438, 218–223. doi: 10.1016/j.bbrc.2013.07.060

Wong, M., and Martin, L. J. (2010). Skeletal muscle-restricted expression of human SOD1 causes motor neuron degeneration in transgenic mice. *Hum. Mol. Genet.* 19, 2284–2230. doi: 10.1093/hmg/ddq106

Yu, Z., Wang, A. M., Adachi, H., Katsuno, M., Sobue, G., Yue, Z., et al. (2011). Macroautophagy is regulated by the UPR-mediator CHOP and accentuates the phenotype of SBMA mice. *PLoS Genet.* 7:e1002321. doi: 10.1371/journal.pgen.1002321

Zhang, X., Li, L., Chen, S., Yang, D., Wang, Y., Zhang, X., et al. (2011). Rapamycin treatment augments motor neuron degeneration in SOD1(G93A) mouse model of amyotrophic lateral sclerosis. *Autophagy* 7, 412–425. doi: 10.4161/auto.7.4.14541

Zhang, X., and Qian, S. B. (2011). Chaperone-mediated hierarchical control in targeting misfolded proteins to aggresomes. *Mol. Biol. Cell* 22, 3277–3288. doi: 10.1091/mbc.E11-05-0388

2

Neuroimmunity dynamics and the development of therapeutic strategies for amyotrophic lateral sclerosis

Melissa Bowerman[1], Thierry Vincent[1,2], Frédérique Scamps[1], Florence E. Perrin[1,3], William Camu[1,4] and Cédric Raoul[1]*

[1] The Neuroscience Institute of Montpellier, INM, INSERM UMR1051, Saint Eloi Hospital, Montpellier, France
[2] Department of Immunology, Saint Eloi Hospital, Montpellier, France
[3] Integrative Biology of Neuroregeneration, Faculty of Science, University of Montpellier 2, Montpellier, France
[4] Department of Neurology, ALS Reference Center, Gui-de-Chauliac Hospital, Montpellier, France

Edited by:
Ricardo Tapia, Instituto de Fisiología Celular, Universidad Nacional Autónoma de México, Mexico

Reviewed by:
Hermona Soreq, The Hebrew University of Jerusalem, Israel
Pamela McCombe, The University of Queensland, Australia

***Correspondence:**
Cédric Raoul, The Neuroscience Institute of Montpellier, INM, INSERM UMR1051, Saint Eloi Hospital, 80 rue Augustin Fliche, 34091 Montpellier, France
e-mail: cedric.raoul@inserm.fr

Amyotrophic lateral sclerosis (ALS) is a fatal paralytic disorder characterized by the progressive and selective loss of both upper and lower motoneurons. The neurodegenerative process is accompanied by a sustained inflammation in the brain and spinal cord. The neuron-immune interaction, implicating resident microglia of the central nervous system and blood-derived immune cells, is highly dynamic over the course of the disease. Here, we discuss the timely controlled neuroprotective and neurotoxic cues that are provided by the immune environment of motoneurons and their potential therapeutic applications for ALS.

Keywords: inflammation, microglia, lymphocytes, astrocytes, hyperexcitability, cytokine, therapy

INTRODUCTION

Amyotrophic lateral sclerosis (ALS) is a neurodegenerative disease characterized by the selective and progressive loss of upper and lower motoneurons, with both genetic and sporadic events contributing to the development of the pathological process (reviewed in Bento-Abreu et al., 2010). The term "neuroinflammation" has been attributed to the inflammatory response that occurs within the central nervous system (CNS) concomitantly to neurodegeneration (reviewed in Glass et al., 2010). Astrocytes, microglia, and immune cells are the key cellular modulators of neuroinflammation and have all been shown to actively participate in ALS pathogenesis (Glass et al., 2010; McCombe and Henderson, 2011; Philips and Robberecht, 2011). Importantly, recent reports have highlighted the presence of both neuroprotective and neurotoxic inflammatory cells in ALS animal models and patients that appear to be mainly dependent on the stage of disease progression. Seeing as reviews on the relationship between astrocytic activation and ALS are numerous, we will focus herein on the dynamic functional changes of microglia and immune cells that take place during ALS pathogenesis. A better understanding of these time-dependent modifications is of utmost importance for the development of ALS therapeutic strategies aimed at targeting the neuroinflammatory process.

A ROLE FOR MICROGLIA IN NEUROINFLAMMATION

ACTIVATION PROFILE IN HUMAN AND ANIMAL MODELS OF ALS

Microglia, the resident immune cells of the CNS, constantly survey the environment and become activated upon alterations resulting from disease or injury eliciting a strong pro-inflammatory response (reviewed in Hanisch and Kettenmann, 2007). In ALS patients, reactive microglia are observed in the motor cortex, motor nuclei of the brainstem, the entire corticospinal tract, the spinal cord, and within the cerebrospinal fluid (CSF; Engelhardt and Appel, 1990; Kawamata et al., 1992; Banati et al., 1995). Given the relationship between astrocytes and microglia and the importance of astrocytosis in ALS (Davalos et al., 2005; Yamanaka et al., 2008), it has been hypothesized that microgliosis may also participate in ALS pathogenesis.

In rodent ALS models, microgliosis occurs in pre-symptomatic and symptomatic $SOD1^{G93A}$ mice (Hall et al., 1998; Alexianu et al., 2001; Petrik et al., 2007; Gerber et al., 2012) and at both onset and early-stage of the disease in $SOD1^{G37R}$ mice (Boillee et al., 2006). An in-depth *in vivo* characterization of microgliosis in $SOD1^{G93A}$ mice shows that microglia are highly reactive in pre-symptomatic stages while they lose their ability to monitor the environment as the disease progresses (Dibaj et al., 2011). Indeed, microglia isolated from either neonatal or early onset $SOD1^{G93A}$ mice display an activated M2 phenotype and enhance motoneuron survival while microglia isolated from either adult or end stage mice have a classically activated M1 phenotype and induce motoneuron death (Weydt et al., 2004; Liao et al., 2012). In the pre-symptomatic and symptomatic $SOD1^{G93A}$ rat model, microglia aggregates are detected in both the spinal cord and brainstem and display a degenerative and apoptotic phenotype at end stage (Fendrick et al., 2007; Graber et al., 2010). Moreover, microglia of pre-symptomatic $SOD1^{H46R}$ rats express the proliferating marker Ki67 and the phagocytic markers ED1 and major histocompatibility complex (MHC) class II (Sanagi et al., 2010; Bataveljic et al., 2011). These data suggest that microgliosis not only typifies ALS but that microglia function changes during disease progression, thus exerting differential effects on motoneurons.

A ROLE FOR MICROGLIA IN ALS PATHOGENESIS

A key finding supporting the contribution of microglia in ALS pathogenesis is the significant extension in lifespan and delay in disease progression when the mutant protein is specifically deleted from macrophages and microglial lineages in both $SOD1^{G37R}$ and $SOD1^{G85R}$ mice (Boillee et al., 2006; Wang et al., 2009). Similarly, bone marrow transplantation (resulting in donor-derived microglia) of $SOD1^{G93A}$ microglia into $PU.1^{-/-}$ mice (that lack CNS microglia at birth) did not induce neurodegeneration whereas wild-type donor-derived microglia transplantation into $SOD1^{G93A}$; $PU.1^{-/-}$ mice improved survival (Beers et al., 2006).

However, phenotypical analysis of microglia in different regions of $SOD1^{G93A}$ spinal cord suggests that both neuroprotective and neurotoxic population of microglial cells may co-exist during the disease and that depletion of proliferative microglia does not prevent motoneuron degeneration (Gowing et al., 2008; Beers et al., 2011b). Together, these studies thus suggest that microglia participates, through a complex balance between neuroprotective and neurotoxic signals, to ALS disease progression.

PROPOSED MECHANISMS OF MICROGLIAL-DERIVED NEUROTOXICITY

Various misregulated pathways within ALS microglia have been identified that may influence motoneuron survival. Endoplasmic reticulum (ER) stress is a characteristic of ALS pathogenesis (reviewed in Lautenschlaeger et al., 2012). In microglia of both sporadic ALS patients and symptomatic $SOD1^{G93A}$ mice, there is an increased expression of C/EBP homologous protein (CHOP; Ito et al., 2009), a member of the apoptotic ER stress pathway (reviewed in Oyadomari and Mori, 2004). It remains unclear if it directly participates in microglial neurotoxicity but exposure of microglia to interferon gamma (IFNγ), which levels are increased in the spinal cord of ALS mice and patients (Aebischer et al., 2011; Aebischer et al., 2012), elicits inducible nitric oxide (NO) synthase (iNOS) expression. The subsequent production of NO can cause an ER stress response that involves CHOP (Kawahara et al., 2001). Interestingly, several SOD1 mouse models show initiation of a specific ER stress response accompanied by microglial activation (Saxena et al., 2009).

Activation of the ligand-dependent CD14 lipopolysaccharide (LPS) receptor located at the microglial surface (Lacroix et al., 1998) initiates a pro-inflammatory Toll-like receptors (TLRs) dependent cascade (Laflamme and Rivest, 2001; Laflamme et al., 2001). Importantly, neurotoxic microglia activation by extracellular $SOD1^{G93A}$ is mediated by the CD14-TLR2 pathway and induces a subsequent release of pro-inflammatory cytokines, including tumor necrosis factor alpha (TNFα) and interleukin (IL)-1β (Liu et al., 2009; Zhao et al., 2010). Moreover, microglia from sporadic ALS patients show an enhanced TLR2 immunoreactivity (Casula et al., 2011). Microglia may thus participate in motoneuron loss following the specific activation of the CD14-TLR pathway by secreted SOD1 mutant, therefore propagating pro-inflammatory stimuli.

The release of extracellular nucleoside di- and tri-phosphates, in particular ATP, by degenerating neurons can elicit microglia activation through the ionotropic P2X and metabotropic P2Y purinergic receptors which can subsequently elicit a pro-inflammatory response, chemotaxis, and phagocytosis (reviewed in Inoue, 2006; Bours et al., 2011). Notably, P2X is increased within spinal cord microglia of ALS patients (Yiangou et al., 2006). Embryonic microglia and neonatal primary microglial cultures from mutant SOD1 mice display an upregulation of $P2X_4$, $P2X_7$, and $P2Y_6$ receptors (D'Ambrosi et al., 2009). Further, activation of $P2X_7$ in $SOD1^{G93A}$ microglia leads to the production of significantly higher levels of TNFα, which has a neurotoxic effect on motoneuron cultures (Ugolini et al., 2003), and of cyclooxygenase-2 (COX-2), which produces the potent inflammatory mediators prostaglandins (D'Ambrosi et al., 2009).

Moreover, a reduced ATP hydrolysis activity in mutant SOD1 microglia, suggests a potentiation of a purinergic-mediated inflammation that can participate to the neuroinflammatory state of microglial cells. Since ATP induces an astrocytic neurotoxic phenotype through $P2X_7$ receptor signaling (Gandelman et al., 2010), one can hypothesize that increased extracellular ATP in ALS, whether exacerbated by motoneurons and/or microglia contributes to the pathogenic microgliosis.

THE POTENTIAL INFLUENCE OF MICROGLIA ON NEURONAL EXCITABILITY

There is presently few assessment of the influence of microglia on motoneuron electrophysiology. However, studies on peripheral nerve or spinal cord injuries show that microglia activation has prominent effects on neuronal inhibitory control and loss of inhibitory control is a contributing mechanism to the motoneuron hyperexcitability that typifies ALS pathogenesis in humans (Bae et al., 2013).

Loss of neuronal inhibitory control occurs by several means including decrease in gamma-aminobutyric acid (GABA)ergic interneurons combined with changes in the expression of the $GABA_A$ receptor messenger RNA subunit (Petri et al., 2003; Maekawa et al., 2004). $GABA_A$ and glycine receptors are chloride (Cl^-) channels and the expression of cation-chloride co-transporter contributes to inhibitory effects of these Cl^- currents (Blaesse et al., 2009). Indeed, the entry of Cl^- following the opening of $GABA_A$ and glycine receptor-gated Cl^- channels inhibits neuron excitability by hyperpolarizing membrane potential. Under physiological condition, low intracellular Cl^- concentration $[Cl^-]_i$ is maintained by the potassium (K^+)-chloride co-transporter KCC2 that extrudes Cl^- from mature neurons (Rivera et al., 1999). Stimulation of spinal microglia following peripheral nerve injury induces a decrease in KCC2 expression among dorsal horn nociceptive neurons (Coull et al., 2003). KCC2 decrease is induced by the brain-derived neurotrophic factor (BDNF) and this is consistent with the previous observation that BDNF can be produced by non-neuronal cells involved in immune responses, including T and B lymphocytes, monocytes, and microglia (Kerschensteiner et al., 1999; Coull et al., 2005). BDNF produces a depolarizing shift in the anion reversal potential of dorsal horn lamina I neurons due to an increase in $[Cl^-]_i$. This shift prompts an inversion of inhibitory GABA currents that contributes to neuropathic pain following nerve injury (Coull et al., 2005). Decrease in KCC2 expression is thus responsible for the excitatory effects of GABA on neurons. Microglia activation and BDNF secretion are mediated through ATP activation of microglial P2X receptors. As discussed earlier, P2X receptors might be involved in ALS pathology since a higher density of $P2X_7$-immunoreactive microglial cells/macrophages are found in affected regions of spinal cords from ALS patients (Yiangou et al., 2006). Furthermore, levels of BDNF have been found to be increased in microglial cells isolated from ALS mice at the onset of disease and KCC2 is decreased in vulnerable motoneurons in $SOD1^{G93A}$ mice (Fuchs et al., 2010; Liao et al., 2012). Additionally, BDNF might play a role in the influence of microglia on motoneuron electric activity as suggested by work on spasticity. Spasticity is characterized by a velocity-dependent increase in muscle tone resulting from hyperexcitable stretch reflexes, spasms and hypersensitivity to normally innocuous sensory stimulations. Spasticity develops following spinal cord injury and is also regarded as an ALS clinical symptom (Rowland and Shneider, 2001). The main mechanism hypothesized to be responsible for spasticity is increased motoneuron excitability and increased synaptic inputs in response to muscle stretch due to reduced inhibitory mechanisms. Recently, it has been demonstrated that, following spinal cord injury, increased levels of BDNF mediated spasticity, due to post-transcriptional downregulation of KCC2 (Boulenguez et al., 2010). Together, these studies suggest that reactive microglia in ALS may exert an aberrant effect on the electrical activity of motoneurons and highlight the importance of furthering our understanding of this functional interaction.

Lastly, a hypothetical scenario relates to the defect in astrocytic glutamate transporter and the neurotoxic accumulation of the excitatory amino acid. It has been demonstrated that TNFα promotes glutamate release by activated microglia through the cystine/glutamate exchanger (Xc; Piani and Fontana, 1994). Though the implication of the Xc system in ALS has not yet been investigated, it may represent a potential mechanism of microglia-mediated excitotoxicity that warrants further study (Qin et al., 2006).

THE DUAL ROLE OF NEUROIMMUNITY IN MOTONEURON DISEASE

PATHOLOGICAL PHENOTYPE OF THE IMMUNE SYSTEM IN ALS

In addition to astrocytes and microglia, blood-derived immune cells may also play synergistic and critical functions during disease progression. Presence of a systemic immune activation is suggested by abnormalities observed in the blood and the CSF of ALS patients such as increased numbers of circulating lymphocytes ($CD4^+$ helper T cells, $CD8^+$ cytotoxic T lymphocytes, CTL, and natural killer, NK cells), increased expression of MHC class II molecules on monocytes as well as higher levels of inflammatory chemokines and cytokines (regulated on activation normal T cell expressed and secreted, RANTES, monocyte chemotactic protein, MCP-1, IL-12, IL-15, IL-17, and IL-23; Zhang et al., 2005; Rentzos et al., 2007, 2010, 2012; McCombe and Henderson, 2011). Further, post-mortem studies of brain and spinal cord lesions from ALS patients show that the activation and proliferation of microglia is associated with an infiltration of activated macrophages, mast cells and T lymphocytes which are found in close proximity to degenerating tissues (Engelhardt et al., 1993; Graves et al., 2004; Lewis et al., 2012). An in-depth autopsy of six ALS patients reveals an enrichment of T-cell receptor Vβ2-positive T cells in the spinal cord and CSF, suggesting an antigen-driven T cell selection (Panzara et al., 1999). Finally, ALS patients with a more rapidly progressing pathology show decreased numbers of regulatory T lymphocytes (Tregs), suggesting that the number of Tregs is inversely correlated with disease progression (Beers et al., 2011a; Rentzos et al., 2012). Tregs secrete anti-inflammatory cytokines such as IL-4, IL-10 and transforming growth factor beta (TGF-β) and has been show to induce the production of the neurotrophic factors glial-derived neurotrophic factor (GDNF) and BDNF by astrocytes (Reynolds et al., 2007). Tregs are also able to dampen a T helper (Th)1 pro-inflammatory response and attenuate toxic microglial responses. Contribution of the innate immune system is also suggested by the presence of immunoglobulins and complement deposition as well as a significant increase of NK cells in the blood of ALS patients (Donnenfeld et al., 1984; Engelhardt and Appel, 1990; Rentzos et al., 2012). While these investigations of ALS samples and tissues do not assess the contributory role of the immune system to disease pathogenesis, they do highlight its active presence.

In support of what is observed in humans, ALS rodent models also display a particular immunological phenotype. Indeed, $SOD1^{G93A}$ mice have allowed the demonstration that the inflammatory cellular subtypes are phenotypicaly and functionally different depending upon the disease stage (Liao et al., 2012). During the initial stages, infiltrating $CD4^+$ T cells are mainly Th2 ($IL\text{-}4^+$) while there is a skew toward Th1 ($IFN\gamma^+$) cells and $CD8^+$ T cells (both IL-17A positive and negative) as the disease progresses (Fiala et al., 2010; Beers et al., 2011b). Alteration in inflammatory cell subtypes is associated with, and maybe driven by, differences in Tregs. Interestingly, early symptomatic $SOD1^{G93A}$ mice have an increased number of Tregs and a decreased proliferation of effectors T lymphocytes (Teffs), whereas a decreased numbers of Tregs and an increased proliferation of Teffs is found in end stage animals (Beers et al., 2011a; Zhao et al., 2012). The innate immune system is also affected in ALS rodents, displayed by the substantial increase of NKT cells firstly in the liver and then in the spinal cord of $SOD1^{G93A}$ mice (Chiu et al., 2008; Finkelstein et al., 2011).

Whether neuroinflammation is a cause or a consequence of motoneuron dysfunction is still debated. It is interesting to note that inflammation is not limited to the CNS but systemic with a correlation between disease evolution and levels of plasma LPS as well as the numbers of activated circulating monocytes and T lymphocytes (Zhang et al., 2005, 2009). A thymic dysfunction also parallels the neurodegenerative process in mutant *SOD1* mice and ALS patients (Seksenyan et al., 2010). In the CNS of ALS patients, TAR DNA-binding protein 43 (TDP-43) displays an increased expression and interacts with nuclear factor kappa B (NF-κB) in glial and neuronal cells. LPS-activation of NF-κB in microglial cells expressing the TDP-43 mutant is associated with the production of pro-inflammatory cytokines, including TNFα, IL-1β, IL-6, and IFNγ (Swarup et al., 2011). NF-κB, is also an important intermediate of the TLR signaling pathway that contribute to the initiation of inflammatory responses (O'Connell et al., 2012). The central role of inflammation and NF-κB in ALS was recently confirmed by the description in familial ALS of mutations in the gene encoding optineurin, a negative regulator of TNF-induced NF-κB activation (Maruyama et al., 2010).

Additional regulators of the neuroinflammatory response are the microRNAs (miRNA), an abundant class of small, non-coding RNA that regulate gene expression in a wide range of biological processes (O'Connell et al., 2012). Recently, a dominantly inherited mutation in the heterogeneous nuclear ribonucleoprotein (hnRNP) A1 has been associated with familial ALS (Kim et al., 2013). hnRNPA1 is a RNA-binding protein involved in RNA metabolism, including the regulation of alternative pre-mRNA splicing, mRNA export, and stability as well as the processing of miRNA (Guil and Caceres, 2007). Interestingly, hnRNPA1 can directly interact with TDP-43 (Buratti et al., 2005), and TDP-43 was proposed to contribute to the post-translational processing of miRNA through interaction with the endonucleases, Drosha and Dicer (Kawahara and Mieda-Sato, 2012). The activity of Dicer, which processes miRNA precursors at the RNA-induced silencing complex (Wilson and Doudna, 2013), is required to maintain motoneuron functional integrity. Indeed, the conditional deletion of *Dicer* in vesicular acetylcholine transporter-expressing cells leads to motoneuron degeneration and denervation atrophy in mice (Haramati et al., 2010). Another intriguing link with the miRNA pathway in the neuro-immune interaction has been recently revealed by the demonstration that the neurotransmitter acetylcholine can inhibit the production of pro-inflammatory cytokines, TNFα and IL-6, through induction of miRNA-124 in macrophages (Sun et al., 2013). In addition, a subset of $CD4^+$ T cells has been described to produce acetylcholine to modulate the inflammatory response taking part of the autonomic homeostatic reflexes (Rosas-Ballina et al., 2011). Regarding ALS pathogenesis, a dysfunction of the cholinergic circuit has been reported in the spinal cord of SOD1 mutant mice, early in the disease course (Casas et al., 2013). Moreover, the choline acetyltransferase mRNA is a target of TDP-43 (Polymenidou et al., 2011), and the decrease in cholinergic input in the neuroinflammatory context of Alzheimer's disease was also shown to lead to the down regulation of hnRNPA1 (Berson et al., 2012). Despite the sequential events implicating miRNAs and the cholinergic signaling needs to be further explored, this evidence concurs toward the contribution of the neuro-immune interaction in the degenerative process.

The information from pre-clinical models and ALS patients suggests that systemic immune activation (innate and adaptive) might play a key role in ALS pathogenesis and may represent an interesting target for the development of novel treatments. However, a better understanding of the specific roles played by the different subtypes of immune cells is of utmost necessity. Indeed, accumulative evidence suggests that inflammatory cells mediate both protective and deleterious effects on motoneuron survival and that these functions vary during disease progression.

THE PROTECTIVE FUNCTION OF THE IMMUNE RESPONSE IN ALS

Protective immunity, a crucial homeostatic phenomenon in the repair of damaged tissues, results from both the clearance of debris and the effects of cytokines and growth factors delivered by inflammatory cells to the site of injury (Hohlfeld et al., 2000; Schwartz and Moalem, 2001). The neuroprotective ability of immune cells is also evident in ALS. Indeed, when *SOD1*^{G93A} mice are bred with mice lacking functional T cells or $CD4^+$ T cells, microglia skew toward an M1 inflammatory phenotype and disease progression accelerates, suggesting that $CD4^+$ T cells provide neuroprotection by suppressing the activation of cytotoxic microglia. Accordingly, reconstitution of T cells following bone marrow transplantation of *SOD1*^{G93A} mice lacking functional T and B cells prolonged their survival and suppressed the activation of M1 microglia (Beers et al., 2008). Further analysis showed that neuroprotection is mainly supported by $CD4^+CD25^+Foxp3^+$ Tregs that secrete IL-4, thus promoting M2 protective microglia and IL-4 secreting Th2 cells, while inhibiting the neurotoxic Th1 response and IFNγ secretion. The passive transfer of Tregs into ALS mice lacking functional T cells results in lengthened disease duration and prolonged survival (Beers et al., 2011a). Accordingly, these neuroprotective Tregs are increased in the peripheral blood of ALS patients during early stages but their numbers decrease as the disease progression accelerates and are thus inversely correlated with disease progression rates (Beers et al., 2011a; Rentzos et al., 2012; Henkel et al., 2013). Furthermore, Foxp3 and CD25 expression is reduced in Tregs from rapidly progressing patients and are also inversely correlated with disease progression rates (Henkel et al., 2013). Co-culture experiments showed that Tregs suppress the expression of cytotoxic factors Nox2 and iNOS from *SOD1*^{G93A} microglia through IL-4 secretion and inhibit the proliferation of *SOD1*^{G93A} Teffs via the combined secretion of IL-4, IL-10, and TGF-β (Zhao et al., 2012). Hence, Tregs enhance the neuroprotective properties of the immune system during the stable disease phase while a switch from a neuroprotective Tregs/M2 to a deleterious Th1/M1 response characterizes disease progression. The key role of this balance between protective and deleterious immune responses in modulating clinical outcome is confirmed by the temporal and regional association between neuroinflammation and motoneuron injury in ALS mice (Beers et al., 2011b). Indeed, initial weakness in the hindlimbs is associated with a Th1 proinflammatory infiltrate in the lumbar spinal cord, while a protective Th2 immune response is observed in the cervical cord and may explain the delayed motor weakness in the forelimbs (Beers et al., 2011b). Therefore, the inflammatory infiltrate observed in ALS lesions appears not simply as a consequence of motoneuron degeneration but is actively involved in the neurodegenerative process. Tregs and Th2 lymphocytes assume the majority of the neuroprotective functions of the immune system and targeting their signaling pathways may be an attractive therapeutic strategy in ALS.

THE NEUROTOXIC FUNCTION OF THE IMMUNE RESPONSE IN ALS

Cytotoxic T lymphocytes and NK cells are important effector cells of the immune system that eliminate aberrant cells, classically virus-infected cells, or tumorigenic cells (Zhang and Bevan, 2011; Kaur et al., 2012). Interestingly, at symptomatic stage, an increased number of $CD8^+$ T and NK cells is observed in the blood and spinal cord of ALS patients (Calvo et al., 2010; Rentzos et al., 2012). Neurotoxic effects might be associated with a Th1-driven CTL pro-inflammatory immune response. Accordingly, mutant *SOD1* Th1 lymphocytes proliferate to a greater extend and produce more

IFNγ during the rapidly progressing phase than Th1 lymphocytes isolated during the slowly progressing phase.

Different death pathways induced by $CD8^{+}$ CTL lymphocytes could potentially lead to motoneuron death in ALS. CTL are antigen-specific effector cells that express the ligand for Fas (FasL) and most potential CTL targets express Fas at their surface. The activation of Fas (CD95) by its cognate ligand FasL commits cells to a death program through a caspase cascade (Peter et al., 2007). Interestingly, the activation of Fas triggers a death pathway in motoneurons that appeared restricted to this cell type (Raoul et al., 1999, 2002, 2006; Bernard-Marissal et al., 2012; Aebischer et al., 2013). Motoneurons expressing ALS-linked SOD1 mutations showed an increased susceptibility to Fas-mediated death through activation of a Fas/NO amplification loop (Raoul et al., 2002, 2006). Accordingly, mutant *SOD1* mice with homozygous loss-of-function FasL mutation present a reduced loss of motoneurons and a prolonged life expectancy (Petri et al., 2006). It remains to be determined whether CTL contribute to Fas-induced motoneuron loss. Another cytotoxic mechanism of CTL-mediated killing of target cells is the perforin-granzyme system. Upon recognition of a target cell by CTL, cytotoxic granules containing perforin and granzyme are released in the extracellular space. Perforin is a pore forming protein allowing the entry in the target cells of granzyme serine proteases that subsequently induce caspase activation and cell death (van Domselaar and Bovenschen, 2011). It is noteworthy that increased levels of granzyme A and B isoforms are increased in the serum of ALS patients (Ilzecka, 2011). However, the functional significance of such an increase remains to be determined. IFNγ, which is produced by CTL cells, can exert both immunostimulatory and immunomodulatory effects during an immune response. IFNγ produced by mutant astrocytes and motoneurons can elicit a death program in motoneurons through the activation of the lymphotoxin beta receptor (LT-βR) by its ligand LIGHT (Aebischer et al., 2011, 2012). The genetic deletion of *Light* in $SOD1^{G93A}$ mice suggests that the LIGHT pathway contributes to the progression phase of the disease. Recently, the intracerebroventicular infusion of neutralizing anti-IFNγ antibody has been shown to delay the motor function decline in $SOD1^{G93A}$ mice, suggesting that IFNγ contributes to ALS pathogenesis (Otsmane et al., 2013). However, The precise contribution of IFNγ in the neuroinflammatory response remains to be investigated.

An infiltration of NK cells has been reported in the spinal cord of symptomatic ALS mice (Chiu et al., 2008). While the role of NK cells in ALS remains unknown, several hypothetical mechanisms can be raised about their pathogenic contribution. Indeed, activated NK cells inhibit neurite outgrowth of cerebellar neurons in a cell contact-dependent manner *in vitro* (Pool et al., 2012). In sensory neurons, IL-2-activated NK cells have a killing activity that requires the perforin-granzyme system (Backstrom et al., 2000). Further, the production of IFNγ by activated NK cells might directly trigger motoneuron death through the LIGHT/LT-βR pathway or potentiate a cytotoxic Th1/CTL response via the combined action of other NK-related cytokines such as IL-17 or IL-22 (Cella et al., 2010). NK cells thus represent an interesting branch of the immunopathology that should be further considered.

Several studies suggest that humoral immunity and immunoglobulins could also contribute to the disease. Autoantibodies to voltage-gated Ca^{2+} or K^{+} channels have been described in ALS patients, which induce specific motoneuron alterations both *in vitro* and *in vivo* after passive transfer in mice (Appel et al., 1991; Engelhardt et al., 1995; Demestre et al., 2005; Pagani et al., 2006; Nwosu et al., 2010). Abnormal levels of anti-Fas antibodies, able to induce neuronal apoptosis *in vitro*, have been detected in the serum of patients with ALS (Yi et al., 2000; Sengun and Appel, 2003). C5a and other complement activation products released after activation of the classical complement pathway by antibodies are elevated in the CSF and spinal cord of ALS mice and patients and specific inhibition of C5a receptor ameliorates disease in $SOD1^{G93A}$ mice (Woodruff et al., 2008; Heurich et al., 2011). Thus, both the innate and adaptive immune system appears to have deleterious consequences on the survival and maintenance of motoneurons in ALS (**Figure 1**).

EXPLOITING THE NEUROPROTECTIVE AND NEUROTOXIC PROPERTIES OF NEUROIMMUNITY FOR THE DEVELOPMENT OF THERAPEUTIC STRATEGIES

In light of the dynamic functional changes of microglia and immune cells discussed above, attempts to develop therapeutic strategies targeting neuroinflammation have only emphasized the importance of understanding the temporal neuroinflammatory events in ALS.

In pre-clinical mouse models, genetic deletion of the $P2X_7$ receptor, which was previously described as being upregulated in ALS microglia (D'Ambrosi et al., 2009), resulted in increased motoneuron loss, increased microgliosis, and accelerated disease progression, thus suggesting an unanticipated protective role for the $P2X_7$ receptor (Apolloni et al., 2013). Similarly, as mentioned earlier, genetic depletion of functional T cells or $CD4^{+}$ cells in $SOD1^{G93A}$ mice lead to increased disease progression, decreased survival as well as promoted production of pro-inflammatory effectors (Beers et al., 2008). Finally, eliminating the expression of galectin-3, a multifunctional immunomodulator that is increased in ALS microglia (Norling et al., 2009), in $SOD1^{G93A}$ mice, also results in aberrant microgliosis and increased disease progression (Lerman et al., 2012). These alterations ($P2X_7$, immune cells and galectin-3) were embryonically and permanently induced, implying that at a certain time-point during the development of the animal and the progression of the disease, these molecular and cellular components are necessary for alleviating certain ALS symptoms and pathological features.

At the clinical level, the failure of certain trials assessing the influence of drugs that directly or indirectly impact neuroinflammation may be due to inappropriate knowledge of the dynamic changes that occur within microglia and immune cells. Indeed, drastic immunosuppressive strategies such as cyclosporine, cyclophosphamide, intravenous immunoglobulin G treatment, and total lymphoid irradiation did not provide any significant benefits to ALS patients (Brown et al., 1986; Drachman et al., 1994; Gourie-Devi et al., 1997). Similarly, drugs used to target specific neuroinflammatory effectors that showed promising

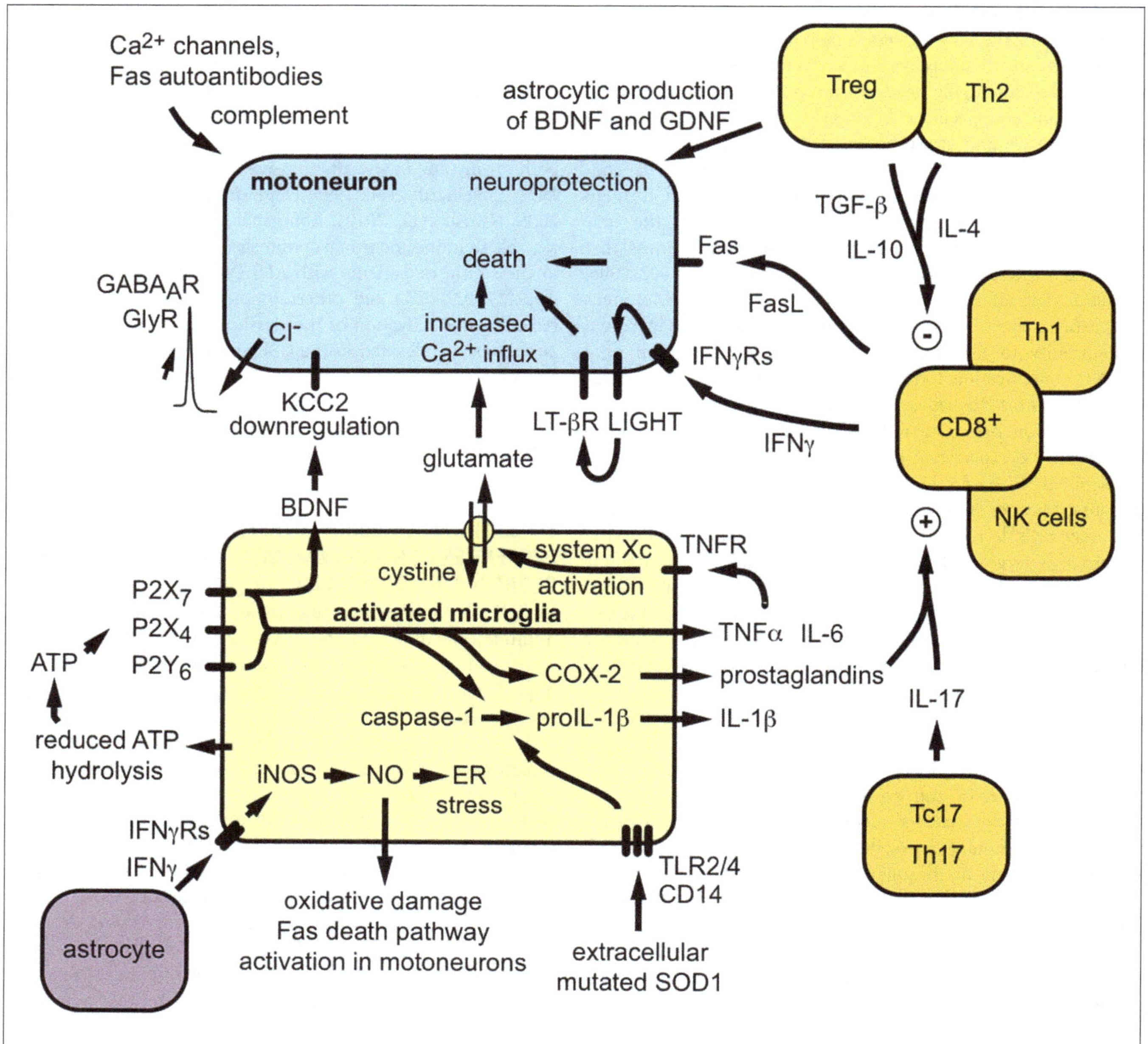

FIGURE 1 | Potential mechanisms by which peripheral and central immunity might contribute to the neurodegenerative process in ALS. Both neuroprotective and neurotoxic functions can be proposed for the involvement of microglia and lymphocytes in ALS pathogenesis.

results in pre-clinical models such as celecoxib and pioglitazone (Drachman et al., 2002; Schutz et al., 2005), proved to be ineffective in improving motor functions and survival in ALS patients (Cudkowicz et al., 2006; Dupuis et al., 2012).

The progressive spreading, extension and diffusion of the neurodegenerative process that typically occurs in ALS patients may result from the concurrent progressive invasion of the CNS by glial cells and most importantly, the functional changes that take place within these cells. Importantly, an incomplete understanding of said changes could lead to undesired and unexpected results. Indeed, both minocycline and thalidomide (an analog of lenalidomide) revealed serious harmful effects in patients during a randomized placebo-controlled phase III trial and a single arm, open label phase II study, respectively (Gordon et al., 2007; Stommel et al., 2009).

As translational therapy targeting neuroinflammatory and immunomodulatory effectors is rapidly progressing, it has become clear that a step backward is presently required to better assess the temporal functional changes that occur within glial and immune cells in ALS pathogenesis. The cellular environment being composed of both neuroprotective and neurotoxic functions, specific therapeutic windows may dictate the choice of drugs and their pathogenic targets. Alternatively, a combinatory therapeutic approach may be more efficient at modulating the contributions of non-neuronal cells to ALS pathology. Thus, while neuroinflammation undoubtedly plays a role in ALS pathogenesis, therapeutic success will be reached in limiting the activation and amplification of toxic glial and immune cells whilst preserving the cellular subtypes that are beneficial to motoneuron survival.

ACKNOWLEDGMENTS

Our work is supported by grants from the Institute National de la Santé et de la Recherche Médicale (INSERM), Association Française Contre les Myopathies (AFM), Association Française Pour la Recherche Sur la SLA (ARSLA), Direction de L'Hospitalisation et de L'Organisation des Soins (DHOS), and the Thierry Latran foundation. Melissa Bowerman is a recipient of a long-term EMBO Marie Curie Fellowship. We apologize to authors whose work could not have been cited due to space limitations.

REFERENCES

Aebischer, J., Benard-Marissal, N., Pettmann, B., and Raoul, C. (2013). Death receptors in the selective degeneration of motoneurons in amyotrophic lateral sclerosis. *J. Neurodegener. Dis.* 2013, 746845. doi: 10.1155/2013/746845

Aebischer, J., Cassina, P., Otsmane, B., Moumen, A., Seilhean, D., Meininger, V., et al. (2011). IFNgamma triggers a LIGHT-dependent selective death of motoneurons contributing to the non-cell-autonomous effects of mutant SOD1. *Cell Death Differ.* 18, 754–768. doi: 10.1038/cdd.2010.143

Aebischer, J., Moumen, A., Sazdovitch, V., Seilhean, D., Meininger, V., and Raoul, C. (2012). Elevated levels of IFNgamma and LIGHT in the spinal cord of patients with sporadic amyotrophic lateral sclerosis. *Eur. J. Neurol.* 19, 752–759. doi: 10.1111/j.1468-1331.2011.03623.x

Alexianu, M. E., Kozovska, M., and Appel, S. H. (2001). Immune reactivity in a mouse model of familial ALS correlates with disease progression. *Neurology* 57, 1282–1289. doi: 10.1212/WNL.57.7.1282

Apolloni, S., Amadio, S., Montilli, C., Volonte, C., and D'Ambrosi, N. (2013). Ablation of P2X7 receptor exacerbates gliosis and motoneuron death in the SOD1-G93A mouse model of amyotrophic lateral sclerosis. *Hum. Mol. Genet.* 22, 4102–4116. doi: 10.1093/hmg/ddt259

Appel, S. H., Engelhardt, J. I., Garcia, J., and Stefani, E. (1991). Immunoglobulins from animal models of motor neuron disease and from human amyotrophic lateral sclerosis patients passively transfer physiological abnormalities to the neuromuscular junction. *Proc. Natl. Acad. Sci. U.S.A.* 88, 647–651. doi: 10.1073/pnas.88.2.647

Backstrom, E., Chambers, B. J., Kristensson, K., and Ljunggren, H. G. (2000). Direct NK cell-mediated lysis of syngenic dorsal root ganglia neurons in vitro. *J. Immunol.* 165, 4895–4900.

Bae, J. S., Simon, N. G., Menon, P., Vucic, S., and Kiernan, M. C. (2013). The puzzling case of hyperexcitability in amyotrophic lateral sclerosis. *J. Clin. Neurol.* 9, 65–74. doi: 10.3988/jcn.2013.9.2.65

Banati, R. B., Gehrmann, J., Kellner, M., and Holsboer, F. (1995). Antibodies against microglia/brain macrophages in the cerebrospinal fluid of a patient with acute amyotrophic lateral sclerosis and presenile dementia. *Clin. Neuropathol.* 14, 197–200.

Bataveljic, D., Stamenkovic, S., Bacic, G., and Andjus, P. R. (2011). Imaging cellular markers of neuroinflammation in the brain of the rat model of amyotrophic lateral sclerosis. *Acta Physiol. Hung.* 98, 27–31. doi: 10.1556/APhysiol.98.2011.1.4

Beers, D. R., Henkel, J. S., Xiao, Q., Zhao, W., Wang, J., Yen, A. A., et al. (2006). Wild-type microglia extend survival in PU.1 knockout mice with familial amyotrophic lateral sclerosis. *Proc. Natl. Acad. Sci. U.S.A.* 103, 16021–16026. doi: 10.1073/pnas.0607423103

Beers, D. R., Henkel, J. S., Zhao, W., Wang, J., and Appel, S. H. (2008). CD4+ T cells support glial neuroprotection, slow disease progression, and modify glial morphology in an animal model of inherited ALS. *Proc. Natl. Acad. Sci. U.S.A.* 105, 15558–15563. doi: 10.1073/pnas.0807419105

Beers, D. R., Henkel, J. S., Zhao, W., Wang, J., Huang, A., Wen, S., et al. (2011a). Endogenous regulatory T lymphocytes ameliorate amyotrophic lateral sclerosis in mice and correlate with disease progression in patients with amyotrophic lateral sclerosis. *Brain* 134, 1293–1314. doi: 10.1093/brain/awr074

Beers, D. R., Zhao, W., Liao, B., Kano, O., Wang, J., Huang, A., et al. (2011b). Neuroinflammation modulates distinct regional and temporal clinical responses in ALS mice. *Brain Behav. Immun.* 25, 1025–1035. doi: 10.1016/j.bbi.2010.12.008

Bento-Abreu, A., Van Damme, P., Van Den Bosch, L., and Robberecht, W. (2010). The neurobiology of amyotrophic lateral sclerosis. *Eur. J. Neurosci.* 31, 2247–2265. doi: 10.1111/j.1460-9568.2010.07260.x

Bernard-Marissal, N., Moumen, A., Sunyach, C., Pellegrino, C., Dudley, K., Henderson, C. E., et al. (2012). Reduced calreticulin levels link endoplasmic reticulum stress and Fas-triggered cell death in motoneurons vulnerable to ALS. *J. Neurosci.* 32, 4901–4912. doi: 10.1523/JNEUROSCI.5431-11.2012

Berson, A., Barbash, S., Shaltiel, G., Goll, Y., Hanin, G., Greenberg, D. S., et al. (2012). Cholinergic-associated loss of hnRNP-A/B in Alzheimer's disease impairs cortical splicing and cognitive function in mice. *EMBO Mol. Med.* 4, 730–742. doi: 10.1002/emmm.201100995

Blaesse, P., Airaksinen, M. S., Rivera, C., and Kaila, K. (2009). Cation-chloride cotransporters and neuronal function. *Neuron* 61, 820–838. doi: 10.1016/j.neuron.2009.03.003

Boillee, S., Yamanaka, K., Lobsiger, C. S., Copeland, N. G., Jenkins, N. A., Kassiotis, G., et al. (2006). Onset and progression in inherited ALS determined by motor neurons and microglia. *Science* 312, 1389–1392. doi: 10.1126/science.1123511

Boulenguez, P., Liabeuf, S., Bos, R., Bras, H., Jean-Xavier, C., Brocard, C., et al. (2010). Down-regulation of the potassium-chloride cotransporter KCC2 contributes to spasticity after spinal cord injury. *Nat. Med.* 16, 302–307. doi: 10.1038/nm.2107

Bours, M. J., Dagnelie, P. C., Giuliani, A. L., Wesselius, A., and Di Virgilio, F. (2011). P2 receptors and extracellular ATP: a novel homeostatic pathway in inflammation. *Front. Biosci.* 3:1443–1456. doi: 10.2741/235

Brown, R. H. Jr., Hauser, S. L., Harrington, H., and Weiner, H. L. (1986). Failure of immunosuppression with a ten- to 14-day course of high-dose intravenous cyclophosphamide to alter the progression of amyotrophic lateral sclerosis. *Arch. Neurol.* 43, 383–384. doi: 10.1001/archneur.1986.00520040063021

Buratti, E., Brindisi, A., Giombi, M., Tisminetzky, S., Ayala, Y. M., and Baralle, F. E. (2005). TDP-43 binds heterogeneous nuclear ribonucleoprotein A/B through its C-terminal tail: an important region for the inhibition of cystic fibrosis transmembrane conductance regulator exon 9 splicing. *J. Biol. Chem.* 280, 37572–37584. doi: 10.1074/jbc.M505557200

Calvo, A., Moglia, C., Balma, M., and Chio, A. (2010). Involvement of immune response in the pathogenesis of amyotrophic lateral sclerosis: a therapeutic opportunity? *CNS Neurol. Disord. Drug Targets* 9, 325–330. doi: 10.2174/187152710791292657

Casas, C., Herrando-Grabulosa, M., Manzano, R., Mancuso, R., Osta, R., and Navarro, X. (2013). Early presymptomatic cholinergic dysfunction in a murine model of amyotrophic lateral sclerosis. *Brain Behav.* 3, 145–158. doi: 10.1002/brb3.104

Casula, M., Iyer, A. M., Spliet, W. G., Anink, J. J., Steentjes, K., Sta, M., et al. (2011). Toll-like receptor signaling in amyotrophic lateral sclerosis spinal cord tissue. *Neuroscience* 179, 233–243. doi: 10.1016/j.neuroscience.2011.02.001

Cella, M., Otero, K., and Colonna, M. (2010). Expansion of human NK-22 cells with IL-7, IL-2, and IL-1beta reveals intrinsic functional plasticity. *Proc. Natl. Acad. Sci. U.S.A.* 107, 10961–10966. doi: 10.1073/pnas.1005641107

Chiu, I. M., Chen, A., Zheng, Y., Kosaras, B., Tsiftsoglou, S. A., Vartanian, T. K., et al. (2008). T lymphocytes potentiate endogenous neuroprotective inflammation in a mouse model of ALS. *Proc. Natl. Acad. Sci. U.S.A.* 105, 17913–17918. doi: 10.1073/pnas.0804610105

Coull, J. A., Beggs, S., Boudreau, D., Boivin, D., Tsuda, M., Inoue, K., et al. (2005). BDNF from microglia causes the shift in neuronal anion gradient underlying neuropathic pain. *Nature* 438, 1017–1021. doi: 10.1038/nature04223

Coull, J. A., Boudreau, D., Bachand, K., Prescott, S. A., Nault, F., Sik, A., et al. (2003). Trans-synaptic shift in anion gradient in spinal lamina I neurons as a mechanism of neuropathic pain. *Nature* 424, 938–942. doi: 10.1038/nature01868

Cudkowicz, M. E., Shefner, J. M., Schoenfeld, D. A., Zhang, H., Andreasson, K. I., Rothstein, J. D., et al. (2006). Trial of celecoxib in amyotrophic lateral sclerosis. *Ann. Neurol.* 60, 22–31. doi: 10.1002/ana.20903

D'Ambrosi, N., Finocchi, P., Apolloni, S., Cozzolino, M., Ferri, A., Padovano, V., et al. (2009). The proinflammatory action of microglial P2 receptors is enhanced in SOD1 models for amyotrophic lateral sclerosis. *J. Immunol.* 183, 4648–4656. doi: 10.4049/jimmunol.0901212

Davalos, D., Grutzendler, J., Yang, G., Kim, J. V., Zuo, Y., Jung, S., et al. (2005). ATP mediates rapid microglial response to local brain injury in vivo. *Nat. Neurosci.* 8, 752–758. doi: 10.1038/nn1472

Demestre, M., Pullen, A., Orrell, R. W., and Orth, M. (2005). ALS-IgG-induced selective motor neurone apoptosis in rat mixed primary spinal cord cultures. *J. Neurochem.* 94, 268–275. doi: 10.1111/j.1471-4159.2005.03184.x

Dibaj, P., Steffens, H., Zschuntzsch, J., Nadrigny, F., Schomburg, E. D., Kirchhoff, F., et al. (2011). In vivo imaging reveals distinct inflammatory activity of CNS microglia versus PNS macrophages in a mouse model for ALS. *PLoS ONE* 6:e17910. doi: 10.1371/journal.pone.0017910

Donnenfeld, H., Kascsak, R. J., and Bartfeld, H. (1984). Deposits of IgG and C3 in the spinal cord and motor cortex of ALS patients. *J. Neuroimmunol.* 6, 51–57. doi: 10.1016/0165-5728(84)90042-0

Drachman, D. B., Chaudhry, V., Cornblath, D., Kuncl, R. W., Pestronk, A., Clawson, L., et al. (1994). Trial of immunosuppression in amyotrophic lateral sclerosis using total lymphoid irradiation. *Ann. Neurol.* 35, 142–150. doi: 10.1002/ana.410350205

Drachman, D. B., Frank, K., Dykes-Hoberg, M., Teismann, P., Almer, G., Przedborski, S., et al. (2002). Cyclooxygenase 2 inhibition protects motor neurons and prolongs survival in a transgenic mouse model of ALS. *Ann. Neurol.* 52, 771–778. doi: 10.1002/ana.10374

Dupuis, L., Dengler, R., Heneka, M. T., Meyer, T., Zierz, S., Kassubek, J., et al. (2012). A randomized, double blind, placebo-controlled trial of pioglitazone in combination with riluzole in amyotrophic lateral sclerosis. *PLoS ONE* 7:e37885. doi: 10.1371/journal.pone.0037885

Engelhardt, J. I., and Appel, S. H. (1990). IgG reactivity in the spinal cord and motor cortex in amyotrophic lateral sclerosis. *Arch. Neurol.* 47, 1210–1216. doi: 10.1001/archneur.1990.00530110068019

Engelhardt, J. I., Siklos, L., Komuves, L., Smith, R. G., and Appel, S. H. (1995). Antibodies to calcium channels from ALS patients passively transferred to mice selectively increase intracellular calcium and induce ultrastructural changes in motoneurons. *Synapse* 20, 185–199. doi: 10.1002/syn.890200302

Engelhardt, J. I., Tajti, J., and Appel, S. H. (1993). Lymphocytic infiltrates in the spinal cord in amyotrophic lateral sclerosis. *Arch. Neurol.* 50, 30–36. doi: 10.1001/archneur.1993.00540010026013

Fendrick, S. E., Xue, Q. S., and Streit, W. J. (2007). Formation of multinucleated giant cells and microglial degeneration in rats expressing a mutant Cu/Zn superoxide dismutase gene. *J. Neuroinflammation* 4, 9. doi: 10.1186/1742-2094-4-9

Fiala, M., Chattopadhay, M., La Cava, A., Tse, E., Liu, G., Lourenco, E., et al. (2010). IL-17A is increased in the serum and in spinal cord CD8 and mast cells of ALS patients. *J. Neuroinflammation* 7, 76. doi: 10.1186/1742-2094-7-76

Finkelstein, A., Kunis, G., Seksenyan, A., Ronen, A., Berkutzki, T., Azoulay, D., et al. (2011). Abnormal changes in NKT cells, the IGF-1 axis, and liver pathology in an animal model of ALS. *PLoS ONE* 6:e22374. doi: 10.1371/journal.pone.0022374

Fuchs, A., Ringer, C., Bilkei-Gorzo, A., Weihe, E., Roeper, J., and Schutz, B. (2010). Downregulation of the potassium chloride cotransporter KCC2 in vulnerable motoneurons in the SOD1-G93A mouse model of amyotrophic lateral sclerosis. *J. Neuropathol. Exp. Neurol.* 69, 1057–1070. doi: 10.1097/NEN.0b013e3181f4dcef

Gandelman, M., Peluffo, H., Beckman, J. S., Cassina, P., and Barbeito, L. (2010). Extracellular ATP and the P2X7 receptor in astrocyte-mediated motor neuron death: implications for amyotrophic lateral sclerosis. *J. Neuroinflammation* 7, 33. doi: 10.1186/1742-2094-7-33

Gerber, Y. N., Sabourin, J. C., Rabano, M., Vivanco, M., and Perrin, F. E. (2012). Early functional deficit and microglial disturbances in a mouse model of amyotrophic lateral sclerosis. *PLoS ONE* 7:e36000. doi: 10.1371/journal.pone.0036000

Glass, C. K., Saijo, K., Winner, B., Marchetto, M. C., and Gage, F. H. (2010). Mechanisms underlying inflammation in neurodegeneration. *Cell* 140, 918–934. doi: 10.1016/j.cell.2010.02.016

Gordon, P. H., Moore, D. H., Miller, R. G., Florence, J. M., Verheijde, J. L., Doorish, C., et al. (2007). Efficacy of minocycline in patients with amyotrophic lateral sclerosis: a phase III randomised trial. *Lancet Neurol.* 6, 1045–1053. doi: 10.1016/S1474-4422(07)70270-3

Gourie-Devi, M., Nalini, A., and Subbakrishna, D. K. (1997). Temporary amelioration of symptoms with intravenous cyclophosphamide in amyotrophic lateral sclerosis. *J. Neurol. Sci.* 150, 167–172. doi: 10.1016/S0022-510X(97)00083-X

Gowing, G., Philips, T., Van Wijmeersch, B., Audet, J. N., Dewil, M., Van Den Bosch, L., et al. (2008). Ablation of proliferating microglia does not affect motor neuron degeneration in amyotrophic lateral sclerosis caused by mutant superoxide dismutase. *J. Neurosci.* 28, 10234–10244. doi: 10.1523/JNEUROSCI.3494-08.2008

Graber, D. J., Hickey, W. F., and Harris, B. T. (2010). Progressive changes in microglia and macrophages in spinal cord and peripheral nerve in the transgenic rat model of amyotrophic lateral sclerosis. *J. Neuroinflammation* 7, 8. doi: 10.1186/1742-2094-7-8

Graves, M. C., Fiala, M., Dinglasan, L. A., Liu, N. Q., Sayre, J., Chiappelli, F., et al. (2004). Inflammation in amyotrophic lateral sclerosis spinal cord and brain is mediated by activated macrophages, mast cells and T cells. *Amyotroph. Lateral Scler. Other Motor Neuron Disord.* 5, 213–219. doi: 10.1080/14660820410020286

Guil, S., and Caceres, J. F. (2007). The multifunctional RNA-binding protein hnRNP A1 is required for processing of miR-18a. *Nat. Struct. Mol. Biol.* 14, 591–596. doi: 10.1038/nsmb1250

Hall, E. D., Oostveen, J. A., and Gurney, M. E. (1998). Relationship of microglial and astrocytic activation to disease onset and progression in a transgenic model of familial ALS. *Glia* 23, 249–256. doi: 10.1002/(SICI)1098-1136(199807)23:3<249::AID-GLIA7>3.0.CO;2-#

Hanisch, U. K., and Kettenmann, H. (2007). Microglia: active sensor and versatile effector cells in the normal and pathologic brain. *Nat. Neurosci.* 10, 1387–1394. doi: 10.1038/nn1997

Haramati, S., Chapnik, E., Sztainberg, Y., Eilam, R., Zwang, R., Gershoni, N., et al. (2010). miRNA malfunction causes spinal motor neuron disease. *Proc. Natl. Acad. Sci. U.S.A.* 107, 13111–13116. doi: 10.1073/pnas.1006151107

Henkel, J. S., Beers, D. R., Wen, S., Rivera, A. L., Toennis, K. M., Appel, J. E., et al. (2013). Regulatory T-lymphocytes mediate amyotrophic lateral sclerosis progression and survival. *EMBO Mol. Med.* 5, 64–79. doi: 10.1002/emmm.201201544

Heurich, B., El Idrissi, N. B., Donev, R. M., Petri, S., Claus, P., Neal, J., et al. (2011). Complement upregulation and activation on motor neurons and neuromuscular junction in the SOD1 G93A mouse model of familial amyotrophic lateral sclerosis. *J. Neuroimmunol.* 235, 104–109. doi: 10.1016/j.jneuroim.2011.03.011

Hohlfeld, R., Kerschensteiner, M., Stadelmann, C., Lassmann, H., and Wekerle, H. (2000). The neuroprotective effect of inflammation: implications for the therapy of multiple sclerosis. *J. Neuroimmunol.* 107, 161–166. doi: 10.1016/S0165-5728(00)00233-2

Ilzecka, J. (2011). Granzymes A and B levels in serum of patients with amyotrophic lateral sclerosis. *Clin. Biochem.* 44, 650–653. doi: 10.1016/j.clinbiochem.2011.02.006

Inoue, K. (2006). The function of microglia through purinergic receptors: neuropathic pain and cytokine release. *Pharmacol. Ther.* 109, 210–226. doi: 10.1016/j.pharmthera.2005.07.001

Ito, Y., Yamada, M., Tanaka, H., Aida, K., Tsuruma, K., Shimazawa, M., et al. (2009). Involvement of CHOP, an ER-stress apoptotic mediator, in both human sporadic ALS and ALS model mice. *Neurobiol. Dis.* 36, 470–476. doi: 10.1016/j.nbd.2009.08.013

Kaur, G., Trowsdale, J., and Fugger, L. (2012). Natural killer cells and their receptors in multiple sclerosis. *Brain* 136(Pt 9), 2657–2676. doi: 10.1093/brain/aws159

Kawamata, T., Akiyama, H., Yamada, T., and McGeer, P. L. (1992). Immunologic reactions in amyotrophic lateral sclerosis brain and spinal cord tissue. *Am. J. Pathol.* 140, 691–707.

Kawahara, Y., and Mieda-Sato, A. (2012). TDP-43 promotes microRNA biogenesis as a component of the Drosha and Dicer complexes. *Proc. Natl. Acad. Sci. U.S.A.* 109, 3347–3352. doi: 10.1073/pnas.1112427109

Kawahara, K., Oyadomari, S., Gotoh, T., Kohsaka, S., Nakayama, H., and Mori, M. (2001). Induction of CHOP and apoptosis by nitric oxide in p53-deficient microglial cells. *FEBS Lett.* 506, 135–139. doi: 10.1016/S0014-5793(01)02898-8

Kerschensteiner, M., Gallmeier, E., Behrens, L., Leal, V. V., Misgeld, T., Klinkert, W. E., et al. (1999). Activated human T cells, B cells, and monocytes produce brain-derived neurotrophic factor in vitro and in inflammatory brain lesions: a neuroprotective role of inflammation? *J. Exp. Med.* 189, 865–870. doi: 10.1084/jem.189.5.865

Kim, H. J., Kim, N. C., Wang, Y. D., Scarborough, E. A., Moore, J., Diaz, Z., et al. (2013). Mutations in prion-like domains in hnRNPA2B1 and hnRNPA1 cause multisystem proteinopathy and ALS. *Nature* 495, 467–473. doi: 10.1038/nature11922

Lacroix, S., Feinstein, D., and Rivest, S. (1998). The bacterial endotoxin lipopolysaccharide has the ability to target the brain in upregulating its membrane CD14 receptor within specific cellular populations. *Brain Pathol.* 8, 625–640. doi: 10.1111/j.1750-3639.1998.tb00189.x

Laflamme, N., and Rivest, S. (2001). Toll-like receptor 4: the missing link of the cerebral innate immune response triggered by circulating gram-negative bacterial cell wall components. *FASEB J.* 15, 155–163. doi: 10.1096/fj.00-0339com

Laflamme, N., Soucy, G., and Rivest, S. (2001). Circulating cell wall components derived from gram-negative, not gram-positive, bacteria cause a profound induction of the gene-encoding Toll-like receptor 2 in the CNS. *J. Neurochem.* 79, 648–657. doi: 10.1046/j.1471-4159.2001.00603.x

Lautenschlaeger, J., Prell, T., and Grosskreutz, J. (2012). Endoplasmic reticulum stress and the ER mitochondrial calcium cycle in amyotrophic lateral sclerosis. *Amyotroph. Lateral Scler.* 13, 166–177. doi: 10.3109/17482968.2011.641569

Lerman, B. J., Hoffman, E. P., Sutherland, M. L., Bouri, K., Hsu, D. K., Liu, F. T., et al. (2012). Deletion of galectin-3 exacerbates microglial activation and accelerates disease progression and demise in a SOD1(G93A) mouse model of amyotrophic lateral sclerosis. *Brain Behav.* 2, 563–575. doi: 10.1002/brb3.75

Lewis, C. A., Manning, J., Rossi, F., and Krieger, C. (2012). The neuroinflammatory response in ALS: the roles of microglia and T cells. *Neurol. Res. Int.* 2012, 803701. doi: 10.1155/2012/803701

Liao, B., Zhao, W., Beers, D. R., Henkel, J. S., and Appel, S. H. (2012). Transformation from a neuroprotective to a neurotoxic microglial phenotype in a mouse model of ALS. *Exp. Neurol.* 237, 147–152. doi: 10.1016/j.expneurol.2012.06.011

Liu, Y., Hao, W., Dawson, A., Liu, S., and Fassbender, K. (2009). Expression of amyotrophic lateral sclerosis-linked SOD1 mutant increases the neurotoxic potential of microglia via TLR2. *J. Biol. Chem.* 284, 3691–3699. doi: 10.1074/jbc.M804446200

Maekawa, S., Al-Sarraj, S., Kibble, M., Landau, S., Parnavelas, J., Cotter, D., et al. (2004). Cortical selective vulnerability in motor neuron disease: a morphometric study. *Brain* 127, 1237–1251. doi: 10.1093/brain/awh132

Maruyama, H., Morino, H., Ito, H., Izumi, Y., Kato, H., Watanabe, Y., et al. (2010). Mutations of optineurin in amyotrophic lateral sclerosis. *Nature* 465, 223–226. doi: 10.1038/nature08971

McCombe, P. A., and Henderson, R. D. (2011). The role of immune and inflammatory mechanisms in ALS. *Curr. Mol. Med.* 11, 246–254. doi: 10.2174/156652411795243450

Norling, L. V., Perretti, M., and Cooper, D. (2009). Endogenous galectins and the control of the host inflammatory response. *J. Endocrinol.* 201, 169–184. doi: 10.1677/JOE-08-0512

Nwosu, V. K., Royer, J. A., and Stickler, D. E. (2010). Voltage gated potassium channel antibodies in amyotrophic lateral sclerosis. *Amyotroph. Lateral Scler.* 11, 392–394. doi: 10.3109/17482960903452283

O'Connell, R. M., Rao, D. S., and Baltimore, D. (2012). microRNA regulation of inflammatory responses. *Annu. Rev. Immunol.* 30, 295–312. doi: 10.1146/annurev-immunol-020711-075013

Otsmane, B., Aebischer, J., Moumen, A., and Raoul, C. (2013). Cerebrospinal fluid-targeted delivery of neutralizing anti-IFNgamma antibody delays motor decline in an ALS mouse model. *Neuroreport* doi: 10.1097/WNR.0000000000000043 [Epub ahead of print].

Oyadomari, S., and Mori, M. (2004). Roles of CHOP/GADD153 in endoplasmic reticulum stress. *Cell Death Differ.* 11, 381–389. doi: 10.1038/sj.cdd.4401373

Pagani, M. R., Reisin, R. C., and Uchitel, O. D. (2006). Calcium signaling pathways mediating synaptic potentiation triggered by amyotrophic lateral sclerosis IgG in motor nerve terminals. *J. Neurosci.* 26, 2661–2672. doi: 10.1523/JNEUROSCI.4394-05.2006

Panzara, M. A., Gussoni, E., Begovich, A. B., Murray, R. S., Zang, Y. Q., Appel, S. H., et al. (1999). T cell receptor BV gene rearrangements in the spinal cords and cerebrospinal fluid of patients with amyotrophic lateral sclerosis. *Neurobiol. Dis.* 6, 392–405. doi: 10.1006/nbdi.1999.0252

Peter, M. E., Budd, R. C., Desbarats, J., Hedrick, S. M., Hueber, A. O., Newell, M. K., et al. (2007). The CD95 receptor: apoptosis revisited. *Cell* 129, 447–450. doi: 10.1016/j.cell.2007.04.031

Petri, S., Kiaei, M., Wille, E., Calingasan, N. Y., and Flint Beal, M. (2006). Loss of Fas ligand-function improves survival in G93A-transgenic ALS mice. *J. Neurol. Sci.* 251, 44–49. doi: 10.1016/j.jns.2006.08.013

Petri, S., Krampfl, K., Hashemi, F., Grothe, C., Hori, A., Dengler, R., et al. (2003). Distribution of GABAA receptor mRNA in the motor cortex of ALS patients. *J. Neuropathol. Exp. Neurol.* 62, 1041–1051.

Petrik, M. S., Wilson, J. M., Grant, S. C., Blackband, S. J., Tabata, R. C., Shan, X., et al. (2007). Magnetic resonance microscopy and immunohistochemistry of the CNS of the mutant SOD murine model of ALS reveals widespread neural deficits. *Neuromol. Med.* 9, 216–229. doi: 10.1007/s12017-007-8002-1

Philips, T., and Robberecht, W. (2011). Neuroinflammation in amyotrophic lateral sclerosis: role of glial activation in motor neuron disease. *Lancet Neurol.* 10, 253–263. doi: 10.1016/S1474-4422(11)70015-1

Piani, D., and Fontana, A. (1994). Involvement of the cystine transport system xc-in the macrophage-induced glutamate-dependent cytotoxicity to neurons. *J. Immunol.* 152, 3578–3585.

Polymenidou, M., Lagier-Tourenne, C., Hutt, K. R., Huelga, S. C., Moran, J., Liang, T. Y., et al. (2011). Long pre-mRNA depletion and RNA missplicing contribute to neuronal vulnerability from loss of TDP-43. *Nat. Neurosci.* 14, 459–468. doi: 10.1038/nn.2779

Pool, M., Rambaldi, I., Darlington, P. J., Wright, M. C., Fournier, A. E., and Bar-or, A. (2012). Neurite outgrowth is differentially impacted by distinct immune cell subsets. *Mol. Cell. Neurosci.* 49, 68–76. doi: 10.1016/j.mcn.2011.09.004

Qin, S., Colin, C., Hinners, I., Gervais, A., Cheret, C., and Mallat, M. (2006). System Xc- and apolipoprotein E expressed by microglia have opposite effects on the neurotoxicity of amyloid-beta peptide 1–40. *J. Neurosci.* 26, 3345–3356. doi: 10.1523/JNEUROSCI.5186-05.2006

Raoul, C., Buhler, E., Sadeghi, C., Jacquier, A., Aebischer, P., Pettmann, B., et al. (2006). Chronic activation in presymptomatic amyotrophic lateral sclerosis (ALS) mice of a feedback loop involving Fas, Daxx, and FasL. *Proc. Natl. Acad. Sci. U.S.A.* 103, 6007–6012. doi: 10.1073/pnas.0508774103

Raoul, C., Estevez, A. G., Nishimune, H., Cleveland, D. W., Delapeyriere, O., Henderson, C. E., et al. (2002). Motoneuron death triggered by a specific pathway downstream of Fas. Potentiation by ALS-linked SOD1 mutations. *Neuron* 35, 1067–1083. doi: 10.1016/S0896-6273(02)00905-4

Raoul, C., Henderson, C. E., and Pettmann, B. (1999). Programmed cell death of embryonic motoneurons triggered through the Fas death receptor. *J. Cell Biol.* 147, 1049–1062. doi: 10.1083/jcb.147.5.1049

Rentzos, M., Evangelopoulos, E., Sereti, E., Zouvelou, V., Marmara, S., Alexakis, T., et al. (2012). Alterations of T cell subsets in ALS: a systemic immune activation? *Acta Neurol. Scand.* 125, 260–264. doi: 10.1111/j.1600-0404.2011.01528.x

Rentzos, M., Nikolaou, C., Rombos, A., Boufidou, F., Zoga, M., Dimitrakopoulos, A., et al. (2007). RANTES levels are elevated in serum and cerebrospinal fluid in patients with amyotrophic lateral sclerosis. *Amyotroph. Lateral Scler.* 8, 283–287. doi: 10.1080/17482960701419232

Rentzos, M., Rombos, A., Nikolaou, C., Zoga, M., Zouvelou, V., Dimitrakopoulos, A., et al. (2010). Interleukin-17 and interleukin-23 are elevated in serum and cerebrospinal fluid of patients with ALS: a reflection of Th17 cells activation? *Acta Neurol. Scand.* 122, 425–429. doi: 10.1111/j.1600-0404.2010.01333.x

Reynolds, A. D., Banerjee, R., Liu, J., Gendelman, H. E., and Mosley, R. L. (2007). Neuroprotective activities of CD4+CD25+ regulatory T cells in an animal model of Parkinson's disease. *J. Leukoc. Biol.* 82, 1083–1094. doi: 10.1189/jlb.0507296

Rivera, C., Voipio, J., Payne, J. A., Ruusuvuori, E., Lahtinen, H., Lamsa, K., et al. (1999). The $K+/Cl^{-}$ co-transporter KCC2 renders GABA hyperpolarizing during neuronal maturation. *Nature* 397, 251–255. doi: 10.1038/16697

Rosas-Ballina, M., Olofsson, P. S., Ochani, M., Valdes-Ferrer, S. I., Levine, Y. A., Reardon, C., et al. (2011). Acetylcholine-synthesizing T cells relay neural signals in a vagus nerve circuit. *Science* 334, 98–101. doi: 10.1126/science.1209985

Rowland, L. P., and Shneider, N. A. (2001). Amyotrophic lateral sclerosis. *N. Engl. J. Med.* 344, 1688–1700. doi: 10.1056/NEJM200105313442207

Sanagi, T., Yuasa, S., Nakamura, Y., Suzuki, E., Aoki, M., Warita, H., et al. (2010). Appearance of phagocytic microglia adjacent to motoneurons in spinal cord tissue from a presymptomatic transgenic rat model of amyotrophic lateral sclerosis. *J. Neurosci. Res.* 88, 2736–2746. doi: 10.1002/jnr.22424.

Saxena, S., Cabuy, E., and Caroni, P. (2009). A role for motoneuron subtype-selective ER stress in disease manifestations of FALS mice. *Nat. Neurosci.* 12, 627–636. doi: 10.1038/nn.2297

Schutz, B., Reimann, J., Dumitrescu-Ozimek, L., Kappes-Horn, K., Landreth, G. E., Schurmann, B., et al. (2005). The oral antidiabetic pioglitazone protects from neurodegeneration and amyotrophic lateral sclerosis-like symptoms in superoxide dismutase-G93A transgenic mice. *J. Neurosci.* 25, 7805–7812. doi: 10.1523/JNEUROSCI.2038-05.2005

Schwartz, M., and Moalem, G. (2001). Beneficial immune activity after CNS injury: prospects for vaccination. *J. Neuroimmunol.* 113, 185–192. doi: 10.1016/S0165-5728(00)00447-1

Seksenyan, A., Ron-Harel, N., Azoulay, D., Cahalon, L., Cardon, M., Rogeri, P., et al. (2010). Thymic involution, a co-morbidity factor in amyotrophic lateral sclerosis. *J. Cell Mol. Med.* 14, 2470–2482. doi: 10.1111/j.1582-4934.2009.00863.x

Sengun, I. S., and Appel, S. H. (2003). Serum anti-Fas antibody levels in amyotrophic lateral sclerosis. *J. Neuroimmunol.* 142, 137–140. doi: 10.1016/S0165-5728(03)00263-7

Stommel, E. W., Cohen, J. A., Fadul, C. E., Cogbill, C. H., Graber, D. J., Kingman, L., et al. (2009). Efficacy of thalidomide for the treatment of amyotrophic lateral sclerosis: a phase II open label clinical trial. *Amyotroph. Lateral Scler.* 10, 393–404. doi: 10.3109/17482960802709416

Sun, Y., Li, Q., Gui, H., Xu, D. P., Yang, Y. L., Su, D. F., et al. (2013). MicroRNA-124 mediates the cholinergic anti-inflammatory action through inhibiting the production of pro-inflammatory cytokines. *Cell Res.* doi: 10.1038/cr.2013.116 [Epub ahead of print].

Swarup, V., Phaneuf, D., Dupre, N., Petri, S., Strong, M., Kriz, J., et al. (2011). Deregulation of TDP-43 in amyotrophic lateral sclerosis triggers nuclear factor kappaB-mediated pathogenic pathways. *J. Exp. Med.* 208, 2429–2447. doi: 10.1084/jem.20111313

Ugolini, G., Raoul, C., Ferri, A., Haenggeli, C., Yamamoto, Y., Salaun, D., et al. (2003). Fas/tumor necrosis factor receptor death signaling is required for axotomy-induced death of motoneurons in vivo. *J. Neurosci.* 23, 8526–8531.

van Domselaar, R., and Bovenschen, N. (2011). Cell death-independent functions of granzymes: hit viruses where it hurts. *Rev. Med. Virol.* doi: 10.1002/rmv.697 [Epub ahead of print].

Wang, L., Sharma, K., Grisotti, G., and Roos, R. P. (2009). The effect of mutant SOD1 dismutase activity on non-cell autonomous degeneration in familial amyotrophic lateral sclerosis. *Neurobiol. Dis.* 35, 234–240. doi: 10.1016/j.nbd.2009.05.002

Weydt, P., Yuen, E. C., Ransom, B. R., and Moller, T. (2004). Increased cytotoxic potential of microglia from ALS-transgenic mice. *Glia* 48, 179–182. doi: 10.1002/glia.20062

Wilson, R. C., and Doudna, J. A. (2013). Molecular mechanisms of RNA interference. *Annu. Rev. Biophys.* 42, 217–239. doi: 10.1146/annurev-biophys-083012-130404

Woodruff, T. M., Costantini, K. J., Crane, J. W., Atkin, J. D., Monk, P. N., Taylor, S. M., et al. (2008). The complement factor C5a contributes to pathology in a rat model of amyotrophic lateral sclerosis. *J. Immunol.* 181, 8727–8734.

Yamanaka, K., Chun, S. J., Boillee, S., Fujimori-Tonou, N., Yamashita, H., Gutmann, D. H., et al. (2008). Astrocytes as determinants of disease progression in inherited amyotrophic lateral sclerosis. *Nat. Neurosci.* 11, 251–253. doi: 10.1038/nn2047

Yi, F. H., Lautrette, C., Vermot-Desroches, C., Bordessoule, D., Couratier, P., Wijdenes, J., et al. (2000). In vitro induction of neuronal apoptosis by anti-Fas antibody-containing sera from amyotrophic lateral sclerosis patients. *J. Neuroimmunol.* 109, 211–220. doi: 10.1016/S0165-5728(00)00288-5

Yiangou, Y., Facer, P., Durrenberger, P., Chessell, I. P., Naylor, A., Bountra, C., et al. (2006). COX-2, CB2 and P2X7-immunoreactivities are increased in activated microglial cells/macrophages of multiple sclerosis and amyotrophic lateral sclerosis spinal cord. *BMC Neurol.* 6:12. doi: 10.1186/1471-2377-6-12

Zhang, N., and Bevan, M. J. (2011). CD8(+) T cells: foot soldiers of the immune system. *Immunity* 35, 161–168. doi: 10.1016/j.immuni.2011.07.010

Zhang, R., Gascon, R., Miller, R. G., Gelinas, D. F., Mass, J., Hadlock, K., et al. (2005). Evidence for systemic immune system alterations in sporadic amyotrophic lateral sclerosis (sALS). *J. Neuroimmunol.* 159, 215–224. doi: 10.1016/j.jneuroim.2004.10.009

Zhang, R., Miller, R. G., Gascon, R., Champion, S., Katz, J., Lancero, M., et al. (2009). Circulating endotoxin and systemic immune activation in sporadic amyotrophic lateral sclerosis (sALS). *J. Neuroimmunol.* 206, 121–124. doi: 10.1016/j.jneuroim.2008.09.017

Zhao, W., Beers, D. R., Henkel, J. S., Zhang, W., Urushitani, M., Julien, J. P., et al. (2010). Extracellular mutant SOD1 induces microglial-mediated motoneuron injury. *Glia* 58, 231–243. doi: 10.1002/glia.20919

Zhao, W., Beers, D. R., Liao, B., Henkel, J. S., and Appel, S. H. (2012). Regulatory T lymphocytes from ALS mice suppress microglia and effector T lymphocytes through different cytokine-mediated mechanisms. *Neurobiol. Dis.* 48, 418–428. doi: 10.1016/j.nbd.2012.07.008

3

The relationship between depressive symptoms, disease state, and cognition in amyotrophic lateral sclerosis

Laura Jelsone-Swain[1], Carol Persad[2], Kristen L. Votruba[2], Sara L. Weisenbach[2], Timothy Johnson[3], Kirsten L. Gruis[4†] and Robert C. Welsh[1,2]*

[1] *Department of Radiology, University of Michigan, Ann Arbor, MI, USA*
[2] *Department of Psychiatry, University of Michigan, Ann Arbor, MI, USA*
[3] *Department of Biostatistics, University of Michigan, Ann Arbor, MI, USA*
[4] *Department of Neurology, The State University of New York Upstate Medical University, Syracuse, NY, USA*

Edited by:
Francesco Pagnini, Catholic University of Milan, Italy

Reviewed by:
Steven E. Mock, University of Waterloo, Canada
Colin M. Bosma, Harvard University, USA

****Correspondence:***
Robert C. Welsh, Department of Radiology, University of Michigan, Room 3208C, Medical Science I, 1301 Catherine Street, Ann Arbor, MI 48109, USA.
e-mail: rcwelsh@med.umich.edu

† Dr. Kirsten Gruis conducted her role in this study while in the Neurology Department at the University of Michigan, Ann Arbor, MI, USA.

Cognitive impairment (CI) in amyotrophic lateral sclerosis (ALS) may present a serious barrier to a patient's wellbeing and significantly decrease quality of life. Although reports of CI in ALS without frank dementia are becoming quite common, questions remain regarding the specific cognitive domains affected, as well as how other psychological and medical factors may impact cognitive functioning in these patients. Additionally, the influence of depressive symptoms on disease processes is not known. We aimed to address these questions by completing extensive neuropsychological tests with 22 patients with ALS and 17 healthy volunteers. A subgroup of these patients also completed questionnaires to measure depressive and vegetative symptoms. We tested for overall cognitive differences between groups, the influence of physical (e.g., bulbar and limb), vegetative (e.g., fatigue), and depressive symptoms on cognitive performance, and the relationship between depressive symptoms and disease severity in ALS. Overall, patients performed more poorly than healthy controls (HCs), most notably on tests of executive functioning and learning and memory. Results suggest that true cognitive performance differences exist between patients with ALS and HCs, as these differences were not changed by the presence of vegetative or depressive symptoms. There was no effect of limb or bulbar symptoms on cognitive functioning. Also, patients were not any more depressed than HCs, however increased depressive scores correlated with faster disease progression and decreased limb function. Collectively, it is suggested that translational advances in psychological intervention for those with CI and depression become emphasized in future research.

Keywords: ALS, motor neuron disease, neuropsychology, depression, ALSFRS-r, cognition, limb symptoms

INTRODUCTION

Until recently, amyotrophic lateral sclerosis (ALS) was still considered by many a pure motor neuron disease (Pongratz, 2000), and the notion of cognitive impairment (CI) in ALS was met with much resistance until just the past several years (Bak and Chandran, 2012). It is now widely accepted that ALS is a multisystem disorder involving CI in approximately 30% of those diagnosed with the disease (Rippon et al., 2006). ALS with CI is now recognized as a subcategory of ALS (Strong et al., 2009) and is denoted as ALS*ci* (Murphy et al., 2007), which entails presentation of CI without frank dementia. Importantly, some experts propose that ALS is not a categorical disease, but rather a spectrum disorder between pure ALS and Frontotemporal Lobar Degenerative diseases, such as Frontotemporal dementia (Abrahams et al., 2000; Grossman et al., 2007; Murphy et al., 2007; Woolley and Katz, 2008; Merrilees et al., 2010).

Recent advances in the field support the need for study into cognitive problems associated with ALS (see Phukan et al., 2007). One critical reason for this research is that cognitive difficulties in patients with ALS negatively impact quality of life, and appear to be even more detrimental to quality of life than physical impairment (Goldstein et al., 2002). Personal communication with patients who believe their cognitive ability has been compromised report being negatively impacted by these symptoms and wanting help, or at least support, in this area. Additionally, CI can influence decision-making (Girardi et al., 2011), treatment compliance (Olney et al., 2005), survival (Olney et al., 2005; Flaherty-Craig et al., 2011), and even the wellbeing of caregivers (Merrilees et al., 2010).

Most studies that have identified CI in patients with ALS have utilized a comprehensive neuropsychological battery to assess performance across multiple modalities. Of these studies, verbal fluency remains one of the most sensitive measures for CI, repeatedly showing poorer performance in those with ALS compared to healthy individuals (Abrahams et al., 1997, 2000; Kilani et al., 2004; Grossman et al., 2007). These findings hold even after correcting for possible verbal production impairment (Abrahams et al., 2004). Other studies have found decreased performance in other areas of executive function (Kilani et al., 2004), memory (Abrahams et al., 1997; Hanagasi et al., 2002), and language (Hillis et al., 2004; Raaphorst et al., 2010). Although reports of CI in ALS are becoming more common, characteristics of ALS*ci* are not well defined due to a number of factors. These include the lack of availability of valid cognitive measures that can be administered to ALS patients with significant motor or speech limitations, as well as minimal research focusing on additional variables that could also impact cognition, such as physical symptoms and mood state.

As previously mentioned, ALS*ci* is not well understood, and the involvement of physical symptoms on CI in ALS is not known. Specifically, previous research has indicated that those with bulbar onset are more likely to have ALS*ci* (Gordon et al., 2011), yet others have not supported this notion (Rusina et al., 2010). Additionally, vegetative physical symptoms of ALS may impact the interpretation of those identified with ALS*ci*. For example, it is known that fatigue, one of the most common vegetative symptoms in ALS, interferes with cognitive test performance in other patient groups (Diamond et al., 2008). For the purpose of this paper, vegetative symptoms collectively refer to changes in concentration, fatigue, appetite, sleeping, and energy level. Although these symptoms can also be specific to depression, ALS patients with physical weakness are likely to have more vegetative symptoms in the performance of daily activities rather than from depression, especially if the patient does not report other symptoms of depression such as hopelessness and guilt. Therefore, it is necessary to differentiate between physical and depressive symptoms in predicting CI in order to obtain a more accurate description of CI in patients with ALS. This may also lead to more streamlined classification of those with true CI who may need or want intervention.

Like CI, research suggests that depressive symptoms in ALS may also have a negative impact on many aspects of quality of life (Tramonti et al., 2012), and could potentially affect cognition. To our knowledge however, no studies have examined the influence of depressive symptoms on cognitive performance in ALS. Like vegetative symptoms, mood status could present a potential confound in the diagnosis of ALS*ci*. Also, depressive symptoms may increase the risk of having CI, or differentially affect cognition in patients with ALS compared to a healthy control population. These situations are likely, as depression can negatively influence cognitive performance in other diseases (Diamond et al., 2008; Sassoon et al., 2012).

The relationship between depression and prognosis or physical symptom presentation in ALS is another area of research that has received little attention, possibly due to the general report of a global positive psychosocial adjustment in these patients (Brown and Mueller, 1970; Lulé et al., 2012). Despite this view, prevalence rates of depression (McLeod and Clarke, 2007) and reports on the effect of depression on ALS are not consistent. For example, Atassi et al. (2011) reported no relationship between disease progression and depression, yet a previous study identified a significant negative impact of psychological distress on mortality outcome (McDonald et al., 1994). Using the ALS Functional Rating Scale (ALSFRS), a group in South Korea found that decreased physical functioning correlated with depressive symptoms (Oh et al., 2012), highlighting the importance of examining this relationship. Patients in this study however were on average both highly physically disabled (ALSFRS mean score of 19) and many were clinically depressed (Beck Depression Inventory mean score of 24.5). If consistent evidence supports the association of depressive symptoms with disease processes (especially while patients are still early in the disease course and without clinical depression), this would bring about new emphasis into the study of depression in ALS, ultimately leading to improved identification of those at highest risk and thus early intervention.

The overall goal of this study was to recognize if cognitive status is affected in patients with ALS early in their disease course and without severe clinical depression. We also examined other variables that may be associated with cognitive performance that could either facilitate in future early screening or confound the diagnosis of ALS*ci*. Specifically, we investigated the relationship of physical impairment, vegetative symptoms, and depressive symptoms on cognitive functioning. In addition, we tested whether depressive symptoms are associated with disease progression or physical impairment. We utilized standard neuropsychological tests to measure these relationships. Based on previous literature, we hypothesized that patients with ALS would perform at a lower level on tests within the neuropsychological battery, especially those targeting executive functioning skills. We predicted that physical, vegetative, and depressive symptoms would negatively influence cognitive performance, but that these would not be confounding variables in performance differences between patients with ALS and healthy volunteers (suggesting true cognitive impairment in the ALS group). We also hypothesized that ALS patients would have more depressive symptoms than healthy controls, and that increased depressive symptoms would be related to disease severity.

MATERIALS AND METHODS

PARTICIPANTS

Twenty-two patients with ALS participated in this study. All patients were recruited through the ALS Clinic at the University of Michigan. Patients were diagnosed by a neuromuscular physician at the University of Michigan using the El Escorial criteria for ALS. Enrolled patients were engaged in a larger longitudinal neuroimaging component of this study; therefore all patients were without any contraindications to magnetic resonance imaging (MRI), were able to lay flat on their back without respiratory distress, were not dependent on artificial ventilation, and were ambulatory. Twenty-three healthy controls (HCs) were recruited through the general community from an internet-based recruitment tool (UMClinicalTrials.org) and from flyers posted around the Ann Arbor, MI area. Participants were excluded from either group if they had a history of alcohol or drug abuse, neurological disease (other than ALS), were ever diagnosed with a psychological disorder, or were severely clinically depressed at the time of their participation. No patient was excluded from the study, and one healthy volunteer was excluded for major depression. Because we aimed to compare cognitive status in patients with ALS to a truly healthy control group, HCs at risk for mild CI (see Statistical Analysis) were also excluded from the final analysis. Participant demographic information for these final groups is displayed in **Table 1**. Signed consent from each participant was obtained, and all aspects of this study were approved by the Institutional Review Board at the University of Michigan.

Table 1 | Means and SD for demographic information by group.

Demographic variables	ALS patients	Healthy controls
Age	59 (6.6)	58 (5.0)
DH	18R*, 4L	15R, 2L
Sex	13M, 9F	5M, 12F
Education years	13.4 (2.0)	16 (2.6)
Symptom onset	17L, 5B	NA
ALSFRS-r total	37.2 (6.9)	NA
ALSFRS-r limb	16.5 (5.3)	NA
ALSFRS-r bulbar	10.0 (2.4)	NA
ALSFRS-r resp.	10.73 (1.9)	NA
MSO	26.2 (35.6)	NA

*DH, dominant hand; Education Years, number of complete years of education, considering degrees obtained; ALSFRS-r Limb, subscore from ALSFRS-r questionnaire assessing limb function (questions 4–9); ALSFRS-r Bulbar, subscore from ALSFRS-r questionnaire assessing bulbar function (questions 1 – 3); ALSFRS-r Resp., subscore from ALSFRS-r questionnaire assessing respiratory function (questions 10 – 12); MSO, months since symptom onset. *Two patients reported current dominant hand as a result of disease processes and not by preference.*

NEUROPSYCHOLOGICAL ASSESSMENTS

All participants completed a 60-min neuropsychological battery designed by a team of neuropsychologists experienced in motor diseases (lead by CP). These tests were selected to assess a broad range of cognitive skills, particularly those commonly associated with frontotemporal dementia, given the reported prevalence of such deficits in patients with ALS. Depressive and vegetative symptoms were also measured using the Geriatric Depression Scale, short version (GDS), and the Beck Depression Inventory (BDI), respectively. Not all participants completed both questionnaires. Nineteen ALS patients and 15 HCs completed the GDS, and 14 patients and 15 HCs completed the BDI. All tests and questionnaires are described below. Reliability coefficients and, when available, construct validity coefficients are given for each measurement (Strauss et al., 2006).

Mini-Mental State Examination (Folstein et al., 1975)

The Mini-Mental State Examination (MMSE) is a brief test of global cognitive function and is often used as a screen for dementia. The scale assesses a subject's orientation to time and place, instantaneous recall, short-term memory, and ability to perform serial subtractions or reverse spelling. The MMSE also measures constructional capacities (the ability to copy a design) and the use of language. Internal consistency of this test ranges between 0.31–0.96, test re-test reliability ranges between 0.80–0.95, and construct validity is modest to high in correlating with other similar tests.

Hopkins Verbal Learning Test (Shapiro et al., 1999)

The Hopkins Verbal Learning Test (HVLT) is a learning and memory test that measures initial recall (test re-test reliability 0.74), delayed recall (20 min, test re-test reliability 0.66), and discrimination recall (test re-test reliability 0.40) for a list of words read by the administrator. The test is available in multiple alternate forms with a moderate to high construct validity with other similar tests.

Faces Subtest: Wechsler Memory Scale (WMS-III; subtests – Faces) (Wechsler, 1997)

Faces is a test of visual learning and recognition memory for pictures of faces. There is an initial recall test (Faces I) and a delayed recall test (Faces II, 30 min after first exposure to the set of faces). Internal reliability for these tests is between 0.60–0.96, internal consistency is between 0.70–0.79, and construct validity is modest.

Boston Diagnostic Aphasia Examination: Complex Ideational Material (Goodglass and Kaplan, 1983)

The Complex Ideational Material (CIM) subtest of the Boston Diagnostic Aphasia Examination (BDAE) measures auditory comprehension. This task requires patients to understand and express agreement or disagreement concerning factual material that are derived from inference. Complex Ideational Material has an internal consistency of 0.80 and a construct validity score between 0.86 and 0.93. This test was originally designed for patients with aphasia, so test-re-test reliability measurements were not provided as test performance is expected to change with this group.

The Boston Naming Test (Kaplan et al., 1978)

The Boston Naming Test (BNT) is a confrontation-naming test that is largely used to measure language processing. The test consists of 60 large pen and ink drawings of items ranging in familiarity. Participants are asked to freely name each item. If the identity of an item is not known, first a stimulus cue is provided, then a phonemic cue if needed. Scores used in this study only include freely identified and stimulus-cued correct responses. Internal consistency coefficients range between 0.78–0.96 and test re-test reliability is high (0.91). Construct validity is also high.

Judgment of Line Orientation (Benton, 1983)

The Judgment of Line Orientation (JOLO) measures visuospatial ability, specifically the ability to estimate angular relationships between line segments by visually matching angled line pairs to numbered radii that form a semicircle. The internal consistency for this test is between 0.84 and 0.91 and the test re-test coefficient is 0.90. Construct validity is high when compared with other visual spatial subtests.

Digit Span (Wechsler Adult Intelligence Scale: WAIS subtest) (Wechsler, 1997)

Digit Span is a subtest from the WAIS measuring auditory working memory. This test consists of two sections measuring immediate recall of a forward and backward digit series. In this study the total cumulative score of number of correct trials was used to measure overall working memory recall. Backward digit span is more challenging and was also used as a measurement in this study. The maximum span of backward digits recalled was used; therefore this measurement was not collinear with the total cumulative score. The generalizeability coefficient for this test is high (0.80–0.89) and the test re-test coefficient for the backward subscore is marginal (0.60–0.69).

Oral Trail-Making Test (Lezak, 1995)

The Oral Trail-Making Tests (OTMT) are tests of processing speed (Trails A) and conceptual ability (Trails B). For Trails A, the subject is required to recite consecutive numbers, from 1–25, as quickly as possible. On Trails B, subjects are asked to alternate between numbers and letters, from 1-A to 13-M. Two scores for each part are obtained – the total time and number of errors. To more accurately measure set-shifting abilities from Oral Trail-Making Test B and partial out motor speed due to possible verbal speed production impairment in patients with ALS (Abrahams et al., 2000), time (in seconds) to complete Oral Trail-Making Test B was divided by time (in seconds) to complete Oral Trail-Making Test A, resulting in an Oral Trails B/Oral Trails A ratio. This ratio results in a more statistically accurate measure to account for processing speed differences between groups. The test re-test reliability is adequate for test A and high for test B. Tests A and B correlate well with each other (0.31).

Controlled Oral Word Association Test (Benton, 1983)

The Controlled Oral Word Association Test (COWAT) is a test of verbal letter fluency using the letters C, F, and L. Participants are asked to name as many words beginning with each letter in 1 min (each). This is largely a test of executive function. The internal consistency for this test, specifically using the letters CFL, is high (0.83). Test re-test reliability is high (0.70) and construct validity is high.

Animal Naming (Sager et al., 2006)

The Animal Naming test is a categorical verbal fluency test and is used as a test of executive function. Participants are asked to name as many animals as they can in 1 min. Test re-test reliability is 0.56 and construct validity is moderately high.

Geriatric Depression Scale-Short Form (Yesavage and Sheikh, 1986)

This 15-(yes/no) questionnaire was developed specifically to measure depression in older adults. Symptoms common to normal aging and those pertaining to feelings of guilt, sexual activity, suicide, and somatic symptoms are not included in this questionnaire. Rather, this questionnaire focuses on the individual's locus of control, "... making this more suitable for subjects in hospital or long-term care" (Strauss et al., 2006, p. 1104). Therefore the Geriatric depression scale-short form (GDS) was deemed as a more valid measure of core depressive symptoms in the ALS group and was used as a measure of depression severity. The short version has a high correlation with the full version, which is moderately to highly correlated with other tests of depression (0.73–0.91). The internal consistency for the full version ranges between 0.71 and 0.84 and test re-test reliability is 0.84.

Beck Depression Inventory (Beck et al., 1996)

This 21-item likert-scale questionnaire is a brief self-report of depression. The BDI contains a number of somatic and vegetative symptoms that can overlap with physical illness, more common in older adults and especially those with motor neuron diseases. Therefore impetus for completing the BDI was to provide a measure of vegetative symptoms to asses show they may contribute to cognitive functioning. Five questions were selected to describe vegetative symptoms: 15. Loss of Energy; 16. Changes in Sleeping Pattern; 18. Changes in Appetite; 19. Concentration Difficulty; 20. Tiredness or Fatigue. The internal consistency coefficient for this questionnaire is high (0.88) and the test re-test reliability is adequate to high (0.74–0.93). The construct validity is also high.

STATISTICAL ANALYSIS

Neuropsychological test results used to compare cognitive performance between groups are listed in **Table 2**. All data is presented in raw scores. All data were examined to check for parametric analysis statistical assumptions. Results from two tests did not meet these assumptions: the Complex Ideational Material (CIM) and Oral Trails-Making Test B/A ratio scores. In the CIM, the majority of participants performed at ceiling level (maximum score of 12 points), with just one person scoring nine points. The CIM was therefore excluded from further statistical models. The Oral Trails B/A ratio score was slightly positively skewed in both groups. Therefore individual scores from the Oral Trails B/A ratio were transformed (using the natural logarithm function), which resulted in a normal distribution for both groups. IBM's statistical software package SPSS, version 19, was used to conduct all analyses.

To assure our control group consisted of truly healthy volunteers, z-scores from neuropsychological tests were examined for mild cognitive impairment (MCI). Using standard criteria established in the literature, controls were excluded for suspected MCI if they scored at or below the fifth percentile on one or more cognitive test (Royall et al., 2004; Aarsland et al., 2010). Five controls were excluded for MCI, resulting in 17 participants in the HC group.

Age and years of education were compared between groups using independent sample t-tests, which showed no age differences ($p = 0.65$) but significantly more years of education in the HC group [$t(37) = -3.65$, $p < 0.01$]. Therefore education was included as a covariate in the following statistical models.

RESULTS

All patients with ALS completed the ALS Functional Rating Scale, revised version (ALSFRS-r). The ALSFRS-r is a 12-question survey measuring physical functioning of patients with ALS and is a strong predictor of progression and survival (Kollewe et al., 2008). Limb, bulbar, and respiratory functioning are measured in this scale and the maximum total score is 48 (lower scores indicate decreased physical function). Mean ALSFRS-r score for this patient group was 37.2 ($SD = 6.9$). Additionally, all participants completed the Oldenfield handedness questionnaire and a head trauma questionnaire (Armon and Nelson, 2012). Demographic information is presented in **Table 1**.

COGNITIVE IMPAIRMENT IN THE ALS PATIENT GROUP

Using the consensus criteria developed by Strong et al. (2009), individual normalized scores were examined for each patient to identify those with possible ALS*ci*. Scores below the fifth percentile, or falling below a z-score of -1.6, were flagged. Individuals whose scores fell below this cut-off on two or more distinct tests were identified as patients with ALS*ci*.

Examining z-scores from each of the tests within the neuropsychological battery, eight of the 22 patients (36.4%) with ALS were identified as having CI. This finding is consistent with previous research showing an estimated 30% of patients with comorbid CI

Table 2 | Neuropsychological test results between patients with ALS and healthy controls.

Cognitive domain	Neuropsychological test measurement	ALS patients ($n=22$)		Healthy controls ($n=17$)		Group differences	
		Mean raw score (SD)	% Impaired	Mean raw score (SD)	% Impaired	*F*-value	*p*-value
Mental status/dementia screen	MMSE total score	27.41 (2.04)	na	27.65 (1.50)	na	0.31	0.58
Executive function	COWAT (CFL) total score	32.77 (9.25)	4.50	49.53 (12.62)	0.0	11.12	<0.01
	Animal Naming total score	15.91 (4.22)	36.36	22.06 (4.59)	5.8	10.04	<0.01
	OTMT B seconds	44.68 (29.62)	4.50	25.56 (15.49)	0.0	na	na
	OTMT transformed ratio (B seconds/A seconds)	1.32 (0.55)	na	1.18 (0.39)	na	1.19	0.28
Memory/learning	HVLT initial recall, trials 1–3	23.86 (5.82)	31.80	27.24 (4.13)	5.8	1.10	0.30
	HVLT delayed recall, trial 4	8.59 (2.40)	27.3	9.94 (1.39)	0.0	1.65	0.21
	HVLT discrimination score	10.18 (1.62)	18.2	11.24 (0.97)	0.0	2.68	0.11
	Faces I total score	34.86 (4.81)	4.5	39.00 (4.47)	0.0	10.390	<0.01
	Faces II total score	37.05 (4.87)	9.0	40.65 (2.78)	0.0	6.81	0.01
Attention/concentration	Digit Span total score	15.68 (3.72)	4.5	18.12 (3.33)	0.0	2.53	0.12
	Digit Span backward span	4.50 (1.06)	0.0	5.24 (1.35)	0.0	0.83	0.37
Visuoperceptual	JOLO total score	23.91 (5.38)	13.63	25.88 (4.26)	5.8	0.05	0.83
Language	BNT total score including semantic cues	56.55 (2.46)	0.0	55.94 (3.15)	0.0	3.95	0.06
Depression	GDS (ALS $n=19$, HC $n=15$)	2.32 (1.97)	na	1.07 (1.16)	na	(t) 2.17	0.04
	BDI (ALS $n=14$, HC $n=15$)	5.57 (3.80)	na	3.00 (2.17)	na	(t) 2.26	0.03
Vegetative symptoms	BDI_veg (ALS $n=14$, HC $n=15$)	2.64 (1.74)	na	1.67 (1.29)	na	(t) 1.73	0.10

MMSE, Mini-Mental State Exam; COWAT, Controlled Oral Word Association Test; OTMT, Oral Trail-Making Test; HVLT, Hopkins Verbal Learning Test; Faces I & II from the Wechsler Memory Scale III; JOLO, Judgment of Line Orientation; BNT, Boston Naming Test; GDS, Geriatric Depression Scale; BDI, Beck Depression Inventory; BDI_veg, five questions measuring vegetative symptoms taken from the BDI; % impaired, percent of participants in each group with a z-score < -1.6. Only tests used in the identification of MCI or ALSci were included. Between group statistics from the primary MANCOVA were Bonferroni corrected for multiple comparisons ($p < 0.05$), education was entered as a covariate and degrees of freedom were 1, 36. Independent sample t-tests were conducted for the GDS, BDI, and BDI_veg. GDS degrees of freedom, 32; BDI degrees of freedom, 27.

(Massman et al., 1996; Lomen-Hoerth et al., 2003; Rippon et al., 2006; Gordon et al., 2010; Raaphorst et al., 2010; Grace et al., 2011). Five of these patients scored at or below the threshold on the Animal Naming test and seven scored at or below the threshold on the HVLT. Scores from the Animal Naming and the HVLT tests were also among the most impaired scores overall in the ALS group, including scores from patients who did not meet criteria for ALS*ci*. **Table 2** indicates the percent of patients who performed below the fifth percentile on each measurement.

A MANCOVA was conducted to test the effect of diagnosis group on cognitive performance, which showed a significant difference between ALS patients and HCs, $F(13, 24) = 4.10, p = 0.001$, $\eta^2 = 0.69$. There was a specific significant difference between groups on Faces I, Faces II, COWAT, and Animal Naming. These statistics are shown in **Table 2**. The overall effect of education was not significant, $F(13, 24) = 1.60, p = 0.15, \eta^2 = 0.46$, however education had an exclusive effect on the BNT, $F(1, 36) = 7.04$, $p = 0.012$.

Because verbal fluency performance can be confounded by speech production impairment in patients with ALS (Abrahams et al., 2004), we examined speed (in seconds) from Oral Trails-Making Test A between groups. An independent sample t-test showed that verbal speed differences approached significance, $t(37) = 1.86$, $p = 0.07$. Therefore a second MANCOVA was performed to evaluate the effect of diagnosis (ALS and HC) and verbal production speed (Oral Trails A seconds) on verbal fluency (COWAT and Animal Naming) performance. There was no main effect of verbal speed, $F(2, 34) = 1.56$, $p = 0.22$, $\eta^2 = 0.08$ and no between-subjects effects of verbal speed on the Animal Naming test, $F(1, 35) = 3.07, p = 0.09$, or COWAT, $F(1, 33) = 1.53$, $p = 0.22$. There was still a main effect of diagnosis, $F(2, 34) = 5.63$, $p < 0.01$. These results suggest that differences in verbal fluency between groups were not confounded by verbal production speed.

PHYSICAL SYMPTOMS OF ALS DID NOT HAVE AN EFFECT ON COGNITIVE PERFORMANCE

Physical dysfunction did not predict global cognitive summary scores

The severity of physical dysfunction in patients with ALS may influence cognitive test performance. Some studies found that physical symptoms affect cognition differentially, specifically that those with more severe bulbar symptoms are more likely to have

CI (Gordon et al., 2011). To test this and the influence of physical functioning on cognition, bulbar (questions 1–3) and limb (questions 4–9) functioning were derived from ALSFRS-r subscores. These were entered into a linear regression analysis with overall cognitive performance as the outcome variable. A cognitive performance summary score was calculated for each individual by taking the summation of z-scores from each of the cognitive test measure ($M = -0.32$, $SD = 6.03$). This model was not significant, $F(2, 19) = 1.50$, $p = 0.25$, $R^2 = 0.05$. Bivariate correlations (Pearson's r) between physical symptoms and overall cognitive performance were also not significant: bulbar $p = 0.45$, limb $p = 0.12$.

Vegetative symptoms did not influence cognitive test scores

Another possible confound in a patient's cognitive status could be attributed to vegetative symptoms common in patients with ALS. We therefore created a subscore of vegetative symptoms measured within the BDI, and examined the effect of these symptoms on cognitive test performance between patients and controls. Five questions from the BDI were used, described previously. A MANCOVA was conducted to test the hypothesis that vegetative symptoms may extraneously influence cognitive test performance. Diagnosis, education, and vegetative symptom subscores were entered as independent variables. Because patients are more likely to be affected by these symptoms due to physical weakness, we predicted that patients with ALS would be more negatively affected compared to HCs; therefore an interaction term between diagnosis group and vegetative symptoms was also included in this model.

This analysis showed no main effect for vegetative symptoms on cognitive performance, $F(13, 12) = 1.31$, $p = 0.33$, $\eta^2 = 0.59$. However, vegetative symptoms did influence test performance on the Digit Span backward scores between groups, $F(1, 24) = 5.25$, $p = 0.03$, $\eta^2 = 0.18$. Even after accounting for the possible effect of vegetative symptoms on cognitive performance, there was still a main effect of diagnosis group, $F(13, 12) = 3.19$, $p = 0.03$, $\eta^2 = 0.78$. As in the original analysis, there was no effect of education, $F(13, 12) = 1.06$, $p = 0.46$, $\eta^2 = 0.54$. Also, there was no interaction effect between vegetative symptoms and diagnosis group, $F(13, 12) = 0.59$, $p = 0.82$, $\eta^2 = 0.39$.

Because only 14 patients completed the BDI, t-tests were conducted to test for demographic variable differences between patients with and without BDI data, and a MANOVA was conducted to test for a main effect on cognitive test performance. Age, education, disease duration, and progression rate (PR) did not differ between groups. There were also no differences between cognitive test scores. ALSFRS-r scores however approached significance, $t(20) = 2.04$, $p = 0.06$. The group who completed the BDI had a mean ALSFRS-r score of 39 ($SD = 4.46$) whereas those without had a mean ALSFRS-r score of 34 ($SD = 8.98$). Given the small sample size, it is possible that there was not an effect for vegetative symptoms on cognition because patients in this analysis were physically higher functioning. However, this importantly shows that patients with less disease severity still have overall poorer cognitive performance than HCs, independent of the effects of vegetative symptoms.

DEPRESSIVE SYMPTOMS IN ALS IN RELATION TO DISEASE SEVERITY AND COGNITION

Patients with ALS were not more clinically depressed than HCs

We tested the hypothesis that patients with ALS were more depressed than the HC group by conducting independent sample t-tests using scores from the GDS. ALS patient mean scores were higher on the GDS than the HC group (see **Table 2**). Although these differences were statistically significant, the mean scores did not fall within clinical range for depression. When examining individual depression scores, two participants in each group met clinical criteria for possible mild depression as measured by the GDS. Vegetative symptoms, measured from the BDI, reported by patients were not different than the HC group.

Depressive scores correlated with progression rate (PR) and limb dysfunction

The fourth major goal of this study was to determine if depressive symptoms are related to disease severity in ALS. A correlation analysis using Pearson's r-coefficient was conducted comparing GDS scores with PR. PR was calculated using the equation:

$$(PR) = \frac{(48 \text{ - ALSFRS-}r\text{ Patients Score})}{\text{Months Since Symptoms Onset}} \text{(Kollewe et al., 2008)}$$

This correlation was significant, $r = 0.52$, $p = 0.02$ (see **Figure 1**). To further examine this relationship, the ALSFRS-r was divided into three subscores measuring bulbar (questions 1–3), limb (questions 4–9), and respiratory (questions 10–12) impairment. Of these models, depression scores negatively correlated with limb dysfunction, $r = -0.72$, $p < 0.001$ (**Figure 2**). Depression scores did not correlate with bulbar ($p = 0.60$) or respiratory symptoms ($p = 0.49$), however it should be noted that the range of bulbar and respiratory symptoms in our group was small.

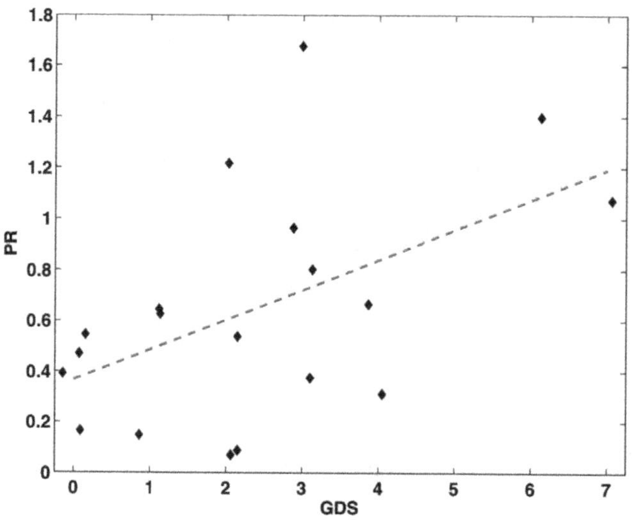

FIGURE 1 | Scatter plot showing the significant correlation between increased depressive scores from the GDS and faster progression rate (calculated by the PR equation, $n = 19$).

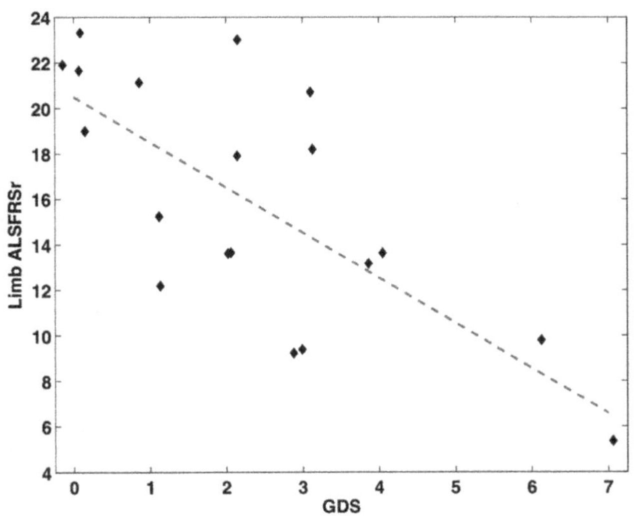

FIGURE 2 | Scatter plot showing the significant correlation between increased depressive scores from the GDS and decreased limb function measured from the ALSFRS-r ($n = 19$).

Depressive symptoms affect cognitive test performance

The final MANCOVA in this study was performed to test the hypothesis that depressive symptoms have an influence on cognitive test performance differentially in patients with ALS. Depression may negatively impact cognition, and we aimed to answer whether ALS patients are more at risk for CI if they have comorbid depressive symptoms. Therefore, an interaction variable between GDS scores and diagnosis group and main effect variables of diagnosis group, GDS scores, and education were entered into the MANCOVA to test for effects on cognitive test measurements from the neuropsychological battery.

In this MANCOVA, there was a significant interaction effect between GDS scores and diagnosis group, $F(13, 17) = 2.90$, $p = 0.02$, $\eta^2 = 0.69$. As expected, there were significant main effects of depressive symptoms, $F(13, 17) = 3.34$, $p = 0.01$, $\eta^2 = 0.72$ and diagnosis group, $F(13, 17) = 4.51$, $p < 0.01$, $\eta^2 = 0.78$. Examining the univariate effects on each cognitive test separately, there was interestingly not a significant main effect of depression on any single cognitive test, although the HVLT delayed recall scores approached significance, $p = 0.07$. There also was not a significant univariate effect of the interaction variable on any single cognitive test. Slopes of univariate analyses were examined to assess which group was more affected by depression on each cognitive test individually. Patients were more negatively affected by depressive symptoms on six of the cognitive test measurements (HVLT delayed recall, Faces II delayed recall, Oral Trails ratio, Animal Naming test, JOLO, and BNT), whereas the HCs were more negatively affected on five of the cognitive test measurements (MMSE, HVLT immediate recall and discrimination, Faces I immediate recall, and COWAT). This indicates there was not a specific pattern of which group was overall more affected by depressive symptoms, rather that the groups were indeed affected differently on individual cognitive domains. For example, patients appear more affected by depressive symptoms on tests of delayed recall whereas HCs appear more affected on tests of immediate recall.

DISCUSSION

There has been a recent push toward psychological intervention for patients with ALS in order to improve overall quality of life (Pagnini et al., 2012). Interventions would be better streamlined if risk factors for psychological distress were identified early, including risks for cognitive dysfunction and depression. In this study, we analyzed cognitive test performance between patients with ALS and a healthy control population. Importantly, we assessed the influence of physical and depressive symptoms on cognitive functioning in ALS, which may lead to better screening of individuals possibly at risk of having ALS*ci*. We also examined depressive symptoms in patients with ALS, and assessed if these depressive symptoms are related to disease progression or the manifestation of physical dysfunction specific to the disease process.

COGNITIVE PERFORMANCE DIFFERENCES BETWEEN PATIENTS WITH ALS AND HEALTHY CONTROLS

Results from our study corroborate previous findings, supporting cognitive performance differences between patients with ALS and HCs (Grossman et al., 2007; Strong et al., 2009). Overall, patients performed more poorly on cognitive testing than HCs, with specific deficits in executive function (verbal fluency) and visual recognition memory. Among patients identified as having ALS*ci*, the majority had impaired scores in semantic fluency and verbal learning and memory. Poorer performance in verbal fluency was not confounded by speech production speed. These findings are consistent with the literature, as verbal fluency remains the most sensitive to ALS cognitive dysfunction, and many others have noted impairment in memory and learning (Massman et al., 1996; Strong et al., 1996, 1999; Abrahams et al., 1997, 2004; Hanagasi et al., 2002; Grossman et al., 2007; Christidi et al., 2012). Utilizing neuropsychological tests that measure these cognitive domains would be most beneficial to screen for cognitive decline in a multidisciplinary ALS clinic setting, and have already been implemented in some clinics (Flaherty-Craig et al., 2009, 2011; Woolley et al., 2010).

THE EFFECT OF PRIMARY AND SECONDARY PHYSICAL SYMPTOMS ON COGNITION IN ALS

Results did not support a unique contribution of limb or bulbar function on cognition. There has been no evidence that limb onset or symptoms are related to CI, and our results support previous research that found no specific effect of bulbar symptoms (Rippon et al., 2006; Gordon et al., 2010; Rusina et al., 2010). However, research on this is not consistent, and several studies have indicated that those with bulbar onset are more likely to be cognitively impaired (Lomen-Hoerth et al., 2003; Gordon et al., 2011). It may be possible that higher reports of CI in these patients are partly due to speech-motor impairment confounds, as a recent meta-analysis of 554 non-demented individuals with ALS did not find a relationship between CI and bulbar onset ALS (Raaphorst et al., 2010). Although we did not find an effect of bulbar symptoms on cognitive function, the number of patients with bulbar onset ALS were disproportionally less than those with limb onset, therefore our study was limited in that we could not conduct a comparative analysis between onset subtypes. Additionally, there was a small range of scores for bulbar symptoms, as measured by questions 1–3 in the ALSFRS-r (see **Table 1**), which may have contributed to our null result. Regardless, the involvement of bulbar symptoms on cognition, if any, should be further investigated to establish consensus.

One of our primary goals was to test whether vegetative symptoms confound or mask the interpretation of CI in ALS. Our results indicate, however, that these symptoms did not contribute to cognitive performance differences between patients with ALS and HCs. Although against our hypothesis, these results suggest that secondary physical symptoms, such as fatigue, collectively do not interfere significantly with test performance in patients with ALS. This finding was from a subgroup of patients in our study with overall high physical functioning, suggesting that CI manifests very early in the disease process. This finding supports ALS*ci* as a true variant of the disease, and increases the importance of understanding CI in ALS.

RELATIONSHIP BETWEEN DEPRESSIVE SYMPTOMS, PHYSICAL SYMPTOMS, AND COGNITION IN ALS

Depression contributes to decreased quality of life in patients with ALS (Tramonti et al., 2012), however our study indicated that as a group patients with ALS were no more likely to be depressed than a HC population. Although these results are consistent with recent reports (Averill et al., 2007; Atassi et al., 2011) that claim prevalence rates of depression are low in ALS, our study was limited by a small sample size and was not representative of a valid prevalence-rate study. Importantly, we found that increased depressive symptoms were associated with both disease progression and the severity of limb dysfunction. Severe global physical dysfunction has been shown to correlate with clinical depression (Oh et al., 2012), and now this effect has been demonstrated in a physically high functioning group without clinical depression (and using the revised version of the ALSFRS). Additionally, this relationship was most sensitive to limb dysfunction, suggesting those with more severe limb impairment may be at most risk. Given these findings, in conjunction with evidence for increased mortality risk in those with psychological distress (McDonald et al., 1994), future research on depression treatment and its association with survival should be emphasized.

Another important finding from our study indicates that depressive symptoms had an effect on cognitive performance. Although novel in the ALS literature, the relationship between depression and cognition has been demonstrated among other diseases (Diamond et al., 2008), and it has even been suggested that depression treatment could lead to improved cognitive performance (Sassoon et al., 2012). Likewise, a recent meta-analysis found that cognition can predict depression status, which could be targeted to increase treatment efficacy for depression (Phillips et al., 2010). Although there are no reports of depression treatment improving cognitive functioning or vise versa in ALS, these could potentially become important avenues for future translational research.

LIMITATIONS AND CONCLUSIONS

Limitations

A major limitation in our study is that we were not able to test other factors that have been found to influence cognitive performance in patients with ALS. For example, Kim et al. (2007) found that patients with reduced forced vital capacity (FCV) performed significantly worse on tasks measuring memory retention/retrieval and verbal fluency than patients with normal vital capacity. Moreover, it has been suggested that impaired cognition might be reversible to some degree with increased vital capacity (Kim et al., 2007; Strutt et al., 2012). We suspect that patients in our study did not have impaired FVC for two reasons: they were enrolled in an MRI study and therefore able to lay flat on their back for more than 1 hour without respiratory distress, and scored near maximum on the ALSFRS-r questions measuring respiratory symptoms. Regardless, we did not explicitly acquire FVC measurements and were therefore unable to take into account this possible confound in our data.

Similarly, pseudobulbar affect is another symptom that may have a differential effect on cognition, and previous research has suggested that those with this symptom may be more at risk for CI (Abrahams et al., 1997). Again, we did not measure pseudobulbar affect symptoms and are therefore unable to account for this possible influence on cognition.

Our study also lacks a causal interpretation. We found that depressive symptoms and cognitive performance are related, but because we were unable to manipulate depressive symptoms or cognitive performance we were unable to identify the exact direction of this relationship. Additionally, our study showed that depressive symptoms are related to disease progression and limb dysfunction, yet it cannot be concluded whether increased depressive symptoms caused or directly influenced disease state. It is suggested that future studies examine depression and cognition intervention in order to identify a directional change in either disease state or cognitive performance.

Another major limitation in our study is the small sample size of groups. It is common for studies examining cognitive performance to include more than 100 participants, yet our study only compared 22 patients to 17 HCs. This is often a limitation in many rare disease population studies, however, and is especially common in the ALS literature. Future research would benefit from multicenter pooling of data, as suggested by Turner et al. (2011), in order to acquire larger sample sizes and gain higher statistical power.

In line with our small sample size, our analysis examining the effect of vegetative symptoms on cognition between groups was especially limited because only 14 patients completed the BDI. Those who completed the BDI were less severe in their disease symptoms. This analysis cannot therefore be generalized to the whole group in our study. However, this importantly shows that patients with less disease severity still have overall poorer cognitive performance than HCs, strengthening the finding that CI is a true symptom of ALS. The role of vegetative symptoms should be further explored, including larger sample sizes and patients with varying degrees of disease severity.

Conclusions

Overall, this study supported previous findings that CI is a symptom in approximately 35% of patients with ALS, and that patients overall perform worse than HCs in tests of executive dysfunction and learning and memory. Cognitive performance differences remained after accounting for variables including vegetative symptoms, physical dysfunction, and depressive symptoms. Additionally, we report that increased depressive symptoms are related to faster disease progression and greater limb dysfunction in patients with ALS. We therefore suggest that future research investigate the effects of depression therapy in patient care.

Although CI can significantly contribute to decreased quality of life for patients with ALS, research in this area is limited and often lacks a translational emphasis. Importantly, there is currently no treatment for patients who suffer from CI in ALS. Research though has highlighted several avenues to pursue in investigating CI intervention, including improving FVC (Kim et al., 2007; Strutt et al., 2012), treating pseudobulbar affect (Abrahams et al., 1997), and now therapy for depressive symptoms. Conversely, CI treatment may also improve depressive symptoms. We emphasize that future research focus on effective psychological or clinical interventions that may improve quality of life caused by CI or depression, and that these interventions be applied in future multidisciplinary ALS clinics.

ACKNOWLEDGMENTS

We thank Claire Eberhart and Rami Arabas for their time in organizing the data and creating databases. We also thank all the participants and their families who dedicated their time to be a part of this study. Funding for this study was provided by NIH RO1-NS052514 (RCW) and Basic Radiological Sciences Award (RCW).

REFERENCES

Aarsland, D., Bronnick, K., Williams- Gray, C., Weintraub, D., Marder, K., Kulisevsky, J., et al. (2010). Mild cog- nitive impairment in Parkinson dis- ease: a multicenter pooled analysis. *Neurology* 75, 1062–1069.

Abrahams, S., Goldstein, L., Simmons, A., Brammer, M., Williams, S., Giampietro, V., et al. (2004). Word retrieval in amyotrophic lateral scle- rosis: a functional magnetic reso- nance imaging study. *Brain* 127, 1507–1517.

Abrahams, S., Goldstein, L. H., Al- Chalabi, A., Pickering, A., Morris, R. G., Passingham, R. E., et al. (1997). Relation between cognitive dysfunction and pseudobulbar palsy in amyotrophic lateral sclerosis. *J. Neurol. Neurosurg. Psychiatr.* 62, 464–472.

Abrahams, S., Leigh, P. N., Harvey, A., Vythelingum, G. N., Grisé, D., and Goldstein, L. H. (2000). Ver- bal fluency and executive dysfunc- tion in amyotrophic lateral scle- rosis (ALS). *Neuropsychologia* 38, 734–747.

Armon, C., and Nelson, L. M. (2012). Is head trauma a risk factor for amyotrophic lateral sclerosis? An evi- dence based review. *Amyotroph. Lat- eral Scler.* 13, 351–356.

Atassi, N., Cook, A., Pineda, C. M. E., Yerramilli-Rao, P., Pulley, D., and Cudkowicz, M. (2011). Depres- sion in amyotrophic lateral scle- rosis. *Amyotroph. Lateral Scler.* 12, 109–112.

Averill, A. J., Kasarskis, E. J., and Segerstrom, S. C. (2007). Psy- chological health in patients with amyotrophic lateral sclerosis. *Amy- otroph. Lateral Scler.* 8, 243–254.

Bak, T. H., and Chandran, S. (2012). What wires together dies together: verbs, actions and neurodegenera- tion in motor neuron disease. *Cortex* 48, 936–944.

Beck, A. T., Steer, R. A., and Brown, G. K. (ed.). (1996). *Beck Depression Inventory*, 2nd Edn. Texas: The Psycho- logical Corporation San Antonio, Texas.

Benton, A. L. (1983). *Multilingual Apha- sia Examination*. Iowa City, IA: AJA Associates.

Brown, W. A., and Mueller, P. S. (1970). Psychological function in individu- als with amyotrophic lateral sclerosis (ALS). *Psychosom. Med.* 32, 141–152.

Christidi, F., Zalonis, I., Smyrnis, N., and Evdokimidis, I. (2012). Selective attention and the three- process memory model for the interpretation of verbal free recall in amyotrophic lateral sclero- sis. *J. Int. Neuropsychol. Soc.* 18, 809–818.

Diamond, B. J., Johnson, S. K., Kauf- man, M., and Graves, L. (2008). Relationships between information processing, depression, fatigue and cognition in multiple sclero- sis. *Arch. Clin. Neuropsychol.* 23, 189–199.

Flaherty-Craig, C., Brothers, A., Dear- man, B., Eslinger, P., and Simmons, Z. (2009). Penn State screen exam for the detection of frontal and temporal dysfunction syndromes: application to ALS. *Amyotroph. Lateral Scler.* 10, 107–112.

Flaherty-Craig, C. V., Brothers, A., Yang, C., Svoboda, R., and Sim- mons, Z. (2011). Declines in prob- lem solving and anosognosia in amyotrophic lateral sclerosis: appli- cation of Guilford's structure of intellect theory. *Cogn. Behav. Neurol.* 24, 26.

Folstein, M. F., Folstein, S. E., and McHugh, P. R. (1975)."Mini-mental state." A practical method for grad- ing the cognitive state of patients for the clinician. *J. Psychiatr. Res.* 12, 189–198.

Girardi, A., MacPherson, S. E., and Abrahams, S. (2011). Deficits in emotional and social cognition in amyotrophic lateral sclerosis. *Neu- ropsychology* 25, 53–65.

Goldstein, L. H., Atkins, L., and Leigh, P. N. (2002). Correlates of Quality of Life in people with motor neuron disease (MND). *Amyotroph. Lateral Scler. Other Motor Neuron Disord.* 3, 123–129.

Goodglass, H., and Kaplan, E. F. (1983). *The Assessment of Aphasia and Related Disorders*. Philadelphia, PA: Lea & Febiger.

Gordon, P. H., Delgadillo, D., Piquard, A., Bruneteau, G., Pradat, P.-F., Salachas, F., et al. (2011). The range and clinical impact of cogni- tive impairment in French patients with ALS: a cross-sectional study of neuropsychological test perfor- mance. *Amyotroph. Lateral Scler.* 12, 372–378.

Gordon, P. H., Goetz, R. R., Rabkin, J. G., Dalton, K., McElhiney, M., Hays, A. P., et al. (2010). A prospective cohort study of neu- ropsychological test performance in ALS. *Amyotroph. Lateral Scler.* 11, 312–320.

Grace, G. M., Orange, J. B., Rowe, A., Findlater, K., Freedman, M., and Strong, M. J. (2011). Neuropsycho- logical functioning in PLS: a com- parison with ALS. *Can. J. Neurol. Sci.* 38, 88–97.

Grossman, A. B., Woolley Levine, S., Bradley, W. G., and Miller, R. G. (2007). Detecting neurobehavioral changes in amyotrophic lateral scle- rosis. *Amyotroph. Lateral Scler.* 8, 56–61.

Hanagasi, H. A., Gurvit, I. H., Ermutlu, N., Kaptanoglu, G., Karamursel, S., Idrisoglu, H. A., et al. (2002). Cognitive impairment in amy- otrophic lateral sclerosis: evidence from neuropsychological investiga- tion and event-related potentials. *Brain Res. Cogn. Brain Res.* 14, 234–244.

Hillis, A. E., Oh, S., and Ken, L. (2004). Deterioration of naming nouns versus verbs in primary pro- gressive aphasia. *Ann. Neurol.* 55, 268–275.

Kaplan, E. F., Goodglass, H., and Wein- traub, S. (1978). *The Boston Naming Test*. Boston, MA: E. Kaplan & H. Goodglass.

Kilani, M., Micallef, J., Soubrouillard, C., Rey-Lardiller, D., Demattei, C., Dib, M., et al. (2004). A longitudi- nal study of the evolution of cog- nitive function and affective state in patients with amyotrophic lateral sclerosis. *Amyotroph. Lateral Scler.* 5, 46–54.

Kim, S.-M., Lee, K.-M., Hong, Y.-H., Park, K. S., Yang, J.-H., Nam, H.-W., et al. (2007). Relation between cog- nitive dysfunction and reduced vital capacity in amyotrophic lateral scle- rosis. *J. Neurol. Neurosurg. Psychiatr.* 78, 1387–1389.

Kollewe, K., Mauss, U., Krampfl, K., Petri, S., Dengler, R., and Moham- madi, B. (2008). ALSFRS-R score and its ratio: a useful predictor for ALS-progression. *J. Neurol. Sci.* 275, 69–73.

Lezak, D. L. (1995). *Neuropsychological Assessment*. New York, NY: Oxford University Press.

Lomen-Hoerth, C., Murphy, J., Lang- more, S., Kramer, J. H., Olney, R. K., and Miller, B. (2003). Are amy- otrophic lateral sclerosis patients cognitively normal? *Neurology* 60, 1094–1097.

Lulé, D., Pauli, S., Altintas, E., Singer, U., Merk, T., Uttner, I., et al. (2012). Emotional adjustment in amyotrophic lateral sclerosis (ALS). *J. Neurol.* 259, 334–341.

Massman, P. J., Sims, J., Cooke, N., Haverkamp, L. J., Appel, V., and Appel, S. H. (1996). Prevalence and correlates of neuropsychological deficits in amyotrophic lateral scle- rosis. *J. Neurol. Neurosurg. Psychiatr.* 61, 450–455.

McDonald, E. R., Wiedenfeld, S. A., Hil- lel, A., Carpenter, C. L., and Wal- ter, R. A. (1994). Survival in amy- otrophic lateral sclerosis. The role of psychological factors. *Arch. Neurol.* 51, 17–23.

McLeod, J. E., and Clarke, D. M. (2007). A review of psychosocial aspects of motor neurone disease. *J. Neurol. Sci.* 258, 4–10.

Merrilees, J., Klapper, J., Murphy, J., Lomen-Hoerth, C., and Miller, B. L. (2010). Cognitive and behavioral challenges in caring for patients with frontotemporal dementia and amyotrophic lateral sclero- sis. *Amyotroph. Lateral Scler.* 11, 298–302.

Murphy, J., Henry, R., and Lomen- Hoerth, C. (2007). Establishing sub- types of the continuum of frontal lobe impairment in amyotrophic lateral sclerosis. *Arch. Neurol.* 64, 330–334.

Oh, H., Sin, M.-K., Schepp, K. G., and Choi-Kwon, S. (2012). Depressive symptoms and functional impair- ment among amyotrophic lateral sclerosis patients in South Korea. *Rehabil. Nurs.* 37, 136–144.

Olney, R. K., Murphy, J., Forshew, D., Garwood, E., Miller, B. L., Langmore, S., et al. (2005). The effects of execu- tive and behavioral dysfunction on the course of ALS. *Neurology* 65, 1774–1777.

Pagnini, F., Simmons, Z., Corbo, M., and Molinari, E. (2012). Amy- otrophic lateral sclerosis: time for research on psychological interven- tion? *Amyotroph. Lateral Scler.* 13, 416–417.

Phillips, W. J., Hine, D. W., and Thorsteinsson, E. B. (2010). Implicit cognition and depression: a meta- analysis. *Clin. Psychol. Rev.* 30, 691–709.

Phukan, J., Pender, N. P., and Hardiman, O. (2007). Cognitive impairment in amyotrophic lateral sclerosis. *Lancet Neurol.* 6, 994–1003.

Pongratz, D. (2000). Treatment of psy- chiatric symptoms in amyotrophic lateral sclerosis (ALS). *Eur. Neu- ropsychopharmacol.* 10, 116–117.

Raaphorst, J., de Visser, M., Linssen, W. H. J. P., de Haan, R. J., and Schmand, B. (2010). The cognitive profile of amyotrophic lateral scle- rosis: a meta-analysis. *Amyotroph. Lateral Scler.* 11, 27–37.

Rippon, G. A., Scarmeas, N., Gordon, P. H., Murphy, P. L., Albert, S. M., Mitsumoto, H., et al. (2006). An observational study of cogni- tive impairment in amyotrophic lateral sclerosis. *Arch. Neurol.* 63, 345–352.

Royall, D. R., Chiodo, L. K., and Polk, M. J. (2004). Misclassification is likely in the assessment of mild cognitive impairment. *Neuroepidemiology* 23, 185–191.

Rusina, R., Ridzon, P., Kulišťák, P., Keller, O., Bartoš, A., Buncová, M., et al. (2010). Relationship between ALS and the degree of cognitive impair- ment, markers of neurodegenera- tion and predictors for poor out- come. A prospective study. *Eur. J. Neurol.* 17, 23–30.

Sager, M. A., Hermann, B. P., La Rue, A., and Woodard, J. L. (2006). Screening for dementia in community-based memory clinics. *WMJ* 105, 25–29.

Sassoon, S. A., Rosenbloom, M. J., Fama, R., Sullivan, E. V., and Pfeffer- baum, A. (2012). Selective neurocog- nitive deficits and poor life function- ing are associated with significant depressive symptoms in alcoholism- HIV infection comorbidity. *Psychia- try Res.* 199, 102–110.

Shapiro, A. M., Benedict, R. H., Schretlen, D., and Brandt, J. (1999). Construct and concurrent valid- ity of the Hopkins Verbal learning test-revised. *Clin. Neuropsychol.* 13, 348–358.

Strauss, E., Sherman, E. M. S., and Spreen, O. (2006). *A Compendium of Neuropsychological Tests: Admin- istration, Norms, and Commentary*, 3rd Edn. New York, NY: Oxford University Press.

Strong, M. J., Grace, G. M., Freed- man, M., Lomen-Hoerth, C., Wool- ley, S., Goldstein, L. H., et al. (2009). Consensus criteria for the diagnosis of frontotemporal cogni- tive and behavioural syndromes in amyotrophic lateral sclerosis. *Amy- otroph. Lateral Scler.* 10, 131–146.

Strong, M. J., Grace, G. M., Orange, J., and Leeper, H. A. (1996). Cogni- tion, language, and speech in amy- otrophic lateral sclerosis: a review. *J. Clin. Exp. Neuropsychol.* 18, 291–303.

Strong, M. J., Grace, G. M., Orange, J. B., Leeper, H. A., Menon, R. S., and Aere, C. (1999). A prospective study of cognitive impairment in ALS. *Neurology* 53, 1665–1670.

Strutt, A. M., Palcic, J., Wager, J. G., Titus, C., MacAdam, C., Brown, J., et al. (2012). Cognition, behavior, and respiratory function in amyotrophic lateral sclerosis. *ISRN Neurol.* 2012, 912123.

Tramonti, F., Bongioanni, P., Di Bernardo, C., Davitti, S., and Rossi, B. (2012). Quality of life of patients with amyotrophic lateral sclerosis. *Psychol. Health Med.* 17, 621–628.

Turner, M. R., Grosskreutz, J., Kas- subek, J., Abrahams, S., Agosta, F., Benatar, M., et al. (2011). Towards a neuroimaging biomarker for amy- otrophic lateral sclerosis. *Lancet neu- rology* 10, 400.

Wechsler, D. (1997). *WMS-III, Wechsler Memory Scale*, 3rd Edn. New York, NY: The Psychological Corporation.

Woolley, S. C., and Katz, J. S. (2008). Cognitive and behavioral impair- ment in *amyotrophic* lateral sclero- sis. *Phys. Med. Rehabil. Clin. N. Am.* 19, 607–617, xi.

Woolley, S. C., York, M. K., Moore, D. H., Strutt, A. M., Murphy, J., Schulz, P. E., et al. (2010). Detecting frontotemporal dysfunction in ALS: utility of the ALS Cognitive Behav- ioral Screen (ALS-CBS). *Amyotroph. Lateral Scler.* 11, 303–311.

Yesavage, J. A., and Sheikh, J. I. (1986). 9/Geriatric Depression Scale (GDS). *Clin. Gerontol.* 5, 165–173.

4

Gacyclidine improves the survival and reduces motor deficits in a mouse model of amyotrophic lateral sclerosis

Yannick N. Gerber[1,2], Alain Privat[1] and Florence E. Perrin[1,2,3*]

[1] Institute for Neurosciences of Montpellier (INM), INSERM U 1051, Montpellier, France
[2] "Integrative Biology of Neurodegeneration," IKERBASQUE Basque Foundation for Science, Neuroscience Department, University of the Basque Country, Bilbao, Spain
[3] "Integrative Biology of Neuroregeneration," Faculty of Science, University of Montpellier 2, Montpellier, France

Edited by:
Ricardo Tapia, Universidad Nacional Autónoma de México, Mexico

Reviewed by:
Patrizia Longone, Fondazione Santa Lucia, Italy
Helene E. Hirbec, Institut of Functional Genomics, France

***Correspondence:**
Florence E. Perrin, Institute for Neurosciences of Montpellier, INSERM U 1051, Saint-Eloi Hospital, 80 av., Augustin Fliche, 34091 Montpellier Cedex 05, France
e-mail: florence.perrin@inserm.fr

Amyotrophic lateral sclerosis (ALS) is a fatal neurodegenerative disorder typified by a massive loss of motor neurons with few therapeutic options. The exact cause of neuronal degeneration is unknown but it is now admitted that ALS is a multifactorial disease with several mechanisms involved including glutamate excitotoxicity. More specifically, *N*-methyl-D-aspartate (NMDA)-mediated cell death and impairment of the glutamate-transport has been suggested to play a key role in ALS pathophysiology. Thus, evaluating NMDAR antagonists is of high therapeutic interest. Gacyclidine, also named GK11, is a high affinity non-competitive NMDAR antagonist that may protect against motor neuron death in an ALS context. Moreover, GK11 presents a low intrinsic neurotoxicity and has already been used in two clinical trials for CNS lesions. In the present study, we investigated the influence of chronic administration of two doses of GK11 (0.1 and 1 mg/kg) on the survival and the functional motor activity of hSOD1^{G93A} mice, an animal model of ALS. Treatment started at early symptomatic age (60 days) and was applied bi-weekly until the end stage of the disease. We first confirmed that functional alteration of locomotor activity was evident in the hSOD1^{G93A} transgenic female mice by 60 days of age. A low dose of GK11 improved the survival of the mice by 4.3% and partially preserved body weight. Improved life span was associated with a delay in locomotor function impairment. Conversely, the high dose treatment worsened motor functions. These findings suggest that chronic administration of GK11 beginning at early symptomatic stage may be beneficial for patients with ALS.

Keywords: GK11, NMDA receptor antagonist, ALS, survival, locomotion

INTRODUCTION

Amyotrophic lateral sclerosis (ALS) is a chronic neurodegenerative disease characterized by neuronal death of both lower and upper motoneurons in the spinal cord, the brain stem and the motor cortex. This chronic motor neuronopathy leads to progressive atrophy of skeletal muscles, paralysis and ultimately to death of the patients mainly due to respiratory failure [for review see (Turner et al., 2013)].

Pathogenesis and mechanisms of selective vulnerability of motoneurons in ALS are still largely unknown although, within the past two decades, it has been demonstrated that ALS is a complex multifactorial disease. Indeed many factors including protein misfolding, glutamate-mediated excitotoxicity, oxidative stress and impaired axonal transport may contribute to motoneuron death in ALS [for review see Robberecht and Philips (2013)]. An excessive stimulation of glutamate receptors induces excitotoxic processes; this phenomenon being largely implicated in both acute and chronic neurodegenerative diseases (Olney, 1989; Plaitakis and Constantakakis, 1993; Mehta et al., 2013), and in particular in ALS (Heath and Shaw, 2002; Bogaert et al., 2010). In the objective of translation to clinics, excitotoxicity is one of the key pharmacological targets as attested by the only FDA-approved drug, riluzole (2-amino-6-trifluoromethoxy benzothiazole) which is a modulator of excitatory neurotransmitters activity (including glutamate) (Bogaert et al., 2010). Glutamate interacts with a large range of specific transporters and receptors such as N-methyl-D-aspartate receptors (NMDARs) (Mehta et al., 2013) and a promising, but so far overlooked therapeutic strategy, is to reduce excitotoxicity using NMDA receptor antagonist [for review see Spalloni et al. (2013)]. The low-affinity non-competitive NMDAR antagonist, memantine displayed encouraging results in hSOD1^{G93A} mice (Wang and Zhang, 2005; Joo et al., 2007), an ALS animal model. Clinical trials have shown that memantine is safe and well tolerated by ALS patients (de Carvalho et al., 2010; Levine et al., 2010) but no evidence of its efficacy had been reported yet.

Gacyclidine (GK11), a phencyclidine, is a non-competitive NMDA receptor antagonist, with a selective affinity for NR2B receptors, that had been shown to prevent glutamate-induced neuronal death *in vitro* and is less neurotoxic than other NMDA receptor antagonists (Hirbec et al., 2001; Vandame et al., 2007). Moreover, *in vivo* GK11 exhibits neuroprotective effects following organophosphorous nerve agents-induced convulsions (Bhagat et al., 2005) and following spinal cord injury (Feldblum et al.,

2000; Gaviria et al., 2000a,b; Kouyoumdjian et al., 2009; Lonjon et al., 2010).

In this study we have evaluated the effect of chronic treatment of two doses of GK11 on the survival and the locomotor function of hSOD1^{G93A} mice. We demonstrate a dose effect of GK11 on the survival of the mice, treatment with a low GK11 dose induced an increase in life span conversely to a high dose that reduced it. Moreover, treatment-induced increase in survival was associated with a reduction of locomotor function impairment whereas high dose treatment worsened the motor phenotype.

MATERIALS AND METHODS

ANIMALS

Transgenic mice carrying the G93A human SOD1 mutation, B6SJL-Tg (SOD1-G93A) 1Gur/J (ALS mice, high copy number) were purchased from The Jackson Laboratory (Bar Harbor, ME, USA) and bred on a B6SJL background. Transgenic mice were identified by PCR and housed in controlled conditions (hygrometry, temperature and 12h light/dark cycle); the environment was not modified over the course of the protocol. Only females were used and litter-matching between groups were done as much as possible. We carried out all animal experiments in accordance with the guidelines approved by the French Ministry of Agriculture and following the European Council directive (2010/63/UE). Every effort was made to minimize the number and suffering of animals. Age of death was defined as functional paralysis of both hindlimbs and a righting reflex >20 s. These criteria follow the commonly accepted guide lines for working on ALS mice (Leitner and Lutz, 2009; Solomon et al., 2011).

GK11 TREATMENTS

Twice a week, mice (transgenic and control) were intraperitoneally injected with either gacyclidine (two different concentrations; 1 mg/kg or 0.1 mg/kg) (Neuréva, Montpellier, France) or NaCl. The treatment doses were determined according to the following criteria: the dose of 1 mg/kg corresponds to the acute therapeutic dose in rat (Feldblum et al., 2000; Gaviria et al., 2000b) and we wanted to test the possible toxic effect of a chronic administration. Repeated administration of low dose of non-competitive NMDA receptor antagonists induces hyperlocomotion in rat (Wolf and Khansa, 1991; Loscher and Honack, 1992; Matsuoka et al., 2005). Injections were thus not done daily not only to reduce the risk of peritonitis but also to prevent possible interference of injections with behavioral tests. Treatment started at 60 days of age and was carried until the death of the animal. Number of mice: controls injected with GK11 (0.1 mg/Kg, $n = 10$; 1 mg/Kg, $n = 5$) or NaCl ($n = 14$); transgenic mice injected with GK11 (0.1 mg/Kg, $n = 15$; 1 mg/Kg, $n = 5$) or NaCl ($n = 21$).

BEHAVIORAL ANALYSIS

Catwalk

We used the CatWalk™ (Noldus, Wageningen, The Netherlands) to study dynamic and voluntarily walking patterns of the mice. As previously described (Gerber et al., 2012a) we selected amongst locomotor patterns, the "relative position" that corresponds to the distance between the placement of front and hind paws over one walking step. For data collection, six runs per animal were performed on a weekly basis from day 60 (just prior the first injection) and until animals were not able to correctly cross the walkway due to hindlimb paralysis. For each mouse, a minimum of three runs crossed at the same speed with 3-full step sequence patterns per run were recorded. To accustom the animals to the environment and thus to avoid bias due to stress, we placed transgenic and control littermates mice on the CatWalk 7 and 3 days prior to the first recording session. Catwalk analyses started before the first injection, the next behavioral session was done at least 72 h after treatment. Recordings were performed until the failure to obtain satisfactory paw patterns with the CatWalk analysis system due to hindlimb paralysis and thus absence of paw detection in the transgenic groups. Data analysis was done in collaboration with InnovationNet (Tiranges, France).

Open field activity

Spontaneous locomotor activity of mice was monitored in an open field test. Animals were placed in an empty test arena (45 × 45 cm box) and movements automatically recorded. We analyzed the total distance (cm) (Bioseb, Open field, Actitrack software, Vitrolles, France). Recording sessions started at P53 and until the end of life of the transgenic mice; analysis correspond to a weekly 8 min' sessions preceded by 2 min without recordings to avoid any bias due to stress. Open field test were performed on a weekly basis, 48 h after the injection. Recording sessions were performed until mice were unable to move in the test arena

STATISTICAL ANALYSIS

Kaplan Meier analysis and log-rank test were applied for survival curves (**Figure 1A**). Two ways ANOVA followed by Tukey-Kramer test was used for all analysis that consist on a combination of a treatment (at three different doses, NaCl, GK11 0.1 mg/kg and GK11 1 mg/kg) on two distinct genotypes over time (**Figures 1B, 2B, 3A–C, 4**). From 116 days onward transgenic and control mice could not be directly compared due to speed differences, moreover due to death GK11 1 mg/kg-treated transgenic mice were not included from P123 onwards. We thus used one way ANOVA followed by Tukey-Kramer test for **Figure 3D** and one way ANOVA followed by Mann-Whitney test for **Figures 3E,F**. For all analysis at P60 i.e., before the treatment started t-test was done (**Figures 1A, A1**). CatWalk data consist on replicates of a minimum of 3 and a maximum of 6 runs (same speed with 3 full step sequence) per animal in all cases these values were averaged. Experiments were designed to reach a 95% power to detect a 10% or greater difference between groups. We used GraphPad Prism version 5.03 (GraphPad software, CA, USA, and Minitab 15, Minitab Inc, USA).

RESULTS

DOSE EFFECT OF GACYCLIDINE ON THE SURVIVAL OF THE MICE

We first assessed the influence of a chronic treatment with GK11 (0.1 mg/kg), a non-competitive NMDA receptor antagonist, on the survival of hSOD^{G93A} female mice. Animals treated with GK11 display an increased survival as compared to animals

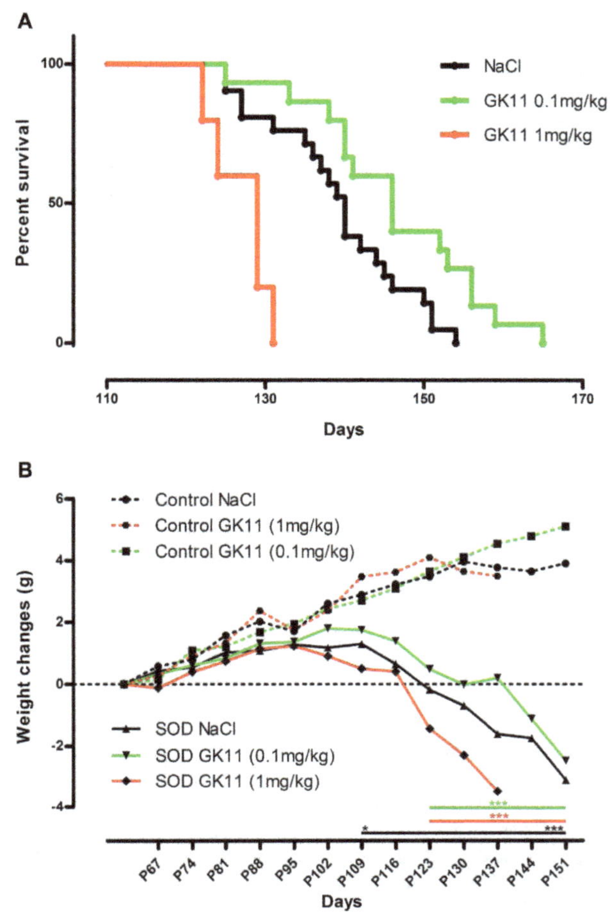

FIGURE 1 | Dose effect of Gacyclidine on hSOD1^{G93A} mice survival and weight. (A)—Kaplan-Meier curves of hSOD1^{G93A} mice injected i.p with NaCl ($n = 21$), GK11 0.1 mg/kg ($n = 15$) or GK11 1 mg/kg ($n = 5$). **(B)**—Weight changes (g) in control (dash line) and transgenic mice (continuous line) injected with NaCl, GK11 0.1 mg/kg or GK11.1 mg/kg. Two-ways ANOVA followed by Tukey-Kramer test [$F_{(10, 695)}=96.18$]. Weight of NaCl treated controls and transgenics significantly differs from P109 whereas weight of GK11 (both doses) treated controls and transgenics significantly differ from P123. $^{*}p < 0.05$ and $^{***}p < 0.001$.

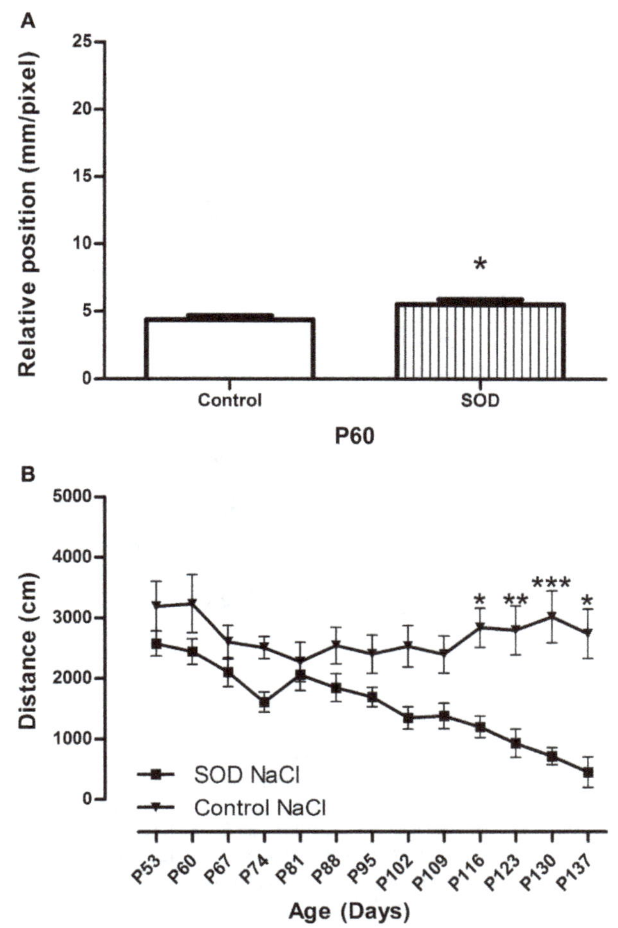

FIGURE 2 | Locomotor function analysis of hSOD1^{G93A} female mice. (A)—CatWalk gait analysis. Graph represent the distance between the front and hind paws on a step sequence ("relative position") of control females ($n = 32$) and hSOD1^{G93A}animals ($n = 41$) before treatment. Statistics: t-test: $^{*}p < 0.05$ **(B)**—Open field test. Spontaneous locomotor activity represented by the mean distance covered by control female and hSOD1^{G93A} mice in a weekly 8 min recording test over disease progression. For Open field test a minimum of 10 animals were used from day 53 to 130, then due to the death of hSOD1^{G93A} mice, a minimum of 5 animals were analyzed (P137). Statistics: two ways ANOVA followed by Tukey Kramer test. $F_{(12, 262)}=95.95$. $^{*}p < 0.05$, $^{**}p < 0.01$ and $^{***}p < 0.001$.

injected with NaCl. Median survivals are indeed of 146 and 140 for mice injected with GK11 and NaCl respectively; this represent a significant 4.3% increase in life span (Kaplan Meier, P-value = 0.0341) (**Figure 1A**).

To evaluate the possible toxicity margin of the molecule, we injected mice with a 1 log higher GK11 concentration (1 mg/kg). Mice chronically injected with this high dose show a significant decrease in lifespan as compared to the littermates injected with NaCl. Median survivals are indeed of 129 and 140 for mice injected with GK11 and NaCl respectively; this represents a significant 7.9% decrease in life span (Kaplan Meier, P-value = 0.006) (**Figure 1A**).

Over the progression of the disease, transgenic mice lost weight due to muscular atrophy. We monitored body weight changes from P60 until death. NaCl injected transgenic mice weight differs significantly from those of the NaCl injected control group from P109 whereas weight of GK11 treated transgenic mice (both doses) is significantly different from GK11 treated control mice from P123 (**Figure 1B**). There is no effect of GK11 treatment on the body weight of control mice.

We thus evidence a beneficial effect of a chronic low dose of GK11 on the survival of hSOD1^{G93A} female mice whereas a high dose of GK11 has a detrimental effect.

LOCOMOTOR FUNCTION IS ALTERED AT 60 DAYS OF AGE IN FEMALE hSOD1^{G93A} MICE

In the perspective of translational studies, it is important to apply the therapeutic strategy at early symptomatic period. Experiments were done on female mice, it was thus mandatory to thoroughly characterize disease onset and progression in female

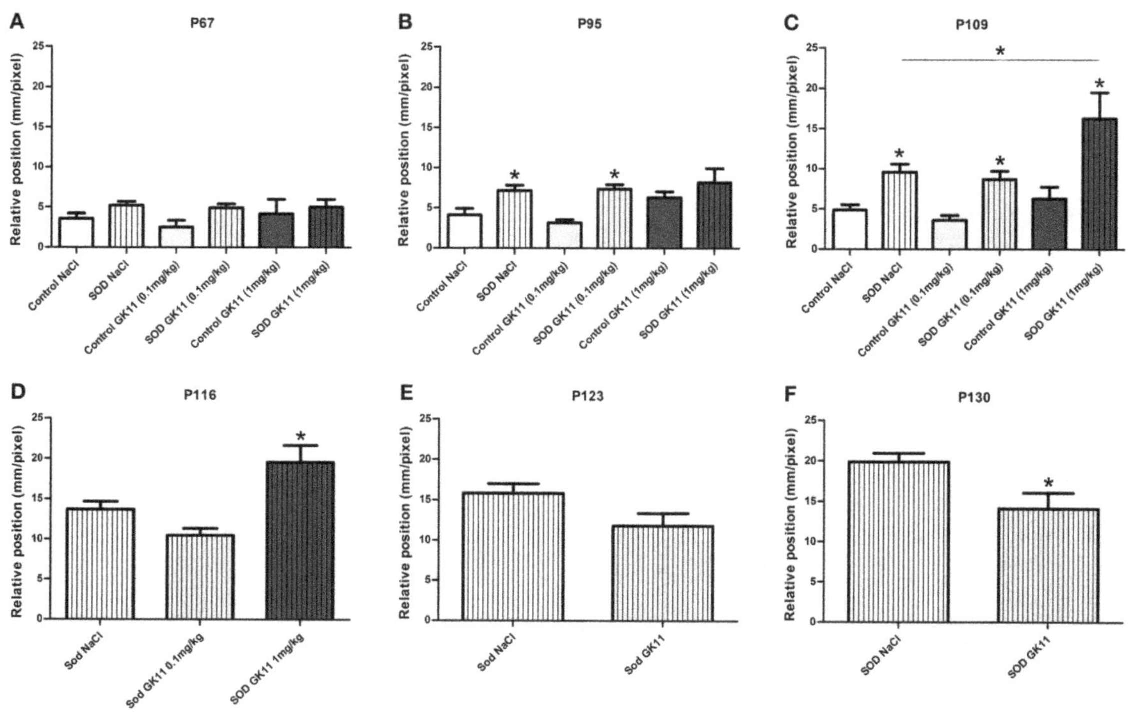

FIGURE 3 | Evaluation of Gacyclidine effects on hSOD1^{G93A} mice motor pattern: CatWalk gait analysis. Graphs represent the distance between the front and hind paws on a step sequence ("relative position"). **(A–C)**—control and hSOD1^{G93A} animals (NaCl, GK11 0.1 mg/kg or GK11 1 mg/kg treated)—Respectively at 67, 95, and, 109 days of age. **(D)**—hSOD1^{G93A} animals (NaCl, GK11 0.1 mg/kg or GK11 1 mg/kg injected) at 116 days. **(E, F)** hSOD1^{G93A} animals (NaCl or GK11 0.1 mg/kg injected) at 123 and 130 days. A minimum of 4 and up to 24 animals per time point were analyzed from 67 to 116 days of age; recording were stopped for GK 11 1 mg/kg after P116 due to hindlimb paralysis. Then due to progression of the paralysis a minimum of 8 and up to 15 animals per time point were analyzed from 123 to 130 days of age. Statistics: **(A–C)**: two ways ANOVA followed by Tukey Kramer test. **D**: one way ANOVA followed by Tukey Kramer test. **(E,F)**: one way ANOVA followed by Mann-Whitney test. *$p < 0.05$.

hSOD1^{G93A} mice. We have used the previously described combination of CatWalk and open field analysis (Gerber et al., 2012a) to evaluate locomotor alterations. To compare with our former motor analysis on male hSOD1^{G93A} mice, we tested the female mice on a weekly basis from 60 days of age and selected the same parameters. We quantified the spontaneous motor activity using the open field system and the "relative position" of the paws (distance between front and hind footprints over a step cycle) using the CatWalk system.

As a prerequisite for accurate CatWalk investigation, we verified if the B6SJL strain is suitable for gait analysis. In that aim, we analyzed the stride of control females from P60 to P130. It had indeed been shown that stride must remain stable in control mice all along the study protocol to avoid any misleading conclusions (Clarke and Still, 1999). The stride remains identical throughout our study (**Table A1**).

At 60 days of age hSOD1^{G93A} female mice present an alteration in gait pattern appearing as the inability to draw their hind limbs up to the previous position of their front limbs (**Figure 2A**) This alteration increased further up to 109 days of age (**Figures 3A–C**, SOD NaCl vs. control NaCl). To evaluate the spontaneous motor activity of hSOD1^{G93A} and control mice, we used the open field system. We evidence a decreased in the mean distance covered by transgenic animals as compared to their control littermate from P116 (**Figure 2B**).

Combination of CatWalk and open field analysis allows an accurate description of motor alterations and permit to identify gait pattern alteration, and thus clinical onset of the disease, at 60 days of age. This is in agreement with our previous results in male hSOD1^{G93A} mice (Gerber et al., 2012a) (**Figure A1**).

INCREASED LIFE SPAN CORRELATED WITH DELAYED MOTOR DEFICITS

We then used the CatWalk system to tentatively correlate the effects of the drug on the lifespan with modification of disease onset and/or progression of the disease; we compared locomotor functions of transgenic hSOD1^{G93A} females injected with either GK11 (0.1 mg/kg or 1 mg/kg) or NaCl. In parallel, we evaluated whether GK11 had an effect on non-transgenic animal by comparing treated versus NaCl injected control mice.

From 67 days to 109 days, the relative position is identical in transgenic groups injected with GK11 0.1 mg/kg or 1 mg/kg compared to transgenic mice injected with NaCl. Controls animals of all groups (GK11 0.1 mg/kg, 1 mg/kg or NaCl) remain stable over the same period. However, transgenic mice (0.1 mg/kg and NaCl) show an alteration of the motor pattern when compared to their respective controls that increased from 95 to 109 days of age. At 109 days, transgenic mice injected with GK11 at high concentration show a critically altered phenotype compared not only to controls but also to the transgenic group injected with NaCl (**Figures 3A–C**). From 116 days onward, due to hindlimb

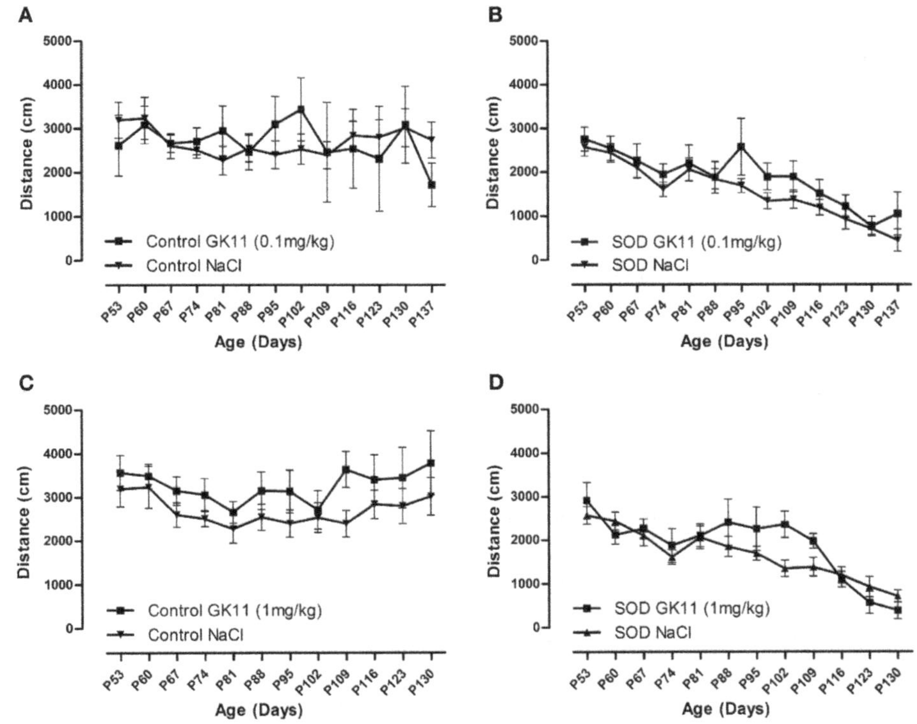

FIGURE 4 | Evaluation of Gacyclidine effects on the spontaneous motor activity of hSOD1^{G93A} mice: Open Field analysis. Spontaneous locomotor activity represented by the mean distance covered by female controls and hSOD1^{G93A} mice in a weekly 8 min recording test over disease progression included. **(A,B)**—Control and hSOD1^{G93A} mice injected with NaCl or GK11 0.1 mg/kg. **(C,D)**—Control and hSOD1^{G93A} mice injected with NaCl or GK11 1 mg/kg. A minimum of 5 animals were analyzed per time point. Statistics: two ways ANOVA followed by Tukey Kramer test.

paralysis, transgenic and control mice do not achieve the CatWalk test at the same speed and thus, referring to Clarke's et al. study (Clarke and Still, 1999), cannot be compared. We thus analyzed separately hSOD1^{G93A} and control mice. At 116 days, mice injected with GK11 1 mg/kg show an altered phenotype compared to the NaCl injected mice (**Figure 3D**). No satisfactory recording sessions were obtained for the GK11 1 mg/kg from P123 onwards (**Figures 3E,F**). GK11 0.1 mg/kg treated mice exhibit a reduction of locomotor function impairment compared to the transgenic NaCl group at P130 (**Figure 3F**). No difference between control groups were seen over the same period (data not shown). These results suggest that treatment with a low dose of GK11 induces a slight but significant delay in hindlimb paralysis progression. Oppositely, treatment with a high dose of GK11 worsened the motor pattern.

We used an open field system to measure the spontaneous locomotor activity of control and transgenic mice. No difference has been noted in the mean crossed distances when we compared both GK11 doses (0.1 and 1 mg/kg) and NaCl injected mice for both control and transgenic groups (**Figures 4A–D**).

DISCUSSION

Glutamate mediated excitotoxicity is involved in ALS pathogenesis (Foran and Trotti, 2009) and several studies have evaluated the pharmacological profile of a number of molecules acting on glutamate release and transport [for review (Corona et al., 2007; Bogaert et al., 2010)]. Gacyclidine (GK11), a non-competitive NMDA receptor antagonist, has already been used in the clinics (Hirbec et al., 2001; Tadie et al., 2003; Lepeintre et al., 2004) and a single GK11 dose of 1 mg/kg has demonstrated neuroprotective effects on a model of photochemical spinal cord injury (Gaviria et al., 2000b). Chronic GK11 administration has never been reported. In view of these data, we decided to analyze the impact of a chronic treatment of GK11 on the survival and locomotor activity of hSOD1^{G93A} mice.

Our study clearly shows a dose response effect; indeed although a high GK11 dose is detrimental by shortening the life span of the mice by 7.9%, a low dose induces a 4.3% increase in survival vs. controls. Moreover, this increased life span is associated with a reduction in walking pattern deficits whereas high dose treatment worsened the motor phenotype.

GENDER EFFECTS ON SURVIVAL AND FUNCTIONAL DEFICITS IN THE SOD1^{G93A} MOUSE MODEL OF ALS

We have recently carried out a thorough analysis analyses of survival and motor function in hSOD1^{G93A} male mice (Gerber et al., 2012a,b). For the present study we have used females. Transgenic females survive significantly longer than males; median survivals were of 129 and 140 days for males and females respectively. Comparison with a previous study (Heiman-Patterson et al., 2005) attests for the stability of this mouse model; indeed reported life span was of 128 and 133 days for males and females respectively.

We have evaluated locomotor function of female hSOD1^{G93A} mice using the same combination of dynamic walking patterns and spontaneous motor activity analysis as previously done with males (Gerber et al., 2012a). As for males, we detect early functional deficits that confirm symptoms onset at 60 days of age, i.e., 20 days earlier than previously described (**Figure A1**). Indeed, dynamic gait analysis using the CatWalk system demonstrates alteration in gait pattern for both males and females from 60 days onwards. Spontaneous motor activity evaluated with an open field highlighted a decrease in the mean distance covered by transgenic animals as compared to their control littermate from 116 days onwards for females as compared to 102 days of age onwards for males (Gerber et al., 2012a). This difference may reflect gender-specific mechanism of synaptic impairment since a recent study demonstrated sexual dimorphism in the decline of the presynaptic machinery at an early symptomatic stage (Naumenko et al., 2011). Mean survival of hSOD1^{G93A} mice is of 140 days for female as compared to 129 days for males (Gerber et al., 2012a), however, even if female mice survive longer than male counterparts, early motor symptoms impairment are detected at 60 days of age in both gender.

ANTIGLUTAMATE DRUGS

One of the popular hypothesis regarding mechanisms involved in ALS is that an excessive activation of glutamate receptors may be responsible for motoneuron death (Corona et al., 2007). NMDA receptors are known for their permeability to cations and in particular to calcium; their over activation leading to excitoxic phenomenon. Recent findings have shown that subtypes of AMPA receptors, that either do not express the GluR2 subunit or express an edited form of this subunit, present a similar permeability to calcium than NMDA receptors (Van Den Bosch et al., 2000; Kawahara et al., 2006; Corona et al., 2007). These AMPA receptor subtypes are widely expressed in motoneurons and are therefore involved in excitotoxic processes (Carriedo et al., 1996; Gerardo-Nava et al., 2013). However, modulating AMPA excitoxicity mediated pathway is mostly ineffective in clinical trials and induce various side effect (such as dizziness and Ataxia) [for review see (Chang et al., 2012)]. Nevertheless, perampanel, a non-competitive AMPA receptor antagonist to AMPAR is very promising in the treatment of epilepsy (Rogawski, 2011). Several antiglutamate drugs have been evaluated in ALS [for review see (Gibson and Bromberg, 2012)]. Riluzole is the only approved treatment and prolongs median survival by about 2 to 3 months in ALS patients (Miller et al., 2012) and by 10.5% in mice (Gurney et al., 1996). Riluzole induces an inhibition of glutamate release and modulation of both alpha-amino-3-hydroxy-5-methyl-4-isoxazolepropionic acid (AMPA) and N-methyl-d-aspartate (NMDA) receptors (Jin et al., 2010; Cifra et al., 2013). However, Riluzole displays other diverse and multiple non-specific pharmacological properties (Cheah et al., 2010) that may cause adverse effects such as nausea, asthenia and raised alanine transferase (Miller et al., 2012). As recently pinpointed (Spalloni et al., 2013) the role of NMDA receptors activation in ALS has not received much attention, even if a low affinity non-competitive NMDAR antagonist, memantine, has shown promising results in an ALS animal model. In this context, evaluations of new therapeutic agents are of utmost importance. GK11, a high affinity uncompetitive NMDAR antagonist, presents a low intrinsic neurotoxicity, paucity of side effects attributed to its selectivity for NR2 B containing receptors (Vandame et al., 2007). No interaction was found with glutamatergic AMPA, kainate, or $\sigma 1$ and $\sigma 2$ receptors (Hirbec et al., 2001).

In our study, early symptomatic (starting at P60) bi-weekly chronic administration of a low dose of GK11 (0.1 mg/kg) yields a 4.3% increase in the life span of the female hSOD1^{G93A} mice. These results are similar to the effects of memantine (Wang and Zhang, 2005; Joo et al., 2007). Conversely to memantine (Joo et al., 2007), increase in survival induced by GK11 is associated with a significant protective effect on locomotor deterioration at the end stage of the disease. Of particular interest is the fact that, to-date, GK11 is the most specific NMDA receptor antagonist efficient in an animal model of ALS, thus definitely pinpointing the involvement of this receptor in the pathogenesis of the disease. High dose GK11 treatment leads to a decrease in the life span of female hSOD1^{G93A} associated to a more abrupt development of motor symptoms and hindlimb paralysis. Importantly, high dose drug treatment has no effect on weight loss, CatWalk or open field performances in the control group as reported in a recent study in rats undergoing an acute treatment (Vandame et al., 2013). This toxic side effect might reflect an induction of specific cascade events in the SOD context.

In conclusion, we demonstrate here that a chronic administration (starting at early symptomatic stage) of a non-competitive NMDA receptors antagonist significantly increases the survival of a mouse model of ALS. Indeed, a chronic low dose of GK11 prolongs the life span and reduces weight loss and motor deficits in hSOD1^{G93A} female mice. These results, combined with those from previous studies on CNS injury, demonstrating in patients a relative efficacy and the absence of side effects (Tadie et al., 2003; Lepeintre et al., 2004), suggest that low dose of GK11 could be used as a new and effective NMDA receptor antagonist for ALS patients.

AUTHOR CONTRIBUTIONS

Yannick N. Gerber: study conception and design, acquisition of data, analysis and interpretation of data and drafting of manuscript. Alain Privat: study conception and design and critical revision. Florence E. Perrin: study conception and design, analysis and interpretation of data and critical revision.

ACKNOWLEDGMENTS

The authors acknowledge J.C. Sabourin for his participation in management of the mouse colony, P. Villette, InnovationNet, for his great contribution in the analysis of the CatWalk data and H. N. Noristani for his contribution in the statistical analysis. This study was supported by the Spanish Government, Plan Nacional de I+D+I 2008–2011 and ISCIII - Subdireccion General de Evaluacion y Fomento de la Investigacion [PI10/00709 to Florence E. Perrin], the Basque Government, Fondo Comun de Cooperacion Aquitania-Euskadi and Proyectos de Investigacion

Sanitaria [to Florence E. Perrin] and the Association "Demain Debout Aquitaine" [to Yannick N. Gerber].

REFERENCES

Bhagat, Y. A., Obenaus, A., Hamilton, M. G., Mikler, J., and Kendall, E. J. (2005). Neuroprotection from soman-induced seizures in the rodent: evaluation with diffusion- and T2-weighted magnetic resonance imaging. *Neurotoxicology* 26, 1001–1013. doi: 10.1016/j.neuro.2005.04.006

Bogaert, E., d'Ydewalle, C., and Van Den Bosch, L. (2010). Amyotrophic lateral sclerosis and excitotoxicity: from pathological mechanism to therapeutic target. *CNS Neurol. Disord. Drug Targets* 9, 297–304. doi: 10.2174/187152710791292576

Carriedo, S. G., Yin, H. Z., and Weiss, J. H. (1996). Motor neurons are selectively vulnerable to AMPA/kainate receptor-mediated injury *in vitro*. *J. Neurosci.* 16, 4069–4079.

Chang, P. K., Verbich, D., and McKinney, R. A. (2012). AMPA receptors as drug targets in neurological disease–advantages, caveats, and future outlook. *Eur. J. Neurosci.* 35, 1908–1916. doi: 10.1111/j.1460-9568.2012.08165.x

Cheah, B. C., Vucic, S., Krishnan, A. V., and Kiernan, M. C. (2010). Riluzole, neuroprotection and amyotrophic lateral sclerosis. *Curr. Med. Chem.* 17, 1942–1199. doi: 10.2174/092986710791163939

Cifra, A., Mazzone, G. L., and Nistri, A. (2013). Riluzole: what it does to spinal and brainstem neurons and how it does it. *Neuroscientist* 19, 137–144. doi: 10.1177/1073858412444932

Clarke, K. A., and Still, J. (1999). Gait analysis in the mouse. *Physiol. Behav.* 66, 723–729. doi: 10.1016/S0031-9384(98)00343-6

Corona, J. C., Tovar-y-Romo, L. B., and Tapia, R. (2007). Glutamate excitotoxicity and therapeutic targets for amyotrophic lateral sclerosis. *Expert Opin. Ther. Targets* 11, 1415–1428. doi: 10.1517/14728222.11.11.1415

de Carvalho, M., Pinto, S., Costa, J., Evangelista, T., Ohana, B., and Pinto, A. (2010). A randomized, placebo-controlled trial of memantine for functional disability in amyotrophic lateral sclerosis. *Amyotroph. Lateral Scler.* 11, 456–460. doi: 10.3109/17482968.2010.498521

Feldblum, S., Arnaud, S., Simon, M., Rabin, O., and D'Arbigny, P. (2000). Efficacy of a new neuroprotective agent, gacyclidine, in a model of rat spinal cord injury. *J. Neurotrauma* 17, 1079–1093. doi: 10.1089/neu.2000.17.1079

Foran, E., and Trotti, D. (2009). Glutamate transporters and the excitotoxic path to motor neuron degeneration in amyotrophic lateral sclerosis. *Antioxid. Redox Signal.* 11, 1587–1602. doi: 10.1089/ars.2009.2444

Gaviria, M., Privat, A., d'Arbigny, P., Kamenka, J., Haton, H., and Ohanna, F. (2000a). Neuroprotective effects of a novel NMDA antagonist, Gacyclidine, after experimental contusive spinal cord injury in adult rats. *Brain Res.* 874, 200–209. doi: 10.1016/S0006-8993(00)02581-6

Gaviria, M., Privat, A., d'Arbigny, P., Kamenka, J. M., Haton, H., and Ohanna, F. (2000b). Neuroprotective effects of gacyclidine after experimental photochemical spinal cord lesion in adult rats: dose-window and time-window effects. *J. Neurotrauma* 17, 19–30. doi: 10.1089/neu.2000.17.19

Gerardo-Nava, J., Mayorenko, I. I., Grehl, T., Steinbusch, H. W., Weis, J., and Brook, G. A. (2013). Differential pattern of neuroprotection in lumbar, cervical and thoracic spinal cord segments in an organotypic rat model of glutamate-induced excitotoxicity. *J. Chem. Neuroanat.* 53, 11–17. doi: 10.1016/j.jchemneu.2013.09.007

Gerber, Y. N., Sabourin, J. C., Rabano, M., Vivanco, M., and Perrin, F. E. (2012a). Early functional deficit and microglial disturbances in a mouse model of amyotrophic lateral sclerosis. *PLoS ONE* 7:e36000. doi: 10.1371/journal.pone.0036000

Gerber, Y. N., Sabourin, J. C., Hugnot, J. P., and Perrin, F. E. (2012b). Unlike physical exercise, modified environment increases the lifespan of SOD1G93A mice however both conditions induce cellular changes. *PLoS ONE* 7:e45503. doi: 10.1371/journal.pone.0045503

Gibson, S. B., and Bromberg, M. B. (2012). Amyotrophic lateral sclerosis: drug therapy from the bench to the bedside. *Semin. Neurol.* 32, 173–178. doi: 10.1055/s-0032-1329193

Gurney, M. E., Cutting, F. B., Zhai, P., Doble, A., Taylor, C. P., Andrus, P. K., et al. (1996). Benefit of vitamin E, riluzole, and gabapentin in a transgenic model of familial amyotrophic lateral sclerosis. *Ann. Neurol.* 39, 147–157. doi: 10.1002/ana.410390203

Heath, P. R., and Shaw, P. J. (2002). Update on the glutamatergic neurotransmitter system and the role of excitotoxicity in amyotrophic lateral sclerosis. *Muscle Nerve* 26, 438–458. doi: 10.1002/mus.10186

Heiman-Patterson, T. D., Deitch, J. S., Blankenhorn, E. P., Erwin, K. L., Perreault, M. J., Alexander, B. K., et al. (2005). Background and gender effects on survival in the TgN(SOD1-G93A)1Gur mouse model of ALS. *J. Neurol. Sci.* 236, 1–7. doi: 10.1016/j.jns.2005.02.006

Hirbec, H., Gaviria, M., and Vignon, J. (2001). Gacyclidine: a new neuroprotective agent acting at the N-methyl-D-aspartate receptor. *CNS Drug Rev.* 7, 172–198. doi: 10.1111/j.1527-3458.2001.tb00194.x

Jin, L. J., Schlesinger, F., Song, Y. P., Dengler, R., and Krampfl, K. (2010). The interaction of the neuroprotective compounds riluzole and phenobarbital with AMPA-type glutamate receptors: a patch-clamp study. *Pharmacology* 85, 54–62. doi: 10.1159/000268641

Joo, I. S., Hwang, D. H., Seok, J. I., Shin, S. K., and Kim, S. U. (2007). Oral administration of memantine prolongs survival in a transgenic mouse model of amyotrophic lateral sclerosis. *J. Clin. Neurol.* 3, 181–186. doi: 10.3988/jcn.2007.3.4.181

Kawahara, Y., Sun, H., Ito, K., Hideyama, T., Aoki, M., Sobue, G., et al. (2006). Underediting of GluR2 mRNA, a neuronal death inducing molecular change in sporadic ALS, does not occur in motor neurons in ALS1 or SBMA. *Neurosci. Res.* 54, 11–14. doi: 10.1016/j.neures.2005.09.006

Kouyoumdjian, P., Lonjon, N., Prieto, M., Haton, H., Privat, A., Asencio, G., et al. (2009). A remotely controlled model of spinal cord compression injury in mice: toward real-time analysis. *J. Neurosurg. Spine* 11, 461–470. doi: 10.3171/2009.4.SPINE0979

Leitner, M. M., and Lutz, S. C. (2009). *Working With ALS Mice in Guidelines for Preclinical Testing and Colony Management*. Bar Harbor, ME: The Jackson Laboratory; Cambridge, MA: Prize 4Life, 1–21.

Lepeintre, J. F., D'Arbigny, P., Mathe, J. F., Vigue, B., Loubert, G., Delcour, J., et al. (2004). Neuroprotective effect of gacyclidine. A multicenter double-blind pilot trial in patients with acute traumatic brain injury. *Neuro-Chirurgie* 50(2–3 Pt 1), 83–95.

Levine, T. D., Bowser, R., Hank, N., and Saperstein, D. A. (2010). Pilot trial of memantine and riluzole in ALS: correlation to CSF biomarkers. *Amyotroph. Lateral Scler.* 11, 514–519. doi: 10.3109/17482968.2010.513052

Lonjon, N., Kouyoumdjian, P., Prieto, M., Bauchet, L., Haton, H., Gaviria, M., et al. (2010). Early functional outcomes and histological analysis after spinal cord compression injury in rats. *J. Neurosurg. Spine* 12, 106–113. doi: 10.3171/2009.7.SPINE0989

Loscher, W., and Honack, D. (1992). The behavioural effects of MK-801 in rats: involvement of dopaminergic, serotonergic and noradrenergic systems. *Eur. J. Pharmacol.* 215, 199–208. doi: 10.1016/0014-2999(92)90029-4

Matsuoka, T., Sumiyoshi, T., Tanaka, K., Tsunoda, M., Uehara, T., Itoh, H., et al. (2005). NC-1900, an arginine-vasopressin analogue, ameliorates social behavior deficits and hyperlocomotion in MK-801-treated rats: therapeutic implications for schizophrenia. *Brain Res.* 1053, 131–136. doi: 10.1016/j.brainres.2005.06.035

Mehta, A., Prabhakar, M., Kumar, P., Deshmukh, R., and Sharma, P. L. (2013). Excitotoxicity: bridge to various triggers in neurodegenerative disorders. *Eur. J. Pharmacol.* 698, 6–18. doi: 10.1016/j.ejphar.2012.10.032

Miller, R. G., Mitchell, J. D., and Moore, D. H. (2012). Riluzole for amyotrophic lateral sclerosis (ALS)/motor neuron disease (MND). *Cochrane Database Syst. Rev.* 3, CD001447. doi: 10.1002/14651858.CD001447.pub3

Naumenko, N., Pollari, E., Kurronen, A., Giniatullina, R., Shakirzyanova, A., Magga, J., et al. (2011). Gender-specific mechanism of synaptic impairment and its prevention by GCSF in a mouse model of ALS. *Front. Cell. Neurosci.* 5:26. doi: 10.3389/fncel.2011.00026

Olney, J. W. (1989). Glutamate, a neurotoxic transmitter. *J. Child Neurol.* 4, 218–226. doi: 10.1177/088307388900400315

Plaitakis, A., and Constantakakis, E. (1993). Altered metabolism of excitatory amino acids, N-acetyl-aspartate and N-acetyl-aspartyl-glutamate in amyotrophic lateral sclerosis. *Brain Res. Bull.* 30, 381–386. doi: 10.1016/0361-9230(93)90269-H

Robberecht, W., and Philips, T. (2013). The changing scene of amyotrophic lateral sclerosis. *Nat. Rev. Neurosci.* 14, 248–264. doi: 10.1038/nrn3430

Rogawski, M. A. (2011). Revisiting AMPA receptors as an antiepileptic drug target. *Epilepsy Curr.* 11, 56–63. doi: 10.5698/1535-7511-11.2.56

Solomon, J. A., Tarnopolsky, M. A., and Hamadeh, M. J. (2011). One universal common endpoint in mouse models of amyotrophic lateral sclerosis. *PLoS ONE* 6:e20582. doi: 10.1371/journal.pone.0020582

Spalloni, A., Nutini, M., and Longone, P. (2013). Role of the N-methyl-d-aspartate receptors complex in amyotrophic lateral sclerosis. *Biochim. Biophys. Acta* 1832, 312–322. doi: 10.1016/j.bbadis.2012.11.013

Tadie, M., Gaviria, M., Mathe, J.-F., Menthonenex, P., Loubert, G., Lagarrigue, J., et al. (2003). Early care and treatment with a neuroprotective drug, gacyclidine, in patients with acute spinal cord injury. *Rachis* 15, 363–376.

Turner, M. R., Hardiman, O., Benatar, M., Brooks, B. R., Chio, A., de Carvalho, M., et al. (2013). Controversies and priorities in amyotrophic lateral sclerosis. *Lancet Neurol.* 12, 310–322. doi: 10.1016/S1474-4422(13)70036-X

Van Den Bosch, L., Vandenberghe, W., Klaassen, H., Van Houtte, E., and Robberecht, W. (2000). Ca(2+)-permeable AMPA receptors and selective vulnerability of motor neurons. *J. Neurol. Sci.* 180, 29–34. doi: 10.1016/S0022-510X(00)00414-7

Vandame, D., Desmadryl, G., Becerril Ortega, J., Teigell, M., Crouzin, N., Buisson, A., et al. (2007). Comparison of the pharmacological properties of GK11 and MK801, two NMDA receptor antagonists: towards an explanation for the lack of intrinsic neurotoxicity of GK11. *J. Neurochem.* 103, 1682–1696. doi: 10.1111/j.1471-4159.2007.04925.x

Vandame, D., Ulmann, L., Teigell, M., Cappelini-Prieto, M., Vignon, J., Privat, A., et al. (2013). Development of NMDARs antagonists with reduced neurotoxic side effects: a study on GK11. *PLoS ONE* 8:e81004. doi: 10.1371/journal.pone.0081004

Wang, R., and Zhang, D. (2005). Memantine prolongs survival in an amyotrophic lateral sclerosis mouse model. *Eur. J. Neurosci.* 22, 2376–2380. doi: 10.1111/j.1460-9568.2005.04431.x

Wolf, M. E., and Khansa, M. R. (1991). Repeated administration of MK-801 produces sensitization to its own locomotor stimulant effects but blocks sensitization to amphetamine. *Brain Res.* 562, 164–168. doi: 10.1016/0006-8993(91)91202-C

APPENDIX

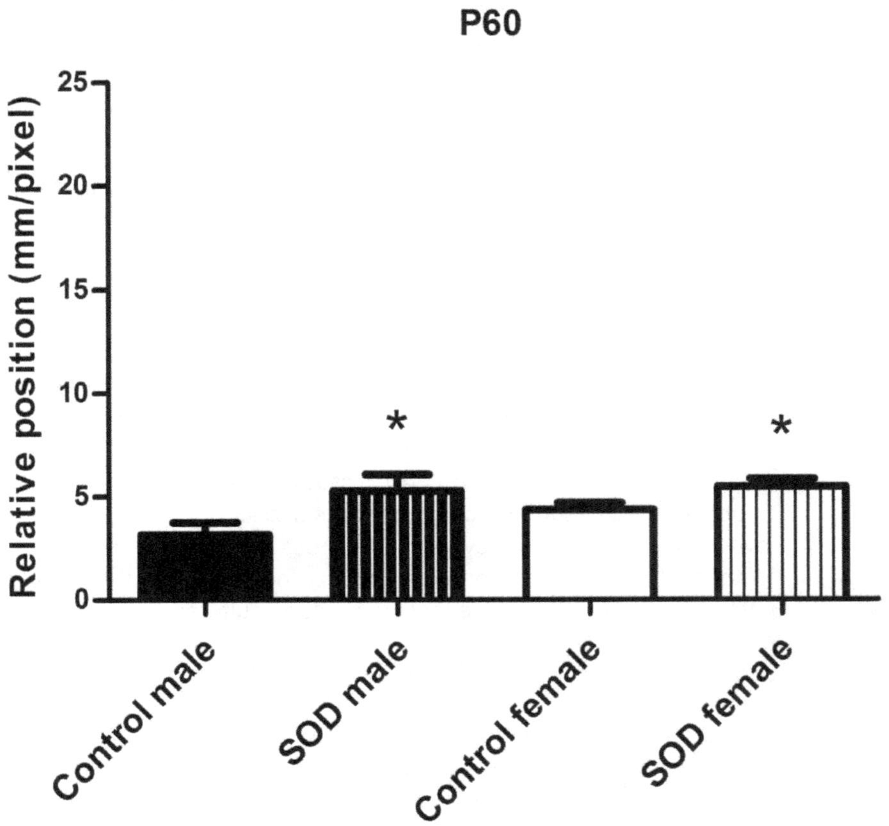

FIGURE A1 | Locomotor function analysis of hSOD1^{G93A} female and male mice. CatWalk gait analysis. Graph represent the distance between the front and hind paws on a step sequence ("relative position") of control males ($n = 16$), hSOD1^{G93A} males ($n = 11$), control females ($n = 32$) and hSOD1^{G93A} animals ($n = 41$) at 60 days of age. Statistics: t-test: $*p < 0.05$.

Table A1 | Frontlimb and hindlimb stride (mm) of control mice at P60 ($n = 22$), Control NaCl at P81 ($n = 12$), P109 ($n = 13$) and P130 ($n = 11$).

Colonne1	P60	P81	P109	P130
Frontlimb (mm)	58.81 ± 1.275	59.00 ± 1.317	59.14 ± 1.549	61.48 ± 2.053
Hindlimb (mm)	59.28 ± 1.393	59.27 ± 1.372	59.14 ± 1.507	61.20 ± 1.945

5

Astrocytes expressing mutant SOD1 and TDP43 trigger motoneuron death that is mediated via sodium channels and nitroxidative stress

Fabiola Rojas, Nicole Cortes, Sebastian Abarzua, Agnieszka Dyrda and Brigitte van Zundert*

Faculty of Biological Sciences and Faculty of Medicine, Center for Biomedical Research, Universidad Andres Bello, Santiago, Chile

Edited by:
Ricardo Tapia, Universidad Nacional Autónoma de México, Mexico

Reviewed by:
Jie Zhang, University of Texas Health Science Center at San Antonio, USA
Daryl A. Bosco, University of Massachusetts Medical Center, USA

****Correspondence:***
Brigitte van Zundert, Faculty of Biological Sciences and Faculty of Medicine, Center for Biomedical Research, Universidad Andres Bello, Avenida Republica 217, 8370816 Santiago, Chile
e-mail: bvanzundert@unab.cl

Amyotrophic lateral sclerosis (ALS) is a fatal paralytic disorder caused by dysfunction and degeneration of motor neurons. Multiple disease-causing mutations, including in the genes for SOD1 and TDP-43, have been identified in ALS. Astrocytes expressing mutant SOD1 are strongly implicated in the pathogenesis of ALS: we have shown that media conditioned by astrocytes carrying mutant $SOD1^{G93A}$ contains toxic factor(s) that kill motoneurons by activating voltage-sensitive sodium (Na_V) channels. In contrast, a recent study suggests that astrocytes expressing mutated TDP43 contribute to ALS pathology, but do so via cell-autonomous processes and lack non-cell-autonomous toxicity. Here we investigate whether astrocytes that express diverse ALS-causing mutations release toxic factor(s) that induce motoneuron death, and if so, whether they do so via a common pathogenic pathway. We exposed primary cultures of wild-type spinal cord cells to conditioned medium derived from astrocytes (ACM) that express SOD1 (ACM-$SOD1^{G93A}$ and ACM-$SOD1^{G86R}$) or TDP43 (ACM-$TDP43^{A315T}$) mutants; we show that such exposure rapidly (within 30–60 min) increases dichlorofluorescein (DCF) fluorescence (indicative of nitroxidative stress) and leads to extensive motoneuron-specific death within a few days. Co-application of the diverse ACMs with anti-oxidants Trolox or esculetin (but not with resveratrol) strongly improves motoneuron survival. We also find that co-incubation of the cultures in the ACMs with Na_V channel blockers (including mexiletine, spermidine, or riluzole) prevents both intracellular nitroxidative stress and motoneuron death. Together, our data document that two completely unrelated ALS models lead to the death of motoneuron via non-cell-autonomous processes, and show that astrocytes expressing mutations in SOD1 and TDP43 trigger such cell death through a common pathogenic pathway that involves nitroxidative stress, induced at least in part by Na_V channel activity.

Keywords: ALS, non-cell-autonomous, motor neuron, degeneration, ROS/RNS, anti-oxidants

INTRODUCTION

Amyotrophic lateral sclerosis (ALS) is a fatal paralytic disorder caused by the progressive degeneration of cranial and spinal motoneurons in adulthood, and leading to death by respiratory failure within 3–5 years of diagnosis. Although the majority of ALS cases are sporadic (SALS), ~10% are familial (FALS) and are generated by mutations in at least 15 identified ALS-associated gene loci (Bento-Abreu et al., 2010; Ferraiuolo et al., 2011). Dominant mutations in superoxide dismutase 1 (SOD1) and transactive response DNA-binding protein 43 (TARDBP gene, TDP43 protein) are common causes of ALS (Cleveland and Rothstein, 2001; Pasinelli and Brown, 2006; Cozzolino et al., 2012)—to date, more than 150 SOD1 mutations and 40 TARDBP mutations are known to be associated with the ALS phenotype (http://alsod.iop.kcl.ac.uk/; Abel et al., 2012).

Although the molecular underpinnings of motoneuron degeneration in ALS have not yet been elucidated, *in vivo* and *in vitro* studies with use of transgenic mice that carry ALS-causing mutants reveal a large number of pathogenic changes in affected motoneurons: these include mitochondrial dysfunction, hyperexcitability, glutamate excitotoxicity, nitroxidative stress from reactive oxygen species (ROS) or reactive nitrogen species (RNS) (collectively leading to nitroxidative stress), protein aggregation and misfolding, proteasome impairment, cytoskeletal disruption, activation of cell death signals, and dysregulation of transcription and RNA processing (Beckman et al., 2001; Cleveland and Rothstein, 2001; Bruijn et al., 2004; Pasinelli and Brown, 2006; Ferraiuolo et al., 2011; Cozzolino et al., 2012; van Zundert et al., 2012). Despite these advances in identifying these cellular alterations, however, the origin(s) and interplay between multiple pathogenic processes of motoneuron death in ALS remain largely unknown.

A large number of studies highlight the importance of dysregulated crosstalk between motoneurons and non-neuronal cells in ALS (Ilieva et al., 2009). The notion that ALS is at least partially a non-cell-autonomous disease originates in a groundbreaking study from Clement et al. (2003) who generated chimeric mice composed of mixtures of normal and SOD1 mutant-expressing cells, and showed that wild-type non-neuronal cells extend the survival of motoneurons carrying mutant SOD1. Additional research has since firmly established the contribution of "deadly neighboring cells" (astrocytes, microglia, oligodendrocytes, and Schwann cells) to the degeneration of motoneurons (Boillée et al., 2006; Yamanaka et al., 2008a,b; Lobsiger et al., 2009; Ilieva et al., 2009). Other findings offer compelling evidence that primary mutant SOD1-expressing astrocytes from mouse (Di Giorgio et al., 2007; Nagai et al., 2007; Castillo et al., 2013; Fritz et al., 2013), rat (Vargas et al., 2006; Cassina et al., 2008), and humans (Marchetto et al., 2008) effectively and selectively kill motoneurons, but spare interneurons. Importantly, astrocytes differentiated from neuronal progenitor cells (NPCs) obtained either from post-mortem spinal cord tissue or from skin biopsies from FALS (SOD1 mutations and hexanucleotide expansion in C9orf72) and SALS patients also display non-cell-autonomous toxicity, and selectively kill motoneurons in a co-culture model system (Haidet-Phillips et al., 2011; Meyer et al., 2014). Moreover, astrocytes that express mutants in SOD1 contribute to the pathogenesis of ALS by releasing into the media a toxic factor(s) that kills motoneurons (Nagai et al., 2007; Cassina et al., 2008; Castillo et al., 2013; Fritz et al., 2013). Little is known regarding the non-cell- autonomous toxicity mediated by mutants other than in SOD1, but a recent study suggests that astrocytes expressing mutated TDP43 (TDP43^{M337V}) lack non-cell-autonomous toxicity and contribute to ALS pathology only through cell-autonomous processes (Serio et al., 2013).

Here we show that conditioned medium derived from astrocytes that were harvested from transgenic mice carrying ALS-causing mutations in SOD1 (SOD1^{G93A} and SOD1^{G86R}) or TDP43 (TDP43^{A315T}) contain toxic factors that trigger motoneuron death. Based on earlier studies which document the involvement of Na$_V$ channel-mediated excitability and nitroxidative stress in the pathogenesis of ALS (Ferraiuolo et al., 2011; Cozzolino et al., 2012; van Zundert et al., 2012), we tested here whether these pathogenic changes are induced in motoneurons via non-cell-autonomous processes. We demonstrate that they do so, and our results indicate that nitroxidative stress within the neurons is mediated by Na$_V$ channel activity.

MATERIALS AND METHODS

ANIMALS

Care and use of rodents was in accordance with the US National Institute of Health guidelines, and was approved by the Institutional Animal Care and Use Committee of Andres Bello University. Hemizygous transgenic mice carrying mutant human SOD1^{G93A} (high copy number; B6SJL; Cat. No. 002726), wild-type human SOD1^{WT} (B6SJL; Cat. No. 002297), mutant mouse SOD1^{G86R} (FVB crossed on B6SJL background; Cat. No. 005110), or mutant mouse TDP43^{A315T} (B6.Cg crossed on C57BL/6J; Cat. No. 010700) were originally obtained from Jackson Laboratories (Bar Harbor, USA). Non-transgenic littermates and transgenic mice over-expressing the gene for human SOD1^{WT} were used as controls. Transgenes were identified by polymerase chain reaction (Wegorzewska et al., 2009; Castillo et al., 2013; Fritz et al., 2013). The SOD1^{G93A} mice, but not the hSOD1^{WT} mice, develop signs of neuromuscular deficits (tremor of the legs and loss of extension reflex of the hind paws) starting at 3 months of age and have an average lifespan of 19–21 weeks (Gurney et al., 1994). Mice carrying SOD1^{G86R} (Ripps et al., 1995) or TDP43^{A315T} (Wegorzewska et al., 2009) develop similar loss of motor function between 3 and 4 months and do not survive to the age of 4 months.

CONDITIONED MEDIA PREPARATION

ACM was prepared as described (Nagai et al., 2007; Castillo et al., 2013; Fritz et al., 2013). Briefly, cultures of astrocytes were prepared from P1-2 wild-type mice and from transgenic mice expressing human SOD1^{G93A}, mouse hSOD1^{G86R}, human SOD1^{WT}, or mouse TDP43^{A315T}. Cultures were maintained in DMEM (Hyclone, Cat. No. SH30081.02) containing 10% FBS (Hyclone, Cat. No. SH30071.03; lot ATC31648) and 1% penicillin-streptomycin (Gibco, Cat. No. 15070-063) at 37°C 5% CO_2. Cultures reached confluence after 2–3 weeks and contained >95% GFAP$^+$ astrocytes. Residual microglia were removed by shaking cultures in an orbital shaker (200 r.p.m. in the incubator) overnight (7 h), at which point media was replaced by spinal culture media (see below). After 7 days, ACM was collected, centrifuged (500 g for 10 min) and stored at −80°C; before use, it was supplemented with 4.5 mg/ml D-glucose (final concentration) and penicillin/streptomycin, and filtered. A chick hindlimb muscle extract was also added to the ACM before use (Sepulveda et al., 2010).

For all experiments the ACM was diluted 8–10-fold. The exact dilution was determined for each new batch of ACM by comparing the motoneuron toxicity of the ACM from transgenic animals carrying the ALS-causing mutants (ACM-SOD1^{G93A}, ACM-SOD1^{G86R}, and ACM-TDP43^{A315T}) to that of ACM generated from mice carrying the wild-type human SOD1 gene (ACM-SOD1^{WT}) or from non-transgenic littermates (ACM-NT-Control); at the selected dilutions the conditioned media derived from the astrocytes expressing the ALS-causing genes robustly killed motoneurons, whereas the ACM-NT-Control and ACM-SOD1^{WT} did not affect motoneuron survival. The ACM was applied to ventral spinal cord cultures derived from rats because better quality motoneurons are obtained from rats than from mice; a number of studies have shown that such mixed species co-cultures (from rat, mice, human) do not appear to induce any side effects (e.g., Pehar et al., 2004; Di Giorgio et al., 2007; Nagai et al., 2007; Castillo et al., 2013; Fritz et al., 2013).

PRIMARY SPINAL CORD NEURONAL CULTURES

Pregnant Sprague–Dawley rats were deeply anesthetized with CO_2, and primary spinal cultures were prepared from E14 pups (Sepulveda et al., 2010; Castillo et al., 2013; Fritz et al., 2013). Briefly, whole spinal cords were excised and placed into ice-cold HBSS (Gibco, Cat. No. 14185-052) containing 50 μg/ml penicillin/streptomycin (Gibco, Cat. No. 15070-063). The dorsal part of the spinal cord was removed using a small razor blade, and the ventral cord was minced and enzymatically treated by incubating in pre-warmed HBSS containing 0.25% trypsin (Gibco, Cat. No. 15090-046) for 20 min at 37°C. Cells were transferred to a 15 ml tube containing neuronal growth media containing 70% MEM (Gibco, Cat. No. 11090-073), 25% Neurobasal media (Gibco, Cat. No. 21103-049), 1% N2 supplement (Gibco, Cat.

No. 17502-048), 1% L-glutamine (Gibco, Cat. No. 25030-081), 1% penicillin-streptomycin (Gibco, Cat. No. 15070-063), 2% horse serum (Hyclone, Cat. No. SH30074.03; lot AQH24495) and 100 mM sodium pyruvate (Gibco, Cat. No. 11360-070); they were precipitated, transferred to a new 15-ml-tube containing 2 ml of growth media, re-suspended by mechanical agitation through fire-polished glass Pasteur pipettes of different tip diameters, and counted; 1×10^6 cells were plated on freshly prepared poly-L-lysine-coated 24-well plates (1 mg/ml; 30.000–70.000 mW; Sigma, Cat. No. P2636). Cells were cultured for 7 days at 37°C under 5% CO_2, and supplemented with 45 μg/ml chick hindlimb muscle extract (Sepulveda et al., 2010); the media was refreshed every 3 days.

PHARMACOLOGICAL TREATMENTS IN CULTURE

Mexiletine (Tocris, Cat. No. 2596) was dissolved in water to 100 mM and used at final concentration of 25 nM. Riluzole (Sigma, Cat. No. R116) was dissolved in distilled water (plus 10% Tween20) at 100 μM, and added to cultures to final concentration of 100 nM. Spermidine (Sigma, Cat. No. S2626) was dissolved in water at 100 mg/ml and added to cultures to a final concentration of 10 μM. Trolox (Sigma, Cat. No. 238813) was dissolved in distilled water at 100 mM and added to cultures to final concentration of 1 μM. Esculetin (Sigma, Cat. No. 17795) was dissolved in dimethyl sulfoxide (DMSO), and added to cultures to final concentration 25 μM. Resveratrol (Tocris, Cat. No. 1418) was dissolved in DMSO (Sigma) at 100 mM and added to cultures to final concentration of 1 μM. All stock solutions were stored at −20°C.

CELL LABELING AND COUNTING

Motoneurons and interneurons were immunolabeled and counted as previously described (Sepulveda et al., 2010; Castillo et al., 2013; Fritz et al., 2013). Briefly, primary spinal cultures were fixed at 7 DIV with 4% paraformaldehyde, and immunostained with an antibody against MAP2 (1:400; Santa Cruz Biotechnology) to label all neurons (interneurons plus motoneurons) and with the SMI-32 antibody (1:1,000, Sternberger Monoclonals) to reveal the presence of unphosphorylated neurofilament-H, which is expressed specifically in motoneurons in spinal cord cultures (Urushitani et al., 2006; Nagai et al., 2007); antibody binding was visualized with the appropriate fluorescent secondary antibodies. Our wild-type primary spinal cord cultures typically contain at least 6–10% motoneurons until 12 DIV (Sepulveda et al., 2010). Immunolabeled neurons were documented on an inverted Nikon Eclipse Ti-U microscope equipped with a SPOT Pursuit™ USB CameraCCD (14-bit), Epi-fl Illuminator, mercury lamp, and Sutter Smart-Shutter with a lambda SC controller. Cells were photographed using a 20× objective; MAP2- and SMI-32-positive neurons were counted offline within 20 randomly chosen fields, and the percentage of SMI-32-positive motoneurons within the total number of MAP2-positive cells was calculated. Each condition was replicated in at least 3 independent cultures, and in duplicate.

NITROXIDATIVE STRESS MEASUREMENTS WITH CM-H_2DCF-DA

The intracellular levels of ROS/RNS were measured with CM-H_2DCF-DA (Invitrogen, Cat. No. C6827). H_2DCF-DA is not a specific probe for a particular oxidant and has been used to monitor certain ROS/RNS (see Discussion). The CM-H_2DCF-DA stock solution (5 mM) was prepared in DMSO and was diluted in the culture medium to a final concentration of 1 μM just before addition to the cells. After application of the diverse ACMs to the spinal cord cultures for different time (minutes-hours-days), cells were washed (PBS 1×) to remove the ACMs and exposed to CM-H_2DCF-DA for 30 min at 37°C in dark, to label both motoneurons and interneurons. To facilitate the CM-H_2DCF-DA membrane penetration, 0.004% Pluronic acid F-127 (Invitrogen, Cat. No. P-3000MP) was added to the culture medium to facilitate dye entry, eliminating possible hydrolysis of dyes by external esterases and maintain better cell integrity (Appaix et al., 2012). After the incubation time, the CM-H_2DCF-DA-cointaing culture medium was removed and cultures were washed twice with PBS 1× and suspended in culture medium (500 μl final volume). Next, cells were immediately imaged using an inverted Nikon Eclipse Ti-U microscope equipped with a SPOT Pursuit™ USB CameraCCD (14-bit), Epi-fl Illuminator, mercury lamp, and Sutter Smart-Shutter with a lambda SC controller. Cells were photographed using a 20× objective. As CM-H_2DCF-DA is a non-fluorescent dye it passively diffuses into cells and is hydrolyzed intracellularly to the DCFH carboxylate anion that is trapped inside; oxidation of DCFH results in the formation of the fluorescent product DCF, with excitation and emission wavelengths $\lambda_{ex}/\lambda_{em} = 492$–495/517–527 nm. The exposure time was kept below 4 s in order to avoid photo-oxidation of the ROS/RNS sensitive dye and for all given treatments fields were exposed for exactly the same amount of time. At least three independent fields were acquired for each condition and at least 10 cells per field were used for quantification of the fluorescence signal. Cells were marked by drawing a region of interest around the cell body, and mean fluorescence intensity was calculated for each cell after subtraction of the background signal using the image analysis module in ImageJ software. Those cells with a relative intensity unit (RIU) of ≥1.5 were counted as positive. Cultures were also incubated with H_2O_2 (200 μM for 20 min) to serve as a positive control and to normalize the number of DCF-positive cells after ACM application.

DATA ANALYSIS

ANOVA, followed by *post-hoc* Tukey tests, was used to detect significant changes. Student's *t*-tests were used to compare the response of two cell populations to individual treatments. Unless otherwise stated, error bars represent the mean ± s.e.m.; $^{*}p < 0.05$, $^{**}p < 0.01$, $^{***}p < 0.001$ vs. control.

RESULTS

ACM-SOD1^{G93A}, ACM-SOD1^{G86R}, OR ACM-TDP43^{A315T} TRIGGERS DEATH OF CULTURED PRIMARY MOTONEURONS

Here we investigated whether astrocytes expressing diverse ALS causing mutants release toxic factor(s) that induce motoneuron death, and if so, whether a common pathogenic pathway is involved. Astrocyte conditioned media (ACM) was derived from astrocytes that were harvested from mice carrying mutant SOD1 (ACM-SOD1^{G93A} and ACM-SOD1^{G86R}) or TDP43 (ACM-TDP43^{A315T}). These media were added at 8–10-fold dilutions (see Materials and Methods) to wild-type primary rat spinal cultures at 4 DIV for 3 days; effects on neuron survival were assessed at 7 DIV (**Figure 1A**). To define the presence of all neurons, an antibody against microtubule-associated protein 2 (MAP2) was used (**Figure 1B**; arrowhead); motoneurons were specifically identified with use of the SMI-32 antibody, which recognizes unphosphorylated neurofilament-H (**Figure 1B**; arrow), as previously described (Urushitani et al., 2006; Nagai et al., 2007; Sepulveda et al., 2010; Castillo et al., 2013; Fritz et al., 2013). Chronic (3 days) exposure (from 4 to 7 DIV) of spinal cultures to ACM-SOD1^{G93A}, ACM-SOD1^{G86R}, or ACM-TDP43^{A315T} induced ~50% motoneuron death (**Figures 1C,D**). The number of interneurons was unchanged after application of ACM-SOD1^{G93A} ($91 \pm 1\%$ vs. control, $p > 0.05$ by t-test), ACM-SOD1^{G86R} ($96 \pm 19\%$ vs. control, $p > 0.05$ by t-test), or ACM-TDP43^{A315T} ($103 \pm 23\%$ vs. control, $p > 0.05$ by t-test). Our findings that ACM-SOD1^{G93A} and ACM-SOD1^{G86R} robustly reduces motoneuron cell survival, while sparing interneurons, are consistent with previous studies (Nagai et al., 2007; Castillo et al., 2013; Fritz et al., 2013). Our results with ACM-TDP43^{A315T} also show for the first time that astrocytes carrying a TDP43 mutant kill motoneurons through non-cell-autonomous processes.

Three types of control media were used throughout this work. (1) "Control" media that was not conditioned by astrocytes. (2) "ACM-NT-Control" media derived from astrocytes that were harvested from littermate mice that were negative for the SOD1 and TDP43 gene. (3) "ACM-SOD1^{WT}" media derived from astrocytes that were harvested from transgenic mice carrying the non-pathological human wild-type SOD1 gene. None of these media caused motoneuron death (**Figure 1E**). In particular, the finding that ACM-SOD1^{WT} was not toxic indicates that the factor inducing motoneuron death is specifically due to the SOD1^{G93A} or SOD1^{G86R} mutation, rather than to overexpression of the human SOD1 protein. By contrast, we can not exclude the possibility that motoneuron death in our spinal cultures is attributable, at least in part, by increased levels of the TDP43 protein itself. In fact, accumulating data with transgenic models have established that excessive levels of even human wild-type TDP43 result in neurodegeneration, likely as a result in the disruption of RNA metabolism (Wegorzewska et al., 2009; Wils et al., 2010; Igaz et al., 2011; Ling et al., 2013).

ACM-SOD1^{G93A}, ACM-SOD1^{G86R}, OR ACM-TDP43^{A315T} LEADS TO INCREASES IN INTRACELLULAR ROS/RNS LEVELS

Increased intracellular levels of nitroxidative stress are widely and consistently observed in ALS patients, and in *in vitro* and *in vivo* mouse models that express SOD1 mutants (Barber and Shaw, 2010). To investigate whether soluble toxic factors released by astrocytes that carry SOD1 and TDP43 mutants induce an oxidative burden in primary neurons, we exposed 4 DIV cultures to the diverse ACMs for 30–120 min, washed cells to remove the ACMs, and subsequently loaded the cells with CM-H_2DCF-DA for 30 min (**Figure 2A**). CM-H_2DCF-DA is a non-fluorescent dye that passively diffuses into cells and is hydrolyzed intracellularly to the DCFH carboxylate anion that is trapped inside; oxidation of DCFH results in the formation of the fluorescent product DCF. Increased intensity in fluorescent DCF could thus reflect detection of certain reactive oxygen and nitrogen species, inducing nitroxidative stress. Combined real-time fluorescence and phase-contrast imaging

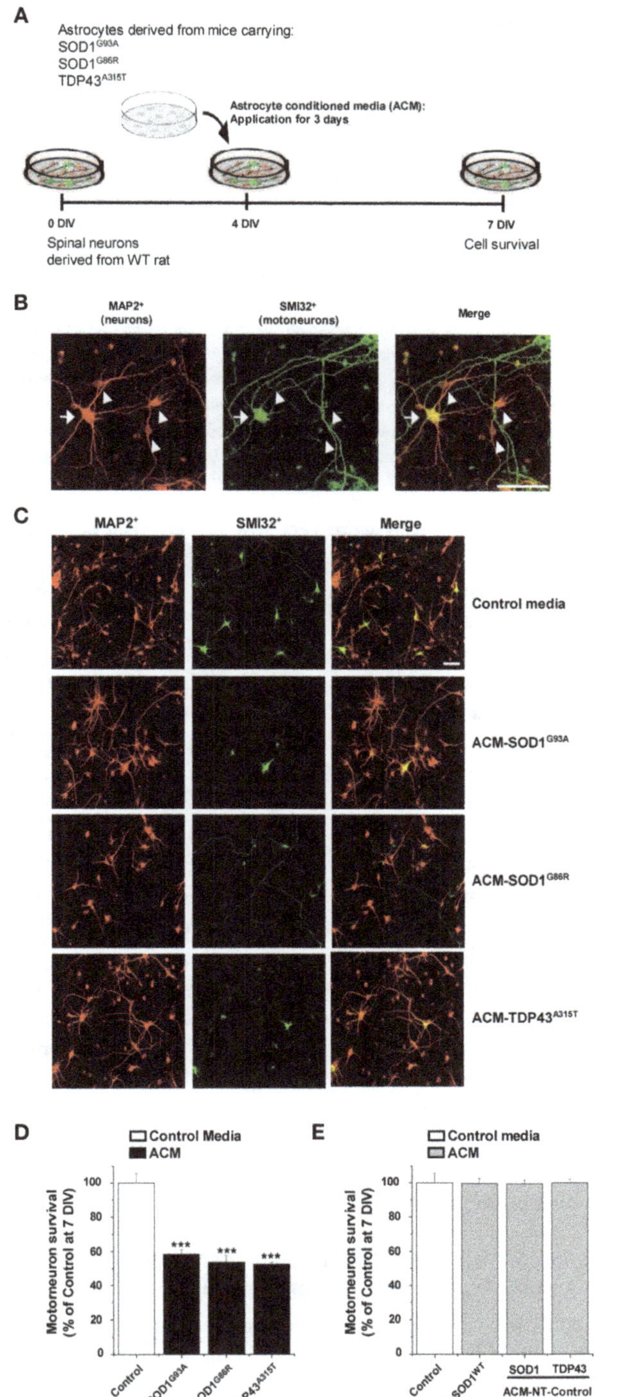

FIGURE 1 | Exposure of primary spinal cord cultures to astrocyte conditioned media (ACM) derived from SOD1^{G93A}, SOD1^{G86R}, and TDP43^{A315T} expressing mice triggers death of motoneurons. (A) Flow diagram of experiment. Primary wild-type (WT) rat spinal cord cultures (4 DIV) were exposed for 3 days to ACM derived from transgenic mice overexpressing SOD1^{G93A} (ACM-SOD1^{G93A}), SOD1^{G86R} (ACM-SOD1^{G86R}), or TDP43^{A315T} (ACM-TDP43^{A315T}). Cells were fixed at 7 DIV, and cell survival was assayed with immunocytochemistry. **(B)** Fixed 7 DIV spinal cord cultures were double-labeled with anti-microtubule-associated

(Continued)

FIGURE 1 | Continued
protein 2 (MAP2) antibody (red) to visualize interneurons (arrowhead) and with the SMI-32 antibody (green) to identify motoneurons (arrow). Scale bar, 25 μm. **(C)** Representative images of $MAP2^+/SMI32^+$-labeled neurons in spinal cultures under control conditions (top image) or treated with the three different ACMs, as indicated in the figure. Scale bar, 200 μm. **(D)** Graph showing the percentage of motoneurons that survived after treatment with ACMs derived from $SOD1^{G93A}$, $SOD1^{G86R}$, and $TDP43^{A315T}$ astrocytes, relative to motoneurons from sister cultures treated with control medium. **(E)** Graph showing the percentage of motoneurons that survived after treatment with media derived from mouse littermates that were negative for the mutated forms of SOD1 and TDP43 (ACM-NT-Control), or with media derived from transgenic mice carrying the non-pathological human wild-type SOD1 gene (ACM-$SOD1^{WT}$). Survival is shown relative to cultures treated with control media. Values represent mean ± s.e.m. from at least 3 independent experiments performed in duplicate, analyzed by One-Way ANOVA followed by a Tukey *post-hoc* test. $^{***}P < 0.001$ relative to control medium at 7 DIV.

showed that DCF levels were very low under basal culture conditions, while application of ACM-$SOD1^{G93A}$ induced both a gradual increase in the intensity and the number of neurons displaying intracellular DCF fluorescence in spinal cord cultures; the fluorescence reached a peak at 30 min (**Figure 2B**). This increase was mimicked by H_2O_2 (**Figure 2B**; 200 μM for 20 min) but was blocked by use of diverse general anti-oxidants (see **Figure 4**). In control experiments, application of ACM-$SOD1^{WT}$ did not change DCF fluorescence over the same exposure times (**Figure 2B$_2$**). Exposure of spinal cord cultures to either ACM-$SOD1^{G86R}$ (**Figure 2C**) or ACM-$TDP43^{A315T}$ (**Figure 2D**) also triggered a gradual increase of intracellular DCF fluorescence in neurons; this fluorescence peaked at 60 and 30 min, respectively. Treatment of neuronal cultures with either ACM-NT-Control (**Figures 2C$_2$–D$_2$**) or control media did not induce significant differences (see **Supplementary Figure 1** for images of all controls). Together, these results indicate that toxic factors released by astrocytes that carry diverse ALS-causing mutants results in increased nitroxidative stress in spinal cord neurons. The increased nitroxidative stress, however, is unable to induce immediate cell death as the number of motoneurons only starts to significantly reduce after 24 h of ACM application (**Supplementary Figure 2**).

ANTI-OXIDANTS PREVENT MOTONEURON DEATH INDUCED BY ACM-$SOD1^{G93A}$, ACM-$SOD1^{G86R}$, OR ACM-$TDP43^{A315T}$

To determine whether the increased nitroxidative stress induced by the diverse ACMs contributes to motoneuron cell death, 4 DIV spinal cord neurons were chronically incubated in a combination of the toxic media plus one of the following anti-oxidants: Trolox, esculetin or resveratrol (**Figure 3A**). These anti-oxidants are reported to reduce intracellular levels of ROS/RNS (also documented in the present study—see **Figure 4** for effects on DCF fluorescence; also see reference citations below). Multiple doses (ranging from 100 nM to 100 μM) of the anti-oxidants were used to assess the survival of motoneurons under control conditions, and after co-application with ACM-$SOD1^{G93A}$ (see **Supplementary Table 1**). For each anti-oxidant drug, the maximum effect in preventing motoneuron death induced by ACM-$SOD1^{G93A}$ is displayed in **Figure 3B**; the same concentrations of anti-oxidants were also used to test whether they could rescue motoneuron death induced by ACM-$SOD1^{G86R}$ (**Figure 3C**) or ACM-$TDP43^{A315T}$ (**Figure 3D**) (see below for details on each anti-oxidant). We also applied these doses of anti-oxidants to cultures incubated with ACM-$SOD1^{WT}$ and found that none of the anti-oxidants were successful in significantly increasing the number of motoneurons (**Figure 3E**); similar results were obtained when anti-oxidants were co-applied to spinal cord culture with control media or ACM-NT-Control (not shown), indicating that the beneficial effects of these compounds are specifically attributable to counterbalancing increased nitroxidative stress induced by the diverse toxic ACMs, rather than to simply increasing overall motoneuron cell survival in the cultures.

We first analyzed use of vitamin E, the most potent naturally occurring scavenger of reactive oxygen and nitrogen species known (Tucker and Townsend, 2005). Extensive studies in ALS patients and mice models have shown, however, that vitamin E application *in vivo* is not capable of significantly prolonging survival (Gurney et al., 1996; Desnuelle et al., 2001; Ascherio et al., 2005; Graf et al., 2005) These disappointing results are likely related to the findings that vitamin E poorly penetrates the blood-brain barrier, leading to insufficient doses of this anti-oxidant in the central nervous system; IC_{50} of vitamin E is between 1.5 and 59 μM while ventricular CSF concentration of this vitamin was found at 0.114 μM (reviewed in Barber and Shaw, 2010). Here we opted to use Trolox, a water-soluble vitamin E analog that neutralizes ROS (Ghiselli et al., 1995; Khaldy et al., 2000; Barber et al., 2009; Distelmaier et al., 2012). Chronic co-application of ACM-$SOD1^{G93A}$ (**Figure 3B**) or ACM-$TDP43^{A315T}$ (**Figure 3D**) with 1 μM of Trolox significantly improved motoneuron survival. In the spinal cord cultures treated with ACM-$SOD1^{G86R}$ plus Trolox improvement of motoneurons survival was even better and comparable with motoneuron survival obtained under control conditions (**Figure 3C**).

Next we analyzed esculetin and resveratrol, two molecules that have anti-oxidant activities (Lin et al., 2000; Kaneko et al., 2003; Baur and Sinclair, 2006; Barber et al., 2009). Esculetin and resveratrol were also identified from a screen of the Spectrum Collection library (consisting of 2000 small compounds) as two of the best-hit molecules, based on their ability to function as effective anti-oxidants by reducing DCF fluorescence and to increase the viability of a mutant $SOD1^{G93A}$-expressing cell line; moreover, *in silico* analysis predicted that these two compounds have specific biochemical properties that allow efficient blood-brain barrier penetration (Barber et al., 2009). We found that chronic co-application of ACM-$SOD1^{G93A}$ (**Figure 3B**) or ACM-$TDP43^{A315T}$ (**Figure 3D**) with 25 μM esculetin significantly improved the survival of motoneurons and, in fact, treatment of spinal cord neurons with esculetin plus ACM-$SOD1^{G86R}$ enhanced motoneuron survival to the level obtained under control conditions (**Figure 3C**).

By contrast, chronic application of resveratrol at 1 μM (**Figure 3B**)—as well as at a wide range of concentrations (100 nM to 10 μM) (**Supplementary Table 1**)—failed to prevent motoneuron death induced by ACM-$SOD1^{G93A}$. Co-application

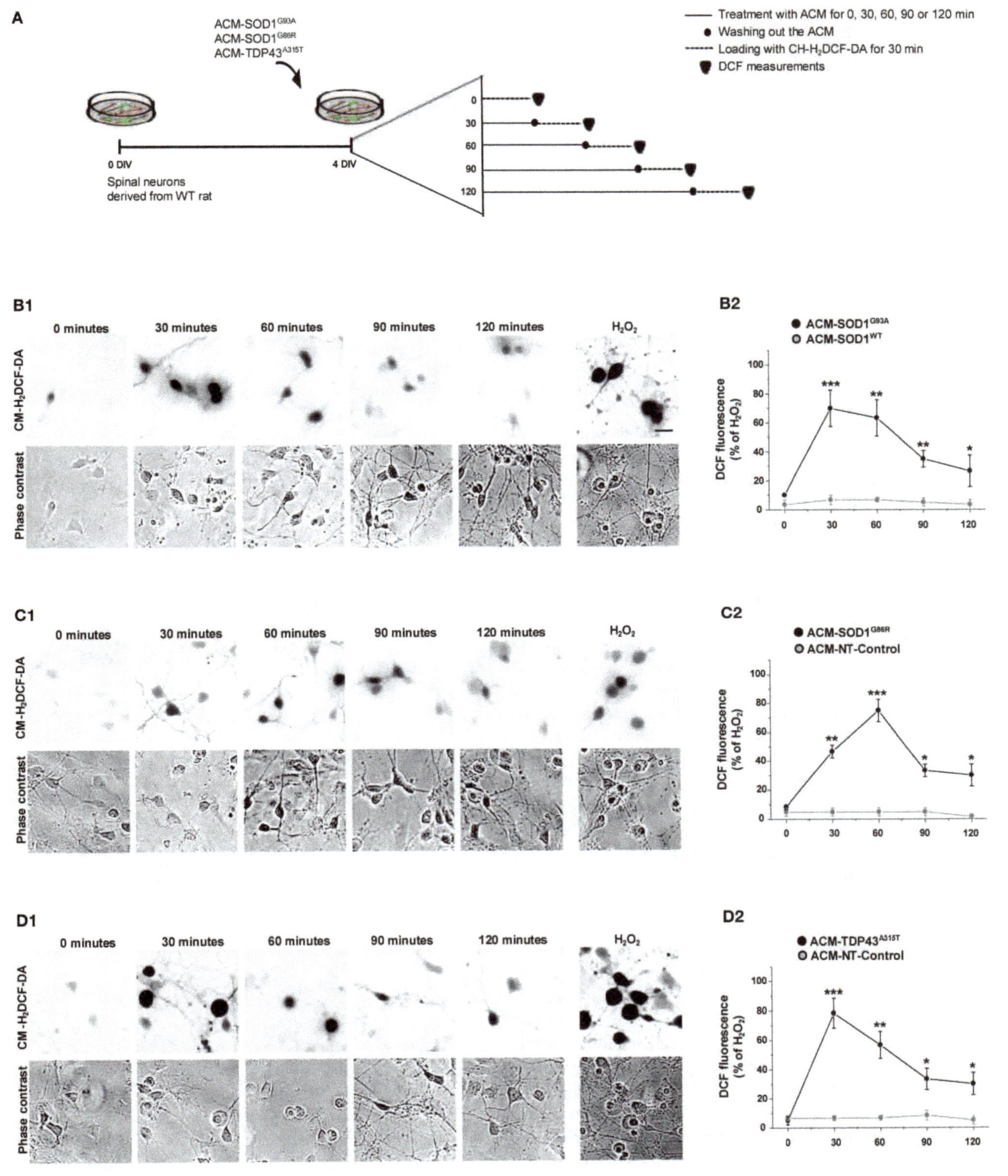

FIGURE 2 | Exposure of primary spinal cord cultures to ACM-SOD1^{G93A}, ACM-SOD1^{G86R}, and ACM-TDP43^{A315T} induces rapid increases in intracellular dichlorofluorescein (DCF) fluorescence. **(A)** Flow diagram of experiment. Primary wild-type spinal cultures (4 DIV) were exposed for 0–120 min with the different ACMs (solid lines), washed to remove the ACMs (filled circles), and loaded for 30 min with the fluorescent membrane permeable ROS/RNS probe CM-H_2DCF-DA (dotted lines). Next cultures were washed and DCF measurements were immediately performed (filled triangles). **(B–D)** Cultures exposed to ACM-SOD1^{G93A} **(B)**, ACM-SOD1^{G86R} **(C)**, or ACM-TDP43^{A315T} **(D)**. **(B$_1$–D$_1$)** The negatives of representative DCF fluorescent images (in which both motoneurons and interneurons are marked) and corresponding phase contrast images of spinal cord cultures photographed at 0, 30, 90 and 120 min after application of ACM-SOD1^{G93A}

(Continued)

FIGURE 2 | Continued
(B$_1$), ACM-SOD1^{G86R} **(C$_1$)**, or ACM-TDP43^{A315T} **(D$_1$)** are shown. In all experiment, H_2O_2 (200 µM for 20 min) served as positive control and to normalize the number of DCF-positive cells after ACM application. Scale bar, 200 µm. **(B$_2$–D$_2$)** Graphs showing the percentage of DCF fluorescent cells (including both motoneurons and interneurons) under the conditions indicated. Results obtained with different controls are included in the graphs: control media, ACM-NT-Control, and ACM-SOD1^{WT}. DCF fluorescence is relative to cultures treated with H_2O_2 (100%). Note that DCF fluorescence peaked after 30 min of incubation of spinal cultures with ACM-SOD1^{G93A} and ACM-TDP43^{A315T} **(B$_2$,D$_2$)**, and after 60 min for incubation with ACM-SOD1^{G86R} **(C$_2$)**. Values represent mean ± s.e.m. from at least 3 independent experiments performed in duplicate, analyzed by *t*-test. $^*p < 0.05$, $^{**}p < 0.01$, $^{***}p < 0.001$ vs. control.

of 1 µM resveratrol also did not significantly improve survival of motoneurons incubated with either ACM-SOD1^{G86R} (**Figure 3C**) or ACM-TDP43^{A315T} (**Figure 3D**). This negative effect was not related to toxicity of this anti-oxidant, as overall motoneuron cell survival in cultures treated with resveratrol was similar to that achieved under control conditions or cultures treated with ACM-SOD1^{WT} (see **Figure 3E** and **Supplementary Table 1**).

As discussed before, the application of the diverse ACMs to spinal cord cultures resulted in a strong DCF signals at 30–60 min which then gradually reduced (**Figure 2**). However, this is only a transient reduction and cells start to steadily increase DCF fluorescence from 24 h after ACM application; 7 DIV neurons treated chronically for 3 days with the diverse ACMs resulted in robust levels of ROS/RNS (~70–80% DCF fluorescence relative to H_2O_2) (**Supplementary Figure 3**). We next analyzed whether the doses of anti-oxidants that effectively increased cell survival (as shown in **Figure 3**) also prevented the increase in ROS/RNS levels induced by the diverse ACMs (**Figure 4A**). Co-application of ACM-SOD1^{G93A} plus Trolox (1 µM) or eculetin (25 µM) to spinal cord cultures decreased intracellular DCF fluorescence to a degree similar to that achieved in control cultures (**Figure 4B**). By contrast, resveratrol (1 µM) slightly, but not significantly, reduced nitroxidative stress induced by ACM-SOD1^{G93A}. We also observed that co-application of Trolox and esculetin with ACM-SOD1^{G86R} (**Figure 4C**) or ACM-TDP43^{A315T} (**Figure 4D**) had similar beneficial effects in preventing nitroxidative stress; however, again, resveratrol was not effective in significantly reducing the DCF signal. This negative effect of resveratrol was not due to the absence of its anti-oxidant capacity; resveratrol reduced DCF fluorescence induced by H_2O_2 (200 µM for 20 min) by ~50% (**Supplementary Figure 4**).

Application of these anti-oxidants to control cultures (not shown), or to spinal cord cultures treated with either ACM-NT-Control (not shown) or with ACM-SOD1^{WT} (**Figure 4E**) revealed that none of these compounds led to significant decreases in basal DCF fluorescence intensity. Together, our data indicate that the favorable effects of Trolox and esculetin on motoneuron survival principally result from counterbalancing the increases in intracellular levels of ROS induced in neurons by the toxic actions of ACM-SOD1^{G93A}, ACM-SOD1^{G86R}, or ACM-TDP43^{A315T}.

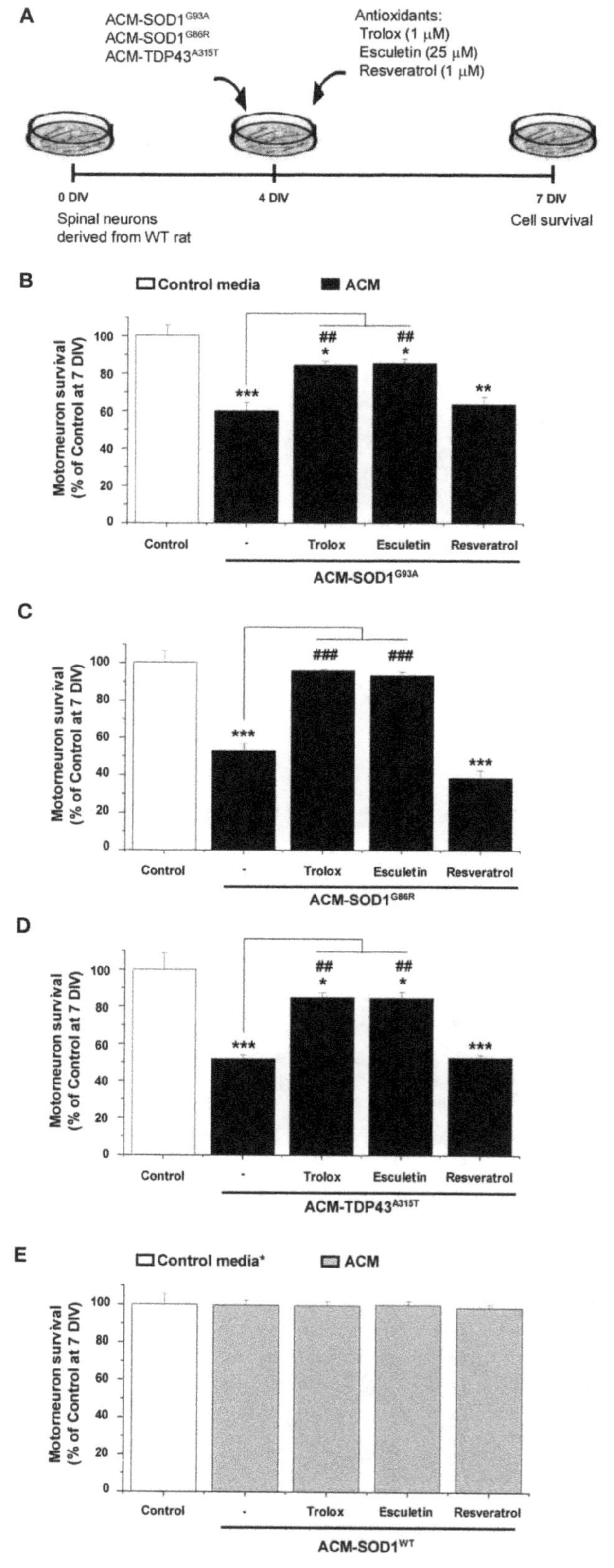

FIGURE 3 | Anti-oxidants Trolox and esculetin prevent motoneurons death induced by ACM-SOD1^{G93A}, ACM-SOD1^{G86R}, and ACM-TDP43^{A315T}. (A) Flow diagram of experiment. ACMs were applied

(Continued)

FIGURE 3 | Continued
chronically starting at 4 DIV alone, or together with the anti-oxidants Trolox (1 μM), esculetin (25 μM), or resveratrol (1 μM). Cell survival was assayed at 7 DIV. **(B–E)** Graphs showing the relative percentage of motoneurons that survived at 7 DIV, after being treated with the diverse anti-oxidants and ACM-SOD1^{G93A} **(B)**, ACM-SOD1^{G86R} **(C)**, ACM-TDP43^{A315T} **(D)**, or ACM-SOD^{WT} **(E)**, relative to motoneurons from sister cultures treated with control medium (indicated with*) or with only the ACM (indicated with#). Note that Trolox and esculetin prevented motoneuron death induced by the diverse ALS-causing ACMs, while resveratrol was ineffective. Note also that none of the compounds improved the survival of control neurons. Values represent means ± s.e.m. from at least 3 independent experiments, analyzed by One-Way ANOVA followed by a Tukey *post-hoc* test. $^{*}P < 0.05$, $^{**}P < 0.01$, $^{***}P < 0.001$ relative to survival with control media at 7 DIV; $^{\#\#}P < 0.01$ and $^{\#\#\#}P < 0.001$ compared to survival with ALS-causing ACM at 7 DIV. See **Supplementary Table 1**. for the effects of a wide range of concentrations of anti-oxidants on motoneuron survival.

Na$_V$ CHANNEL BLOCKERS RESCUE MOTONEURON DEATH INDUCED BY ACM-SOD1^{G93A}, OR ACM-TDP43^{A315T}

To gain insights into the mechanism whereby astrocytes expressing diverse ALS-causing mutant proteins increase intracellular ROS/RNS levels and kill motoneurons, we argued that if the conditioned media from the SOD1 and TDP43 mutant astrocytes share a toxic factor(s), then this toxicity must converge to a common target. We recently reported that ACM-SOD1^{G93A} rapidly (within 30 min) increases neuronal Na$_V$ channel mediated excitability; moreover, the application of several blockers of the Na$_V$ channel activity (including use of mexiletine, spermidine, and riluzole) reduced the hyperexcitability and prevented motoneuron death induced by ACM-SOD1^{G93A} (Fritz et al., 2013). Hence we tested whether the Na$_V$ channel blocker mexiletine (an orally active lidocaine analog that is a local anesthetic and an antiarrhytmic drug that targets the "local anesthetic receptor site" of Na$_V$ channels (Ragsdale et al., 1994; Catterall et al., 2005; Olschewski et al., 2009), spermidine (a polyamine that affects the gating of varies ion channels and serves as an endogenous, activity-dependent Na$_V$ channel blocker (Williams, 1997; Fleidervish et al., 2008) and riluzole which has multiple effects, but at low concentrations (e.g., 100 nM in spinal cord cultures) suppresses neuronal excitability by affecting Na$_V$ channels (Kuo et al., 2005; Theiss et al., 2007; Bellingham, 2011; Fritz et al., 2013) can also rescue motoneuron cell death induced by ACM-SOD1^{G86R} or ACM-TDP43^{A315T} (**Figure 5A**). We used the same concentrations of these Na$_V$ channel blockers as described previously: 25 nM mexiletine, 10 μM spermidine and 100 nM riluzole (Fritz et al., 2013)—these doses were chosen based on earlier determinations that at these concentrations the Na$_V$ channel blockers reduced excitability and also effectively prevented motoneuron cell death induced by ACM-SOD1^{G93A}, without affecting overall motoneuron cell survival in control cultures (Fritz et al., 2013; and see also **Figures 5B,E**).

To directly compare the beneficial effect of co-application of mexiletine, spermidine or riluzole on the diverse toxic ACMs, we first analyzed motoneuronal survival when these sodium channel blockers were co-applied with ACM-SOD1^{G93A} (**Figure 5B**). As expected, chronic application (from 4 to 7 DIV) of mexiletine together with ACM-SOD1^{G93A} to spinal cord cultures prevented motoneuron death in those cultures (**Figure 5B**),

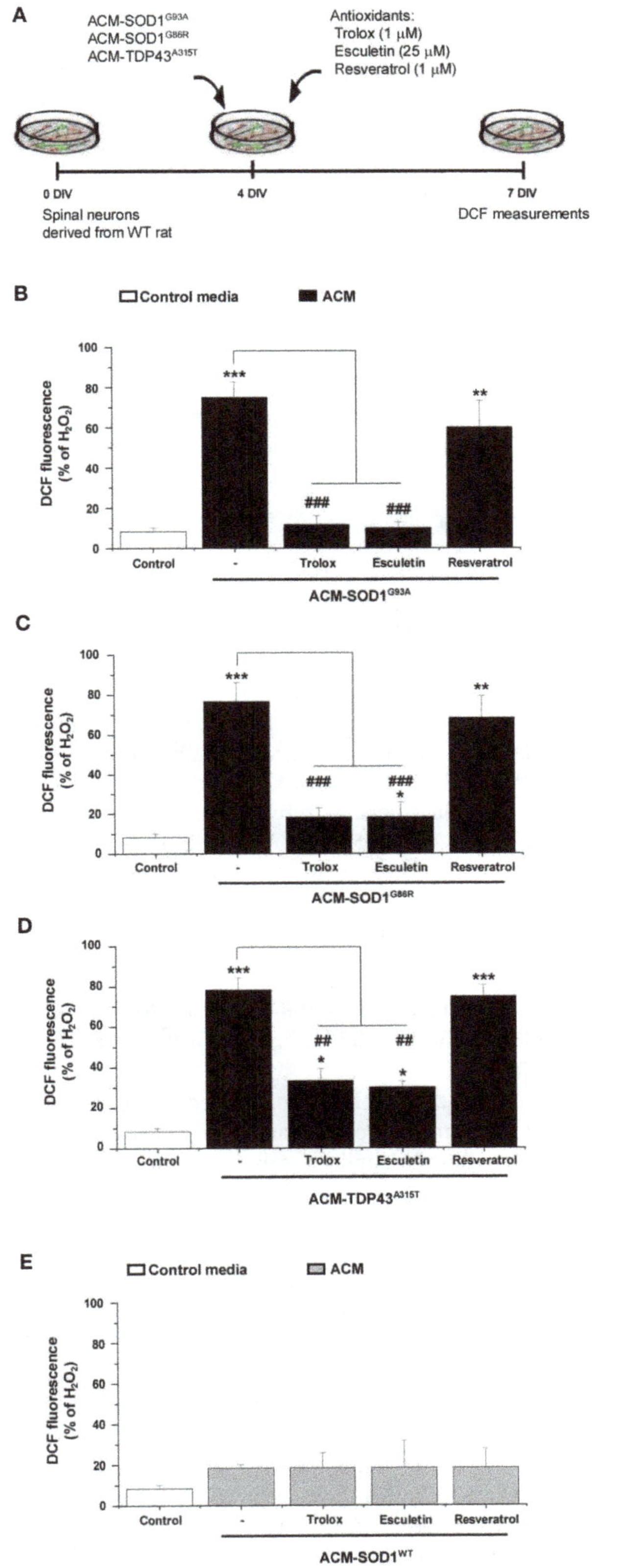

FIGURE 4 | The effect of anti-oxidants on DCF fluorescence in spinal cord cultures exposed to the diverse ACMs. (A) Flow diagram of experiment. ACMs were applied chronically starting at 4 DIV alone, or *(Continued)*

FIGURE 4 | Continued
together with the anti-oxidants Trolox (1 μM), esculetin (25 μM), or resveratrol (1 μM). At 7 DIV, cultures were incubated with the membrane permeable ROS/RNS probe CM-H_2DCF-DA and DCF fluorescence was measured 30 min later. **(B–E)** Graphs showing the percentage of DCF fluorescent cells after being treated with the diverse anti-oxidants and ACM-SOD1^{G93A} **(B)**, ACM-SOD1^{G86R} **(C)**, ACM-TDP43^{A315T} **(D)**, or ACM-SOD^{WT} **(E)**, In all experiment, H_2O_2 (200 μM for 20 min) served as positive control and to normalize the number of DCF-positive cells after ACM application. The graphs indicate statistics relative to motoneurons from sister cultures treated with control medium (indicated with*) or with only the ACM (indicated with#). Note that co-application of the diverse ACMs with Trolox or esculetin resulted in significant lower DCF fluorescent intensities, whereas resveratrol was not effective. Values represent means ± s.e.m. from at least 3 independent experiments, analyzed by One-Way ANOVA followed by a Tukey *post-hoc* test. $^{**}P < 0.01$, $^{***}P < 0.001$ relative to DCF fluorescence with control media at 7 DIV; $^{\#\#}P < 0.01$ and $^{\#\#\#}P < 0.001$ compared to DCF fluorescence with ALS-causing ACM at 7 DIV.

as we have shown earlier (Fritz et al., 2013). Addition of mexiletine to spinal cord cultures exposed to ACM-SOD1^{G86R} (**Figure 5C**) and ACM-TDP43^{A315T} (**Figure 5D**) was also very beneficial and resulted in partially or complete prevention of motoneuron cell death, respectively. Spermidine (10 μM) also completely rescued motoneuron from death induced by ACM-SOD1^{G93A} (**Figure 5B**), ACM-SOD1^{G86R} (**Figure 5C**), or ACM-TDP43^{A315T} (**Figure 5D**). And furthermore chronic co-incubation of spinal cord cultures with 100 nM riluzole and ACM-SOD1^{G93A} (**Figure 5B**) or ACM-SOD1^{G86R} (**Figure 5C**) completely prevented motoneuron death. The beneficial effects of this drug were less apparent on motoneurons incubated with ACM-TDP43^{A315T} (**Figure 5D**).

Na$_V$ CHANNEL BLOCKERS PREVENT INCREASES IN NITROXIDATIVE STRESS INDUCED BY ACM-SOD1^{G93A}, ACM-SOD1^{G86R}, OR ACM-TDP43^{A315T}

To determine whether the Na$_V$ channel-mediated hyperexcitability occurs upstream or downstream of the nitroxidative stress detected by DCF, we co-applied the diverse ACMs with Na$_V$ channel blockers to 4 DIV cultures and measured the intensity of DCF fluorescence (**Figure 6A**). The incubation time of the Na$_V$ channel blockers with the ACMs was chosen based on the maximum peak in the established time-course of DCF fluorescence for each conditioned media (see **Figure 2**): ACM-SOD1^{G93A} and ACM-TDP43^{A315T} were tested at 30 min, whereas ACM-SOD1^{G86R} was tested at 60 min. We found that all three Na$_V$ channel blockers significantly reduced DCF fluorescence induced by the diverse ACMs, but to different degrees: mexiletine and spermidine reduced the DCF fluorescent signal induced by ACMs-SOD1^{G93A} to a level similar to that achieved in untreated cultures, while riluzole decreased DCF fluorescence to below basal levels (**Figure 6B**). Similar effects were observed when these Na$_V$ channel blockers were co-applied with ACM-SOD1^{G86R} (**Figure 6C**), ACM-TDP43^{A315T} (**Figure 6D**), or ACM-SOD1^{WT} (**Figure 6E**). Collectively, these data indicate that astrocytes expressing diverse ALS-causing mutant genes, including in the alleles SOD1 and TDP43, secrete soluble factors that kill wild-type motoneurons

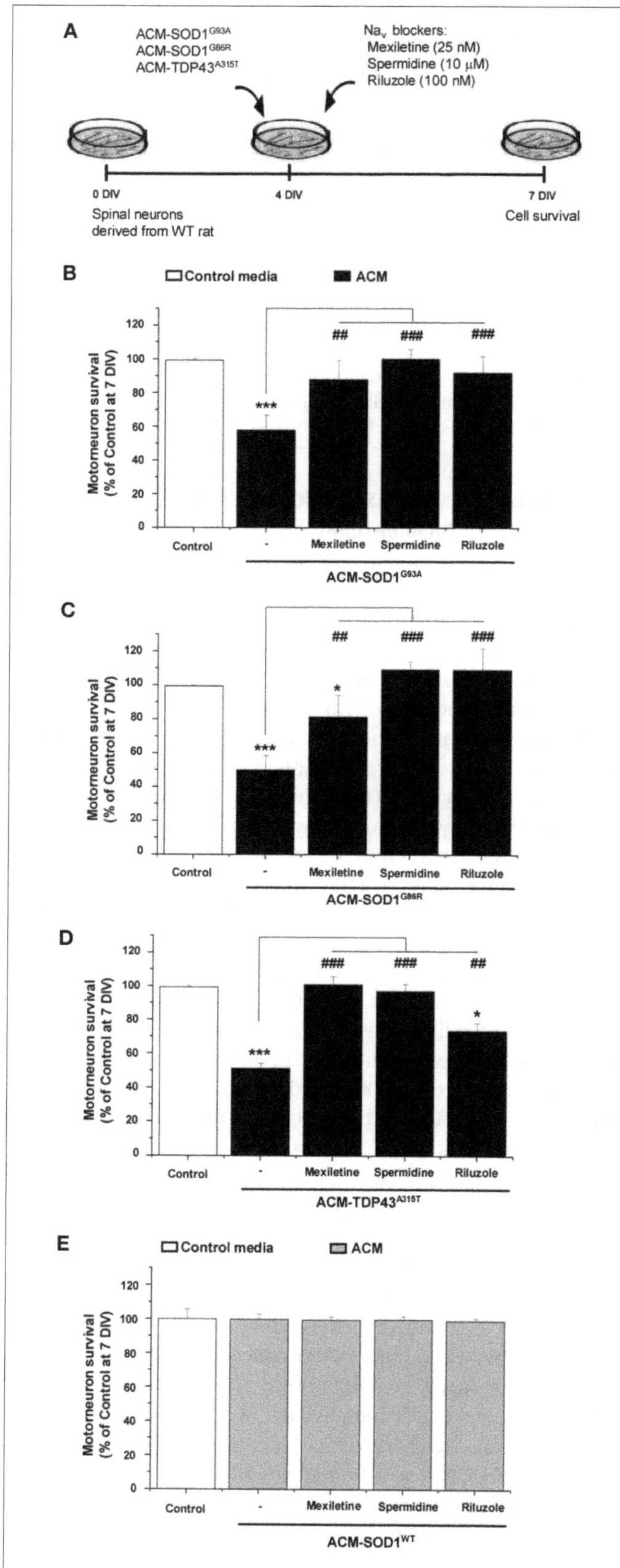

FIGURE 5 | Na$_V$ channel blockers prevent motoneuron death induced by ACM-SOD1^{G93A}, ACM-SOD1^{G86R}, and ACM-TDP43^{A315T}. (A) Flow diagram of experiment. ACMs were applied chronically starting at 4 DIV *(Continued)*

FIGURE 5 | Continued
alone, or together with the Na_V channel blockers mexiletine (25 nM), spermidine (10 μM), or riluzole (100 nM). Cell survival was assayed at 7 DIV. **(B–E)** Graphs showing the relative percentage of motoneurons that survived at 7 DIV, after being treated with the diverse Na_V channel blockers and ACM-SOD1^{G93A} **(B)**, ACM-SOD1^{G86R} **(C)**, ACM-TDP43^{A315T} **(D)**, or ACM-SOD1^{WT} **(E)**, relative to motoneurons from sister cultures treated with control medium (indicated with*) or with only the ACM (indicated with#). Values represent means ± s.e.m. from at least 3 independent experiments, analyzed by One-Way ANOVA followed by a Tukey *post-hoc* test. $^{*}P < 0.05$, $^{***}P < 0.001$ relative to survival with control media at 7 DIV; $^{\#\#}P < 0.01$ and $^{\#\#\#}P < 0.001$ compared to survival with ALS-causing ACM at 7 DIV.

through a common pathway that involves increased nitroxidative stress, mediated at least in part by Na_V channel activity.

DISCUSSION

We provide evidence to demonstrate that astrocytes expressing mutations in SOD1 and TDP43 genes trigger motoneuron pathology and death through non-cell-autonomous processes mediated by the release of soluble toxic factor(s). We show that conditioned media derived from astrocytes that express ALS-causing mutations in SOD1 (SOD1^{G93A} and SOD1^{G86R}) and TDP43 (TDP43^{A315T}) enhance ROS/RNS levels in neurons, and reduce motoneuron survival. We also document that application of anti-oxidants to spinal cord cultures prevents the increases in intracellular nitroxidative stress induced by diverse ACMs, and counteracts motoneuron death induced by the toxins in these media. Our finding that addition of Na_V channel blockers to spinal cord cultures also strongly diminish ACM-induced enhancement of DCF fluorescence and motoneuron death further indicates that Na_V channel-mediated excitability occurs upstream of nitroxidative stress and is required for the generation of a certain type of such stress. Collectively, these results indicate that astrocytes that express ALS-causing mutants in SOD1 and TDP43 contribute to ALS pathogenesis by activating a common molecular pathway that involves nitroxidative stress mediated, at least in part, by Na_V channel activity.

MUTATIONS IN SOD1 AND TDP43 CAUSE MOTONEURON PATHOLOGY AND DEATH BY NON-CELL-AUTONOMOUS PROCESSES

Ample evidence reveals that astrocytes expressing SOD1 mutants contribute to the pathogenesis of ALS: we and others have also demonstrated that such astrocytes release neurotoxic factors that kill primary motoneurons in culture (Nagai et al., 2007; Cassina et al., 2008; Castillo et al., 2013; Fritz et al., 2013). In agreement with these studies, we show here that ACM-SOD1^{G93A} and ACM-SOD1^{G86R} also extensively and selectively kill primary motoneurons. Additionally, we also examined whether mutants in TDP43 contribute to disease pathogenesis by non-cell-autonomous processes. As for ACM-SOD1^{G93A} and ACM-SOD1^{G86R}, we document that exposure of wild-type spinal cord cultures to conditioned media generated by astrocytes derived from transgenic mice that express mutant TDP43^{A315T} suffices to trigger robust death of motoneurons. These data indicate that astrocytes harboring mutant TDP43^{A315T} release soluble toxic factor(s) into the media and thereby contribute to disease pathogenesis via non-cell-autonomous processes.

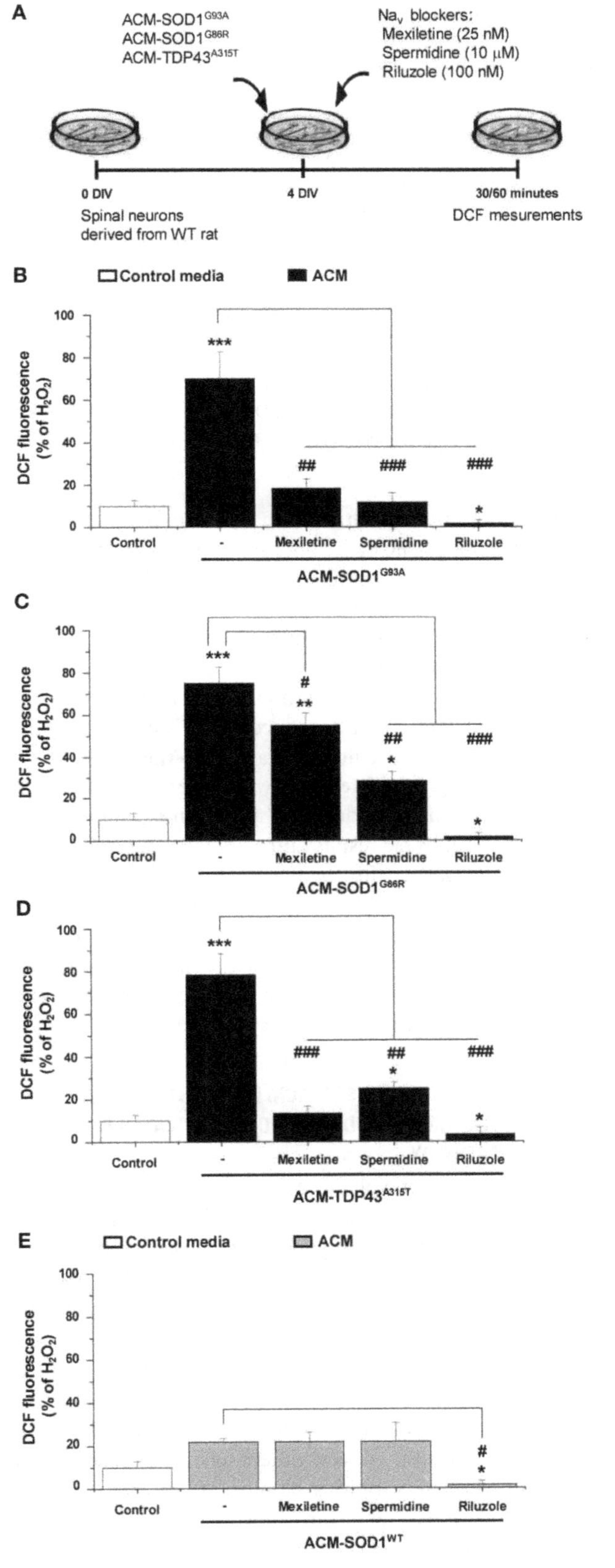

FIGURE 6 | Na_V channel blockers reduce DCF fluorescence induced by ACM-SOD1^{G93A}, ACM-SOD1^{G86R}, and ACM-TDP43^{A315T}. (A) Flow diagram of experiment. Spinal cultures (4 DIV) were exposed for 30 *(Continued)*

FIGURE 6 | Continued
(ACM-SOD1^{G93A} or ACM-TDP43^{A315T}) or 60 (ACM-SOD1^{G86R}) minutes (see **Figure 2** for peak of DCF fluorescence), alone or together with Na$_V$ channel blockers mexiletine (25 nM), spermidine (10 μM), or riluzole (100 nM). Next, cultures were incubated with the membrane permeable ROS/RNS probe CM-H_2DCF-DA and DCF fluorescence was measured 30 min later. **(B–E)** Graphs showing the percentage of DCF fluorescent cells after being treated with the diverse Na$_V$ channel blockers and Na$_V$ channel blockers and ACM-SOD1^{G93A} **(B)**, ACM-SOD1^{G86R} **(C)**, ACM-SOD^{WT} **(D)**, ACM-TDP43^{A315T} **(E)**. In all experiment, H_2O_2 (200 μM for 20 min) served as positive control and to normalize the number of DCF-positive cells after ACM application. The graphs indicate statistics relative to motoneurons from sister cultures treated with control medium (indicated with*) or with only the ACM (indicated with#). Values represent means ± s.e.m. from at least 3 independent experiments, analyzed by One-Way ANOVA followed by a Tukey *post-hoc* test. $^{*}P < 0.05$, $^{**}P < 0.01$, $^{***}P < 0.001$ relative to DCF fluorescence with control media at 7 DIV; $^{\#\#}P < 0.01$ and $^{\#\#\#}P < 0.001$ compared to DCF fluorescence with ALS-causing ACM at 7 DIV.

Our findings are in contrast to a recent publication by Serio et al. (2013), who showed that astrocytes expressing mutant TDP43^{M337V}contribute to ALS pathology exclusively via cell-autonomous processes, and do not via non-cell-autonomous toxicity. These authors generated astrocytes from induced pluripotent stem cells (IPSCs) derived from a human ALS patient carrying the TDP43^{M337V} mutation. They report that expression of the TDP43 mutant reduced survival of the human astrocytes, but that co-culturing layers of these TDP43^{M337V} mutant containing astrocytes with wild-type motoneurons does not lead to motoneuron death. The reason(s) underlying the difference between their results and ours may be related to technical issues associated with the generation of astrocyte populations from human IPSCs, or to the particular TDP43 mutant involved. Additional experiments on the effects that diverse TDP43 mutants expressed in primary rodent astrocytes, as well as in human IPSCs cell lines, have on motoneurons are needed to resolve this discrepancy.

EXPOSURE OF MOTONEURONS TO ACM FROM ASTROCYTES CARRYING MUTATIONS IN SOD1 AND TDP43 ACTIVATES A COMMON PATHOGENIC PATHWAY

Several hypotheses, involving the influence of nitroxidative stress, glutamate excitotoxicity, hyperexcitability, formation of high-molecular-weight aggregates, mitochondrial dysfunction, cytoskeletal disruption, and activation of cell death signals, have been proposed to explain the toxic effect of mutated SOD1 (Beckman et al., 2001; Cleveland and Rothstein, 2001; Bruijn et al., 2004; Pasinelli and Brown, 2006; Cozzolino et al., 2012; van Zundert et al., 2012). Our results point to critical roles for nitroxidatve stress as well as Na$_V$ channel activity in inducing motoneuron death. We and others have previously used cell cultures and slice preparations obtained from transgenic mice expressing mutations in SOD1 to report that Na$_V$ channel activity and/or excitability is increased in motoneurons (Kuo et al., 2005; van Zundert et al., 2008; Pambo-Pambo et al., 2009; Pieri et al., 2009; Schuster et al., 2011; Quinlan et al., 2011 and reviewed in ElBasiouny et al., 2010 and van Zundert et al., 2012). Moreover, using the ACM-SOD1^{G93A} model system, we recently found that neuronal hyperexcitability, mediated at least in part through elevated Na$_V$ channel activity, is essential for inducing motoneuron death. And furthermore, the data presented here indicate that soluble factor(s) secreted by astrocytes carrying other ALS-causing mutations in SOD1 (SOD^{G86R}), and moreover in TDP43 (TDP43^{A315T}), kill motoneurons via activation of Na$_V$ channels.

Soluble mediator(s) secreted by astrocytes with mutations in SOD1 and TDP43 rapidly enhance neuronal nitroxidative stress, and lead to extensive motoneuron death within a matter of days. The rapid elevation in ROS/RNS levels observed in neurons exposed to the toxic ACMs could be due to diffusion of nitroxidative stress generated outside the cell into the motoneurons, or via intracellular *de novo* generation of ROS/RNS. We favor the second option, as the robust increase in the intensity of DCF fluorescence in motoneurons upon application of toxic ACMs is abolished when Na$_V$ channel blockers are applied to the spinal neuron cultures. Note, however, that it has been documented that DCF detects only particular types of reactive species, including hydrogen peroxide (H_2O_2; in combination with cellular peroxidases), hydroxyl radicals ($^{\bullet}OH$), and peroxynitrite ($ONOO^-$) (Estévez et al., 1999; Myhre et al., 2003; Gomes et al., 2005; Martin et al., 2007; Kalyanaraman et al., 2012), while it is seems insensitive to nitric oxide (NO) and superoxide ($O_2^{\bullet-}$) (Myhre et al., 2003). It is thus possible that neurons are targets of certain ROS/RNS, including external NO or $O_2^{\bullet-}$, that contribute to neuronal nitroxidative stress without being detected by the DCF probe.

With regard to this idea, amply evidence indicates that NO and $O_2^{\bullet-}$ are produced by ALS glial cells—as a result of either mitochondrial dysfunction, increased NADPH oxidase activity, or inflammation—and play a pivotal role in motoneuron pathology and death (Carter et al., 2009; Drechsel et al., 2012). For example, Barbeito and collaborators (Vargas et al., 2006; Cassina et al., 2008) report that 40% of motoneurons are lost when they are co-cultured on astrocytes carrying mutated SOD1^{G93A} and that these astrocytes were found to produce excessive levels of NO and mitochondrial $O_2^{\bullet-}$. Moreover, cell death is abrogated when these astrocytes are pre-treated with either anti-oxidants capable of reducing $O_2^{\bullet-}$ production, or with inhibitors of NO synthase (NOS) (Vargas et al., 2006; Cassina et al., 2008). Additional studies also indicate that astrocytes and microglia that express mutated SOD1 can generate NO and NADPH oxidase (Nox)-derived ROS (Harraz et al., 2008; Marchetto et al., 2008). Also, *in vivo* production of harmful Nox-derived $O_2^{\bullet-}$ is reported in human SALS patients as well as in the SOD1^{G93A} transgenic mouse model (Wu et al., 2006; Marden et al., 2007; Harraz et al., 2008). And finally, recent studies indicate that even extracellular mutant SOD1 and oxidized/misfolded SOD1 protein (both of which are likely to be secreted by cells) can activate microglia and induce nitroxidative stress (Urushitani et al., 2006; Ezzi et al., 2007; Zhao et al., 2010). Based on these studies, it is plausible that wild-type neurons are targets of external NO or $O_2^{\bullet-}$ that (1) accumulates in media conditioned by astrocytes carrying ALS mutants, or (2) is generated by surrounding wild-type glial cells (astrocytes and/or microglia) within the spinal cord culture via the action of factors present in the ACM (such as mutated or oxidized/misfolded SOD1 that is secreted by the ALS astrocytes). The presence of these RNS/ROS not necessarily affects externally positioned molecules located in or on the cell membranes of neurons: Thus, NO freely diffuses across cell membranes, and whereas membranes are relatively impermeable to $O_2^{\bullet -}$, recent studies indicate that this oxidative specie could permeate across redoxosomal membranes through undefined chloride channels (Mumbengegwi et al., 2008; Carter et al., 2009). On the basis of our findings presented here and in previous studies, we support the view that induction of Na_V channel activation by toxic ACMs is a central factor in initiating motoneuron death in ALS (van Zundert et al., 2012; Fritz et al., 2013). Na_V channel activity can be increased directly by different oxidative species (Hammarström and Gage, 2000; Kassmann et al., 2008; Nani et al., 2010), but also indirectly by other factors such kinases (e.g., PKC) and the Na_V channel β-subunits (Franceschetti et al., 2000; Goldin, 2003; Aman et al., 2009). It would be interesting to define by mutagenesis whether oxidation of particular amino acids residues (especially methionines and cysteines) influence Na_V channel activation; these types of experiments, however, are beyond the scope of this study.

Here we present the following hypothesis to reconcile the studies by others and the data we have present here and previously (Fritz et al., 2013) showing that ACM-SOD1^{G93A} rapidly (30 min) increases the frequency of calcium transients in cultured spinal cord neurons. Conditioned media derived from astrocytes carrying SOD1 and TDP43 mutants contains NO and/or leads to the generation of NO in spinal cord cultures. This NO in turn induces the activation of Na_V channels, leading to excessive calcium influxes through activated Ca_V channels; the calcium-mediated activation of mitochondrial respiratory chain complexes and/or Nox complexes will produce intracellular $O_2^{\bullet -}$ that can interact with NO to spontaneously generate $ONOO^-$ that hence can be detected by DCF and promotes intracellular damage, including protein nitration (Beckman et al., 2001; Cleveland and Rothstein, 2001; Martin et al., 2007). This hypothesis is supported by the fact that limiting the levels of $O_2^{\bullet -}$ by either reducing Nox activity (Wu et al., 2006; Harraz et al., 2007) or by application of compounds such as Trolox and esculetin (in this study), which have antioxidant and free radical scavenger capacities (Barber et al., 2009), prevented motoneuron death in diverse ALS models. The finding that the antioxidant resveratrol, unlike Trolox and esculetin, was unable to significantly prevent ACM-induced motoneuron death can be explained by the fact that this compound is a poor free radical scavenger compared to the other two compounds (Barber et al., 2009).

DO SOLUBLE TOXIC FACTOR(S) RELEASED BY ALS ASTROCYTES SPECIFICALLY TARGET MOTONEURONS?

Data presented here and previously (Vargas et al., 2006; Di Giorgio et al., 2007; Nagai et al., 2007; Cassina et al., 2008; Marchetto et al., 2008; Castillo et al., 2013; Fritz et al., 2013) show compelling evidence that whereas astrocytes expressing ALS-linked mutations kill motoneurons in spinal cord cultures, they do not affect the survival of spinal cord interneurons. Data shown here and previously (Castillo et al., 2013; Fritz et al., 2013) indicate that independent of neuronal degeneration exposure of spinal cord cultures to toxic ACMs causes pathophysiological changes—including increases in nitroxidative stress, Na_V channel activity, neuronal excitability, and intracellular calcium transients—in both motoneurons and interneurons. Moreover, detailed analyses in SOD1-ALS mice also indicate that several pathological changes can be detected in interneurons, and importantly, much before the onset of disease symptoms (Martin et al., 2007; van Zundert et al., 2008, 2012; Ramírez-Jarquín et al., 2013; Wootz et al., 2013). If both types of neurons are affected in ALS, why then are motoneurons killed and interneurons spared? Using electrophysiological recordings, we recently showed (Fritz et al., 2013) that application of ACM-SOD1^{G93A} significantly increased the persistent sodium inward current (PC_{Na}) of neurons; this PC_{Na} is mediated by Na_V channels (PC_{Na} is greater for $Nav_{1.1}$ and $Nav_{1.6}$ as compared to $Nav_{1.2}$ and $Nav_{1.3}$), and small increases can have important effects on neuronal excitability, leading to excessive influxes of calcium and sodium (ElBasiouny et al., 2010; van Zundert et al., 2012). Interestingly, we found that neurons with a large soma (>20 μm diameter) and expressing ≥5 primary dendrites (typical for motoneurons) displayed a larger PC_{Na} compared to neurons with a smaller soma (<20 μm diameter) and expressing ≤4 primary dendrites (typical for interneurons). Moreover, application of ACM-SOD1^{G93A} further increased the PC_{Na} of neurons, especially of motoneurons. The expression of specific Na_V channel subtypes, and subsequent activation of these channels by soluble toxic factor(s) released by ALS astrocytes, will thus induce larger PC_{Na} and in turn cause more sustained calcium influxes in motoneurons compared to interneurons. In addition, because motoneurons have a limited cytosolic calcium-buffering capacity, excessive uptake of calcium by mitochondria would be an initial step in a cascade of events that impair mitochondrial function, thereby likely producing excessive $O_2^{\bullet -}$ that ultimately leads to motoneuron death (von Lewinski and Keller, 2005; Bento-Abreu et al., 2010; van Zundert et al., 2012).

In summary, we have elucidated critical roles for both nitroxidative stress and Na_V channel activation in the death of motoneuron that is induced in diverse ALS models. Finally, because patients with SALS and FALS display a similar pathology, have comparable clinical symptoms that include hyperexcitability, and experience a beneficial effect of riluzole, it is possible that diverse Na_V channel blockers will show benefit in both forms of ALS.

AUTHOR CONTRIBUTIONS

Fabiola Rojas, Nicole Cortes, and Sebastian Abarzua performed MN survival experiments. Nicole Cortes and Fabiola Rojas performed DCF measurement. All (Fabiola Rojas, Nicole Cortes, Sebastian Abarzua, Agnieszka Dyrda, and Brigitte van Zundert) analyzed the data and wrote the manuscript.

ACKNOWLEDGMENTS

We thank Luis Melo for technical support. This work was supported by ALS Therapy Alliance-CVS Pharmacy, Fondecyt 1101012, and Anillo ACT1114 (to Brigitte van Zundert).

SUPPLEMENTARY MATERIAL

Supplementary Figure 1 | Exposure of primary spinal cord cultures to Control media or ACM-NT-Control media does not induce increases in intracellular DCF fluorescence. (A) Flow diagram of experiment. Primary wild-type spinal cultures (4 DIV) were exposed for 0–120 min with the different medias (solid lines), washed to remove the ACMs (filled circles), and loaded for 30 min with the fluorescent membrane permeable ROS/RNS probe CM-H_2DCF-DA (dotted lines). Next, cultures were washed and DCF measurements were immediately performed (filled triangles). **(B–D)** Cultures were exposed to three types of control media: "Control" media that was not conditioned by astrocytes **(B)**, "ACM-SOD1^{WT}" media derived from astrocytes that were harvested from transgenic mice carrying the non-pathological human wild-type SOD1 gene **(C)**, and "ACM-NT-Control" media derived from astrocytes that were harvested from littermate mice that were negative for the mutant SOD1 or TDP43 gene; here we show media from TDP43$^{A315T-/-}$ astrocytes. Similar results were obtained after application of media from SOD1$^{G93A-/-}$ or SOD1$^{G86R-/-}$ astrocytes **(D)**. The negatives of representative DCF fluorescent images (in which both motoneurons and interneurons are marked) and corresponding phase contrast images of spinal cord cultures photographed at the different indicated time points of media application are shown. Note that unlike H_2O_2 (200 μM for 20 min), which served as a positive control (shown in **B** in the right), none of the control media induced increases in intracellular DCF fluorescence. Scale bar, 200 μm.

Supplementary Figure 2 | Time-course of motoneuron survival in primary spinal cord cultures exposed to ACM-SOD1^{G93A}. Primary wild-type (WT) rat spinal cord cultures (4 DIV) were exposed for 2, 8, 24, and 72 h to ACM derived from transgenic mice overexpressing SOD1^{G93A} (ACM-SOD1^{G93A}) and fixed immediately afterwards. Cell survival was assayed with immunocytochemistry. Graph showing the percentage of motoneurons that survived after treatment with ACMSOD1^{G93A}, relative to control medium and with media derived from transgenic mice carrying the non-pathological human wild-type SOD1 gene (ACM-SOD1^{WT}). Survival is shown relative to cultures treated with control media. Values represent mean ± s.e.m. from at least 3 independent experiments performed in duplicate, analyzed by One-Way ANOVA followed by a Tukey *post-hoc* test. $^{***}P < 0.001$ relative to control medium at 7 DIV.

Supplementary Figure 3 | Time-course of DCF fluorescence in spinal cord cultures exposed to ACM-SOD1^{G93A}, ACM-SOD1^{G86R}, or ACM-TDP43^{A315T}. (A) Flow diagram of experiment. Primary wild-type spinal cultures (4 DIV) were exposed for 0, 30, 60, 90, and 120 min and 6, 24, 48, and 72 h with the different ACMs (solid lines), washed to remove the ACMs (filled circles), and loaded for 30 min with the fluorescent membrane permeable ROS/RNS probe CM-H_2DCF-DA (dotted lines). Next, cultures were washed and DCF measurements were immediately performed (filled triangles). **(B–D)** Graphs showing the percentage of DCF fluorescent cells (including both motoneurons and interneurons) in cultures exposed to ACM-SOD1^{G93A} **(B)**, ACM-SOD1^{G86R} **(C)**, or ACM-TDP43^{A315T} **(D)**. Results obtained with different controls are included in the graphs: ACMSOD1^{WT} **(B)**, ACM-NT-Control from SOD1$^{G86R-/-}$astrocytes **(C)**, and ACM-NT-Control from TDP43$^{A314T-/-}$ astrocytes **(D)**. DCF fluorescence is relative to cultures treated with H_2O_2, 200 μM for 20 min (100%). Note that application of toxic ACMs resulted in an initial peak of DCF fluorescence at 30–60 min that was followed by a decline in the DCF signal which then started to steadily increase from 24 h on. Values represent mean ± s.e.m. from at least 3 independent experiments performed in duplicate, analyzed by *t*-test. $^{*}p < 0.05$, $^{**}p < 0.01$, $^{***}p < 0.001$ vs. control.

Supplementary Figure 4 | Anti-oxidant resveratrol is as effective as Trolox and esculetin in reducing DCF fluorescence induced by H_2O_2. (A) Flow diagram of experiment. Primary spinal cord cultures (4 DIV) were exposed to 200 μM H_2O_2 for 20 min in the presence or absence of anti-oxidants. Cells were washed and then loaded with the membrane permeable ROS/RNS probe CM-H_2DCF-DA for 30 min. After washing, DCF fluorescence was measured immediately. **(B)** Graphs showing the percentage of DCF fluorescent cells (including motoneurons and interneurons) in cultures exposed to H_2O_2 and Trolox (1 μM), esculetin (25 μM), or resveratrol (1 μM). Values represent means ± s.e.m. from at least 3 independent experiments, analyzed by One-Way ANOVA followed by a Tukey *post-hoc* test. $^{##}P < 0.01$, $^{###}P < 0.001$ relative to DCF fluorescence in H_2O_2 treated cultures.

Supplementary Table 1 | Effects of a wide range of concentrations of antioxidants on the survival of control motoneurons and those exposed to ACM-SOD1^{G93A}. (A) Analysis of survival of motoneurons at 7 DIV in primary cultures after incubation for 4 days with multiple doses of the anti-oxidants Trolox, esculetin, and resveratrol. **(B)** Analysis of surviving motoneurons at 7 DIV in primary cultures after incubation for 4 days with ACM-hSOD1^{G93A} alone (no drug), or with ACM plus different doses of the anti-oxidants. In bold are indicated concentrations at which concentration the anti-oxidant was selected for further analysis on preventing the toxicity induced by the diverse ACMs; those results are displayed in **Figure 3**. Values represent mean ± s.e.m. from at least 3 independent experiments performed in duplicate, analyzed by *t*-test vs. control.

REFERENCES

Abel, O., Powell, J. F., Andersen, P. M., and Al-Chalabi, A. (2012). ALSoD: a user-friendly online bioinformatics tool for amyotrophic lateral sclerosis genetics. *Hum. Mutat.* 33, 1345–1351. doi: 10.1002/humu.22157

Aman, T. K., Grieco-Calub, T. M., Chen, C., Rusconi, R., Slat, E. A., Isom, L. L., et al. (2009). Regulation of persistent Na current by interactions between beta subunits of voltage-gated Na channels. *J. Neurosci.* 29, 2027–2042. doi: 10.1523/JNEUROSCI.4531-08.2009

Appaix, F., Girod, S., Boisseau, S., Romer, J., Vial, J. C., Albrieux, M., et al. (2012). Specific *in vivo* staining of astrocytes in the whole brain after intravenous injection of sulforhodamine dyes. *PLoS ONE* 7:e35169. doi: 10.1371/journal.pone.0035169

Ascherio, A., Weisskopf, M. G., O'reilly, E. J., Jacobs, E. J., McCullough, M. L., Calle, E. E., et al. (2005). Vitamin E intake and risk of amyotrophic lateral sclerosis. *Ann. Neurol.* 57, 104–110. doi: 10.1002/ana.20316

Barber, S. C., Higginbottom, A., Mead, R. J., Barber, S., and Shaw, P. J. (2009). An *in vitro* screening cascade to identify neuroprotective antioxidants in ALS. *Free Radic. Biol. Med.* 46, 1127–1138. doi: 10.1016/j.freeradbiomed.2009.01.019

Barber, S. C., and Shaw, P. J. (2010). Oxidative stress in ALS: key role in motor neuron injury and therapeutic target. *Free Radic. Biol. Med.* 48, 629–641. doi: 10.1016/j.freeradbiomed.2009.11.018

Baur, J. A., and Sinclair, D. A. (2006). Therapeutic potential of resveratrol: the *in vivo* evidence. *Nat. Rev. Drug Discov.* 5, 493–506. doi: 10.1038/nrd2060

Beckman, J. S., Estévez, A. G., Crow, J. P., and Barbeito, L. (2001). Superoxide dismutase and the death of motoneurons in ALS. *Trends Neurosci.* 24, S15–S20. doi: 10.1016/S0166-2236(00)01981-0

Bellingham, M. C. (2011). A review of the neural mechanisms of action and clinical efficiency of riluzole in treating amyotrophic lateral sclerosis: what have we learned in the last decade? *CNS Neurosci. Ther.* 17, 4–31. doi: 10.1111/j.1755-5949.2009.00116.x

Bento-Abreu, A., van Damme, P., van Den Bosch, L., and Robberecht, W. (2010). The neurobiology of amyotrophic lateral sclerosis. *Eur. J. Neurosci.* 31, 2247–2265. doi: 10.1111/j.1460-9568.2010.07260.x

Boillée, S., Yamanaka, K., Lobsiger, C. S., Copeland, N. G., Jenkins, N. A., Kassiotis, G., et al. (2006). Onset and progression in inherited ALS determined by motor neurons and microglia. *Science* 312, 1389–1392. doi: 10.1126/science.1123511

Bruijn, L. I., Miller, T. M., and Cleveland, D. W. (2004). Unraveling the mechanisms involved in motor neuron degeneration in ALS. *Annu. Rev. Neurosci.* 27, 723–749. doi: 10.1146/annurev.neuro.27.070203.144244

Carter, B. J., Anklesaria, P., Choi, S., and Engelhardt, J. F. (2009). Redox modifier genes and pathways in amyotrophic lateral sclerosis. *Antioxid. Redox Signal.* 11, 1569–1586. doi: 10.1089/ARS.2008.2414

Cassina, P., Cassina, A., Pehar, M., Castellanos, R., Gandelman, M., de León, A., et al. (2008). Mitochondrial dysfunction in SOD1G93A-bearing astrocytes promotes motor neuron degeneration: prevention by mitochondrial-targeted antioxidants. *J. Neurosci.* 28, 4115–4122. doi: 10.1523/JNEUROSCI.5308-07.2008

Castillo, K., Nassif, M., Valenzuela, V., Rojas, F., Matus, S., Mercado, G., et al. (2013). Trehalose delays the progression of amyotrophic lateral sclerosis by enhancing autophagy in motoneurons. *Autophagy* 9, 1308–1320. doi: 10.4161/auto.25188

Catterall, W. A., Goldin, A. L., and Waxman, S. G. (2005). International Union of Pharmacology. XLVII. Nomenclature and structure-function relationships of voltage-gated sodium channels. *Pharmacol. Rev.* 57, 397–409. doi: 10.1124/pr.57.4.4

Clement, A. M., Nguyen, M. D., Roberts, E. A., Garcia, M. L., Boillée, S., Rule, M., et al. (2003). Wild-type nonneuronal cells extend survival of SOD1 mutant motor neurons in ALS mice. *Science* 302, 113–117. doi: 10.1126/science.1086071

Cleveland, D. W., and Rothstein, J. D. (2001). From Charcot to Lou Gehrig: deciphering selective motor neuron death in ALS. *Nat. Rev. Neurosci.* 2, 806–819. doi: 10.1038/35097565

Cozzolino, M., Pesaresi, M. G., Gerbino, V., Grosskreutz, J., and Carrì, M. T. (2012). Amyotrophic lateral sclerosis: new insights into underlying molecular mechanisms and opportunities for therapeutic intervention. *Antioxid. Redox Signal.* 17, 1277–1330. doi: 10.1089/ars.2011.4328

Desnuelle, C., Dib, M., Garrel, C., and Favier, A. (2001). A double-blind, placebo-controlled randomized clinical trial of alpha-tocopherol (vitamin E) in the treatment of amyotrophic lateral sclerosis. ALS riluzole-tocopherol Study Group. *Amyotroph. Lateral Scler. Other Motor Neuron Disord.* 2, 9–18. doi: 10.1080/146608201300079364

Di Giorgio, F. P., Carrasco, M. A., Siao, M. C., Maniatis, T., and Eggan, K. (2007). Non-cell autonomous effect of glia on motor neurons in an embryonic stem cell-based ALS model. *Nat. Neurosci.* 10, 608–614. doi: 10.1038/nn1885

Distelmaier, F., Valsecchi, F., Forkink, M., van Emst-de Vries, S., Swarts, H. G., Rodenburg, R. J., et al. (2012). Trolox-sensitive reactive oxygen species regulate mitochondrial morphology, oxidative phosphorylation and cytosolic calcium handling in healthy cells. *Antioxid. Redox Signal.* 17, 1657–1669. doi: 10.1089/ars.2011.4294

Drechsel, D. A., Estévez, A. G., Barbeito, L., and Beckman, J. S. (2012). Nitric oxide-mediated oxidative damage and the progressive demise of motor neurons in ALS. *Neurotox. Res.* 22, 251–264. doi: 10.1007/s12640-012-9322

ElBasiouny, S. M., Schuster, J. E., and Heckman, C. J. (2010). Persistent inward currents in spinal motoneurons: important for normal function but potentially harmful after spinal cord injury and in amyotrophic lateral sclerosis. *Clin. Neurophysiol.* 121, 1669–1679. doi: 10.1016/j.clinph.2009.12.041

Estévez, A. G., Crow, J. P., Sampson, J. B., Reiter, C., Zhuang, Y., Richardson, G. J., et al. (1999). Induction of nitric oxide - dependent apoptosis in motor neurons by zinc-deficient superoxide dismutase. *Science* 286, 2498–2500.

Ezzi, S. A., Urushitani, M., and Julien, J. P. (2007). Wild-type superoxide dismutase acquires binding and toxic properties of ALS-linked mutant forms through oxidation. *J. Neurochem.* 102, 170–178. doi: 10.1111/j.1471-4159.2007.04531.x

Ferraiuolo, L., Kirby, J., Grierson, A. J., Sendtner, M., and Shaw, P. J. (2011). Molecular pathways of motor neuron injury in amyotrophic lateral sclerosis. *Nat. Rev. Neurol.* 7, 616–630. doi: 10.1038/nrneurol.2011.152

Fleidervish, I. A., Goldberg, Y., and Ovsyshcher, I. E. (2008). Bolus injection of acetylcholine terminates atrial fibrillation in rats. *Eur. J. Pharmacol.* 579, 326–329. doi: 10.1016/j.ejphar.2007.11.010

Franceschetti, S., Taverna, S., Sancini, G., Panzica, F., Lombardi, R., and Avanzini, G. (2000). Protein kinase C-dependent modulation of Na^+currents increases the excitability of rat neocortical pyramidal neurons. *J. Physio.* 528, 291–304. doi: 10.1111/j.1469-7793.2000.00291.x

Fritz, E., Izaurieta, P., Weiss, A., Mir, F. R., Rojas, P., Gonzalez, D., et al. (2013). Mutant SOD1-expressing astrocytes release toxic factors that trigger motoneuron death by inducing hyperexcitability. *J. Neurophysiol.* 109, 2803–2814. doi: 10.1152/jn.00500.2012

Ghiselli, A., Serafini, M., Maiani, G., Azzini, E., and Ferro-Luzzi, A. (1995). A fluorescence-based method for measuring total plasma antioxidant capability. *Free Radic. Biol. Med.* 18, 29–36. doi: 10.1016/0891-5849(94)00102-P

Goldin, A. L. (2003). Mechanisms of sodium channel inactivation. *Curr. Opin. Neurobiol.* 13, 284–290. doi: 10.1016/S0959-4388(03)00065-5

Gomes, A., Fernandes, E., and Lima, J. L. (2005). Fluorescence probes used for detection of reactive oxygen species. *J. Biochem. Biophys. Methods* 65, 45–80. doi: 10.1016/j.jbbm.2005.10.003

Graf, M., Ecker, D., Horowski, R., Kramer, B., Riederer, P., Gerlach, M., et al. (2005). High dose vitamin E therapy in amyotrophic lateral sclerosis as add-on therapy to riluzole: results of a placebo-controlled double-blind study. *J. Neural Transm.* 112, 649–660. doi: 10.1007/s00702-004-0220-1

Gurney, M. E., Cutting, F. B., Zhai, P., Doble, A., Taylor, C. P., Andrus, P. K., et al. (1996). Benefit of vitamin E, riluzole, and gabapentin in a transgenic model of familial amyotrophic lateral sclerosis. *Ann. Neurol.* 39, 147–157. doi: 10.1002/ana.410390203

Gurney, M. E., Pu, H., Chiu, A. Y., Dal Canto, M. C., Polchow, C. Y., Alexander, D. D., et al. (1994). Motor neuron degeneration in mice that express a human Cu, Zn superoxide dismutase mutation. *Science* 264, 1772–1775. doi: 10.1126/science.8209258

Haidet-Phillips, A. M., Hester, M. E., Miranda, C. J., Meyer, K., Braun, L., Frakes, A., et al. (2011). Astrocytes from familial and sporadic ALS patients are toxic to motor neurons. *Nat. Biotechnol.* 29, 824–828. doi: 10.1038/nbt.1957

Hammarström, A. K., and Gage, P. W. (2000). Oxygen-sensing persistent sodium channels in rat hippocampus. *J. Physiol.* 529, 107–118. 10.1111/j.1469-7793.2000.00107.x

Harraz, M. M., Marden, J. J., Zhou, W., Zhang, Y., Williams, A., Sharov, V. S., et al. (2008). SOD1 mutations disrupt redox-sensitive Rac regulation of NADPH oxidase in a familial ALS model. *J. Clin. Invest.* 118, 659–670. doi: 10.1172/JCI34060

Harraz, M. M., Park, A., Abbott, D., Zhou, W., Zhang, Y., and Engelhardt, J. F. (2007). MKK6 phosphorylation regulates production of superoxide by enhancing Rac GTPase activity. *Antioxid. Redox Signal.* 9, 1803–1813. doi: 10.1089/ars.2007.1579

Ilieva, H., Polymenidou, M., and Cleveland, D. W. (2009). Non-cell autonomous toxicity in neurodegenerative disorders: ALS and beyond. *J. Cell Biol.* 187, 761–772. doi: 10.1083/jcb.200908164

Kalyanaraman, B., Darley-Usmar, V., Davies, K. J., Dennery, P. A., Forman, H. J., Grisham, M. B., et al. (2012). Measuring reactive oxygen and nitrogen species with fluorescent probes: challenges and limitations. *Free Radic. Biol. Med.* 52, 1–6. doi: 10.1016/j.freeradbiomed.2011.09.030

Kaneko, T., Tahara, S., and Takabayashi, F. (2003). Suppression of lipid hydroperoxide-induced oxidative damage to cellular DNA by esculetin. *Biol. Pharm. Bull.* 26, 840–844. doi: 10.1248/bpb.26.840

Kassmann, M., Hansel, A., Leipold, E., Birkenbeil, J., Lu, S. Q., Hoshi, T., et al. (2008). Oxidation of multiple methionine residues impairs rapid sodium channel inactivation. *Pflugers Arch.* 456, 1085–1095. doi: 10.1007/s00424-008-0477-6

Khaldy, H., Escames, G., León, J., Vives, F., Luna, J. D., and Acuña-Castroviejo, D. (2000). Comparative effects of melatonin, L-deprenyl, Trolox and ascorbate in the suppression of hydroxyl radical formation during dopamine autoxidation *in vitro*. *J. Pineal Res.* 29, 100–107. doi: 10.1034/j.1600-079X.2000.290206.x

Kuo, J. J., Siddique, T., Fu, R., and Heckman, C. J. (2005). Increased persistent Na+ current and its effect on excitability in motoneurones cultured from mutant SOD1 mice. *J. Physiol.* 563, 843–854. doi: 10.1113/jphysiol.2004.074138

Igaz, L. M., Kwong, L. K., Lee, E. B., Chen-Plotkin, A., Swanson, E., Unger, T., et al. (2011). Dysregulation of the ALS-associated gene TDP-43 leads to neuronal death and degeneration in mice. *J. Clin. Invest.* 121, 726–738. doi: 10.1172/JCI44867

Lin, W. L., Wang, C. J., Tsai, Y. Y., Liu, C. L., Hwang, J. M., and Tseng, T. H. (2000). Inhibitory effect of esculetin on oxidative damage induced by t-butyl hydroperoxide in rat liver. *Arch. Toxicol.* 74, 467–472. doi: 10.1007/s002040000148

Ling, S. C., Polymenidou, M., and Cleveland, D. W. (2013). Converging mechanisms in ALS and FTD: disrupted RNA and protein homeostasis. *Neuron* 79, 416–438. doi: 10.1016/j.neuron.2013.07.033

Lobsiger, C. S., Boillee, S., McAlonis-Downes, M., Khan, A. M., Feltri, M. L., Yamanaka, K., et al. (2009). Schwann cells expressing dismutase active mutant SOD1 unexpectedly slow disease progression in ALS mice. *Proc. Natl. Acad. Sci. U.S.A.* 106, 4465–4470. doi: 10.1073/pnas.0813339106

Marchetto, M. C., Muotri, A. R., Mu, Y., Smith, A. M., Cezar, G. G., and Gage, F. H. (2008). Non-cell-autonomous effect of human SOD1G37R astrocytes on motor neurons derived from human embryonic stem cells. *Cell Stem Cell* 3, 649–657. doi: 10.1016/j.stem.2008.10.001

Marden, J. J., Harraz, M. M., Williams, A. J., Nelson, K., Luo, M., Paulson, H., et al. (2007). Redox modifier genes in amyotrophic lateral sclerosis in mice. *J. Clin. Invest.* 117, 2913–2319. doi: 10.1172/JCI31265

Martin, L. J., Liu, Z., Chen, K., Price, A. C., Pan, Y., Swaby, J. A., et al. (2007). Motor neuron degeneration in amyotrophic lateral sclerosis mutant superoxide dismutase-1 transgenic mice: mechanisms of mitochondriopathy and cell death. *J. Comp. Neurol.* 500, 20–46. doi: 10.1002/cne.21160

Meyer, K., Ferraiuolo, L., Miranda, C. J., Likhite, S., McElroy, S., Renusch, S., et al. (2014). Direct conversion of patient fibroblasts demonstrates non-cell autonomous toxicity of astrocytes to motor neurons in familial and sporadic ALS. *Proc. Natl. Acad. Sci. U.S.A.* 111, 829–832. doi: 10.1073/pnas.1314085111

Mumbengegwi, D. R., Li, Q., Li, C., Bear, C. E., and Engelhardt, J. F. (2008). Evidence for a superoxide permeability pathway in endosomal membranes. *Mol. Cell. Biol.* 28, 3700–3712. doi: 10.1128/MCB.02038-07

Myhre, O., Andersen, J. M., Aarnes, H., and Fonnum, F. (2003). Evaluation of the probes 2',7'-dichlorofluorescin diacetate, luminol, and lucigenin as indicators of reactive species formation. *Biochem. Pharmacol.* 65, 1575–1582. doi: 10.1016/S0006-2952(03)00083-2

Nagai, M., Re, D. B., Nagata, T., Chalazonitis, A., Jessell, T. M., Wichterle, H., et al. (2007). Astrocytes expressing ALS-linked mutated SOD1 release factors selectively toxic to motor neurons. *Nat. Neurosci.* 10, 615–622. doi: 10.1038/nn1876

Nani, F., Cifra, A., and Nistri, A. (2010). Transient oxidative stress evokes early changes in the functional properties of neonatal rat hypoglossal motoneurons *in vitro*. *Eur. J. Neurosci.* 31, 951–966. doi: 10.1111/j.1460-9568.2010.07108.x

Olschewski, A., Schnoebel-Ehehalt, R., Li, Y., Tang, B., Bräu, M. E., and Wolff, M. (2009). Mexiletine and lidocaine suppress the excitability of dorsal horn neurons. *Anesth. Analg.* 109, 258–264. doi: 10.1213/ane.0b013e3181a3d5d8

Pambo-Pambo, A., Durand, J., and Gueritaud, J. P. (2009). Early excitability changes in lumbar motoneurons of transgenic SOD1G85R and SOD1G(93A-Low) mice. *J. Neurophysiol.* 102, 3627–3642. doi: 10.1152/jn.00482.2009

Pasinelli, P., and Brown, R. H. (2006). Molecular biology of amyotrophic lateral sclerosis: insights from genetics. *Nat. Rev. Neurosci.* 7, 710–723. doi: 10.1038/nrn1971

Pehar, M., Cassina, P., Vargas, M. R., Castellanos, R., Viera, L., Beckman, J. S., et al. (2004). Astrocytic production of nerve growth factor in motor neuron apoptosis: implications for amyotrophic lateral sclerosis. *J. Neurochem.* 89, 464–473. doi: 10.1111/j.1471-4159.2004.02357.x

Pieri, M., Carunchio, I., Curcio, L., Mercuri, N. B., and Zona, C. (2009). Increased persistent sodium current determines cortical hyperexcitability in a genetic model of amyotrophic lateral sclerosis. *Exp Neurol.* 215, 368–379. doi: 10.1016/j.expneurol.2008.11.002

Quinlan, K. A., Schuster, J. E., Fu, R., Siddique, T., and Heckman, C. J. (2011). Altered postnatal maturation of electrical properties in spinal motoneurons in a mouse model of amyotrophic lateral sclerosis. *J. Physiol.* 589, 2245–2260. doi: 10.1113/jphysiol.2010.200659

Ragsdale, D. S., McPhee, J. C., Scheuer, T., and Catterall, W. A. (1994). Molecular determinants of state-dependent block of Na+ channels by local anesthetics. *Science* 265, 1724–1728. doi: 10.1126/science.8085162

Ramírez-Jarquín, U. N., Lazo-Gómez, R., Tovar-Y-Romo, L. B., and Tapia, R. (2013). Spinal inhibitory circuits and their role in motor neuron degeneration. *Neuropharmacology*. doi: 10.1016/j.neuropharm.2013.10.003. [Epub ahead of print].

Ripps, M. E., Huntley, G. W., Hof, P. R., Morrison, J. H., and Gordon, J. W. (1995). Transgenic mice expressing an altered murine superoxide dismutase gene provide an animal model of amyotrophic lateral sclerosis. *Proc. Natl. Acad. Sci. U.S.A.* 92, 689–693. doi: 10.1073/pnas.92.3.689

Schuster, J. E., Fu, R., Siddique, T., and Heckman, C. J. (2011). Effect of prolonged riluzole exposure on cultured motoneurons in a mouse model of ALS. *J. Neurophysiol.* 107, 484–492. doi: 10.1152/jn.00714.2011

Sepulveda, F. J., Bustos, F. J., Inostroza, E., Zúñiga, F. A., Neve, R. L., Montecino, M., et al. (2010). Differential roles of NMDA receptor subtypes NR2A and NR2B in dendritic branch development and requirement of RasGRF1. *J Neurophysiol.* 103, 1758–1770. doi: 10.1152/jn.00823.2009

Serio, A., Bilican, B., Barmada, S. J., Ando, D. M., Zhao, C., Siller, R., et al. (2013). Astrocyte pathology and the absence of non-cell autonomy in an induced pluripotent stem cell model of TDP-43 proteinopathy. *Proc. Natl. Acad. Sci. U.S.A.* 110, 4697–4702. doi: 10.1073/pnas.1300398110

Theiss, R. D., Kuo, J. J., and Heckman, C. J. (2007). Persistent inward currents in rat ventral horn neurones. *J. Physiol.* 580, 507–522. doi: 10.1113/jphysiol.2006.124123

Tucker, J. M., and Townsend, D. M. (2005). Alpha-tocopherol: roles in prevention and therapy of human disease. *Biomed. Pharmacother.* 59, 380–387. doi: 10.1016/j.biopha.2005.06.005

Urushitani, M., Sik, A., Sakurai, T., Nukina, N., Takahashi, R., and Julien, J. P. (2006). Chromogranin-mediated secretion of mutant superoxide dismutase proteins linked to amyotrophic lateral sclerosis. *Nat. Neurosci.* 9, 108–118. doi: 10.1038/nn1603

van Zundert, B., Izaurieta, P., Fritz, E., and Alvarez, F. J. (2012). Early pathogenesis in the adult-onset neurodegenerative disease amyotrophic lateral sclerosis. *J. Cell Biochem.* 113, 3301–3312. doi: 10.1002/jcb.24234

van Zundert, B., Peuscher, M. H., Hynynen, M., Chen, A., Neve, R. L., Brown, R. H. Jr., et al. (2008). Neonatal neuronal circuitry shows hyperexcitable disturbance in a mouse model of the adult-onset neurodegenerative disease amyotrophic lateral sclerosis. *J. Neurosci.* 28, 10864–1 0874. doi: 10.1523/JNEUROSCI.1340-08.2008

Vargas, M. R., Pehar, M., Cassina, P., Beckman, J. S., and Barbeito, L. (2006). Increased glutathione biosynthesis by Nrf2 activation in astrocytes prevents p75NTR-dependent motor neuron apoptosis. *J. Neurochem.* 97, 687–696. doi: 10.1111/j.1471-4159.2006.03742.x

von Lewinski, F., and Keller, B. U. (2005). Ca2+, mitochondria and selective motoneuron vulnerability: implications for ALS. *Trends Neurosci.* 28, 494–500. doi: 10.1016/j.tins.2005.07.001

Wegorzewska, I., Bell, S., Cairns, N. J., Miller, T. M., and Baloh, R. H. (2009). TDP-43 mutant transgenic mice develop features of ALS and frontotemporal lobar degeneration. *Proc. Natl. Acad. Sci. U.S.A.* 106, 18809–18814. doi: 10.1073/pnas.0908767106

Wils, H., Kleinberger, G., Janssens, J., Pereson, S., Joris, G., Cuijt, I., et al. (2010). TDP-43 transgenic mice develop spastic paralysis and neuronal inclusions characteristic of ALS and frontotemporal lobar degeneration. *Proc. Natl. Acad. Sci. U.S.A.* 107, 3858–3863. doi: 10.1073/pnas.0912417107

Williams, K., (1997). Modulation and block of ion channels: a new biology of polyamines. *Cell Signal.* 9, 1–13. doi: 10.1016/S0898-6568(96)00089-7

Wootz, H., Fitzsimons-Kantamneni, E., Larhammar, M., Rotterman, T. M., Enjin, A., Patra, K., et al. (2013). Alterations in the motor neuron-renshaw cell circuit in the Sod1(G93A) mouse model. *J. Comp. Neurol.* 521, 1449–1469. doi: 10.1002/cne.23322

Wu, D. C., Re, D. B., Nagai, M., Ischiropoulos, H., and Przedborski, S. (2006). The inflammatory NADPH oxidase enzyme modulates motor neuron degeneration in amyotrophic lateral sclerosis mice. *Proc. Natl. Acad. Sci. U.S.A.* 103, 12132–12137. doi: 10.1073/pnas.0603670103

Yamanaka, K., Chun, S. J., Boillee, S., Fujimori-Tonou, N., Yamashita, H., Gutmann, D. H., et al. (2008a). Astrocytes as determinants of disease progression in inherited amyotrophic lateral sclerosis. *Nat. Neurosci.* 11, 251–253. doi: 10.1038/nn2047

Yamanaka, K., Boillee, S., Roberts, E. A., Garcia, M. L., McAlonis-Downes, M., Mikse, O. R., et al. (2008b). Mutant SOD1 in cell types other than motor neurons and oligodendrocytes accelerates onset of disease in ALS mice. *Proc. Natl. Acad. Sci. U.S.A.* 105, 7594–7599. doi: 10.1073/pnas.08025 56105

Zhao, W., Beers, D. R., Henkel, J. S., Zhang, W., Urushitani, M., Julien, J. P., et al. (2010). Extracellular mutant SOD1 induces microglial-mediated motoneuron injury. *Glia* 58, 231–243. doi: 10.1002/glia.20919

6

Investigating cell death mechanisms in amyotrophic lateral sclerosis using transcriptomics

Paul R. Heath*, Janine Kirby and Pamela J. Shaw

Sheffield Institute for Translational Neuroscience, University of Sheffield, Sheffield, UK

Edited by:
Ricardo Tapia, Universidad Nacional Autónoma de México, Mexico

Reviewed by:
Brian K. Kaspar, The Research Institute at Nationwide Children's Hospital, USA
Roger Pamphlett, The University of Sydney, Australia

****Correspondence:***
Paul R. Heath, Sheffield Institute for Translational Neuroscience, University of Sheffield, 385a Glossop Road, Sheffield S10 2HQ, UK
e-mail: p.heath@sheffield.ac.uk

Amyotrophic lateral sclerosis (ALS) is a motor neuron disease characterized by degeneration and loss of upper and lower motor neurons from the motor cortex, brainstem and spinal cord although evidence is suggesting that there is further involvement of other cell types in the surrounding tissue. Transcriptomic analysis by gene expression profiling using microarray technology has enabled the determination of patterns of cell death in the degenerating tissues. This work has examined gene expression at the level of the tissue and individual cell types in both sporadic and familial forms of the disease. In addition, further studies have examined the differential vulnerability of neuronal cells in different regions of the central nervous system. Model systems have also provided further information to help unravel the mechanisms that lead to death of the motor neurons in disease and also provided novel insights. In this review we shall describe the methods that have been used in these investigations and describe how they have contributed to our knowledge of the cell death mechanisms in ALS.

Keywords: transcriptomics, cell death, amyotrophic lateral sclerosis, microarray

INTRODUCTION

Amyotrophic lateral sclerosis (ALS) is described as a degenerative disease involving loss of the upper and lower motor neurons from motor cortex, brain stem and spinal cord leading to muscle denervation, wasting and death. There is now increasing evidence that other cell types are involved and the precise pattern of degeneration is unclear (Ince et al., 2011). Multiple mutually compatible mechanisms have been implicated in the pathogenesis of the disease including oxidative stress, excitotoxicity, ubiquitin and proteasome dysfunction, inflammatory activation, RNA processing dysregulation, mitochondrial dysfunction, cytoskeletal abnormalities and activation of apoptosis (Ferraiuolo et al., 2011). However, there remain many unanswered questions as to the origins of the disease and the precise pathogenetic mechanism. The use of microarray technology to explore gene expression at a particular time point and in particular cells is enabling us to unpick some of the specific changes undergone by cells or tissues involved in the disease and also to determine what processes act to protect cells from degeneration. The technology for different array types has been described and reviewed previously and we will not at this time extend this (Clark et al., 2007; Kirby et al., 2007). Whilst there are inconsistencies between the findings of transcriptomic studies and the precise biological mechanisms involved in a disease situation there is no doubt that properly designed studies which generate functionally verifiable results can be invaluable in assisting in the description of the disease process (Bolstad et al., 2004; Rosenfeld, 2010; Henriques and Gonzalez De Aguilar, 2011). For the purposes of this review we concentrated our attention upon articles that were found from a PubMed search using the search terms microarray and ALS.

RNA QUALITY

A recurring dilemma in studies of gene expression in post mortem tissue has been the residual debate concerning the quality of RNA derived from such tissue and whether it is appropriate for these studies. However, it is now accepted that gene expression studies in post mortem tissue are possible as long as appropriate quality control measures are followed (Harrison et al., 1995; Trabzuni et al., 2011). For most model studies standardized procedures can be set in place in order to reduce potential factors that might cause RNA degradation but even in an established and well organized human brain banking situation there are variables relating to post mortem delay, agonal state and cause of death all of which can affect RNA quality (Tomita et al., 2004; Popova et al., 2008; Durrenberger et al., 2009; Trabzuni et al., 2011). As indicated a number of studies have examined the effect of multiple potential RNA degrading features but the overall consensus is that providing adequate care is taken and good experimental design is incorporated in order to eliminate gross differences between the material being used then a reliable study can be carried out. In order to monitor these potential confounding factors it is important to control for any RNase introduction by carrying out all experimental work in a clean and tidy environment using RNase free materials. In addition it is essential that quality control steps should be included to measure both quantity and quality of the RNA being extracted and used (Copois et al., 2007; Wilkes et al., 2010; Trabzuni et al., 2011). Spectrophotometric methods can be used to measure nucleic acid quantity by examining absorbance at 260 nm. This can give an indication of RNA quality and the 260/280 ratio provides a measure of protein contamination whilst the 260/230 ratio provides a measure of organic solvent carryover. However, these metrics do not give a clear idea of RNA quality. For this, electrophoretic methods are required to examine the RNA directly. In the past a denaturing agarose gel (including formamide in the gel matrix) allowed the RNA to be visualized following staining with ethidium bromide. However, these methods required a large input of total RNA and have now been largely superseded by capillary based methodology such as the Agilent Bioanalyser and/or the TapeStation. In effect, both these devices drive the RNA sample through a capillary and over a laser which monitors absorbance at 260 nm over time hence providing a profile of the absorbance which can be compared to the profile of a molecular weight ladder run at the same time. If total RNA is the test sample then one would expect a small series of peaks at low molecular weight followed by the two ribosomal RNA peaks (the smaller peaks might be removed if a column based separation method is used). Software integral to the machine is then able to calculate an RNA integrity number (RIN) which is scaled from 0 to 10 and depends upon the ratio of the 28S to 18S rRNA peaks and the amount of degraded material that is present. It should be expected that for material derived from tissue culture experiments that a high RIN value is routinely achieved. However, post mortem human material is often quite degraded and RIN values of around 4 might be measured. It has been demonstrated in microarray, RNASeq and qRT-PCR that these values do not preclude a valid experiment (Preece et al., 2003). However, it is important to maintain equivalence in the experimental material and endeavor to compare samples of similar quality as well as support findings through appropriate validation methodologies.

HUMAN STUDIES IN WHOLE TISSUE

Microarray studies on whole tissue generate an overview of the gene expression profile of the whole tissue at the time of the RNA collection. There have been a number of microarray studies which were designed to examine some aspect of gene expression changes in ALS by examining a particular tissue. A very early study by Malaspina et al. (2001), used gridded cDNA membrane arrays to examine the expression of 18,400 genes in the anterior horn of lumbar spinal cord from four ALS cases and four controls (with a further four patients and controls used as verification subjects). Fourteen transcripts were identified as being significantly differentially expressed, and these were shown to belong to processes relevant to ALS including; oxidative stress and neuro-protection, motor neuron function, lipid metabolism, neuroinflammation and anti-apoptotic factors. This was an important demonstration of the potential of this sort of study and whilst it depended upon a predefined group of cDNAs that were present upon the array, the results gave an overview of gene expression in the anterior horn of the lumbar spinal cord. It also confirmed that post mortem tissue could be used in such a study. Ishigaki et al. (2002) took a different approach. Using lumbar spinal cord from 8 sporadic ALS cases and controls they initially used one case and control for molecular indexing which identified 576 cDNA fragments in the sALS material that could be compared to the control to select identifiers for further analysis. In this way spotted microarrays were prepared for 84 cDNAs deemed to be differentially expressed between the sALS and control individuals that were further examined on a wider group of patients and controls. Ultimately six differentially expressed genes were identified; four corresponded to previously known genes, 30-kDa TATA-binding protein-associated factor (*TAFII30*), macrophage-inhibiting factor-related protein-8 (*MRP8*), metallothionein-3 (*MT-3*) and ubiquitin-like protein 5 (*UBL5*) whilst the remaining two were uncharacterized expressed sequence tags. This was an interesting approach but the limited numbers of genes identified made it difficult to identify processes related to cell death.

An early study by Dangond et al. (2004), used Affymetrix FL arrays to compare the expression profile of grey matter from the lumbar spinal cord of seven ALS cases and four controls. A robust analytical process identified 93 genes which discriminated between the two groups. There was some attempt to differentiate between sporadic and familial disease, however, the numbers in the familial group made this analysis less robust. The 93 significant genes were subdivided into groupings defined by known biological functions giving some 10 sub-groups including; transcription and RNA binding, excitotoxicity, cell survival and growth, neuronal function, inflammation, cell receptors and signaling and stress response. Wang et al. (2006), examined the motor cortex in five ALS cases compared to three controls using the newer Affymetrix U133A Gene Chips containing 14,500 genes for microarray analysis. They identified 275 significantly differentially expressed genes, of which 265 were downregulated and they were able to verify the changes in 22 of these genes by quantitative real time polymerase chain reaction (QRT-PCR). Interestingly different groups of genes seemed to be important in sALS motor cortex compared to the spinal cord, but there were similarities in that stress response and excitoxicity were featured in both groups, as were features of mitochondrial metabolism. Unfortunately, the different cell populations of the two regions might be having a profound impact upon the data. A further study of motor cortex (Lederer et al., 2007), used 11 sALS cases and 9 controls in an Agilent slide array based study. Fifty-seven genes were identified as differentially expressed following the filtering and pathway based analysis; 40 down and 17 upregulated. Such a small group of genes were readily verifiable by alternative methods and the list was compared to previous studies including that of Dangond et al. (2004), and 14 genes showed a similar response. Overall a very thorough analysis produced an interesting interacting pathway diagram examining the interplay of differentially expressed genes in the motor cortex of sALS individuals. It is important to note that without describing individual genes it is possible to discern similar patterns in the lists of genes differentially expressed in the whole tissue experiments described here. Recurrent themes are mitochondrial metabolism, excitotoxicity, calcium homeostasis, protein turnover and neuronal maintenance and signaling.

Using a different approach Offen et al. (2009) examined the gene expression profile in spinal cord of sALS patients and compared some of the changes to the Glycine 93 to Alanine (G93A) SOD1 mouse model of fALS. In the study of four sALS cases compared to four matched controls using the Clontech membrane arrays, 60 gene changes were identified in the 1176 probe sets available to be examined. On this occasion the genes identified were grouped into biological processes such as; apoptosis, protein turnover, cell cycle functions, extracellular carrier/transport functions, cytoskeletal and intracellular proteins and proteins relating to transcription and translation. Six genes were further investigated in the G93A *SOD1* mouse model of fALS to determine if the changes seen post mortem were recapitulated during the lifespan of the mouse. These genes were; cathepsins *B* and *D*, apolipoprotein *E*, epidermal growth factor receptor (*EFGR*), ferritin and lysosomal trafficking regulator (*LYST*). These transcripts did seem to increase with disease progression in the mouse model suggesting some overlap between the human situation and the mouse model which does add some credence to the use of the model for human ALS.

Two recent studies have taken a quite different approach. Bernardini et al. (2013), concentrated upon mitochondrial related genes and Figueroa-Romero et al. (2012), tried to relate gene expression changes to methylation events in the genome. The Figueroa-Romero study was focussed on relating genome methylation events to gene expression changes found in sALS spinal cord. 12 sALS cases and 11 age and sex matched controls were used to determine the methylated genetic regions using Illumina Methylation 27 Bead Chips, whilst gene expression analysis was carried out using the Affymetrix Human U133 Plus 2 GeneChips. In the methylation chip assay 3574 regions associated with genes were found to be differentially regulated. In the gene expression study some 1182 genes were found to be differentially expressed in the sALS spinal cord. When comparing the two datasets 51 genes that were hypomethylated were upregulated and 61 genes that were hypermethylated were downregulated. These concordant "epigenes" could be functionally grouped into categories such as; immune response, defence response, neuron adhesion and plasma membrane. Overall this work suggested an epigenetic, or environmental, influence upon the pathogenesis of sALS which may be relevant to the process of cell survival. In the Bernardini study they concentrated upon skeletal muscle which was a new, but potentially relevant, tissue to examine. They hypothesized that muscle degeneration might be functionally important in the process of neurodegeneration and that differentially expressed genes in this tissue could be key in the pathogenic process. They examined quadriceps or biceps muscles in seven sALS cases and seven age and sex-matched controls. A focussed Affymetrix GeneChip array was used and using a fold change cutoff of 1 and *p*-value cutoff of 0.05, 96 differentially expressed genes were identified. Unlike in previous studies on this occasion more genes (80), were seen in the upregulated group. In total 13 genes related to muscle structure were distinguished and when ontology relationships were investigated using the DAVID software (Huang da et al., 2009) platform, other genes were found to be grouped in areas such as the actin cytoskeleton and glycogenesis, with mitochondrial function also identified. Further studies would be needed to determine the relevance of this work particularly with regard to further subtyping of the ALS cases. A study by Shtilbans et al. (2011) also looked at gene expression differences in muscle biopsies from ALS cases and controls. The study was hampered in that mixed groups of familial and sporadic cases were examined and different muscle groups were included in mixed proportions in each comparative group. The differences they found were in genes related to muscle structure, the cytoskeleton and cellular metabolism.

Two studies have used peripheral blood to look for gene expression differences with the underlying hypothesis that changes found in this tissue might reflect changes associated with the disease as has been seen in other neurodegenerative diseases. Saris et al. (2009) used whole blood and a designed analysis tool to uncover disease specific differences whereas Mougeot et al. (2011) isolated lymphocytes and examined these directly. In the Saris study, the weighted co-expression analysis found that genes in pathways related to apoptosis, the mitochondrion, stress response, calcium binding ubiquitination and vesicle transport were differentially expressed between the ALS patients and controls. In contrast, Mougeot used an ontology relationship tool called SAFE and found that a set of genes previously grouped into an ALS related KEGG pathway were differentially expressed in the lymphocytes. Genes in this pathway related to motor neuron degeneration in ALS (KEGG:05014), and included SOD1, caspases 1,3,9, neurofilament light, medium and heavy (*NFL, NFM* and *NFH*), and N-methyl-D-Aspartate receptors *GRIN 1, 2A, 2B, 2C* and *2D*. In addition, an ontology analysis based upon individual genes identified changes in pathways related to DNA metabolism, RNA splicing, mitochondrial function, oxidation, endoplasmic reticulum,ubiquitin proteasome system, post-transcriptional modification and neurological function. The overall conclusion to be drawn from both studies in blood is that although it is a peripheral tissue, it does show gene expression changes and pathways previously implicated by the use of central nervous system (CNS) material, including apoptosis, mitochondria, RNA splicing and, surprisingly, neurological function.

The studies of whole tissue have reached different conclusions, perhaps as a result of using tissue from different stages of disease and location, but there are common themes involved in the processes that are found to be differentially expressed in the ALS tissue which have been associated to motor neuronal cell death. In particular these are apoptosis, oxidative stress, protein processing, mitochondrial function and the cytoskeleton.

SINGLE CELL ANALYSIS OF HUMAN MOTOR NEURONS

The previous studies are valuable but they make it difficult to determine the precise input of each cell. In order to obviate this, several methods have been developed to examine the gene expression profile of individual cells isolated from tissue. Two recent reviews have discussed the available methods for cell specific transcriptome analysis (Kannanayakal and Eberwine, 2005; Okaty et al., 2011), and we shall not discuss these further. In terms of ALS, most studies seem to have adopted a laser capture microdissection approach. In 2005, Jiang et al. carried out a microarray study of laser captured motor neurons from the lumbar region of 14 sporadic ALS cases and 13 controls (Jiang et al., 2005). They used a PALM microdissector and applied the labeled RNA to BD Atlas glass microarrays. They found 52 up and 144 down regulated genes from the 4845 interrogated. Owing to the fact that they compared the isolated spinal motor neurons data to ventral horn spinal cord tissue data they were able to distinguish genes whose differential expression was restricted to the motor neurons and which was not detected when the whole tissue was examined. It was found that genes associated with cell death and cell signaling were upregulated in the disease related motor neurons whereas those associated with the cytoskeleton and transcription were downregulated. This study provided information concerning gene expression changes that were specific to the spinal cord motor neurons and demonstrated the value of this approach over whole tissue studies. Our group has carried out a number of published studies examining the gene expression profile of motor neurons isolated by laser capture microdissection in several models. In her study in 2010, Cox et al. (2010) examined the differences between three individuals who had charged multivesicular body protein 2B (*CHMP2B)* mutations leading to an ALS phenotype and 7 matched normal controls. Following gene expression analysis using Affymetrix Human U133 Plus 2 GeneChips, 890 genes were downregulated and 55 upregulated at a fold change cutoff of 2 and *p*-value 0.05. These were categorized using DAVID software into ontological groupings and groups associated with axon guidance, regulation of actin cytoskeleton and soluble NSF attachment protein receptor (SNARE) interactions in vesicular transport, mammalian target of rapamycin (*mTOR*) signaling and regulation of autophagy, mitogen activated kinase (*MAPK*) signaling, calcium signaling, and cell cycle and apoptosis were found to be the most enriched. Further functional studies were able to confirm a dysfunction in the autophagy pathway in an *in vitro* model. A further study (Kirby et al., 2011), examined gene expression differences in cervical spinal motor neurons between three fALS cases carrying SOD1 mutations and seven normal controls using the Affymetrix Human U133 Plus 2 arrays. In total, 524 probe sets were found to be increased and 646 decreased. These were characterized using the DAVID software package and the major enriched categories were transcription, signaling and metabolism. Importantly further investigations demonstrated the relevance of the cell survival pathway involving *PTEN/AKT* in the motor neurons with anti-apoptotic genes being downregulated in the surviving motor neurons indicating an attempt by these cells to mount a pro-survival response. Comparison of these studies indicates that the different genetic variants have distinct gene expression changes which ultimately lead to motor neuron death.

In contrast to the case control scenario, Brockington et al. (2013), examined features that distinguish the motor neurons from the oculomotor nucleus and the lumbar spinal cord in normal individuals to determine those features that enable the oculomotor motor neurons to be selectively resistant to the cell death undergone by spinal motor neurons in ALS. Tissue from four neurologically normal individuals was collected and laser capture microdissection used to isolate motor neurons from the oculomotor nucleus and lumbar spinal cord. The labeled RNA from these was applied to the Affymetrix Human U133 Plus 2 GeneChip. 1521 gene expression differences were identified as being differentially expressed in the oculomotor neurons. Gene ontology analysis determined that genes involved in synaptic transmission, ubiquitin mediated protein degradation and mitochondrial oxidative phosphorylation were upregulated in oculomotor motor neurons; these pathways had shown decreased expression in the ALS spinal cord and motor cortex in previous studies. This work was supplemented by carrying out comparison studies with other gene expression data derived from an online database and the analysis showed that the differences observed in human oculomotor neurons were also found in two other species confirming that the oculomotor motor neurons had a particular profile of synaptic neurotransmitter receptors, particularly gamma aminobutyric acid (*GABA)* and glutamate which made them less vulnerable to excitotoxic cell death. Electrophysiological studies complemented and supported this conclusion.

Again some common features can be derived that seem to associate the differential expression of genes related to the mechanisms of cell death. These include; cell signaling, autophagy, phosphatase and tensin homologue/protein kinase B (*PTEN/AKT)* cell signaling pathway, ubiquitin and mitochondrial function, cytoskeleton, transcription and apoptosis.

ANIMAL MODELS USING WHOLE TISSUE

Whilst human tissue can only be accessed at end stage, the use of animal models allows progression of the disease to be monitored. An early study by Yoshihara et al. (2002) examined the gene expression differences between tissue homogenates of lumbar spinal cord of G93A SOD1 versus non-transgenic littermates at three ages; 7, 14 and 17 weeks corresponding to presymptomatic, onset and end stage of disease. Using mouse Atlas arrays from Clontech they found an upregulation of inflammatory related genes associated with activated microglia and astrocytes. This was induced by 11 weeks of age and continued to advance up to the 17 week time point.

Fukada et al. (2007) examined the gene expression profile of whole spinal cord from two time points, presymptomatic (98 days) and post symptomatic (154/176 days), in a different mutant SOD1 transgenic model carrying the L126delTT mutation. They used the AceGeneMouse Oligo Chip. At the presymptomatic stage 11 genes were upregulated and two downregulated at a fold change of greater than two whilst at the post-symptomatic stage 54 were upregulated and four downregulated. With such small numbers of differences ontological relationships were hard to carry out and since whole spinal cord was examined the precise relationship of the gene changes to the disease process is difficult to disentangle.

It is thought that physical exercise might have a beneficial effect upon disease progression in ALS and two studies investigated this using microarrays and mouse models (Ferraiuolo et al., 2009; Hashimoto et al., 2009). Hashimoto et al. (2009) examined the response to exercise in normal mice by subjecting the mice to two exercise regimes; a single burst of 30 min exercise or 2 weeks of 30 min exercise per day on a treadmill. Whole spinal cord RNA was examined using the OpArray Mouse V4 array from Operon. Only a small number of changes in gene expression were identified; after the single burst of exercise 3 genes were upregulated and 29 downregulated whilst following the extended exercise regime 1 gene was found to be increased and 13 decreased. As seen in some previous studies the numbers are rather small for pathway analysis and since whole tissue has been studied it is difficult to dissect out precise effects. Ferraiuolo et al. (2009) examined the gene expression changes in gastrocnemius muscle as well as motor neurons isolated from lumbar spinal cord of three female mice subjected to a voluntary exercise regime of 21 days on a running wheel compared to three sedentary mice. Data were also collected concerning the exercise behavior of the mice. In the muscle tissue, 194 genes were upregulated and 176 downregulated using the same parameters. These genes were functionally found to be associated with vascularization and myogenic processes involved with extracellular matrix reorganization. The profiles exhibited by the gastrocnemius muscle are representative of the mixed cell population of the whole tissue and indicate some overall changes in the muscle as a response to the exercise regime. Overall, 203 genes were upregulated and 241 down at a fold change of at least two and p-value of 0.05 or less in the motor neurons. Functionally these genes were categorized into signaling, cytoskeleton and transcription regulation. The response of the motor neurons to exercise was similar to that of hippocampal neurons to repetitive stimulation, akin to a long term potentiation. There is a body of evidence that links exercise to the processes of cell death observed in ALS. This work goes some way to highlight similarities between the physiological response of MNs and skeletal muscle to exercise and the pathophysiology of ALS.

Two recent studies from the same group (Chen et al., 2010; Hu et al., 2013), have used Mouse Exon 1 arrays from Affymetrix to examine gene expression changes and alternative splicing in the G93A SOD1 mouse model. In the first study they examined animals at onset versus litter mate controls and in the second study 30 day transgenic mice were compared to litter mate controls of the same age and 120 day transgenic mice. They examined both differential expression and alternative splicing events. There were only 202 differentially expressed genes with a p-value cutoff of 0.05 found when comparing the 30 day old transgenic to nontransgenic mice but only one of these was at a fold change of > 2. There were in total 2869 differentially expressed genes events found when comparing the 120–30 day transgenic mice with 263 up and 71 down when a fold change of two and p-value of < 0.05 was imposed. Gene ontology analysis of the differentially expressed genes revealed that pathways involving cytokine receptor, cell adhesion, haematopoesis, and cell signaling included the most genes. In the onset group 322 transcripts were differentially expressed with 309 upregulated in the transgenic group when of a fold change of two and $p < 0.05$ was applied. Similar pathways were identified in this study to the previous one. In both studies a splicing index analysis was carried out in order to determine the levels of alternatively spliced transcripts. Comparing the 120 day transgenic to 30 day control 563 transcripts were alternatively spliced, of which 537 were considered as exon inclusion events, whilst only 85 alternative splicing events were identified in the 30 transgenic versus 30 day control comparison and on this occasion 61 were classified as exon inclusion. When the splicing data was examined by pathway analysis it was interesting that similar pathways were highlighted as found in the differentially expressed genes analysis. The data was interpreted to demonstrate that as the disease progressed then an increased number of splicing changes were seen. To some extent this is borne out by the onset study where 333 probe sets showed an altered splicing index indicating possible alternative splicing. However, the comparison of 120 day transgenic mice versus controls is missing which would allow a better comparison relative to normal ageing effects. Whilst some qRTPCR validation was completed the studies represent early work in using the exon arrays to examine the changes invoked by the presence of the G93A *SOD1* mutation on alternative splicing events.

The studies discussed thus far have used mouse models but Hedlund et al. (2010) used the G93A SOD1 rat model for a study of selective motor neuron vulnerability. They quantified the extent of motor neuron loss in different motor neuron nuclei; oculomotor and trochlear (CN3/4), facial (CN7), trigeminal (CN5), hypoglossal (CN12) and cervical spinal cord in the transgenic model. This directed the laser capture studies where motor neurons were collected from the CN3/4, CN12 and cervical spinal cord of normal rats and applied the isolated RNA to whole genome rat microarrays (Rat 230 2 Affymetrix). The microarray analysis showed that the more vulnerable motor neurons of the cervical spinal cord and hypoglossal nerve were more similar than either group compared to the less vulnerable CN3/4 motor neurons. There were interesting differences in Hox gene expression between the motor neuronal groups which were concomitant to the relative positions of the neurons in the anterior to posterior axis. There were also differences in RNA processing between the groups which also seemed to relate to the known association of RNA processing genes with ALS (Baumer et al., 2010). This report highlighted the usefulness of alternative animal models for the study of ALS and took an interesting approach to uncovering some of the underlying differences between selectively vulnerable and resistant motor neurons.

Dupuis and Loeffler (2009) examined neuromuscular changes in transgenic models of ALS. This led from the observation that the first event in the disease process seen in the transgenic mouse model of ALS is the destruction of the neuromuscular junction. Hence, studies concentrating upon the motor neurons may be identifying effects rather than cause of disease. However, it must be borne in mind that the SOD1 mouse model represents an overexpression model of disease and that SOD1 mutations correspond to only 2% of all ALS.

Finally in this section, Kumimoto et al. (2013) have undertaken to study ALS in a Drosophila model. They used a GAL4-UAS promoter to drive expression of wild type Drosophila SOD1 or the human SOD1 mutation glycine 85 to arginine (G85R) in motor neurons and glia. They carried out microarray analysis upon whole flies 5 days old (young), and 45 days (old), using the Drosophila 2 GeneChips from Affymetrix. They used several analyses to examine gene expression changes at the different ages and in the different cell types as well as a meta-analysis to uncover general changes. The mutant *SOD1* G85R in motor neurons alone caused 58 gene expression changes (33 up) at 5 days and 102 transcripts (73 up) at 45 days whereas in glia alone these numbers were 65 (33 up) and 105 (57 up) respectively. When the transgene was expressed in both cell types simultaneously the numbers were; 70 (34 up), and 83 (38 up). The overexpression of G85R SOD1 in the cells of the Drosophila caused changes in gene expression in oxidative stress, mitochondria, lipid metabolism and neurodevelopmental and signaling genes. Since the microarray analysis was carried out upon whole flies it is again difficult to determine the precise cellular effect of the overexpression strategy but there were commonalities in the pathways implicated with previous microarray studies and the impression is that the study offers a new model approach to understanding ALS. Since these studies were somewhat varied in the animal models, the tissue being investigated and the number of genetic changes identified it is difficult to describe common themes in the gene expression changes being seen and their relationship to cell death. However, cell signaling, mitochondrial dysfunction and oxidative stress continue to be implicated in the pathogenesis of ALS in animal models.

SINGLE CELL ANALYSIS OF NON-HUMAN MODEL MOTOR NEURONS

Perrin et al. (2005) combined laser capture dissection with microarray to examine gene expression in the spinal cord motor neurons of the G93A *SOD1* mice. Lumbar spinal motor neurons from male mice at presymptomatic (60 days), onset (90 days) and end stage of disease (120 days) were analyzed using the Mouse 430 2 GeneChip from Affymetrix. At 60 days only 27 genes were differentially expressed with this number increasing to 150 at 90 days and more than 400 by 120 days. At all the time points more genes were found to be upregulated in the G93A SOD1 mice; 17, 95 and 389 respectively. Thirteen of these transcripts were found to be differentially expressed at all stages. A similar study from our group (Ferraiuolo et al., 2007), looked at the effect of both the G93A SOD1 and the wild type SOD1 compared to non-transgenic littermate controls on a homogeneous background of C57bl6. Few changes were seen in motor neurons isolated from the WTSOD1 mice but 252 genes were differentially expressed at 60 days (234 upregulated), 51 at 90 days (32 up) and 167 at 120 days (81 up), in the G93A SOD1 mice. These changes at the presymptomatic, symptomatic and end stage of the disease process in the mice indicate that at an early time point the motor neurons try to mount a metabolic response to the burgeoning disease process by upregulating several pathways. However, by the endstage, this process having failed, the cells appear to try to re-enter the cell cycle which is a doomed response. There are notable differences between the two studies in terms of the overall changes in gene expression profile, although both groups do see changes in the intermediate filament protein vimentin, it is likely that the differences might relate to the actual genetic background of the mice being used, the transgene copy number and also the analytical processes used in examining the data. A study by Saxena et al. (2009) took a different approach to examine the matter of selective vulnerability of motor neurons. They injected RITC-dextran into the gastrocnemius or soleus muscles and following retrograde transport they were able to identify and selectively isolate the motor neurons associated with the vulnerable phenotype which project to the fast fibre gastrocnemius muscle and those that are relatively resistant and project to the soleus muscle which has fatigue resistant or slow fibres. The RNA isolated from the selectively microdissected motor neurons was applied to the Mouse 430 2 arrays from Affymetrix. The longitudinal study showed that the vulnerable motor neurons are selectively prone to endoplasmic reticulum stress and a progressive failure to mount a proper unfolded protein clearance response.

This group of studies are more focussed and underline the importance of the single cell analysis at different stages of disease progression.

SINGLE CELL ANALYSIS OF NON-HUMAN NON-MOTOR NEURON CELL TYPES

Using the G93A Mutant SOD1 mouse model Ferraiuolo et al. (2011) attempted to examine the relationship between motor neurons and astrocytes in this model of disease (Ferraiuolo et al., 2011). Astrocytes were collected from lumbar spinal cord of three male 60 day old mice and three non transgenic litter mate controls, and the labeled RNA applied to Mouse 430 2 Gene Chips from Affymetrix. 583 transcripts were found to be upregulated 526 downregulated in the G93A SOD1 astrocytes. Ontological analysis showed that multiple transcripts associated with carbohydrate metabolism were differentially expressed and an overall decline in the activity of the lactate shuttle was described in the mutant astrocytes indicating an inability to support the metabolic requirements of the motor neurons. The altered metabolism was further investigated and it was shown that non-transgenic motor neurons grown on G93A SOD1 astrocytes demonstrated an increase in the ratio between pro- nerve growth factor and mature nerve growth factor (NGF) which was associated with an over-expression of the p75 receptor for NGF. Hence it was shown that the G93A SOD1astrocytes provided reduced metabolic support to the motor neurons as a result of the downregulation of the lactate shuttle and the activation of the p75 receptor and these factors contributed to the toxicity of the mutant astrocytes to the co-cultured motor neurons.

CELL CULTURE MODEL STUDIES

Two studies have examined the gene expression profile of the NSC 34 cells carrying different human SOD1 mutations. The first study (Kirby et al., 2002), utilized a designed membrane microarray from Clontech with cDNAs for just 588 genes. The experiment was carried out on cells carrying G93A, G85R or isoleucine 113 to threonine (I113T) SOD1 mutations at basal conditions and cells which had undergone stress exerted by serum withdrawal. At the basal condition differences were seen in the numbers of differentially expressed genes for the different SOD1 mutation but a combined analysis showed only 29 genes to be differentially expressed as a result of the SOD1 mutation with seven being downregulated. Very few genes were found to be differentially expressed following the induction of a stress imposed by serum withdrawal which might be a result of the analytical stringency being applied. In a subsequent study (Kirby et al., 2005), a comparison was made between NSC34 cells expressing G93A mutant SOD1 and those expressing wild type human SOD1. On this occasion the mouse U74Av2A GeneChip from Affymetrix was used. At a fold change of two with a p-value of 0.05, 268 transcripts were differentially regulated in the presence of mutant SOD1, of which 197 were downregulated. Following thorough ontological analysis it was found that the presence of the mutant SOD1 caused a significant down-regulation of the cells capacity to deal with oxidative stress. In particular the group of genes with an antioxidant response element in their promoter, termed programmed cell life genes, which would be activated by the transcription factor nuclear factor (erythroid-derived) like 2 *(Nrf2)* were downregulated indicating a failure of the cells to mount a proper therapeutic antioxidant stress response. Subsequent work by Mead et al. (2013) has demonstrated that induction of the *Nrf2* response by S(+)-Apomorphine improves the motor function of the G93A *SOD1* mice underlining the importance of increasing the expression of the programmed cell life genes in a therapeutic strategy to treat ALS.

Vargas et al. (2008) isolated primary astrocytes from both G93A SOD1 mutant and normal littermate control embryonic rats and examined the profile of gene expression using Rat genome 230 2 arrays from Affymetrix. A total of 81 transcripts were differentially expressed by the mutant SOD1 bearing astrocytes with 55 being upregulated. The genes were characterized according to their biological function and were separated into groups; extracellular matrix and cell migration, signaling and receptor activity, transcription, cell proliferation, response to stress, oxidoreductase activity, catalytic activity and unknown. It is interesting to note that despite the fact that different cell types are being investigated there are some similarities in the effect of the *SOD1* mutation in astrocytes and motor neurons from mice and rats.

In the study by Boutahar et al. (2011) they derived primary cortical motor neurons from transgenic mice either with or lacking the G93A *SOD1* mutation. The cells were derived from E14 embryos and maintained in culture for a brief period until the presence of the transgene was confirmed. Some cultures were subjected to stress with hydrogen peroxide or NMDA treatment. Microarrays using Mouse 430 2 GeneChips from Affymetrix were carried out and the results analyzed to determine fold changes of two or more. In the untreated cells 260 transcripts were differentially regulated with 70 upregulated. Following hydrogen peroxide treatment the number was 163 with 59 upregulated and following NMDA treatment 181 with 62 upregulated. Few genes were shared between the three treatments. Gene ontological analysis showed an increase in transcripts associated with the proteasome, some associated with autophagy and cytoskeletal organization and axonal transport. There was some downregulation in transcripts associated with ion transport. It was noted that the presence of the transgene alone increased cell death but this process was mitigated when the additional stresses, hydrogen peroxide or NMDA, were introduced. Hence they identified a small group of genes which were upregulated in the untreated G93A cells but downregulated following the introduction of an additional stress. These genes were; Cathepsin H,(*CSTH*) and Autophagy related 4 homolog D (*ATG4D*) which are involved in protein degradation, tubulin beta-4B chain (*TUBB2C*) and Rho guanine nucleotide exchange factor 11 (*ARHGEF11*) which are cytoskeletal, cell division cycle 25 homolog (*CDC25*) which is involved in cell cycle regulation, solute carrier 7 (*SLC7A12*), DEAD box 43 (*DDX43*) and leucine rich recognition motif 4 (*LRRTM4*) which are involved in the transmembrane domain and transcripts *ACN9, SSBP9* and *TRIM36* involved in transcription regulation.

The studies in cellular culture models all seem to underline the importance of oxidative stress in the pathogenesis of ALS and the difficulty that cells containing mutant SOD1 have in dealing with this metabolic insult.

SYSTEMS BIOLOGY

Some studies have taken a more broad brush approach to the analysis of microarray data and attempted to incorporate data from a number of sources. Kudo et al. (2010) developed an integrative approach to examine post mortem human material, mouse models and microarray methods. They used the mouse models of ALS, G93A SOD1 and frontotemporal dementia (FTD), P30L Tau and isolated both motor neurons and glia for microarray analysis. Using Agilent whole mouse genome microarrays 251 transcripts were identified as being differentially expressed in at least one of the four comparisons. Of these 186 corresponded to known genes and ontological analysis revealed that the most enriched biological processes were associated with protein modification/phosphorylation, signaling, regulation of muscle contraction, stress response, the immune system and cell communication. The data were confirmed both in further murine tissue by semi-quantitative PCR and in human tissue from sALS cases with tissue microarrays. Hence they used complementary methodology to identify common mechanisms in the SOD1 and TAU mouse models of motor neuron degeneration and human sALS. The genes *CNGA3, CRB1* and *OTUB2* were common to all the models and *CNGA3, CRB1, OTUB2, SLK, DDX58, RSPO2* and *MMP14* were related to sALS. In addition, 13 transcripts found differentially regulated in the SOD1 motor neurons were also found to be altered in their expression in the blood of G93A SOD1 mice.

Baciu et al. (2012) adopted a reanalysis approach where they performed an in depth analysis of a microarray experiment carried out using purified peripheral blood lymphocytes from 11 ALS patients and 11 age matched controls. The RNA had been interrogated using Agilent 4 $\times$ 44k human arrays and the authors used a modified BaFL pipeline and at the same time a severe TM4 statistical analysis to remove potential confounding probes sets and "purify" the dataset. The methodology was validated using a previous dataset carried out using similar microarrays and a coronary heart disease study. By carrying out the two different analytical methods the authors attempted to account for errors that might be inherent to either alone. Ultimately, a series of seven genes was identified as being upregulated in the sALS patients, were common to both methods and were verifiable by qRTPCR. These genes were; *B2M, ACTG1, DYNLT1, SKIV2L2, C12orf35, TARDBP* and *ILKAP* (which cross-hybridises with TARDBP).

A recent meta-analysis from Saris et al. (2013) looked to examine the datasets from a number of different microarray studies of both murine and human material. They included seven human studies; three of lumbar cord, two cervical cord and two motor cortex. In addition there were nine studies of transgenic mouse model material; seven of G93A SOD1, one L126delTT SOD1 and one study of the progressive motor neuropathy and wobbler mice. As the authors conclude, despite the variety of input material and different array platforms used, there was a level of consistency in the altered gene expression output. Hence they found altered gene expression in the areas of protein turnover, immune response and apoptosis in both human and murine studies. The mouse studies also showed consistent differences in genes involved in the lysosome, metal ion binding and mitochondrial function. This study is an interesting new approach to attempt to summate all the data that has been produced thus far. There are likely to be further assays of this type which will take advantage of the large datasets in order to generate informative data with greater statistical power owing to the larger numbers of samples being included.

CONCLUDING REMARKS

This short review has attempted to summarize the depth of study that has been carried out using transcriptomic technology to examine the gene expression changes that can be identified in comparisons of ALS tissue and controls. With the variety of studies that have been done it is quite difficult to accurately summarize the information but some overall differences can be seen. In terms of mechanisms that have been uncovered in these studies that are influential in the processes that underlie cell death in ALS it can be seen that certain pathways are repeatedly enriched as a consequence of the disease process. These include; oxidative stress, mitochondrial function, apoptosis, cytoskeleton, neuroinflammation and protein processing. It is interesting to note that when peripheral tissues have been used similar processes have been identified as distinguishing the material from individuals with disease. Whilst many of the studies delineated differences between disease and control at the level of the transcriptome an important development has been developing functional studies to demonstrate the validity of the identified changes and then subsequent studies to investigate mechanisms to ameliorate them.

It is likely that the use of the microarray technology is likely to become more of an adjunct to support a body of work as seen in the study from Egawa et al. (2012). In this case the transcriptomic element of the work was used to characterize human induced pluripotent stem cells derived from dermal fibroblasts of normal individuals and several TDP43 mutants. In the past we have seen the transcriptomic study as being the lead in the experimental approach but on this occasion the development of the induced stem cells was the primary goal and the microarray analysis was simply a tool to assist in the characterization of derived cells and define potential routes for drug intervention. It is likely that with the maturity and confidence that several years of transcriptomic research have generated this type of approach will become more widespread.

A further development in the examination of gene expression differences between tissues is going to be the use of next generation sequencing to examination gene expression directly rather than as an indirect measure based upon manufactured probes. The next generation sequencing methodology provides a more detailed examination of the transcriptome which allows for a more in depth examination of novel transcripts, splice junctions and non-coding RNAs in a single step rather than having to carry out multiple different array experiments. As with the early microarray work there is not yet a defined analytical pathway for interpreting the data from RNA Seq experiments but this is progressing rapidly. There is evidence that the two tools are being used in a combinatorial approach (Kogenaru et al., 2012).

Transcriptomics has been used successfully to investigate the mechanisms underlying the processes of cell death and has provided insights into the pathways that may be dysregulated. As the tools are becoming more established it is likely that more studies will use them to assist in the functional studies needed to develop new treatments for ALS.

AUTHOR CONTRIBUTIONS

Paul R. Heath devised and produced the manuscript, Janine Kirby and Pamela J. Shaw contributed editing and revising of the manuscript.

ACKNOWLEDGMENTS

Paul R. Heath is supported by funding from the BBSRC. Pamela J. Shaw and Janine Kirby are supported by funding from the European Union: Seventh Framework Programme (FP7/2007-2013) under the Euro-MOTOR project (No: 259867, http://www.euromotorproject.eu/) and Pamela J. Shaw and Janine Kirby by the EU Joint Programme–Neurodegenerative Disease Research (JPND), Sampling and biomarker OPtimization and Harmonization In ALS and other motor neuron diseases (SOPHIA). This is an EU Joint Programme—Neurodegenerative Disease Research (JPND) project. The project is supported through the following funding organizations under the aegis of JPND—www.jpnd.eu: France, Agence Nationale de la Recherche (ANR); Germany, Bundesministerium für Bildung und Forschung (BMBF); Ireland, Health Research Board (HRB); Italy, Ministero della Salute; The Netherlands, The Netherlands Organization for Health Research and Development (ZonMw); Poland, Narodowe Centrum Badań i Rozwoju; Portugal, Fundação a Ciência e a Tecnologia; Spain, Ministerio de Ciencia e Innovación; Switzerland, Schweizerischer Nationalfonds zur Förderung der wissenschaftlichen Forschung (SNF); Turkey, Tübitak; United Kingdom, Medical Research Council (MRC). Pamela J. Shaw is supported as an NIHR Senior Investigator.

REFERENCES

Baciu, C., Thompson, K. J., Mougeot, J. L., Brooks, B. R., and Weller, J. W. (2012). The LO-BaFL method and ALS microarray expression analysis. *BMC Bioinformatics* 13:244. doi: 10.1186/1471-2105-13-244

Baumer, D., Ansorge, O., Almeida, M., and Talbot, K. (2010). The role of RNA processing in the pathogenesis of motor neuron degeneration. *Expert Rev. Mol. Med.* 12, e21. doi: 10.1017/S1462399410001523

Bernardini, C., Censi, F., Lattanzi, W., Barba, M., Calcagnini, G., Giuliani, A., et al. (2013). Mitochondrial network genes in the skeletal muscle of amyotrophic lateral sclerosis patients. *PLoS One* 8:e57739. doi: 10.1371/journal.pone.0057739

Bolstad, B. M., Collin, F., Simpson, K. M., Irizarry, R. A., and Speed, T. P. (2004). Experimental design and low-level analysis of microarray data. *Int. Rev. Neurobiol.* 60, 25–58. doi: 10.1016/s0074-7742(04)60002-x

Boutahar, N., Wierinckx, A., Camdessanche, J. P., Antoine, J. C., Reynaud, E., and Lassabliere, F. (2011). Differential effect of oxidative or excitotoxic stress on the transcriptional profile of amyotrophic lateral sclerosis-linked mutant SOD1 cultured neurons. *J. Neurosci. Res.* 89, 1439–1450. doi: 10.1002/jnr.22672

Brockington, A., Ning, K., Heath, P. R., Wood, E., Kirby, J., Fusi, N., et al. (2013). Unravelling the enigma of selective vulnerability in neurodegeneration: motor neurons resistant to degeneration in ALS show distinct gene expression characteristics and decreased susceptibility to excitotoxicity. *Acta Neuropathol.* 125, 95–109. doi: 10.1007/s00401-012-1058-5

Chen, H., Guo, Y., Hu, M., Duan, W., Chang, G., and Li, C. (2010). Differential expression and alternative splicing of genes in lumbar spinal cord of an amyotrophic lateral sclerosis mouse model. *Brain Res.* 1340, 52–69. doi: 10.1016/j.brainres.2010.03.075

Clark, T. A., Schweitzer, A. C., Chen, T. X., Staples, M. K., Lu, G., Wang, H., et al. (2007). Discovery of tissue-specific exons using comprehensive human exon microarrays. *Genome Biol.* 8, R64. doi: 10.1186/gb-2007-8-4-r64

Copois, V., Bibeau, F., Bascoul-Mollevi, C., Salvetat, N., Chalbos, P., Bareil, C., et al. (2007). Impact of RNA degradation on gene expression profiles: assessment of different methods to reliably determine RNA quality. *J. Biotechnol.* 127, 549–559. doi: 10.1016/j.jbiotec.2006.07.032

Cox, L. E., Ferraiuolo, L., Goodall, E. F., Heath, P. R., Higginbottom, A., Mortiboys, H., et al. (2010). Mutations in CHMP2B in lower motor neuron predominant amyotrophic lateral sclerosis (ALS). *PLoS One* 5:e9872. doi: 10.1371/journal.pone.0009872

Dangond, F., Hwang, D., Camelo, S., Pasinelli, P., Frosch, M. P., Stephanopoulos, G., et al. (2004). Molecular signature of late-stage human ALS revealed by expression profiling of postmortem spinal cord gray matter. *Physiol. Genomics* 16, 229–239. doi: 10.1152/physiolgenomics.00087.2001

Dupuis, L., and Loeffler, J. P. (2009). Neuromuscular junction destruction during amyotrophic lateral sclerosis: insights from transgenic models. *Curr. Opin. Pharmacol.* 9, 341–346. doi: 10.1016/j.coph.2009.03.007

Durrenberger, P. F., Filiou, M. D., Moran, L. B., Michael, G. J., Novoselov, S., Cheetham, M. E., et al. (2009). DnaJB6 is present in the core of Lewy bodies and is highly up-regulated in parkinsonian astrocytes. *J. Neurosci. Res.* 87, 238–245. doi: 10.1002/jnr.21819

Egawa, N., Kitaoka, S., Tsukita, K., Naitoh, M., Takahashi, K., Yamamoto, T., et al. (2012). Drug screening for ALS using patient-specific induced pluripotent stem cells. *Sci. Transl. Med.* 4, 145ra104. doi: 10.1126/scitranslmed.3004052

Ferraiuolo, L., De Bono, J. P., Heath, P. R., Holden, H., Kasher, P., Channon, K. M., et al. (2009). Transcriptional response of the neuromuscular system to exercise training and potential implications for ALS. *J. Neurochem.* 109, 1714–1724. doi: 10.1111/j.1471-4159.2009.06080.x

Ferraiuolo, L., Heath, P. R., Holden, H., Kasher, P., Kirby, J., and Shaw, P. J. (2007). Microarray analysis of the cellular pathways involved in the adaptation to and progression of motor neuron injury in the SOD1 G93A mouse model of familial ALS. *J. Neurosci.* 27, 9201–9219. doi: 10.1523/jneurosci.1470-07.2007

Ferraiuolo, L., Higginbottom, A., Heath, P. R., Barber, S., Greenald, D., Kirby, J., et al. (2011). Dysregulation of astrocyte-motoneuron cross-talk in mutant superoxide dismutase 1-related amyotrophic lateral sclerosis. *Brain* 134, 2627–2641. doi: 10.1093/brain/awr193

Figueroa-Romero, C., Hur, J., Bender, D. E., Delaney, C. E., Cataldo, M. D., Smith, A. L., et al. (2012). Identification of epigenetically altered genes in sporadic amyotrophic lateral sclerosis. *PLoS One* 7:e52672. doi: 10.1371/journal.pone.0052672

Fukada, Y., Yasui, K., Kitayama, M., Doi, K., Nakano, T., Watanabe, Y., et al. (2007). Gene expression analysis of the murine model of amyotrophic lateral sclerosis: studies of the Leu126delTT mutation in SOD1. *Brain Res.* 1160, 1–10. doi: 10.1016/j.brainres.2007.05.044

Harrison, P. J., Heath, P. R., Eastwood, S. L., Burnet, P. W., Mcdonald, B., and Pearson, R. C. (1995). The relative importance of premortem acidosis and postmortem interval for human brain gene expression studies: selective mRNA vulnerability and comparison with their encoded proteins. *Neurosci. Lett.* 200, 151–154. doi: 10.1016/0304-3940(95)12102-a

Hashimoto, K., Honda, A., Hayashi, Y., Inuzuka, T., Satoh, M., and Hozumi, I. (2009). DNA microarray analysis of transcriptional responses of mouse spinal cords to physical exercise. *J. Toxicol. Sci.* 34, 445–448. doi: 10.2131/jts.34.445

Hedlund, E., Karlsson, M., Osborn, T., Ludwig, W., and Isacson, O. (2010). Global gene expression profiling of somatic motor neuron populations with different vulnerability identify molecules and pathways of degeneration and protection. *Brain* 133, 2313–2330. doi: 10.1093/brain/awq167

Henriques, A., and Gonzalez De Aguilar, J. L. (2011). Can transcriptomics cut the gordian knot of amyotrophic lateral sclerosis? *Curr. Genomics* 12, 506–515. doi: 10.2174/138920211797904043

Hu, M., Guo, Y., Chen, H., Duan, W., and Li, C. (2013). Exon array analysis of alternative splicing of genes in SOD1G93A transgenic mice. *Appl. Biochem. Biotechnol.* 170, 301–319. doi: 10.1007/s12010-013-0155-9

Huang da, W., Sherman, B. T., and Lempicki, R. A. (2009). Systematic and integrative analysis of large gene lists using DAVID bioinformatics resources. *Nat. Protoc.* 4, 44–57. doi: 10.1038/nprot.2008.211

Ince, P. G., Highley, J. R., Kirby, J., Wharton, S. B., Takahashi, H., Strong, M. J., et al. (2011). Molecular pathology and genetic advances in amyotrophic lateral sclerosis: an emerging molecular pathway and the significance of glial pathology. *Acta Neuropathol.* 122, 657–671. doi: 10.1007/s00401-011-0913-0

Ishigaki, S., Niwa, J., Ando, Y., Yoshihara, T., Sawada, K., Doyu, M., et al. (2002). Differentially expressed genes in sporadic amyotrophic lateral sclerosis spinal cords—screening by molecular indexing and subsequent cDNA microarray analysis. *FEBS Lett.* 531, 354–358. doi: 10.1016/s0014-5793(02)03546-9

Jiang, Y. M., Yamamoto, M., Kobayashi, Y., Yoshihara, T., Liang, Y., Terao, S., et al. (2005). Gene expression profile of spinal motor neurons in sporadic amyotrophic lateral sclerosis. *Ann. Neurol.* 57, 236–251. doi: 10.1002/ana.20379

Kannanayakal, T. J., and Eberwine, J. (2005). mRNA methods used in dissecting gene expression of the brain. *Ageing Res. Rev.* 4, 513–528. doi: 10.1016/j.arr.2005.09.001

Kirby, J., Halligan, E., Baptista, M. J., Allen, S., Heath, P. R., Holden, H., et al. (2005). Mutant SOD1 alters the motor neuronal transcriptome: implications for familial ALS. *Brain* 128, 1686–1706. doi: 10.1093/brain/awh503

Kirby, J., Heath, P. R., Shaw, P. J., and Hamdy, F. C. (2007). Gene expression assays. *Adv. Clin. Chem.* 44, 247–292. doi: 10.1016/s0065-2423(07)44008-2

Kirby, J., Menzies, F. M., Cookson, M. R., Bushby, K., and Shaw, P. J. (2002). Differential gene expression in a cell culture model of SOD1-related familial motor neurone disease. *Hum. Mol. Genet.* 11, 2061–2075. doi: 10.1093/hmg/11.17.2061

Kirby, J., Ning, K., Ferraiuolo, L., Heath, P. R., Ismail, A., Kuo, S. W., et al. (2011). Phosphatase and tensin homologue/protein kinase B pathway linked to motor neuron survival in human superoxide dismutase 1-related amyotrophic lateral sclerosis. *Brain* 134, 506–517. doi: 10.1093/brain/awq345

Kogenaru, S., Qing, Y., Guo, Y., and Wang, N. (2012). RNA-seq and microarray complement each other in transcriptome profiling. *BMC Genomics* 13:629. doi: 10.1186/1471-2164-13-629

Kudo, L. C., Parfenova, L., Vi, N., Lau, K., Pomakian, J., Valdmanis, P., et al. (2010). Integrative gene-tissue microarray-based approach for identification of human disease biomarkers: application to amyotrophic lateral sclerosis. *Hum. Mol. Genet.* 19, 3233–3253. doi: 10.1093/hmg/ddq232

Kumimoto, E. L., Fore, T. R., and Zhang, B. (2013). Transcriptome profiling following neuronal and glial expression of ALS-linked SOD1 in Drosophila. *G3 (Bethesda).* doi: 10.1534/g3.113.005850. [Epub ahead of print].

Lederer, C. W., Torrisi, A., Pantelidou, M., Santama, N., and Cavallaro, S. (2007). Pathways and genes differentially expressed in the motor cortex of patients with sporadic amyotrophic lateral sclerosis. *BMC Genomics* 8:26. doi: 10.1186/1471-2164-8-26

Malaspina, A., Kaushik, N., and De Belleroche, J. (2001). Differential expression of 14 genes in amyotrophic lateral sclerosis spinal cord detected using gridded cDNA arrays. *J. Neurochem.* 77, 132–145. doi: 10.1046/j.1471-4159.2001.00231.x

Mead, R. J., Higginbottom, A., Allen, S. P., Kirby, J., Bennett, E., Barber, S. C., et al. (2013). S[+] Apomorphine is a CNS penetrating activator of the Nrf2-ARE pathway with activity in mouse and patient fibroblast models of amyotrophic lateral sclerosis. *Free Radic. Biol. Med.* doi: 10.1016/j.freeradbiomed.2013.04.018. [Epub ahead of print].

Mougeot, J. L., Li, Z., Price, A. E., Wright, F. A., and Brooks, B. R. (2011). Microarray analysis of peripheral blood lymphocytes from ALS patients and the SAFE detection of the KEGG ALS pathway. *BMC Med. Genomics* 4:74. doi: 10.1186/1755-8794-4-74

Offen, D., Barhum, Y., Melamed, E., Embacher, N., Schindler, C., and Ransmayr, G. (2009). Spinal cord mRNA profile in patients with ALS: comparison with transgenic mice expressing the human SOD-1 mutant. *J. Mol. Neurosci.* 38, 85–93. doi: 10.1007/s12031-007-9004-z

Okaty, B. W., Sugino, K., and Nelson, S. B. (2011). Cell type-specific transcriptomics in the brain. *J. Neurosci.* 31, 6939–6943. doi: 10.1523/jneurosci.0626-11.2011

Perrin, F. E., Boisset, G., Docquier, M., Schaad, O., Descombes, P., and Kato, A. C. (2005). No widespread induction of cell death genes occurs in pure motoneurons in an amyotrophic lateral sclerosis mouse model. *Hum. Mol. Genet.* 14, 3309–3320. doi: 10.1093/hmg/ddi357

Popova, T., Mennerich, D., Weith, A., and Quast, K. (2008). Effect of RNA quality on transcript intensity levels in microarray analysis of human post-mortem brain tissues. *BMC Genomics* 9:91. doi: 10.1186/1471-2164-9-91

Preece, P., Virley, D. J., Costandi, M., Coombes, R., Moss, S. J., Mudge, A. W., et al. (2003). An optimistic view for quantifying mRNA in post-mortem human brain. *Brain Res. Mol. Brain Res.* 116, 7–16. doi: 10.1016/s0169-328x(03)00208-0

Rosenfeld, S. (2010). Do DNA microarrays tell the story of gene expression? *Gene Regul. Syst. Bio.* 4, 61–73. doi: 10.4137/grsb.s4657

Saris, C. G., Groen, E. J., Koekkoek, J. A., Veldink, J. H., and Van Den Berg, L. H. (2013). Meta-analysis of gene expression profiling in amyotrophic lateral sclerosis: a comparison between transgenic mouse models and human patients. *Amyotroph. Lateral Scler. Frontotemporal Degener.* 14, 177–189. doi: 10.3109/21678421.2012.729842

Saris, C. G., Horvath, S., Van Vught, P. W., Van Es, M. A., Blauw, H. M., Fuller, T. F., et al. (2009). Weighted gene co-expression network analysis of the peripheral blood from amyotrophic lateral sclerosis patients. *BMC Genomics* 10:405. doi: 10.1186/1471-2164-10-405

Saxena, S., Cabuy, E., and Caroni, P. (2009). A role for motoneuron subtype-selective ER stress in disease manifestations of FALS mice. *Nat. Neurosci.* 12, 627–636. doi: 10.1038/nn.2297

Shtilbans, A., Choi, S. G., Fowkes, M. E., Khitrov, G., Shahbazi, M., Ting, J., et al. (2011). Differential gene expression in patients with amyotrophic lateral sclerosis. *Amyotroph. Lateral Scler.* 12, 250–256. doi: 10.3109/17482968.2011.560946

Tomita, H., Vawter, M. P., Walsh, D. M., Evans, S. J., Choudary, P. V., Li, J., et al. (2004). Effect of agonal and postmortem factors on gene expression profile: quality control in microarray analyses of postmortem human brain. *Biol. Psychiatry* 55, 346–352. doi: 10.1016/j.biopsych.2003.10.013

Trabzuni, D., Ryten, M., Walker, R., Smith, C., Imran, S., Ramasamy, A., et al. (2011). Quality control parameters on a large dataset of regionally dissected human control brains for whole genome expression studies. *J. Neurochem.* 119, 275–282. doi: 10.1111/j.1471-4159.2011.07432.x

Vargas, M. R., Pehar, M., Diaz-Amarilla, P. J., Beckman, J. S., and Barbeito, L. (2008). Transcriptional profile of primary astrocytes expressing ALS-linked mutant SOD1. *J. Neurosci. Res.* 86, 3515–3525. doi: 10.1002/jnr.21797

Wang, X. S., Simmons, Z., Liu, W., Boyer, P. J., and Connor, J. R. (2006). Differential expression of genes in amyotrophic lateral sclerosis revealed by profiling the post mortem cortex. *Amyotroph. Lateral Scler.* 7, 201–210. doi: 10.1080/17482960600947689

Wilkes, T. M., Devonshire, A. S., Ellison, S. L., and Foy, C. A. (2010). Evaluation of a novel approach for the measurement of RNA quality. *BMC Res. Notes* 3:89. doi: 10.1186/1756-0500-3-89

Yoshihara, T., Ishigaki, S., Yamamoto, M., Liang, Y., Niwa, J., Takeuchi, H., et al. (2002). Differential expression of inflammation- and apoptosis-related genes in spinal cords of a mutant SOD1 transgenic mouse model of familial amyotrophic lateral sclerosis. *J. Neurochem.* 80, 158–167. doi: 10.1046/j.0022-3042.2001.00683.x

7

Beta-2 microglobulin is important for disease progression in a murine model for amyotrophic lateral sclerosis

Kim A. Staats[1,2,3,4†], Susann Schönefeldt[3,4†], Marike Van Rillaer[3,4], Annelies Van Hoecke[1,2], Philip Van Damme[1,2,5], Wim Robberecht[1,2,5], Adrian Liston[3,4*†] and Ludo Van Den Bosch[1,2*†]

[1] KU Leuven Laboratory of Neurobiology and Leuven Research Institute for Neuroscience and Disease (LIND), Leuven, Belgium
[2] VIB Vesalius Research Center, KU Leuven, Leuven, Belgium
[3] VIB Autoimmune Genetics Laboratory, KU Leuven, Leuven, Belgium
[4] Department of Microbiology and Immunology, University of Leuven, Leuven, Belgium
[5] Neurology, University Hospitals Leuven, Leuven, Belgium

Edited by:
Ricardo Tapia, Universidad Nacional Autónoma de México, Mexico

Reviewed by:
Luis H. Barbeito, Institut Pasteur de Montevideo, Uruguay
Moses Rodriguez, Mayo Clinic, USA

****Correspondence:***
Adrian Liston, VIB Autoimmune Genetics Laboratory, KU Leuven, Campus Gasthuisberg O&N2, Herestraat 49 - PB 1026, B-3000 Leuven, Belgium
e-mail: adrian.liston@vib-kuleuven.be
Ludo Van Den Bosch, Laboratory of Neurobiology, Campus Gasthuisberg O&N4, Herestraat 49 - PB 1026, B-3000 Leuven, Belgium
e-mail: ludo.vandenbosch@vib-kuleuven.be
† These authors have contributed equally to the work.

Beta-2 microglobulin (*β2m*) is an essential component of the major histocompatibility complex (MHC) class I proteins and in the nervous system *β2m* is predominantly expressed in motor neurons. As *β2m* can promote nerve regeneration, we investigated its potential role in amyotrophic lateral sclerosis (ALS) by investigating its expression level as well as the effect of genetically removing *β2m* on the disease process in mutant superoxide dismutase 1 ($SOD1^{G93A}$) mice, a model of ALS. We observed a strong upregulation of *β2m* in motor neurons during the disease process and ubiquitous removal of *β2m* dramatically shortens the disease duration indicating that *β2m* plays an essential and positive role during the disease process. We hypothesize that *β2m* contributes to plasticity that is essential for muscle reinnervation. Absence of this plasticity will lead to faster muscle denervation and counteracting this process could be a relevant therapeutic target.

Keywords: beta-2 microglobulin, amyotrophic lateral sclerosis, motor neuron, neurodegeneration, motor neuron disease

INTRODUCTION

Major histocompatibility complex (MHC) class I proteins were originally discovered based on their critical role in the immune system, however immune-independent functions in the nervous system have recently been identified (Huh et al., 2000; Elmer and Mcallister, 2012). Beta-2 microglobulin (*β2m*) is an essential component of MHC class I molecules, being required for expression of all MHC class I on the cell surface. Within the central nervous system *β2m* has a predominantly motor neuronal expression pattern (Linda et al., 1998, 1999; Thams et al., 2009). This protein is therefore a candidate to contribute to the selective vulnerability of such motor neurons during amyotrophic lateral sclerosis (ALS).

ALS is a progressive neurodegenerative disease, characterized by the selective loss of motor neurons and the denervation of muscle fibers, resulting in muscle weakness and paralysis. In Europe, the disease has an annual incidence of 2.7 cases per 100,000 people (Logroscino et al., 2010) and the disease duration post-diagnosis is 3–5 years. In 10% of patients, ALS is a familial disease and 20% of these familial ALS patients contain mutations in the gene encoding superoxide dismutase 1 (*SOD1*). Based on these mutations, ALS rodent models have been generated that predictably mimic the patient disease process (Julien and Kriz, 2006). As the disease progression is indistinguishable between familial and sporadic ALS, common disease mechanisms are predicted. One of these mechanisms is decreased (peripheral) neuronal plasticity that can influence the ability of neuronal networks to compensate for a loss of (motor) neurons in the network. *β2m* is expressed in motor neurons in the lumbar spinal cord (Linda et al., 1999) as well as in motor axons (Thams et al., 2009). Additionally, *β2m* promotes recovery after axotomy (Linda et al., 1998; Oliveira et al., 2004) and sciatic nerve crush (Oliveira et al., 2004), which implies that it may be of importance in ALS too.

In this study, we investigated the role of *β2m* in ALS mice. To this end, we assessed the gene expression of *β2m* and interbred mice genetically lacking *β2m* with $SOD1^{G93A}$ mice and assessed survival and disease pathology.

MATERIALS AND METHODS

ANIMAL EXPERIMENTS

Mice overexpressing human wild-type *SOD1* ($SOD1^{WT}$) or human $SOD1^{G93A}$ and *β2m* knockout mice were purchased from The Jackson Laboratories (Bar Harbor, USA) and maintained on a C57BL/6 background. The $SOD1^{G93A}$ and *β2m* knockout were interbred allowing for approx. 50% of the mice to be littermate controlled in this study. Chow and water were provided *ad libitum* and mice were housed in the specific pathogen free animal facility of the KU Leuven under standard conditions according to the guidelines of the KU Leuven. End stage was defined as the age at which mice could no longer right themselves within 30 s when placed on their back. End stage is used as a measurement of survival and is the condition at which mice are euthanized to prevent further suffering. Disease onset was defined as the age at which mouse weight dropped below 90% of the average day 90–105 weight. The animal caretakers and scientists were blinded to the genotypes of the mice when assessing "end stage". All animal experiments were performed with the approval of the Animal Ethical Committee of KU Leuven (020/2010).

LASER DISSECTION MICROSCOPY

Murine spinal cords were snap-frozen in Tissue-Tec (Sakura Finetek Europe, Alphen aan de Rijn, The Netherlands) to make cryostat sections of 20-μm thickness. Then, cresyl violet–stained motor neurons, located in the ventral horn of the lumbar spinal cord, were collected on membrane slides 1.0 PEN (Carl Zeiss AG, Oberkochen, Germany), using dissection by a laser-dissection microscope (Carl Zeiss AG) and capturing in Adhesive Cap 500 opaque (Carl Zeiss AG). Only motor neurons in which the nucleus was visible and with soma area > 250 μm^2, were collected. At least 1,500 motor neurons were dissected for each animal.

QUANTITATIVE PCR

Isolation of mRNA was performed using the TriPure (Roche, Basel, Switzerland) method and the RNeasy kit (Qiagen, Venlo, The Netherlands). Reverse transcriptase polymerase chain reaction (PCR) used random hexamers (Life Technologies, Carlsbad, USA) and Moloney Murine Leukemia Virus Reverse Transcriptase (MMLV RT; Invitrogen, Carlsbad, USA). Quantitative PCR (qPCR) was performed with the StepOnePlus (Life Technologies) and TaqMan Universal PCR Master Mix (Life Technologies). Gene expression assays were purchased from Life Technologies and IDT DNA (Coralville, USA): *gapdh* (Mm.PT.39a.1), *β2m* (Mm00437762_m1) and *cd8b1* (Mm.PT49a.10182911). For this analysis, presymptomatic tissue was collected at 90 days of age and symptomatic at 120 days of age. The scientist performing the qPCR was blinded to the genotypes of the samples.

NISSL STAINING

To visualize neurons, Nissl staining was performed on 4% formaldehyde fixed spinal cords sections. Sections were briefly immersed in a cresyl violet solution and subsequently in a 70% ethanol with 10% acetic acid. Slides were dehydrated by an increased ethanol concentration series and mounted with PerTex® (Histolab AB, Goteborg, Sweden). Images were collected by Zeiss Axio Imager M1 microscope (Carl Zeiss AG) with AxioCam Mrc5 camera (Carl Zeiss AG). The number of (motor) neurons was quantified by measurement of the soma area as visualized by cresyl violet staining in ImageJ (National Institute of Health) on multiple 40 μm thick sections in the ventral horn of the lumbar spinal cord. Characterisation of motor neurons occurred as previously (Fischer et al., 2004) of at least 5–10 ventral horns of the lumbar spinal cord of 2–4 mice per group. The scientist performing the Nissl staining and neuron quantification was blinded to the genotypes of the samples.

IMMUNOHISTOCHEMISTRY

Mice were transcardially perfused with phosphate buffered saline (PBS) and subsequently with 4% formaldehyde. Spinal cords were post-fixed with 4% formaldehyde overnight at 4°C and transferred to 30% sucrose for an additional night. After snap freezing, tissue was sectioned by cryostat at 40 μm thickness and stained with a polyclonal antibody directed against ubiquitin (Dako, Glostrup, Denmark). Images were collected by Zeiss Axio Imager M1 microscope (Carl Zeiss AG) with AxioCam Mrc5 camera (Carl Zeiss AG). Ubiquitin immunopositive aggregates were counted per ventral horn using ImageJ of 2–6 ventral horns of the lumbar spinal cord of 2–4 mice per group and presented as the average of the number of aggregates per ventral horn. The scientist performing the immunohistochemistry and aggregate quantification was blinded to the genotypes of the samples.

STATISTICAL ANALYSIS

Analysis was performed with the statistical software package Prism Origin (GraphPad Software, La Jolla, USA). Survival was analyzed by Log-Rank testing. Differences between two groups were analyzed using a Student's *t*-test. Differences between more than two groups were analyzed by ANOVA with Bonferroni correction for multiple testing. Significance was assumed at $p < 0.05$. Error bars represent the standard deviation.

RESULTS

To assess the potential for *β2m* to have a functional role in ALS pathogenesis, we assessed gene expression in the spinal cords of non-transgenic, $SOD1^{WT}$ and $SOD1^{G93A}$ mice. We observed a strong increase in *β2m* gene expression during disease progression in $SOD1^{G93A}$ mice (**Figure 1A**). This increase is at least partly due to the increased neuron-specific gene expression of *β2m*, as a greater level of upregulation (10-fold) was identified by qPCR on neurons from $SOD1^{G93A}$ mice compared to neurons from $SOD1^{WT}$ mice isolated by laser dissection microscopy (**Figure 1B**). As we do not observe an increase of $CD8^+$ T cells in the spinal cord of end stage $SOD1^{G93A}$ mice, as assessed by the gene expression analysis of *CD8b1* (**Figure 1C**), these data indicate potential for a neuronal role for *β2m* in ALS.

To determine whether *β2m* has an effect in ALS, we interbred $\beta 2m^{-/-}$ mice with $SOD1^{G93A}$ mice and assessed disease progression in $\beta 2m^{-/-}$ $SOD1^{G93A}$, $\beta 2m^{+/-}$ $SOD1^{G93A}$ and $\beta 2m^{+/+}$ $SOD1^{G93A}$ mice. The survival of $\beta 2m^{+/-}$ $SOD1^{G93A}$ mice did not differ from $\beta 2m^{+/+}$ $SOD1^{G93A}$ littermates (data not shown). The complete genetic ablation of *β2m* did not affect onset of disease (data not shown), but significantly decreased average survival of $SOD1^{G93A}$ mice by 8.9 days (**Figure 2A**) and reduced disease duration by approximately 50% (**Figure 2B**). The decrease of survival in $\beta 2m^{-/-}$ $SOD1^{G93A}$ mice demonstrated a protective role for *β2m* in ALS mice.

To assess whether genetic ablation of *β2m* alters pathology of $SOD1^{G93A}$ mice, we analyzed pathology in the spinal cords of end stage mice. Decreased numbers of motor neurons were

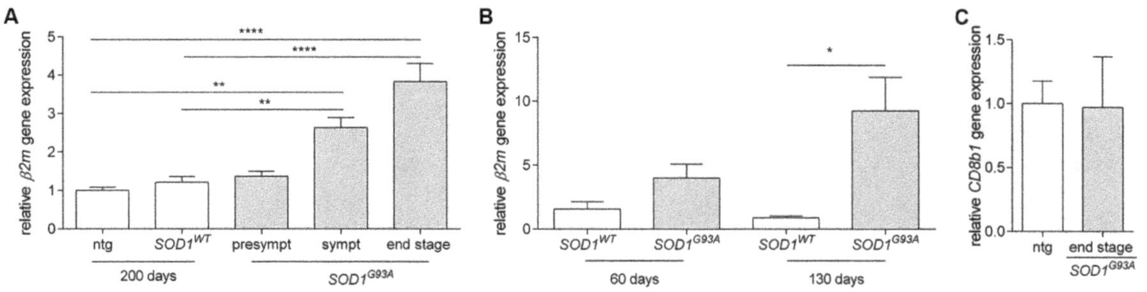

FIGURE 1 | Increased $\beta 2m$ gene expression in ALS mice. **(A)** Relative $\beta 2m$ gene expression in spinal cord of non-transgenic (ntg, $n = 6$) and $SOD1^{WT}$ controls ($n = 6$) compared to presymtomatic (presympt, $n = 6$), symptomatic (sympt, $n = 6$) and end stage ($n = 6$) $SOD1^{G93A}$ mice (ANOVA, Bonferroni post hoc). **(B)** Relative $\beta 2m$ gene expression in neurons isolated by laser dissection microscopy from the spinal cord of $SOD1^{WT}$ controls at 60 days ($n = 2$) and 130 days of age ($n = 3$) compared to neurons from $SOD1^{G93A}$ mice at 60 days ($n = 3$) and 130 days of age ($n = 3$; Student's *t*-test). **(C)** Relative *CD8b1* gene expression in the spinal cord of 150 day old non-transgenic mice (ntg, $n = 5$) and end stage ($n = 5$) $SOD1^{G93A}$ mice. $^{*}p < 0.05$, $^{**}p < 0.01$, $^{****}p < 0.0001$.

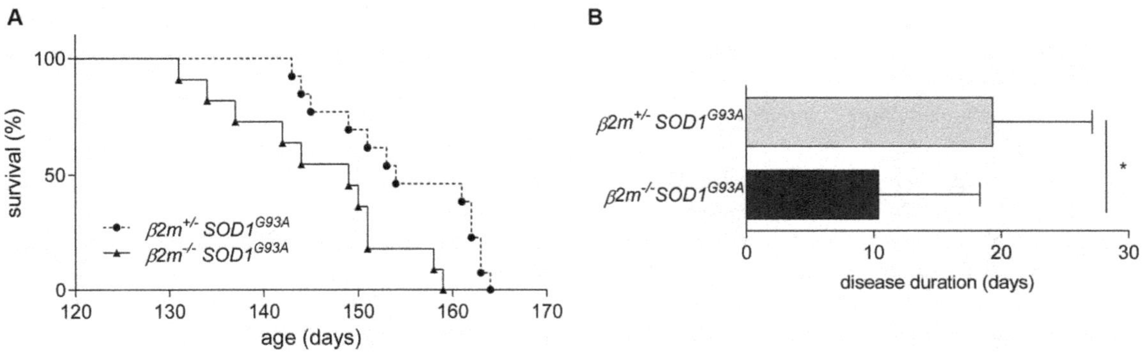

FIGURE 2 | Decreased survival in $\beta 2m$ knockout ALS mice. **(A)** Survival analysis of $\beta 2m^{+/-}$ $SOD1^{G93A}$ ($n = 13$, 154.9 ± 7.7 days) and $\beta 2m^{-/-}$ $SOD1^{G93A}$ mice ($n = 11$, 146.0 ± 8.8 days; Log-Rank $p = 0.009$). **(B)** Disease duration of $\beta 2m^{+/-}$ $SOD1^{G93A}$ ($n = 9$) and $\beta 2m^{-/-}$ $SOD1^{G93A}$ mice ($n = 8$). $^{*}p < 0.05$.

observed in the end stage spinal cord of $SOD1^{G93A}$ and $\beta 2m^{-/-}$ $SOD1^{G93A}$ mice (**Figures 3A–C**, quantified in **Figure 3D**), as were increased ubiquitin-positive aggregates (**Figures 3E–G**, quantified in **Figure 3H**). No differences were observed between the end stage pathology of $SOD1^{G93A}$ and $\beta 2m^{-/-}$ $SOD1^{G93A}$ mice for motor neurons (**Figures 3B, C**) or ubiquitin immunoreactivity (**Figures 3F, G**). This shows that end stage $\beta 2m^{-/-}$ $SOD1^{G93A}$ mice show the same extent of motor neuron loss and aggregate formation as end stage $SOD1^{G93A}$ mice, although disease progression is faster.

DISCUSSION

Here we show that $\beta 2m$ is important in ALS mouse survival and that it is upregulated during disease in the spinal cord and by motor neurons. Upregulation of $\beta 2m$ in neuronal tissues has been reported previously when comparing spinal cord (Edstrom et al., 2004) and brain (VanGuilder Starkey et al., 2012) expression of aged rats to adult controls and in the spinal cord of axotomised rats (Maehlen et al., 1988; Olsson et al., 1989; Linda et al., 1998), which may suggest that stressed neurons increase $\beta 2m$ gene expression to increase plasticity. This concept fits well with reports of the role of $\beta 2m$ in neurons during development and plasticity (Huh et al., 2000; Bilousova et al., 2012), of the hippocampus and visual system (Huh et al., 2000) but not of the cerebellum (Letellier et al., 2008), and the delayed or impaired recovery of $\beta 2m$ knockout mice post axotomy (Linda et al., 1998; Oliveira et al., 2004) and sciatic nerve crush (Oliveira et al., 2004).

Impaired (peripheral) plasticity by $\beta 2m$ knockout may explain the decrease in survival detected in ALS mice in this study, as increased plasticity is protective in ALS mice and rats (Van Hoecke et al., 2012). A number of plasticity-promoting genetic or pharmacological strategies have proven successful in the past in ALS models, such as EphA4 knockdown and inhibition (Van Hoecke et al., 2012), and vascular endothelial growth factor (VEGF) administration in ALS rodents (Storkebaum et al., 2005).

With the use of a ubiquitous $\beta 2m$ knockout mouse we cannot exclude that the decrease of survival of ALS mice lacking $\beta 2m$ may be due to the effect of removing $\beta 2m$ in the immune system. $\beta 2m$ is necessary for the differentiation of $CD8^{+}$ T cells and natural killer T (NKT) cells (Koller et al., 1990). The role of these cell types is not yet fully understood in ALS, as varying results are obtained for ALS mouse survival when mature lymphocytes are not present (Beers et al., 2008; Tada et al., 2011). Additionally, NKT cells may be associated to ALS disease pathology as impairments in NKT cells are reported in ALS mice (Finkelstein et al., 2011). That being said, qPCR analysis of $CD8^{+}$ T cells does not suggest a role for

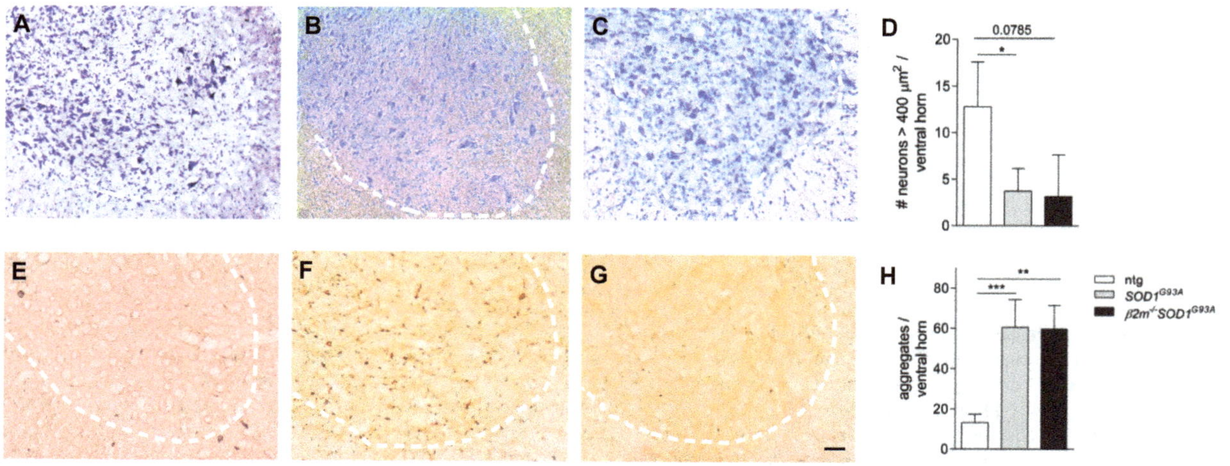

FIGURE 3 | Unaltered end stage pathology in *β2m*-deficient *SOD1*^{G93A} mice. Ventral horns of spinal cord sections of non-transgenic (ntg, $n = 4$; **A** and **E**) and *SOD1*^{G93A} ($n = 4$; **B** and **F**) and $\beta 2m^{-/-}$ *SOD1*^{G93A} ($n = 2$; **C** and **G**) *SOD1*^{G93A} mice. Nissl staining was used to visualize the (motor) neurons **(A–C)**. The number of > 250 μm^2 neurons and > 400 μm^2 motor neurons per ventral horn are quantified in **(D)** Ubiquitin immunoreactivity in spinal cord sections of non-transgenic, *SOD1*^{G93A} and $\beta 2m^{-/-}$ *SOD1*^{G93A} mice are quantified in **(H)** Dashed lines delineate the ventral horn. Scale bar = 100 μm. $*p < 0.05$, $**p < 0.01$, $***p < 0.001$.

these cells as *CD8b1* gene expression is not increased in ALS spinal cords. Additionally, a role for CD8$^+$ T cells may be predicted to be detrimental in contrast to our data demonstrating a detrimental role for *β2m* upon removal in ALS mice. Interestingly, *β2m* has been assessed previously as a biomarker in cerebrospinal fluid or venous blood samples from ALS patients, but with variable results (Brettschneider et al., 2008; Mitchell et al., 2009; Baciu et al., 2012).

The mechanism to which *β2m* contributes to neuronal plasticity is not fully understood, though it is proposed that it may be through paired-immunoglobulin like receptor-B (PirB) (VanGuilder Starkey et al., 2012). This receptor is located on axons, dendrites and neuronal somata (VanGuilder Starkey et al., 2012) and could thus easily facilitate plasticity. Additionally, *β2m* is localized at synapses and in synaptosomes (Shatz, 2009). Alternatively, *β2m* and PirB are associated with decreased plasticity and recovery in other neurodegenerative conditions such as stroke (Adelson et al., 2012), experimental autoimmune encephalomyelitis (EAE; Denic et al., 2012) and ischemia (Wang et al., 2012). These paradigms are largely affected by the immune system and the beneficial effect of *β2m* or PirB in these models may be due to the role of the immune system. This notion is supported by work by Linker et al. that show that reconstitution of CD8$^+$ cells in *β2m* knockout mice delays the effect of EAE compared to *β2m* knockout littermates (Linker et al., 2005).

In conclusion, this work shows the detrimental effect of *β2m* knockout in ALS and identifies *β2m* signaling as a potential new direction for the development of therapeutic strategies counteracting ALS.

AUTHOR CONTRIBUTIONS

Kim A. Staats and Susann Schönefeldt performed the murine behavioral analyses. Kim A. Staats and Marike Van Rillaer conducted the staining experiments. Kim A. Staats and Annelies Van Hoecke analyzed gene expression of motor neurons excised by laser dissection microscopy. Philip Van Damme, Wim Robberecht, Adrian Liston and Ludo Van Den Bosch supervised and designed the experiments. Kim A. Staats, Adrian Liston and Ludo Van Den Bosch wrote the manuscript. All authors approved the final version of the manuscript.

ACKNOWLEDGMENTS

This work was supported by grants from the "Fund for Scientific Research Flanders" (FWO-Vlaanderen), the University of Leuven (KU Leuven), the Belgian Government Interuniversity Attraction Poles, programme P7/16 of the Belgian Federal Science Policy Office) and the European Community's Health Seventh Framework Programme (FP7/2007-2013 under grant agreement 259867). Philip Van Damme holds a clinical investigatorship of the FWO-Vlaanderen. Wim Robberecht is supported through the E. von Behring Chair for Neuromuscular and Neurodegenerative Disorders.

REFERENCES

Adelson, J. D., Barreto, G. E., Xu, L., Kim, T., Brott, B. K., Ouyang, Y. B., et al. (2012). Neuroprotection from stroke in the absence of MHCI or PirB. *Neuron* 73, 1100–1107. doi: 10.1016/j.neuron.2012.01.020

Baciu, C., Thompson, K. J., Mougeot, J. L., Brooks, B. R., and Weller, J. W. (2012). The LO-BaFL method and ALS microarray expression analysis. *BMC Bioinformatics* 13:244. doi: 10.1186/1471-2105-13-244

Beers, D. R., Henkel, J. S., Zhao, W., Wang, J., and Appel, S. H. (2008). CD4$^+$ T cells support glial neuroprotection, slow disease progression and modify glial morphology in an animal model of inherited ALS. *Proc. Natl. Acad. Sci. U S A* 105, 15558–15563. doi: 10.1073/pnas.0807419105

Bilousova, T., Dang, H., Xu, W., Gustafson, S., Jin, Y., Wickramasinghe, L., et al. (2012). Major histocompatibility complex class I molecules modulate embryonic neuritogenesis and neuronal polarization. *J. Neuroimmunol.* 247, 1–8. doi: 10.1016/j.jneuroim.2012.03.008

Brettschneider, J., Mogel, H., Lehmensiek, V., Ahlert, T., Sussmuth, S., Ludolph, A. C., et al. (2008). Proteome analysis of cerebrospinal fluid in amyotrophic lateral sclerosis (ALS). *Neurochem. Res.* 33, 2358–2363. doi: 10.1007/s11064-008-9742-5

Denic, A., Pirko, I., Wootla, B., Bieber, A., Macura, S., and Rodriguez, M. (2012). Deletion of beta-2-microglobulin ameliorates spinal cord lesion load and promotes recovery of brainstem NAA levels in a murine model of multiple sclerosis. *Brain Pathol.* 22, 698–708. doi: 10.1111/j.1750-3639.2012.00576.x

Edstrom, E., Kullberg, S., Ming, Y., Zheng, H., and Ulfhake, B. (2004). MHC class I, beta2 microglobulin and the INF-gamma receptor are upregulated in aged motoneurons. *J. Neurosci. Res.* 78, 892–900. doi: 10.1002/jnr.20341

Elmer, B. M., and Mcallister, A. K. (2012). Major histocompatibility complex class I proteins in brain development and plasticity. *Trends Neurosci.* 35, 660–670. doi: 10.1016/j.tins.2012.08.001

Finkelstein, A., Kunis, G., Seksenyan, A., Ronen, A., Berkutzki, T., Azoulay, D., et al. (2011). Abnormal changes in NKT cells, the IGF-1 axis and liver pathology in an animal model of ALS. *PLoS One* 6:e22374. doi: 10.1371/journal.pone.0022374

Fischer, L. R., Culver, D. G., Tennant, P., Davis, A. A., Wang, M., Castellano-Sanchez, A., et al. (2004). Amyotrophic lateral sclerosis is a distal axonopathy: evidence in mice and man. *Exp. Neurol.* 185, 232–240. doi: 10.1016/j.expneurol.2003.10.004

Huh, G. S., Boulanger, L. M., Du, H., Riquelme, P. A., Brotz, T. M., and Shatz, C. J. (2000). Functional requirement for class I MHC in CNS development and plasticity. *Science* 290, 2155–2159. doi: 10.1126/science.290.5499.2155

Julien, J. P., and Kriz, J. (2006). Transgenic mouse models of amyotrophic lateral sclerosis. *Biochim. Biophys. Acta* 1762, 1013–1024. doi: 10.1016/j.bbadis.2006.03.006

Koller, B. H., Marrack, P., Kappler, J. W., and Smithies, O. (1990). Normal development of mice deficient in beta 2M, MHC class I proteins and $CD8^+$ T cells. *Science* 248, 1227–1230. doi: 10.1126/science.2112266

Letellier, M., Willson, M. L., Gautheron, V., Mariani, J., and Lohof, A. M. (2008). Normal adult climbing fiber monoinnervation of cerebellar Purkinje cells in mice lacking MHC class I molecules. *Dev. Neurobiol.* 68, 997–1006. doi: 10.1002/dneu.20639

Linda, H., Hammarberg, H., Cullheim, S., Levinovitz, A., Khademi, M., and Olsson, T. (1998). Expression of MHC class I and beta2-microglobulin in rat spinal motoneurons: regulatory influences by IFN-gamma and axotomy. *Exp. Neurol.* 150, 282–295. doi: 10.1006/exnr.1997.6768

Linda, H., Hammarberg, H., Piehl, F., Khademi, M., and Olsson, T. (1999). Expression of MHC class I heavy chain and beta2-microglobulin in rat brainstem motoneurons and nigral dopaminergic neurons. *J. Neuroimmunol.* 101, 76–86. doi: 10.1016/s0165-5728(99)00135-6

Linker, R. A., Rott, E., Hofstetter, H. H., Hanke, T., Toyka, K. V., and Gold, R. (2005). EAE in beta-2 microglobulin-deficient mice: axonal damage is not dependent on MHC-I restricted immune responses. *Neurobiol. Dis.* 19, 218–228. doi: 10.1016/j.nbd.2004.12.017

Logroscino, G., Traynor, B. J., Hardiman, O., Chio, A., Mitchell, D., Swingler, R. J., et al. (2010). Incidence of amyotrophic lateral sclerosis in Europe. *J. Neurol. Neurosurg. Psychiatry.* 81, 385–390. doi: 10.1136/jnnp.2009.183525

Maehlen, J., Schroder, H. D., Klareskog, L., Olsson, T., and Kristensson, K. (1988). Axotomy induces MHC class I antigen expression on rat nerve cells. *Neurosci. Lett.* 92, 8–13. doi: 10.1016/0304-3940(88)90733-1

Mitchell, R. M., Freeman, W. M., Randazzo, W. T., Stephens, H. E., Beard, J. L., Simmons, Z., et al. (2009). A CSF biomarker panel for identification of patients with amyotrophic lateral sclerosis. *Neurology* 72, 14–19. doi: 10.1212/01.wnl.0000333251.36681.a5

Oliveira, A. L., Thams, S., Lidman, O., Piehl, F., Hokfelt, T., Karre, K., et al. (2004). A role for MHC class I molecules in synaptic plasticity and regeneration of neurons after axotomy. *Proc. Natl. Acad. Sci. U S A* 101, 17843–17848. doi: 10.1073/pnas.0408154101

Olsson, T., Kristensson, K., Ljungdahl, A., Maehlen, J., Holmdahl, R., and Klareskog, L. (1989). Gamma-interferon-like immunoreactivity in axotomized rat motor neurons. *J. Neurosci.* 9, 3870–3875.

Shatz, C. J. (2009). MHC class I: an unexpected role in neuronal plasticity. *Neuron* 64, 40–45. doi: 10.1016/j.neuron.2009.09.044

Storkebaum, E., Lambrechts, D., Dewerchin, M., Moreno-Murciano, M. P., Appelmans, S., Oh, H., et al. (2005). Treatment of motoneuron degeneration by intracerebroventricular delivery of VEGF in a rat model of ALS. *Nat. Neurosci.* 8, 85–92. doi: 10.1038/nn1360

Tada, S., Okuno, T., Yasui, T., Nakatsuji, Y., Sugimoto, T., Kikutani, H., et al. (2011). Deleterious effects of lymphocytes at the early stage of neurodegeneration in an animal model of amyotrophic lateral sclerosis. *J. Neuroinflammation* 8:19. doi: 10.1186/1742-2094-8-19

Thams, S., Brodin, P., Plantman, S., Saxelin, R., Karre, K., and Cullheim, S. (2009). Classical major histocompatibility complex class I molecules in motoneurons: new actors at the neuromuscular junction. *J. Neurosci.* 29, 13503–13515. doi: 10.1523/jneurosci.0981-09.2009

VanGuilder Starkey, H. D., Van Kirk, C. A., Bixler, G. V., Imperio, C. G., Kale, V. P., Serfass, J. M., et al. (2012). Neuroglial expression of the MHCI pathway and PirB receptor is upregulated in the hippocampus with advanced aging. *J. Mol. Neurosci.* 48, 111–126. doi: 10.1007/s12031-012-9783-8

Van Hoecke, A., Schoonaert, L., Lemmens, R., Timmers, M., Staats, K. A., Laird, A. S., et al. (2012). EPHA4 is a disease modifier of amyotrophic lateral sclerosis in animal models and in humans. *Nat. Med.* 18, 1418–1422. doi: 10.1038/nm.2901

Wang, H., Xiong, Y., and Mu, D. (2012). PirB restricts neuronal regeneration in developing rat brain following hypoxia-ischemia. *Mol. Med. Rep.* 6, 339–344. doi: 10.3892/mmr.2012.907

8

Histone deacetylases and their role in motor neuron degeneration

Rafael Lazo-Gómez, Uri N. Ramírez-Jarquín, Luis B. Tovar-y-Romo and Ricardo Tapia*

División de Neurociencias, Instituto de Fisiología Celular, Universidad Nacional Autónoma de México, D. F., México

Edited by:
Manoj K. Jaiswal, Center for Neuroscience and Regenerative Medicine, USA

Reviewed by:
Thomas G. Oertner, University of Hamburg, Germany
John Weiss, University of California, Irvine, USA

****Correspondence:***
Ricardo Tapia, División de Neurociencias, Instituto de Fisiología Celular, Universidad Nacional Autónoma de México, 04510, D. F., México
e-mail: rtapia@ifc.unam.mx

Amyotrophic lateral sclerosis (ALS) is a fatal neurodegenerative disease, characterized by the progressive loss of motor neurons. The cause of this selective neuronal death is unknown, but transcriptional dysregulation is recently emerging as an important factor. The physical substrate for the regulation of the transcriptional process is chromatin, a complex assembly of histones and DNA. Histones are subject to several post-translational modifications, like acetylation, that are a component of the transcriptional regulation process. Histone acetylation and deacetylation is performed by a group of enzymes (histone acetyltransferases (HATs) and deacetylases, respectively) whose modulation can alter the transcriptional state of many regions of the genome, and thus may be an important target in diseases that share this pathogenic process, as is the case for ALS. This review will discuss the present evidence of transcriptional dysregulation in ALS, the role of histone deacetylases (HDACs) in disease pathogenesis, and the novel pharmacologic strategies that are being comprehensively studied to prevent motor neuron death, with focus on sirtuins (SIRT) and their effectors.

Keywords: amyotrophic lateral sclerosis, neurodegeneration, neuroprotection, transcription dysregulation, histone deacetylases, sirtuins

INTRODUCTION

Amyotrophic lateral sclerosis (ALS) is a fatal neurodegenerative disease characterized by the death of upper and lower motor neurons. There are two type of ALS based on the presence of an identified mutation as a cause of the disease. The familial type (fALS) is most commonly caused by mutations in the superoxide dismutase type 1 (SOD1) gene, for which there is a widely studied transgenic mouse model; however fALS represents only about 10% of cases. The most common type of ALS is called sporadic (sALS), but because there are no identified etiologic factors, validated experimental models lack for this type of the disease. Nevertheless, disease progression and pathologic characteristics in both, fALS and sALS, are similar. Also, in both types of the disease, motor neuron degeneration has been associated with the same mechanisms, such as glutamate-mediated excitotoxicity, inflammatory events, axonal transport deficits, oxidative stress and mitochondrial dysfunction (for recent reviews see Corona et al., 2007; Santa-Cruz et al., 2012).

Besides these factors, a novel mechanism that may be involved in motor neuron death and other neurodegenerative diseases is transcriptional dysfunction, which consists of aberrations of the molecular machinery that regulates gene expression, especially at the transcriptional levels through the manipulation of epigenetic marks (Robberecht and Philips, 2013). These marks are covalent modifications of the chromatin components, DNA and histone proteins, carried out by several key enzymes that finely modulate the status of these marks. Among these marks, histone acetylation has been characterized as an important mechanism in the regulation of the opening of chromatin configuration leading to increased transcription (Kouzarides, 2007). The status of histone acetylation strongly depends on the activity of histone deacetylases (HDACs), a widely conserved family of enzymes that catalyze the removal of acetyl groups from histones and from other proteins. This family, which includes sirtuins (SIRT), has been shown to be important for several cellular processes, such as cell death and stress responses, which makes them attractive for the study of their pathogenic role and as potential therapeutic targets (Haigis and Sinclair, 2010).

This paper will review, first the evidence of transcriptional dysregulation in ALS, then the role of the different members of the HDACs family in disease pathogeny and as therapeutic candidates, and finally the role of SIRT and their effectors in ALS.

RELEVANCE OF HISTONE ACETYLATION IN GENE EXPRESSION

Protein acetylation is an important postranslational modification that regulates numerous cellular functions, such as microtubule dynamics and intracellular transport (Hubbert et al., 2002), development (Bhaumik et al., 2007), metabolism (Cantó et al., 2009), and transcriptional regulation through chromatin remodeling (Kouzarides, 2007).

In eukaryotic cells, including neurons, the genome is organized through the association of DNA with protein complexes, an assembly called chromatin. The most abundant proteins are histones, and these proteins assemble themselves into octamers, composed of two copies of the histones types H2A, H2B, H3 and H4. Around the octamer, ~147 bp of DNA is wrapped, forming the basic unit of chromatin, the nucleosome. Nucleosomes further organize themselves in increasingly complex structures, all of which are subject to modulation, by changing the accessibility of the regulatory regions of DNA (such as promoters, enhancers, silencers or insulators) to the transcriptional machinery, ultimately affecting gene expression (Zhou et al., 2011). This regulation can be accomplished through covalent modifications of the chromatin components: in the DNA it occurs through cytosine methylation and hydroxymethylation, and in the histones through methylation, ubiquitinylation, sumoylation, phosphorylation and acetylation of selected aminoacid residues (Kouzarides, 2007). In general terms, gene expression is directly proportional the level of histone acetylation; because of this, the regulation of this postranslational modification is essential for gene homeostasis. Such regulation depends on two groups of enzymes: histone acetyltransferases (HATs) and HDACs, and drastic alterations to this control of gene expression can be deleterious, as has been proven in various tumor cell models (Frew et al., 2009). Therefore, the upregulation of the expression of a given gene can be accomplished by stimulating the activity of HATs or by inhibiting the activity of HDACs (Kazantsev and Thompson, 2008). Currently, research on HATs and on their possible protective effects on neurodegenerative processes is scarce and no specific activators are known, whereas information on HDACs has become the subject of many studies (Selvi et al., 2010). Although histones are not the only target of these enzymes, and in some instances they are not a target at all, the name HDACs is preserved for historical reasons. They constitute a family integrated in a complex network of intracellular signaling participating through acetylation/deacetylation reactions, with numerous protein substrates and multiple physiological consequences depending on the protein involved (de Ruijter et al., 2003; Kazantsev and Thompson, 2008).

EVIDENCE OF TRANSCRIPTIONAL DYSREGULATION IN ALS

There is evidence that transcriptional dysregulation could contribute to, and possibly be the cause of, some neurodegenerative disorders. This was first proposed for Huntington's disease (Cha, 2000) and relevant findings have been encountered in experimental in vitro and in vivo models of Alzheimer's (Robakis, 2003) and Parkinson's diseases (Yacoubian et al., 2008). In the case of ALS, there is also evidence of transcriptional dysregulation and alterations in the transcriptome in both the sporadic (Figueroa-Romero et al., 2012) and the familial (Kirby et al., 2005) types of the disease. Although the mechanisms and causal relationships have yet to be elucidated, it has been proposed that neuronal protein inclusions, such as those formed by mutated SOD1 or TDP43 (43-kDa transactivator response region (TAR) DNA-binding domain protein) which have been found in ALS and in frontotemporal dementia, could cause their toxicity by acting as surface attractants that sequester vital components of the transcriptional machinery, as was first proved for huntingtin (Cha, 2000). For example, in a screening study to identify targets that disrupt SOD1 aggresome in cultured cells, HDAC inhibition was shown to prevent aggresome formation (Corcoran et al., 2004).

Transcription might also be altered indirectly by modifications of other regulatory components of the transcriptional process, such as HDAC activity. For example, in a *Drosophila* model of polyglutamine neurodegeneration, it was shown that the upregulation of HDACs can ameliorate neuronal death due to a selective transcriptional repression of the CGG repeat-containing gene (Todd et al., 2010). Also, HDAC inhibition is protective for cultured motor neurons against excitotoxicity, a mechanism known to be involved in ALS pathophysiology, due to their ability to modulate gene expression (Kanai et al., 2004). Hence, although the role of transcriptional dysfunction in neurodegenerative diseases is still under study, there is increasing evidence for a role of HDACs in the neurodegenerative processes through the modulation of transcriptional machinery.

HISTONE DEACETYLASES: ROLE OF CLASSES I AND II IN MOTOR NEURON DEGENERATION

Based on structural, localization and functional criteria, HDAC superfamily is composed of five classes. First, in the next paragraphs, we will focus on the "typical" HDACs (11 enzymes, classified in classes I, IIa, IIb and IV), their distribution and the evidence of their role in ALS. The role of SIRT (seven enzymes that constitute class III or "atypical" HDACs) will be addressed later.

Class I and II HDACs are Zn^{2+}-dependent enzymes. Class I include HDAC1, HDAC2, HDAC3 and HDAC8, which are localized in the nucleus and ubiquitously expressed in mammalian tissues (except HDAC8, which is muscle-specific). Broadly speaking, these enzymes are involved in the regulation of gene-specific transcription through the formation of stable transcriptional complexes (de Ruijter et al., 2003). Of these, HDAC2 and HDAC3 seem to have a more important role in the physiology of the central nervous system. Broide et al. (2007) described the distribution of 11 HDACs mRNAs in 50 screened areas of the rat brain, using high-resolution in situ hybridization; HDAC2 and HDAC3 were widely expressed in all areas, especially those of the limbic system (amygdala, piriform cortex, olfactory bulb and hippocampus) and in the granule cell layer of cerebellum, and at the cellular level were found in neurons and oligodendrocytes. In a recent report, a similar distribution of HDAC2 was found in the mouse brain, as well as a moderate expression in primary and secondary motor cortices, and Rexed's laminae 4–9 of the cervical spinal cord (where motor neurons reside). Again, HDAC2 was noted only in neurons and oligodendrocytes, within the nucleus (Yao et al., 2013). Due to their ubiquitous expression in brain and spinal cord, these HDACs have also been implicated in ALS. Janssen et al. (2010) found in ALS patients that HDAC2 expression was upregulated in motor cortex (in layers III–V, where upper motor neuron are located) and in spinal cord grey matter, particularly in the nuclei of motor neurons; they interpreted this result as a protective role of HDAC2 in ALS pathogenesis, although the mechanisms of this effect were not detailed. Regarding this issue, in an in vitro study Kernochan et al. (2005) reported that HDAC inhibition increased promoter activity of the survival motor neuron 2 gene, and this was associated with HDAC2 levels.

Class IIa –HDACs 4, 5, 7 and 9– shuffle between the nucleus and the cytoplasm, and their substrates have not been defined; they have histone deacetylase activity only by interacting with HDAC3 (de Ruijter et al., 2003). HDAC4 and 5 expressions were high in all screened areas, and their locations mimic that of class I HDACs (Broide et al., 2007).

Class IIb is composed of HDAC6 and HDAC10. Again, HDAC10 substrates have not been defined, but it is known that it associates with HDAC3 (de Ruijter et al., 2003). HDAC6 is an unusual enzyme, in the sense that it has two catalytic domains and functions in the cytoplasm where it deacetylates α-tubulin and alters microtubule stability (Hubbert et al., 2002). Furthermore, inhibition of this enzyme stimulates autophagy and the proteasome system in a *Drosophila* model of spinal muscular atrophy (a neurodegenerative disease of spinal motor neurons) resulting in increased survival (Pandey et al., 2007). In the rat brain, its expression is low (Broide et al., 2007) and no changes were noted in ALS patients (Janssen et al., 2010). Nevertheless, evidence of the role of HDAC6 in ALS is emerging. In a recent work it was found that TDP43 and fused in sarcoma/translated in liposarcoma (FUS/TLS), which are proteins that regulate RNA processing and have been found to be mutated in some cases of ALS, interact with each other forming a ribonucleoprotein complex that regulates the expression of HDAC6 through its mRNA stability (Kim et al., 2010).

Class IV HDAC only member, HDAC11, is localized in the cell nucleus and is structurally different from the other classes (Kazantsev and Thompson, 2008). Although its functions are poorly understood, recent reports indicate that this HDAC is abundantly and almost exclusively expressed in the mammalian nervous system, within oligodendrocytes (Liu et al., 2008), and also plays an important role in the maturation of this cell type (Liu et al., 2009b). In other study in the rat brain, HDAC11 expression was found to be ubiquitously distributed, in both neurons and oligodendrocytes; in fact, this HDAC displayed the highest levels of expression of all HDACs (Broide et al., 2007). In nervous tissue of ALS patients, including the ventral horn of the spinal cord, the nucleus and the cytoplasm of motor neurons showed decreased HDAC11 mRNA levels (Janssen et al., 2010).

PROTECTIVE EFFECTS OF HDAC INHIBITION

Chen et al. (2012) addressed the role of class I and II HDACs in an experimental model of acute stroke in rodents. There was progressive decline of mRNA levels of HDACs 1, 2, 5 and 9 in cerebral cortex, while HDACs 3, 6 and 11 mRNA levels were transiently increased. In addition, in an in vitro model of glucose-oxygen deprivation, they reported that selective inhibition of HDAC3 and HDAC6 promoted neuronal survival.

Currently there is an ample battery of small-molecule HDACs inhibitors, that were initially developed to halt cell proliferation in cancer experimental models; HDACs inhibitors are classified as hydroxamate-based (vorinostat, valproic acid (VPA), sodium butyrate, trichostatin A, 4-phenyl butyrate, MC1568 –class II selective–, and tubucin –HDAC6 specific–), and benzamide-based (MS275, compound 106). Their potencies and selectivities vary, but most of them can be considered pan-HDACs inhibitors (Kazantsev and Thompson, 2008).

Several of these compounds have been studied in the transgenic SOD1 mouse model. Trichostatin A induced a modest improvement in motor function and survival as well as protection against motor neuron death, axonal degeneration, muscle atrophy and neuromuscular junction denervation; these effects were attributed to reduced gliosis and upregulation of the glutamate transporter (GLT-1) in the spinal cord (Yoo and Ko, 2011).

VPA is a drug currently in clinical use for other neurological disorders (such as epilepsy and bipolar disorder) due to its numerous mechanisms of action, including HDAC inhibition (Monti et al., 2009). VPA was tested in vivo in the transgenic ALS SOD1 mice, where it did not improve survival or motor performance, but it did improve the acetylation status in the spinal cord through the restoration of the cAMP response element binding protein (CREB) levels in motor neurons and slightly prevented motor neuron death (Rouaux et al., 2007). VPA has already been tested in ALS patients in one clinical trial, showing no benefits in survival or in disease progression in doses commonly used to treat epilepsy (Piepers et al., 2009).

Sodium phenylbutyrate (SPB), another pan-HDAC inhibitor, was shown to extend survival and motor performance in the transgenic ALS SOD1 animal model, and these effects were attributed to an upregulation in the expression of nuclear factor κB (NF-κB), the active form of the inhibitory subunit of NF-κB (i-κB) and of beta cell lymphoma 2 (bcl-2) proteins, all involved in survival and stress responses (Ryu et al., 2005). SPB efficacy has been tested also in combinations with other agents with different mechanisms of action, in the same experimental model. For example, the combination of SPB with riluzole potentiated the beneficial effects of SPB on survival and motor performance, although the authors did not address the possible mechanisms (Del Signore et al., 2009). SPB has also been tested in combination with an antioxidant agent (AEOL 10150), where it was found that this combination extended survival more than either treatment alone (Petri et al., 2006). Finally, it is worth to emphasize that SPB has already been tested in a phase 2 clinical trial, where its effects on histone acetylation status, safety and tolerability were addressed; no toxic effects were noted, and significant increases were observed in the blood histone acetylation status, but the therapeutic efficacy of such treatment was not studied (Cudkowicz et al., 2009).

HISTONE DEACETYLASES: ROLE OF SIRTUINS IN MOTOR NEURON DEGENERATION

Class III HDACs, also called SIRT, are the most divergent class from the rest of the family. This class includes seven members (SIRT1 to SIRT7) with various cellular localizations and preferred enzymatic targets, but what makes unique this class is the dependence of nicotine adenine dinucleotide (NAD^+) to perform their catalytic deacetylation and mono-ADP-ribosyl transferase activities (Michan and Sinclair, 2007). SIRT1, SIRT2, SIRT3 and SIRT5 have predominant histone deacetylase activity (Haigis and Sinclair, 2010). SIRT1, SIRT6 and SIRT7 are located in the nucleus. SIRT1 has a preference for euchromatin and can be shuttled to the cytoplasm, depending on the cell type and the developmental stage (Tanno et al., 2007). SIRT6 tends to associate with heterochromatin and SIRT7 is located in the nucleolus.

SIRT2 resides mostly in the cytoplasm, having an important role in regulation cytoskeletal dynamics. SIRT3, SIRT4 and SIRT5 are mitochondrial (Michan and Sinclair, 2007).

SIRT are named after the silent information regulator 2 (sir2) gene in yeast. When overexpressed, the product of this gene extended the lifespan of budding yeast by repressing genomic instability (Kaeberlein et al., 1999). After that discovery, it was learned that SIR2-like genes or SIRT are found in most organisms, where they regulate basic vital functions. In mammals, sirtuin activation or overexpression do not extend lifespan, but appear to be involved in the benefits of calorie restriction, are responsive to environmental stimuli (e.g., daylight and cell stress), and play important roles in numerous human diseases, such as cancer, diabetes, cardiovascular disease and neurodegeneration (Haigis and Sinclair, 2010).

The catalytic deacetylase activity of SIRT is performed on histones and on other proteins, and this ability place SIRT in a privileged position to exert their actions on the genome through direct and indirect pathways. Among the non-histone protein substrates, the peroxisome proliferator-activated receptor gamma coactivator 1 alpha (PGC1-α; Cantó and Auwerx, 2009) and the forkhead box O3a (FoxO3a) transcription factor (Zhao et al., 2011b) are two of the most studied, and their relation to ALS will be discussed below. Also, SIRT play an important role as cellular energy sensors (Smith et al., 2000), due to their dependence on NAD^+ as a substrate (Imai et al., 2000); in humans, SIRT1-3 and 5 have shown in vitro NAD^+-dependent deacetylating activity (Smith et al., 2000). Therefore, SIRT provide a connection between cellular energy states and transcriptional control (Li, 2013).

SIRT have a widespread distribution in the mammalian tissues, including the nervous system. In the mouse, rat and human CNS, SIRT1 mRNA localization was found to be ubiquitous and prominent in various tissues (such as all regions of spinal cord, hippocampus, basal ganglia, brain stem and cerebellum); SIRT1 expression is confined to the neuronal nucleus in parvalbumin (GABAergic) and tyrosine hydroxylase (dopaminergic) neurons (Zakhary et al., 2010). SIRT1 expression was increased in cerebral cortex (especially in the pyramidal cell layer), hippocampus, thalamus and spinal cord in symptomatic SOD1 G93A mice, but spinal motor neurons were not studied in detail; these changes were interpreted as a stress response to the neurotoxic form of SOD1 (Lee et al., 2012).

PROTECTIVE EFFECTS OF SIRTUINS ACTIVATION

In contrast to other HDACs, the activity of SIRT in the CNS results in neuroprotection. Among the agents with protective action are the polyphenols (vegetal compounds that serve hormonal and protective function in these organisms), particularly resveratrol, which is present in grapes and in red wine, and SRT1720, a synthetic compound derived from resveratrol. These compounds activate selectively both SIRT1 and SIRT2, whereas activators of the remaining SIRT have not yet been described (Kazantsev and Thompson, 2008).

There is a paucity of studies that address SIRT role in ALS pathology. In primary cortical cultures of transgenic SOD1 G93A mice, resveratrol protected against neuron death, and this protection was due to the activation of SIRT1 (Kim et al., 2007). In agreement with these results, in another in vitro study of SOD1 G93A murine motor neurons, it was found that SIRT1 expression was downregulated, and resveratrol prevented neuronal death (Wang et al., 2011). However, the neuroprotection exerted by resveratrol may be due to the stimulation of the activities of other enzymes such as AMP protein kinase (Dasgupta and Milbrandt, 2007). In our laboratory we have recently found that the administration of resveratrol directly in the lumbar spinal cord in rats delays the progress of motor deficits induced by chronic AMPA (α-amino-3-hydroxy-5-methyl-4-isoxazol-propionate) infusion in the lumbar spinal cord (Lazo-Gómez and Tapia, in preparation, an in vivo model of excitotoxic motor neuron death (Tovar-y-Romo et al., 2007).

The downstream effectors of SIRT that confer protection in neurodegenerative settings are beginning to be elucidated. For example, in a transgenic mouse model of Huntington's disease, SIRT1 overexpression exerted its beneficial effects through the deacetylation of FoxO3a and p53 (Jiang et al., 2012). This relation has not been explicitly addressed in ALS experimental models, but there is evidence of the role of SIRT1 effectors in motor neuron death. FoxO3a is a transcriptional factor involved in determining cell fate (survival or apoptosis) in stressful situations, such as starvation and oxidative stress. It has been shown that SIRT1 modulates FoxO3a activities through the deacetylation of specific lysine residues, resulting in activation or inhibition, and this depends on the deacetylated lysine position or on FoxO3a cellular location (nucleus or cytoplasm) (Eijkelenboom and Burgering, 2013). In an in vitro study of motor neuron death induced by several insults (excitotoxicity, the overexpression of mutant SOD1, of mutant $p150^{glued}$ or of poly-glutamin expanded androgen receptor), targeted expression of FoxO3a to the nucleus (where it can modulate the transcription of its target genes) by genetic or pharmacologic means prevented neuron death (Mojsilovic-Petrovic et al., 2009). This is in contrast with other in vitro studies, where motor neuron cultures deprived of trophic support were found to overexpress Fas ligand (FasL), due to FoxO3a translocation to the nucleus, thus resulting in cell death (Barthélémy et al., 2004). The reason for this discrepancy is not clear, but it could be due to differences in the death process triggered by the various insults used, which might be regulated in different ways by FoxO3a.

Another well studied SIRT1 effector is PGC1-α, a transcriptional coactivator involved in the modulation of the responses necessary to overcome cellular energetic deficiencies, such as the stimulation of mitochondrial biogenesis and the respiratory rate, and the increase of the uptake and metabolism of energy substrates. SIRT1 physically interacts with, deacetylates and activates PGC1-α (Cantó and Auwerx, 2009). It has been shown that PGC1-α plays a role in ALS pathology, because decreased mRNA and protein levels of this coactivator were found in both transgenic mice and in patients with the sporadic form of the disease, in muscle and in spinal cord tissues (Thau et al., 2012). Moreover, PGC1-α may play a therapeutic role, as shown by two studies in the transgenic mouse model. Zhao et al. (2011a) used a targeted overexpression of PGC1-α in neurons of SOD1 transgenic mice, which modestly increased survival and significantly improved motor performance; these changes were due to the restoration of mitochondrial activities. This is in contrast to the findings of other study in a double transgenic mouse overexpressing PGC1-α and mutant SOD1 in all tissues, showing that survival was not increased albeit motor performance improved and motor neuron loss was ameliorated. An augmentation of the excitatory amino acid transporter protein 2 (EAAT2) in astrocytes was noted in the double transgenic, suggesting that PGC1-α could exert its beneficial effects through other mechanisms (Liang et al., 2011). Regarding other sirtuin isoforms, such as SIRT3, a mitochondrial sirtuin, Song et al. (2013) showed, in primary spinal motor neuronal cell cultures of transgenic SOD1 G93A mice, that the overexpression of SIRT3 and of PGC1-α protected against mitochondrial fragmentation and neuronal cell death, although the authors did not demonstrate the relation between SIRT3 and PGC1-α.

These findings indicate that sirtuin activation protects against motor neuron degeneration, although some findings in different experimental models suggest that activators may protect through other mechanisms (Tang, 2010) or even that sirtuin inhibition may be protective. For example, in a model of brain ischemia sirtuin inhibition through nicotinamide administration conferred neuroprotection by preserving NAD^+ cellular levels (Liu et al., 2009a).

CONCLUSION

The opportunities for a really effective therapy for ALS are scarce, and therefore HDAC inhibition and sirtuin activation merit further investigation. Studies on the modification of the activity of these enzymes in in vitro and in vivo experimental models of neurodegeneration, including ALS, have given valuable information suggesting potential therapeutic opportunities for this disease. Nevertheless, the mechanisms underlying such effects are poorly understood and their clarification is necessary for designing more specific and potent treatment strategies. Accumulated evidence on sirtuin activation has provided valuable information about the molecular pathways that could be relevant to halt motor neuron degeneration, such as those related to cellular energetic state and PGC1-α. Not all types of HDACs have been evaluated in ALS models and the effects, toxicity, dosage, timing, and mode of administration of specific drugs that inhibit HDAC or activate SIRT have not been established. Of note is the fact that the most widely used model of ALS in which these strategies have been studied is the transgenic rodent with mutations in the human SOD1 gene, but this represent only about 2% of all ALS cases. Novel experimental models of motor neuron degeneration in vivo are clearly needed before safely moving these drugs to clinical trials for a disorder that has proved recalcitrant to all, past and current, therapeutic procedures.

ACKNOWLEDGMENTS

This work was supported by Dirección General de Asuntos del Personal Académico, UNAM (project IN201013) and Consejo Nacional de Ciencia y Tecnología (CONACYT), México (project 128229). Rafael Lazo-Gómez and Uri N. Ramírez-Jarquín are recipients of a CONACyT scholarship.

REFERENCES

Barthélémy, C., Henderson, C. E., and Pettmann, B. (2004). Foxo3a induces motoneuron death through the Fas pathway in cooperation with JNK. *BMC Neurosci.* 5:48. doi: 10.1186/1471-2202-5-48

Bhaumik, S. R., Smith, E., and Shilatifard, A. (2007). Covalent modifications of histones during development and disease pathogenesis. *Nat. Struct. Mol. Biol.* 14, 1008–1016. doi: 10.1038/nsmb1337

Broide, R. S., Redwine, J. M., Aftahi, N., Young, W., Bloom, F. E., and Winrow, C. J. (2007). Distribution of histone deacetylases 1–11 in the rat brain. *J. Mol. Neurosci.* 31, 47–58. doi: 10.1007/bf02686117

Cantó, C., and Auwerx, J. (2009). PGC-1alpha, SIRT1 and AMPK, an energy sensing network that controls energy expenditure. *Curr. Opin. Lipidol.* 20, 98–105. doi: 10.1097/mol.0b013e328328d0a4

Cantó, C., Gerhart-Hines, Z., Feige, J. N., Lagouge, M., Noriega, L., Milne, J. C., et al. (2009). AMPK regulates energy expenditure by modulating NAD+ metabolism and SIRT1 activity. *Nature* 458, 1056–1060. doi: 10.1038/nature07813

Cha, J. H. (2000). Transcriptional dysregulation in Huntington's disease. *Trends Neurosci.* 23, 387–392. doi: 10.1016/s0166-2236(00)01609-x

Chen, Y. T., Zang, X. F., Pan, J., Zhu, X. L., Chen, F., Chen, Z. B., et al. (2012). Expression patterns of histone deacetylases in experimental stroke and potential targets for neuroprotection. *Clin. Exp. Pharmacol. Physiol.* 39, 751–758. doi: 10.1111/j.1440-1681.2012.05729.x

Corcoran, L. J., Mitchison, T. J., and Liu, Q. (2004). A novel action of histone deacetylase inhibitors in a protein aggresome disease model. *Curr. Biol.* 14, 488–492. doi: 10.1016/j.cub.2004.03.003

Corona, J. C., Tovar-y-Romo, L. B., and Tapia, R. (2007). Glutamate excitotoxicity and therapeutic targets for amyotrophic lateral sclerosis. *Expert Opin. Ther. Targets* 11, 1415–14128. doi: 10.1517/14728222.11.11.1415

Cudkowicz, M. E., Andres, P. L., Macdonald, S. A., Bedlack, R. S., Choudry, R., Brown, R. H., et al. (2009). Phase 2 study of sodium phenylbutyrate in ALS. *Amyotroph. Lateral Scler.* 10, 99–106. doi: 10.1080/17482960802320487

Dasgupta, B., and Milbrandt, J. (2007). Resveratrol stimulates AMP kinase activity in neurons. *Proc. Natl. Acad. Sci. U S A* 104, 7217–7222. doi: 10.1073/pnas.0610068104

de Ruijter, A. J., van Gennip, A. H., Caron, H. N., Kemp, S., and van Kuilenburg, A. B. (2003). Histone deacetylases (HDACs): characterization of the classical HDAC family. *Biochem. J.* 370, 737–749. doi: 10.1042/bj20021321

Del Signore, S. J., Amante, D. J., Kim, J., Stack, E. C., Goodrich, S., Cormier, K., et al. (2009). Combined riluzole and sodium phenylbutyrate therapy in transgenic amyotrophic lateral sclerosis mice. *Amyotroph. Lateral Scler.* 10, 85–94. doi: 10.1080/17482960802226148

Eijkelenboom, A., and Burgering, B. M. (2013). FOXOs: signalling integrators for homeostasis maintenance. *Nat. Rev. Mol. Cell Biol.* 14, 83–97. doi: 10.1038/nrm3507

Figueroa-Romero, C., Hur, J., Bender, D. E., Delaney, C. E., Cataldo, M. D., Smith, A. L., et al. (2012). Identification of epigenetically altered genes in sporadic amyotrophic lateral sclerosis. *PLoS One* 7:e52672. doi: 10.1371/journal.pone.0052672

Frew, A. J., Johnstone, R. W., and Bolden, J. E. (2009). Enhancing the apoptotic and therapeutic effects of HDAC inhibitors. *Cancer Lett.* 280, 125–133. doi: 10.1016/j.canlet.2009.02.042

Haigis, M. C., and Sinclair, D. A. (2010). Mammalian sirtuins: biological insights and disease relevance. *Annu. Rev. Pathol.* 5, 253–295. doi: 10.1146/annurev.pathol.4.110807.092250

Hubbert, C., Guardiola, A., Shao, R., Kawaguchi, Y., Ito, A., Nixon, A., et al. (2002). HDAC6 is a microtubule-associated deacetylase. *Nature* 417, 455–458. doi: 10.1038/417455a

Imai, S., Armstrong, C. M., Kaeberlein, M., and Guarente, L. (2000). Transcriptional silencing and longevity protein Sir2 is an NAD-dependent histone deacetylase. *Nature* 403, 795–800. doi: 10.1038/35001622

Janssen, C., Schmalbach, S., Boeselt, S., Sarlette, A., Dengler, R., and Petri, S. (2010). Differential histone deacetylase mRNA expression patterns in amyotrophic lateral sclerosis. *J. Neuropathol. Exp. Neurol.* 69, 573–581. doi: 10.1097/nen.0b013e3181ddd404

Jiang, M., Wang, J., Fu, J., Du, L., Jeong, H., West, T., et al. (2012). Neuroprotective role of Sirt1 in mammalian models of Huntington's disease through activation of multiple Sirt1 targets. *Nat. Med.* 18, 153–158. doi: 10.1038/nm.2558

Kaeberlein, M., McVey, M., and Guarente, L. (1999). The SIR2/3/4 complex and SIR2 alone promote longevity in Saccharomyces cerevisiae by two different mechanisms. *Genes Dev.* 13, 2570–2580. doi: 10.1101/gad.13.19.2570

Kanai, H., Sawa, A., Chen, R. W., Leeds, P., and Chuang, D. M. (2004). Valproic acid inhibits histone deacetylase activity and suppresses excitotoxicity-induced GAPDH nuclear accumulation and apoptotic death in neurons. *Pharmacogenomics J.* 4, 336–344. doi: 10.1038/sj.tpj.6500269

Kazantsev, A. G., and Thompson, L. M. (2008). Therapeutic application of histone deacetylase inhibitors for central nervous system disorders. *Nat. Rev. Drug Discov.* 7, 854–868. doi: 10.1038/nrd2681

Kernochan, L. E., Russo, M. L., Woodling, N. S., Huynh, T. N., Avila, A. M., Fischbeck, K. H., et al. (2005). The role of histone acetylation in SMN gene expression. *Hum. Mol. Genet.* 14, 1171–1182. doi: 10.1093/hmg/ddi130

Kim, D., Nguyen, M. D., Dobbin, M. M., Fischer, A., Sananbenesi, F., Rodgers, J. T., et al. (2007). SIRT1 deacetylase protects against neurodegeneration in models for Alzheimer's disease and amyotrophic lateral sclerosis. *EMBO J.* 26, 3169–3179. doi: 10.1038/sj.emboj.7601758

Kim, S. H., Shanware, N. P., Bowler, M. J., and Tibbetts, R. S. (2010). Amyotrophic lateral sclerosis-associated proteins TDP-43 and FUS/TLS function in a common biochemical complex to co-regulate HDAC6 mRNA. *J. Biol. Chem.* 285, 34097–34105. doi: 10.1074/jbc.m110.154831

Kirby, J., Halligan, E., Baptista, M. J., Allen, S., Heath, P. R., Holden, H., et al. (2005). Mutant SOD1 alters the motor neuronal transcriptome: implications for familial ALS. *Brain* 128, 1686–1706. doi: 10.1093/brain/awh503

Kouzarides, T. (2007). Chromatin modifications and their function. *Cell* 128, 693–705. doi: 10.1016/j.cell.2007.02.005

Lee, J. C., Shin, J. H., Park, B. W., Kim, G. S., Kim, J. C., Kang, K. S., et al. (2012). Region-specific changes in the immunoreactivity of SIRT1 expression in the central nervous system of SOD1(G93A) transgenic mice as an in vivo model of amyotrophic lateral sclerosis. *Brain Res.* 1433, 20–28. doi: 10.1016/j.brainres.2011.11.019

Li, X. (2013). SIRT1 and energy metabolism. *Acta Biochim. Biophys. Sin. (Shanghai)* 45, 51–60. doi: 10.1093/abbs/gms108

Liang, H., Ward, W. F., Jang, Y. C., Bhattacharya, A., Bokov, A. F., Li, Y., et al. (2011). PGC-1alpha protects neurons and alters disease progression in an amyotrophic lateral sclerosis mouse model. *Muscle Nerve* 44, 947–956. doi: 10.1002/mus.22217

Liu, D., Gharavi, R., Pitta, M., Gleichmann, M., and Mattson, M. P. (2009a). Nicotinamide prevents NAD^+ depletion and protects neurons against excitotoxicity and cerebral ischemia: NAD^+ consumption by SIRT1 may endanger energetically compromised neurons. *Neuromolecular Med.* 11, 28–42. doi: 10.1007/s12017-009-8058-1

Liu, H., Hu, Q., D'Ercole A, J., and Ye, P. (2009b). Histone deacetylase 11 regulates oligodendrocyte-specific gene expression and cell development in OL-1 oligodendroglia cells. *Glia* 57, 1–12. doi: 10.1002/glia.20729

Liu, H., Hu, Q., Kaufman, A., D'Ercole, A. J., and Ye, P. (2008). Developmental expression of histone deacetylase 11 in the murine brain. *J. Neurosci. Res.* 86, 537–543. doi: 10.1002/jnr.21521

Michan, S., and Sinclair, D. (2007). Sirtuins in mammals: insights into their biological function. *Biochem. J.* 404, 1–13. doi: 10.1042/bj20070140

Mojsilovic-Petrovic, J., Nedelsky, N., Boccitto, M., Mano, I., Georgiades, S. N., Zhou, W., et al. (2009). FOXO3a is broadly neuroprotective in vitro and in vivo against insults implicated in motor neuron diseases. *J. Neurosci.* 29, 8236–8247. doi: 10.1523/jneurosci.1805-09.2009

Monti, B., Polazzi, E., and Contestabile, A. (2009). Biochemical, molecular and epigenetic mechanisms of valproic acid neuroprotection. *Curr. Mol. Pharmacol.* 2, 95–109. doi: 10.2174/1874-470210902010095

Pandey, U. B., Nie, Z., Batlevi, Y., McCray, B. A., Ritson, G. P., Nedelsky, N. B., et al. (2007). HDAC6 rescues neurodegeneration and provides an essential link between autophagy and the UPS. *Nature* 447, 859–863. doi: 10.1038/nature05853

Petri, S., Kiaei, M., Kipiani, K., Chen, J., Calingasan, N. Y., Crow, J. P., et al. (2006). Additive neuroprotective effects of a histone deacetylase inhibitor and a catalytic antioxidant in a transgenic mouse model of amyotrophic lateral sclerosis. *Neurobiol. Dis.* 22, 40–49. doi: 10.1016/j.nbd.2005.09.013

Piepers, S., Veldink, J. H., de Jong, S. W., van der Tweel, I., van der Pol, W. L., Uijtendaal, E. V., et al. (2009). Randomized sequential trial of valproic acid in amyotrophic lateral sclerosis. *Ann. Neurol.* 66, 227–234. doi: 10.1002/ana.21620

Robakis, N. K. (2003). An Alzheimer's disease hypothesis based on transcriptional dysregulation. *Amyloid* 10, 80–85. doi: 10.3109/13506120309041729

Robberecht, W., and Philips, T. (2013). The changing scene of amyotrophic lateral sclerosis. *Nat. Rev. Neurosci.* 14, 248–264. doi: 10.1038/nrn3430

Rouaux, C., Panteleeva, I., Rene, F., Gonzalez de Aguilar, J. L., Echaniz-Laguna, A., Dupuis, L., et al. (2007). Sodium valproate exerts neuroprotective effects in vivo through CREB-binding protein-dependent mechanisms but does not improve survival in an amyotrophic lateral sclerosis mouse model. *J. Neurosci.* 27, 5535–5545. doi: 10.1523/jneurosci.1139-07.2007

Ryu, H., Smith, K., Camelo, S. I., Carreras, I., Lee, J., Iglesias, A. H., et al. (2005). Sodium phenylbutyrate prolongs survival and regulates expression of anti-apoptotic genes in transgenic amyotrophic lateral sclerosis mice. *J. Neurochem.* 93, 1087–1098. doi: 10.1111/j.1471-4159.2005.03077.x

Santa-Cruz, L. D., Ramírez-Jarquín, U. N., and Tapia, R. (2012). "Role of mitochondrial dysfunction in motor neuron degeneration in ALS," in *Amyotrophic Lateral Sclerosis*, ed M. H. Maurer (In Tech, Rijeka, Croatia). 197–224.

Selvi, B. R., Cassel, J. C., Kundu, T. K., and Boutillier, A. L. (2010). Tuning acetylation levels with HAT activators: therapeutic strategy in neurodegenerative diseases. *Biochim. Biophys. Acta* 1799, 840–853. doi: 10.1016/j.bbagrm.2010.08.012

Smith, J. S., Brachmann, C. B., Celic, I., Kenna, M. A., Muhammad, S., Starai, V. J., et al. (2000). A phylogenetically conserved NAD+-dependent protein deacetylase activity in the Sir2 protein family. *Proc. Natl. Acad. Sci. U S A* 97, 6658–6663. doi: 10.1073/pnas.97.12.6658

Song, W., Song, Y., Kincaid, B., Bossy, B., and Bossy-Wetzel, E. (2013). Mutant SOD1G93A triggers mitochondrial fragmentation in spinal cord motor neurons: neuroprotection by SIRT3 and PGC-1alpha. *Neurobiol. Dis.* 51, 72–81. doi: 10.1016/j.nbd.2012.07.004

Tang, B. L. (2010). Resveratrol is neuroprotective because it is not a direct activator of Sirt1- A hypothesis. *Brain Res. Bull.* 81, 359–361. doi: 10.1016/j.brainresbull.2009.12.007

Tanno, M., Sakamoto, J., Miura, T., Shimamoto, K., and Horio, Y. (2007). Nucleocytoplasmic shuttling of the NAD+-dependent histone deacetylase SIRT1. *J. Biol. Chem.* 282, 6823–6832. doi: 10.1074/jbc.m609554200

Thau, N., Knippenberg, S., Korner, S., Rath, K. J., Dengler, R., and Petri, S. (2012). Decreased mRNA expression of PGC-1alpha and PGC-1alpha-regulated factors in the SOD1G93A ALS mouse model and in human sporadic ALS. *J. Neuropathol. Exp. Neurol.* 71, 1064–1074. doi: 10.1097/nen.0b013e318275df4b

Todd, P. K., Oh, S. Y., Krans, A., Pandey, U. B., Di Prospero, N. A., Min, K. T., et al. (2010). Histone deacetylases suppress CGG repeat-induced neurodegeneration via transcriptional silencing in models of fragile X tremor ataxia syndrome. *PLoS Genet.* 6:e1001240. doi: 10.1371/journal.pgen.1001240

Tovar-y-Romo, L. B., Zepeda, A., and Tapia, R. (2007). Vascular endothelial growth factor prevents paralysis and motoneuron death in a rat model of excitotoxic spinal cord neurodegeneration. *J. Neuropathol. Exp. Neurol.* 66, 913–922. doi: 10.1097/nen.0b013e3181567c16

Wang, J., Zhang, Y., Tang, L., Zhang, N., and Fan, D. (2011). Protective effects of resveratrol through the up-regulation of SIRT1 expression in the mutant hSOD1–G93A-bearing motor neuron-like cell culture model of amyotrophic lateral sclerosis. *Neurosci. Lett.* 503, 250–255. doi: 10.1016/j.neulet.2011.08.047

Yacoubian, T. A., Cantuti-Castelvetri, I., Bouzou, B., Asteris, G., McLean, P. J., Hyman, B. T., et al. (2008). Transcriptional dysregulation in a transgenic model of Parkinson disease. *Neurobiol. Dis.* 29, 515–528. doi: 10.1016/j.nbd.2007.11.008

Yao, Z. G., Zhang, L., Huang, L., Zhu, H., Liu, Y., Ma, C. M., et al. (2013). Regional and cell-type specific distribution of HDAC2 in the adult mouse brain. *Brain Struct. Funct.* 218, 563–573. doi: 10.1007/s00429-012-0416-3

Yoo, Y. E., and Ko, C. P. (2011). Treatment with trichostatin A initiated after disease onset delays disease progression and increases survival in a mouse model of amyotrophic lateral sclerosis. *Exp. Neurol.* 231, 147–159. doi: 10.1016/j.expneurol.2011.06.003

Zakhary, S. M., Ayubcha, D., Dileo, J. N., Jose, R., Leheste, J. R., Horowitz, J. M., et al. (2010). Distribution analysis of deacetylase SIRT1 in rodent and human nervous systems. *Anat. Rec. (Hoboken)* 293, 1024–1032. doi: 10.1002/ar.21116

Zhao, W., Varghese, M., Yemul, S., Pan, Y., Cheng, A., Marano, P., et al. (2011a). Peroxisome proliferator activator receptor gamma coactivator-1alpha (PGC-1alpha) improves motor performance and survival in a mouse model of amyotrophic lateral sclerosis. *Mol. Neurodegener.* 6:51. doi: 10.1186/1750-1326-6-51

Zhao, Y., Wang, Y., and Zhu, W. G. (2011b). Applications of post-translational modifications of FoxO family proteins in biological functions. *J. Mol. Cell Biol.* 3, 276–282. doi: 10.1093/jmcb/mjr013

Zhou, V. W., Goren, A., and Bernstein, B. E. (2011). Charting histone modifications and the functional organization of mammalian genomes. *Nat. Rev. Genet.* 12, 7–18. doi: 10.1038/nrg2905

9

Well-being in amyotrophic lateral sclerosis: a pilot experience sampling study

Ruben G. L. Real[1]*, Thorsten Dickhaus[2], Albert Ludolph[3], Martin Hautzinger[4] and Andrea Kübler[1,5]

[1] *Department of Psychology I, Institute of Psychology, University of Würzburg, Würzburg, Germany*
[2] *Weierstrass Institute for Applied Analysis and Stochastics, Research Group "Stochastic Algorithms and Nonparametric Statistics", Berlin, Germany*
[3] *Department of Neurology, University of Ulm, Ulm, Germany*
[4] *Department of Clinical Psychology and Psychotherapy, University of Tübingen, Tübingen, Germany*
[5] *Institute for Medical Psychology and Behavioural Neurobiology, University of Tübingen, Tübingen, Germany*

Edited by:
Francesco Pagnini, Catholic University of Milan, Italy

Reviewed by:
Michelle Dow Keawphalouk, Harvard/MIT, USA
Donatella Mattia, IRCCS Fondazione Santa Lucia, Italy
Eleonora Volpato, Fondazione Don Gnocchi, Milan, Italy

****Correspondence:***
Ruben G. L. Real, Department of Psychology I, Insitute of Psychology, University of Würzburg, Marcusstr. 9-11, 97070 Würzburg, Germany
e-mail: ruben.real@uni-wuerzburg.de

Objective: The aim of this longitudinal study was to identify predictors of instantaneous well-being in patients with amyotrophic lateral sclerosis (ALS). Based on flow theory well-being was expected to be highest when perceived demands and perceived control were in balance, and that thinking about the past would be a risk factor for rumination which would in turn reduce well-being.

Methods: Using the experience sampling method, data on current activities, associated aspects of perceived demands, control, and well-being were collected from 10 patients with ALS three times a day for two weeks.

Results: Results show that perceived control was uniformly and positively associated with well-being, but that demands were only positively associated with well-being when they were perceived as controllable. Mediation analysis confirmed thinking about the past, but not thinking about the future, to be a risk factor for rumination and reduced well-being.

Discussion: Findings extend our knowledge of factors contributing to well-being in ALS as not only perceived control but also perceived demands can contribute to well-being. They further show that a focus on present experiences might contribute to increased well-being.

Keywords: amyotrophic lateral sclerosis, ALS, coping, well-being, experience sampling, ESM, reminiscence, rumination

1. INTRODUCTION

Amyotrophic Lateral Sclerosis (ALS) is a rare neurodegenerative disease characterized by progressive paralysis (Logroscino et al., 2008). In the absence of a cure (Logroscino et al., 2008, 2010) the treatment of ALS focuses on the alleviation of symptoms and the maintenance of the best possible degree of functioning (Clarke et al., 2001). A rich literature exists on factors influencing quality of life and coping with the disease (c.f. Pagnini, 2013). For example, different styles of coping (Matuz et al., 2010; Montel et al., 2012a), spirituality (McLeod and Clarke, 2007), or care-giver relations (Chiò et al., 2004) have all been related to psychosocial well-being in patients with ALS. In line with psychological theories on subjective quality of life (e.g., Rapkin and Schwartz, 2004) the great physical burden of ALS shows no simple relationship to well-being, with many studies showing small and insignificant correlations (Robbins et al., 2001; Pagnini, 2013) or even positive associations (Lulé et al., 2009). However, many of the questionnaires used in research on well-being and quality of life in patients with ALS require participants to generate aggregate statements about their experiences, e.g., by asking them how they felt (on average) during the past days (Cohen et al., 1995; Robbins et al., 2001) or even weeks (Hammer et al., 2008). Thus, little is known about the factors which are associated with instantaneous well-being, i.e., well-being as it fluctuates from moment to moment throughout the day.

In this study, therefore, the experience sampling method (ESM) was used (Larson and Csikszentmihalyi, 1983; Stone et al., 2003) to analyze possible predictors of well-being. Experience sampling, originally developed because of concerns of how accurate people are in "reconstructing their experience[s] after the fact" (Larson and Csikszentmihalyi, 1983, p. 42), asks participants to record their experiences directly at the moment of sampling. By randomizing sampling times throughout the study period, it is possible to collect representative data on the participants' experiences, such as well-being, and possible influencing factors (Shiffman et al., 2008; Scollon et al., 2009).

At its most basic level, flow theory assumes that the physical and mental activities people engage in, influence their well-being. More specifically, it predicts that well-being is highest if perceived control and perceived demands match in a given situation (Csikszentmihalyi, 1990). Any imbalance between demands and abilities results in reduced well-being, e.g., feelings of frustration, when demands exceed abilities, or of boredom, when abilities exceed situational demands (Csikszentmihalyi, 1990). Given that the progressive loss of motor functions requires constant adaptation and change (King et al., 2009), we hypothesized that finding this balance would be of crucial importance in patients with ALS. A second prediction of flow theory is that well-being depends on the extent to which thoughts are focused on present experiences (Schmidt et al., 2007). However, the little data available from patients with ALS is heterogeneous. Support comes from a study by Plahuta et al. (2002), which found that hopelessness, a future oriented direction of thought, is related to increased suffering and higher intentions of suicide in patients with ALS. However, the use of the coping strategy "planning" (Carver, 1997), an arguably more direct and less negatively valenced indicator of "thoughts directed toward the future" does not seem to be strongly related to well-being (Montel et al., 2012b). Qualitative findings from interviews with patients are also mixed (Fanos et al., 2008). On the one hand, several subjects indicated the use of "living in the moment" as a successful coping strategy while others sought consolation in remembering positive past experiences. The constant adaptation and change required for coping with ALS (King et al., 2009), necessitates disengaging from goals no longer attainable, or anticipating disengagement from goals which may become unattainable in the future. Generally, confrontation with unattainable goals—even more so when the factors which make a goal unattainable are essentially uncontrollable as is the case in ALS (Nolen-Hoeksema et al., 2008)—has been shown to be a risk factor for rumination, and, thus, decreased well-being (Nolen-Hoeksema, 1991; Martin and Tesser, 1996). Therefore, we hypothesized that thinking about the past and future would be associated with reduced well-being, and that rumination would mediate this effect.

2. METHODS

2.1. PATIENTS

A convenience sample of ten patients (seven male; see **Table 1**) fulfilling the revised El Escorial criteria for clinically definite ALS (Brooks et al., 2000) was recruited via the Institute for Medical Psychology and Behavioral Neurobiology of the University of Tübingen and the Department of Neurology of the University of Ulm. All participants contacted for inclusion agreed to participate in this study. Mean time since diagnosis was 38.10 months ($SD = 35.96$, range = 12–129). One patient had a percutaneous endoscopic gastrostomy (PEG), and three were non-invasively ventilated. The study was approved by the Ethical Review Board of the Medical Faculty, University of Tübingen. Written informed consent was obtained from all participants.

Table 1 | Patients' Characteristics.

	ALSFRS-R	ADI-12	well-being	*M*	*SD*	Range
Age (years)	0.52	0.32	−0.09	52.30	11.56	35–71
ALSFRS-R		$0.59^{\#}$	-0.75^{*}	19.20	10.57	1–35
ADI-12			$-0.63^{\#}$	20.70	7.41	12–34
well-being				4.79	0.69	3.93–5.86

Intercorrelations, means, and standard correlations.

Note: $N = 10$. $^{\#}p < 0.10$, $^{*}p < 0.05$.

2.2. PROCEDURE

We collected data on well-being, perceived demands, perceived control, temporal direction of thoughts and rumination over the course of two weeks at three randomly chosen times per day using the ESM. Patients were provided with a pager that beeped when they should record their experiences using a standardized questionnaire. To avoid interference with morning and evening caring routines, sampling was restricted to between 10 a.m. and 6 p.m. Patients were instructed to answer the ESM-questionnaires immediately after the beep and while answering the questions to refer only to the situation in which the beep occurred. At the beginning of the two weeks study period, patients were visited at their homes and the procedure was explained in full detail and questions concerning the study protocol were answered.

2.3. MEASURES

Functional status was assessed with the revised ALS Functional Rating Scale (ALSFRS-R) (Cedarbaum et al., 1999), and the extent of depressive symptoms with the ALS specific ALS Depression Inventory (ADI-12) (Hammer et al., 2008). These standardized measures were collected once at the beginning of the two week study period.

The ESM-questionnaire used in this study was previously used by Csikszentmihalyi and Larson (1987) and assessed the extent of perceived demands and control with two items, "How challenging was your activity?" and "Was the situation under your control?" To minimize participants' burden in terms of time and effort, rumination was measured with the single item "Did your thoughts turn round in circles?" (Jong-Meyer et al., 2009) and temporal direction of thoughts with two face-valid items ("Did you look ahead/to the past?"). Each item was scored on a 10-point Likert-type scale ranging from 0 (low) to 9 (high). Patients' well-being was measured with 13 well-being-related items developed by Larson and Csikszentmihalyi (1983). Each item was scored on a 7-point Likert-type scale, and a composite score reflecting well-being was derived by averaging ESM-items of the well-being category. To determine the reliability of this scale while taking the inter-correlation of repeated measurements into account Cronbach's α was calculated across subjects for every time point during the 2-week study period, yielding 42 coefficients. Reliability of the well-being scale was satisfactory (median $\alpha = 0.86$).

Patients completed an average of 33.30 assessments (range 13–43). Fifty percent of all questionnaires were answered within 10 min and 75% within 45 min after the beep. Further analysis revealed that without the most disabled participant (one male who used a personal computer to answer the questionnaires) 75% of all questionnaires were answered within 30 min after the beep. One patient was excluded from the following analyses because of excessive numbers of missing items, leading to a final sample size of $N = 9$.

2.4. STATISTICAL ANALYSES

Random intercept multiple regression analysis was used to test the hypothesis that well-being depended on the balance of demands and control (Edwards and Cooper, 1990; Edwards, 1994, also see Supplementary Material). The analysis was also performed with functional status included as a covariate, which indicated that the results we report here were independent of functional status. Mediation analysis (MacKinnon et al., 2002; Kenny et al., 2003) was used to test the hypothesis that thinking about the past would have a negative effect on well-being and that this effect would be mediated by rumination. We report 95% confidence intervals for the mediated effect (Tofighi and MacKinnon, 2011). The same analysis was repeated for thinking about the future. Analyses were performed in R (R Development Core Team, 2011). Cohen's f^2 was calculated as a measure of the effect size (Selya et al., 2012).

3. RESULTS

Average well-being (see **Table 1**) was marginally negatively associated with symptoms of depression, but significantly positively associated with functional status. Functional status was marginally positively associated with symptoms of depression. Patient's age was not associated with functional status, symptoms of depression, or well-being.

Our first hypothesis suggested that well-being would depend on the balance of perceived control and demands. However, no support was found for this prediction (see Supplementary Material). Instead, results indicated that perceived control was associated with increased well-being ($b = 0.18$, $SE = 0.03$, $p < 0.001$, $f^2 = 0.22$), regardless of the level of perceived demands. In contrast, the effect of perceived demands depended on whether these demands were perceived as controllable: Only, if demands were perceived as *controllable*, they were associated with increased well-being ($b = 0.09$, $SE = 0.02$, $p < 0.001, f^2 = 0.17$). If demands were perceived as *uncontrollable*, the positive effect of demands was significantly reduced ($b = -0.14$, $SE = 0.05, p < 0.01, f^2 = 0.03$), rendering the effect of demands on well-being non-significant ($b = 0.02$, $SE = 0.05$, $p > 0.70$, $f^2 = 0.01$).

Our second hypothesis proposed that thinking about the past would lead to increased rumination which in turn would reduce well-being. **Table 2** shows that thinking about the past (Row 1), thinking about the future (Row 2), and rumination (Row 3) were associated with lower well-being, and that thinking about the past (Row 4) was significantly and thinking about the future (Row 5) was marginally associated with higher rumination. Mediation analysis confirmed a negative effect of thinking about the past on well-being via rumination ($b = -0.03$, 95% CI [−0.05 −0.02]). No evidence was found that the negative effect of thinking about the future on well-being was mediated via increased rumination ($b = -0.01$, 95% CI [−0.02 0.001]).

4. DISCUSSION

Little is known about how patients with ALS cope with their disease from moment to moment in daily life. Thus, in this study the ESM was used to record patients' experiences throughout the day. Despite their severe physical disability, patients were able to complete the ESM-questionnaires within a short time after the scheduled signal. These results provide evidence that even a potentially demanding procedure such as the ESM may be a valuable tool in assessing patients' thoughts, well-being and cognitive state. The relationships between functional status, presence of depressive symptoms and well-being indicated that depressive symptoms were more present and well-being was lower in early stages of the disease. This result mirrors findings of better quality of life in patients who are longer affected by the disease (Lulé et al., 2008, 2009).

Flow theory predicts that well-being depends on finding the optimal balance between perceived demands and control (Csikszentmihalyi, 1990), and we hypothesized that finding this balance would be of crucial importance in patients with ALS. However, our data did not support this hypothesis. Instead, but in line with previous findings (Plahuta et al., 2002), perceived control was associated with increased well-being, regardless of the level of perceived demands. However, our results extend this idea, by showing that increased demands can also contribute to increased well-being, as long as they are perceived as controllable. While flow theory is primarily concerned with experiences related to activities in the present, experiences may also differ in their temporal orientation. We hypothesized that if attention is not focused on the here and now, but directed toward the past or the future, this would increase the risk for rumination, which in turn would reduce well-being. Our results indicate that thinking about the past was indeed associated with decreased well-being and that this effect was mediated by rumination. While some patients may find solace in remembering the good times they have had (Fanos

Table 2 | Results of mediation analysis.

	Predicted	Predictor	*b*	*SE*	*DF*	*t*	*p*	f^2
PREDICTORS OF WELL-BEING								
1	Well-being	Thinking about the past	−0.03	0.01	250.83	−2.73	0.01	0.02
2	Well-being	Thinking about the future	−0.03	0.01	250.97	−2.08	0.04	0.01
3	Well-being	Rumination	−0.08	0.01	255.84	−5.60	<0.001	0.10
PREDICTORS OF RUMINATION								
4	Rumination	Thinking about the past	0.41	0.04	252.89	10.34	<0.001	0.40
5	Rumination	Thinking about the future	0.09	0.05	252.50	1.70	0.09	0.01
MEDIATION MODELS								
6	Well-being	Thinking about the past	0.00	0.01	247.77	0.17	0.87	
7		Rumination	−0.08	0.02	254.12	−4.79	<0.001	
8	Well-being	Thinking about the future	−0.02	0.01	250.30	−1.66	0.10	
9		Rumination	−0.08	0.01	254.83	−5.43	<0.001	

et al., 2008), reminiscing may also introduce the risk of being reminded of unattainable goals, thus, in turn, increasing the risk of reduced well-being. Likewise, thinking about the future was negatively associated with well-being; however, it was only loosely related to rumination, and no support was found for rumination mediating a negative effect of thinking about the future on well-being. We may thus speculate that thoughts about the future are not necessarily ruminative, possibly only in patients experiencing hopelessness (Plahuta et al., 2002).

4.1. LIMITATIONS AND CONSIDERATIONS FOR FUTURE STUDIES

4.1.1. Sampling

Several limiting factors of the current study deserve attention. To minimize interruption of daily routine, time slots in which patients had pre-set appointments (e.g., occupational therapy) were excluded from the experience sampling and sampling was restricted to the time between 10 a.m. and 6 p.m. This restriction may have prevented us from sampling several activities of daily living, e.g., personal hygiene, which may be very demanding and frustrating for severely ill patients (Foley et al., 2014).

4.1.2. Economic considerations

From a research perspective it is often desirable to use longer rather than shorter instruments, if only to increase reliability (Spearman, 1910). However, in a repeated measures context, this desire needs to be balanced with economic considerations, especially in a sample in which motor difficulties, e.g., when holding a pen, are common. Thus, to avoid spurious results, e.g., low well-being due to the frustrating experience of having to repeatedly answer a long questionnaire, and to reduce the risk of high levels of non-reponse (Iglesias and Torgerson, 2000) the questionnaires we used were kept as short as possible. Yet it is clear, that assessing rumination with only one item is a simplification of a complex construct. However, both empirical (Jong-Meyer et al., 2009) as well as theoretical accounts (Carver, 1996) suggest, that the item we used possesses high face validity for assessing rumination.

4.1.3. Sample size and generalizability

Finally, although not uncommon in ESM studies (e.g., Teuchmann et al., 1999), the small sample size limits generalization of results, until future studies can replicate our findings. Further, our analyses focused on within-subject variables, but between-subject factors and their interactions could also play an important role. For example, care-givers tend to underestimate the patient's quality of life (Trail et al., 2003), and it might be interesting to know, whether this is accompanied by a tendency to shield the patient from demanding activities, which according to our findings, might actually improve the patient's well-being. To the best of our knowledge, our study is the first to employ the ESM in patients with ALS. Thus, little information on appropriate sample sizes was available beforehand, demonstrating the pilot character of this study. Judging from the obtained effect sizes, mainly small to medium according to Cohen (1992), we suggest increasing sample sizes in future studies. Results from simulation studies (Snijders and Bosker, 1993) suggest, that an increase in the number of participants might be of greater interest than increasing the number of observations per participant. Further, if a research question focused primarily on between-subject factors (see above) a larger sample size would also be recommended. Thus, it should be kept in mind, that the optimal balance between number of participants and the number of observations per participant is dependent on the particular research question.

The ESM methodology has been applied in a variety of chronic diseases, e.g., in patients with cancer, chronic pain, cardiovascular diseases, or patients requiring hemodialysis (c.f. Smyth and Stone, 2003), testifying to the wide applicability of the method (c.f. Christensen et al., 2003). However, depending on the research questions, sophisticated data analysis methods, and technical equipment, e.g., electronic paging and recording devices with a user-friendly and unobstrusive interface, may be needed. Given the large challenge of living with ever progressing motor impairments, we suggest that future studies may take full advantage of the widespread availability of smartphones which lend themselves to ESM-studies (e.g., Runyan et al., 2013). Using such a system it might even become possible to densely track the evolution of coping with ALS over prolonged periods of time. However, apart from generating valuable data for research purposes, such a procedure might also affect patients' well-being, e.g., by making relations between certain situations and well-being transparent to the patient.

4.2. SUMMARY

Our results suggest that the ESM may be a valuable tool to elucidate components of coping and well-being in daily life in patients with ALS. Perceived control over challenging situations seems to be of major importance for maintaining high well-being. We further show that well-being may not only depend on perceived control, but that it also depends on the level of perceived demands. Encouraging patients to pursue, within limits, potentially demanding activities might help to improve their well-being.

Both thoughts directed toward the past and the future may negatively affect well-being, whereas rumination mediates this effect when thoughts are directed toward the past. We speculate that patients who experience poor well-being and may even be depressed might benefit from interventions which not only strengthen an internal locus of control (Nonnenmacher et al., 2013; Foley et al., 2014) but also encourage living in the present.

On a more global perspective the flow-theoretical approach and our results correspond well with recent work aiming at evaluating mindfulness-based (Kocovski et al., 2009) interventions in patients with ALS (Pagnini et al., 2014a,b). These interventions aim to help focusing on the experiences in the here and now, and thus to reduce the risk of reactive, e.g., ruminative, thoughts, which may otherwise reduce well-being or even lead to depression (Bishop et al., 2004). Our results provide further evidence for this promising approach, by highlighting the importance of the temporal direction of thoughts and the importance of perceived demands and control for the experience of well-being in patients with ALS.

FUNDING

Funding for this study was provided by a grant to Ruben G. L. Real of the research training group 1253/1 which is supported by the German Research Foundation (Deutsche Forschungsgemeinschaft, DFG) by Federal and Länder funds. The study sponsor had no role in the study design, collection, analysis or interpretation of the data, writing the manuscript, or the decision to submit the paper for publication.

ACKNOWLEDGMENTS

We thank Petra Nedele who assisted in data collection. This publication was funded by the German Research Foundation (DFG) and the University of Wuerzburg in the funding programme Open Access Publishing.

REFERENCES

Bishop, S. R., Lau, M., Shapiro, S., Carlson, L., Anderson, N. D., Carmody, J., et al. (2004). Mindfulness: a proposed operational definition. *Clin. Psychol. Sci. Pract.* 11, 230–241. doi: 10.1093/clipsy.bph077

Brooks, B. R., Miller, R. G., Swash, M., Munsat, T. L., and for the World Federation of Neurology Research Group on Motor Neuron Diseases. (2000). El escorial revisited: revised criteria for the diagnosis of amyotrophic lateral sclerosis. *Amyotroph. Lateral Scler. Other Motor Neuron Disord.* 1, 293–299. doi: 10.1080/146608200300079536

Carver, C. S. (1996). "Goal engagement and the human experience," in *Ruminative Thoughts*, Volume IX of *Advances in Social Cognition*, ed R. S. Wyer (Mahwah, NJ: Lawrence Erlbaum), 49–59.

Carver, C. S. (1997). You want to measure coping but your protocol's too long: consider the brief cope. *Int. J. Behav. Med.* 4, 92–100. doi: 10.1207/s15327558ijbm0401_6

Cedarbaum, J. M., Stambler, N., Malta, E., Fuller, C., Hilt, D., Thurmond, B., et al. (1999). The alsfrs-r: a revised als functional rating scale that incorporates assessments of respiratory function. *J. Neurol. Sci.* 169, 13–21. doi: 10.1016/S0022-510X(99)00210-5

Chiò, A., Gauthier, A., Montuschi, A., Calvo, A., Di Vito, N., and Mutani, R. (2004). A cross sectional study on determinants of quality of life in als. *J. Neurol. Neurosurg. Psychiatry* 75, 1597–1601. doi: 10.1136/jnnp.2003.033100

Christensen, T., Barrett, L., Bliss-Moreau, E., Lebo, K., and Kaschub, C. (2003). A practical guide to experience-sampling procedures. *J. Happiness Stud.* 4, 53–78. doi: 10.1023/A:1023609306024

Clarke, S., Hickey, A., O'Boyle, C., and Hardiman, O. (2001). Assessing individual quality of life in amyotrophic lateral sclerosis. *Qual. Life Res.* 10, 149–158. doi: 10.1023/A:1016704906100

Cohen, J. (1992). A power primer. *Psychol. Bull.* 112, 155–159. doi: 10.1037/0033-2909.112.1.155

Cohen, S. R., Mount, B. M., Strobel, M. G., and Bul, F. (1995). The mcgill quality of life questionnaire: a measure of quality of life appropriate for people with advanced disease. a preliminary study of validity and acceptability. *Palliative Med.* 9, 207–219. doi: 10.1177/026921639500900306

Csikszentmihalyi, M. (1990). *Flow: The Psychology of Optimal Experience*. New York, NY: Harper and Row.

Csikszentmihalyi, M., and Larson, R. (1987). Validity and reliability of the experience-sampling method. *J. Nerv. Ment. Dis.* 175, 526–536. doi: 10.1097/00005053-198709000-00004

Edwards, J. R. (1994). The study of congruence in organizational behavior research: critique and a proposed alternative. *Organ. Behav. Hum. Decis. Process.* 58, 51–100. doi: 10.1006/obhd.1994.1029

Edwards, J. R., and Cooper, C. L. (1990). The person-environment fit approach to stress: recurring problems and some suggested solutions. *J. Organ. Behav.* 11, 293–307. doi: 10.1002/job.4030110405

Fanos, J. H., Gelinas, D. F., Foster, R. S., Postone, N., and Miller, R. G. (2008). Hope in palliative care: From narcissism to self-transcendence in amyotrophic lateral sclerosis. *J. Palliative Care* 11, 470–475. doi: 10.1089/jpm.2007.0098

Foley, G., Timonen, V., and Hardiman, O. (2014). Exerting control and adapting to loss in amyotrophic lateral sclerosis. *Soc. Sci. Med.* 101, 113–119. doi: 10.1016/j.socscimed.2013.11.003

Hammer, E. V., Häcker, S., Hautzinger, M., Meyer, T. D., and Kübler, A. (2008). Validity of the als-depression-inventory (adi-12): a new screening instrument for depressive disorders in patients with amyotrophic lateral sclerosis. *J. Affect. Disord.* 109, 213–219. doi: 10.1016/j.jad.2007.11.012

Iglesias, C., and Torgerson, D. (2000). Does length of questionnaire matter? a randomised trial of response rates to a mailed questionnaire. *J. Health Serv. Res. Policy* 5, 219–221. doi: 10.1177/135581960000500406

Jong-Meyer, R. D., Parthe, T., and Projektgruppe (2009). Einfluss von achtsamkeitsübung und dezentrierung auf rumination und spezifität autobiographischer erinnerungen. *Z. Klin. Psychol. Psych.* 38, 240–249. doi: 10.1026/1616-3443.38.4.240

Kenny, D. A., Bolger, N., and Korchmaros, J. D. (2003). Lower level mediation in multilevel models. *Psychol. Methods* 8, 115–128. doi: 10.1037/1082-989X.8.2.115

King, S. J., Duke, M. M., and O'Connor, B. A. (2009). Living with amyotrophic lateral sclerosis/motor neurone disease (als/mnd): decision-making about 'ongoing change and adaptation'. *J. Clin. Nurs.* 18, 745–754. doi: 10.1111/j.1365-2702.2008.02671.x

Kocovski, N. L., Segal, Z. V., and Battista, S. R. (2009). "Mindfulness and psychopathology: problem formulation," in *Clinical Handbook of Mindfulness*, ed F. Didonna (New York, NY: Springer New York), 85–98.

Larson, R., and Csikszentmihalyi, M. (1983). "The experience sampling method," in *Naturalistic Approaches to Studying Social Interaction*, Vol. 15, ed H. T. Reis (San Francisco, CA: Jossey-Bass), 41–46.

Logroscino, G., Traynor, B. J., Hardiman, O., Chiò, A., Couratier, P., Mitchell, J. D., et al. (2008). Descriptive epidemiology of amyotrophic lateral sclerosis: new evidence and unsolved issues. *J. Neurol. Neurosurg. Psychiatry* 79, 6–11. doi: 10.1136/jnnp.2006.104828

Logroscino, G., Traynor, B. J., Hardiman, O., Chio, A., Mitchell, D., Swingler, R. J., et al. (2010). Incidence of amyotrophic lateral sclerosis in europe. *J. Neurol. Neurosurg. Psychiatry* 81, 385–390. doi: 10.1136/jnnp.2009.183525

Lulé, D., Häcker, S., Ludolph, A., Birbaumer, N., and Kübler, A. (2008). Depression and quality of life in patients with amyotrophic lateral sclerosis. *Deutsch. Ärztebl. Int.* 105, 397–403. doi: 10.3238/arztebl.2008.0397

Lulé, D., Zickler, C., Häcker, S., Bruno, M. A., Demertzi, A., Pellas, F., et al. (2009). Life can be worth living in locked-in syndrome. *Prog. Brain Res.* 177, 339–351. doi: 10.1016/S0079-6123(09)17723-3

MacKinnon, D. P., Lockwood, C. M., Hoffman, J. M., West, S. G., and Sheets, V. (2002). A comparison of methods to test mediation and other intervening variable effects. *Psychol. Methods* 7, 83–104. doi: 10.1037/1082-989X.7.1.83

Martin, L. L., and Tesser, A. (1996). "Some ruminative thoughts," in *Ruminative Thoughts*, Vol. IX of *Advances in Social Cognition*, ed R. S. Wyer (Mahwah, NJ: Lawrence Erlbaum), 1–47.

Matuz, T., Birbaumer, N., Hautzinger, M., and Kübler, A. (2010). Coping with amyotrophic lateral sclerosis: an integrative view. *J. Neurol. Neurosurg. Psychiatry* 81, 893–898. doi: 10.1136/jnnp.2009.201285

McLeod, J. E., and Clarke, D. M. (2007). A review of psychosocial aspects of motor neurone disease. *J. Neurol. Sci.* 258, 4–10. doi: 10.1016/j.jns.2007.03.001

Montel, S., Albertini, L., and Spitz, E. (2012a). Coping strategies as related to medical and demographic data in amyotrophic lateral sclerosis. *Acta Neurol. Scand.* 125, 136–141. doi: 10.1111/j.1600-0404.2011.01513.x

Montel, S., Albertini, L., and Spitz, E. (2012b). Coping strategies in relation to quality of life in amyotrophic lateral sclerosis. *Muscle Nerve* 45, 131–134. doi: 10.1002/mus.22270

Nolen-Hoeksema, S. (1991). Responses to depression and their effects on the duration of depressive episodes. *J. Abnorm. Psychol.* 100, 569–582. doi: 10.1037/0021-843X.100.4.569

Nolen-Hoeksema, S., Wisco, B. E., and Lyubomirsky, S. (2008). Rethinking rumination. *Perspect. Psychol. Sci.* 3, 400–424. doi: 10.1111/j.1745-6924.2008.00088.x

Nonnenmacher, S., Hammer, E. M., Lulé, D., Hautzinger, M., and Kübler, A. (2013). Psychische störungen und individuelle lebensqualität bei der chronisch progredient-terminalen erkrankung amyotrophe lateralsklerose (als). *Z. Klin. Psychol. Psych.* 42, 55–63. doi: 10.1026/1616-3443/a000186

Pagnini, F. (2013). Psychological wellbeing and quality of life in amyotrophic lateral sclerosis: a review. *Int. J. Psychol.* 48, 194–205. doi: 10.1080/00207594.2012.691977

Pagnini, F., Di Credico, C., Gatto, R., Fabiani, V., Rossi, G., Lunetta, C., et al. (2014a). Meditation training for people with amyotrophic lateral sclerosis and their caregivers. *J. Altern. Complement. Med.* 20, 272–275. doi: 10.1089/acm.2013.0268

Pagnini, F., Phillips, D., and Langer, E. (2014b). A mindful approach with end-of-life thoughts. *Front. Psychol.* 5:138. doi: 10.3389/fpsyg.2014.00138

Plahuta, J. M., McCulloch, B. J., Kasarskis, E. J., Ross, M. A., Walter, R. A., and McDonald, E. R. (2002). Amyotrophic lateral sclerosis and hopelessness: psychosocial factors. *Soc. Sci. Med.* 55, 2131–2140. doi: 10.1016/S0277-9536(01)00356-2

Rapkin, B. D., and Schwartz, C. E. (2004). Toward a theoretical model of quality-of-life appraisal: implications of findings from studies of response shift. *Health Qual. Life Out.* 2:14. doi: 10.1186/1477-7525-2-14

R Development Core Team (2011). *R: A Language and Environment for Statistical Computing.* Vienna: R Foundation for Statistical Computing.

Robbins, R. A., Simmons, Z., Bremer, B. A., Walsh, S. M., and Fisher, S. (2001). Quality of life in als is maintained as physical function declines. *Neurology* 56, 442–444. doi: 10.1212/WNL.56.4.442

Runyan, J. D., Steenbergh, T. A., Bainbridge, C., Daugherty, D. A., Oke, L., and Fry, B. N. (2013). A smartphone ecological momentary assessment - intervention app for collecting real-time data and promoting self-awareness. *PLoS ONE* 8:e71325. doi: 10.1371/journal.pone.0071325

Schmidt, J. A., Shernof, D. J., and Csikszentmihalyi, M. (2007). "Individual and situational factors related to the experience of flow in adolescence," in *Oxford Handbook of Methods in Positive Psychology, Series in Positive Psychology*, eds A. D. Ong and M. H. M. Van Dulmen (Oxford; New York, NY: Oxford University Press), 542–558.

Scollon, C. N., Prieto, C. K., and Diener, E. (2009). "Experience sampling: promises and pitfalls, strength and weaknesses," in *Assessing Well-Being*, Volume 39 of *Social Indicators Research Series*, ed E. Diener (Dordrecht: Springer), 157–180.

Selya, A. S., Rose, J. S., Dierker, L. C., Hedeker, D., and Mermelstein, R. J. (2012). A practical guide to calculating cohen's f2, a measure of local effect size, from proc mixed. *Front. Psychol.* 3:111. doi: 10.3389/fpsyg.2012.00111

Shiffman, S., Stone, A. A., and Hufford, M. R. (2008). Ecological momentary assessment. *Annu. Rev. Clin. Psychol.* 4, 1–32. doi: 10.1146/annurev.clinpsy.3.022806.091415

Smyth, J. M., and Stone, A. A. (2003). Ecological momentary assessment research in behavioral medicine. *J. Happiness Stud.* 4, 35–52. doi: 10.1023/A:1023657221954

Snijders, T. A. B., and Bosker, R. J. (1993). Standard errors and sample sizes for two-level research. *J. Educ. Behav. Stat.* 18, 237–259. doi: 10.3102/10769986018003237

Spearman, C. (1910). Correlation calculated from faulty data. *Br. J. Psychol.* 3, 271–295.

Stone, A. A., Shiffman, S. S., and DeVries, M. W. (2003). "Ecological momentary assessment," in *Well-Being*, eds D. Kahneman, E. Diener, and N. Schwarz (New York, NY: Russell Sage Foundation), 26–39.

Teuchmann, K., Totterdell, P., and Parker, S. K. (1999). Rushed, unhappy, and drained: an experience sampling study of relations between time pressure, perceived control, mood, and emotional exhaustion in a group of accountants. *J. Occup. Health Psychol.* 4, 37–54. doi: 10.1037/1076-8998.4.1.37

Tofighi, D., and MacKinnon, D. P. (2011). Rmediation: an r package for mediation analysis confidence intervals. *Behav. Res. Methods* 43, 692–700. doi: 10.3758/s13428-011-0076-x

Trail, M., Nelson, N. D., Van, J. N., Appel, S. H., and Lai, E. C. (2003). A study comparing patients with amyotrophic lateral sclerosis and their caregivers on measures of quality of life, depression, and their attitudes toward treatment options. *J. Neurol. Sci.* 209, 79–85. doi: 10.1016/S0022-510X(03)00003-0

10

Redox environment is an intracellular factor to operate distinct pathways for aggregation of Cu, Zn-superoxide dismutase in amyotrophic lateral sclerosis

Yoshiaki Furukawa*

Laboratory for Mechanistic Chemistry of Biomolecules, Department of Chemistry, Keio University, Yokohama, Japan

Edited by:
Ricardo Tapia, Universidad Nacional Autónoma de México, Mexico

Reviewed by:
Nobuhiro Harada, Fujita Health University School of Medicine, Japan
Salvador Ventura, Universitat Autonoma de Barcelona, Spain

***Correspondence:**
Yoshiaki Furukawa, Laboratory for Mechanistic Chemistry of Biomolecules, Department of Chemistry, Keio University, 3-14-1 Hiyoshi, Kohoku, Yokohama, Kanagawa 223-8522, Japan
e-mail: furukawa@chem.keio.ac.jp

Dominant mutations in Cu,Zn-superoxide dismutase (SOD1) cause a familial form of amyotrophic lateral sclerosis (fALS). Misfolding and aggregation of mutant SOD1 proteins are a pathological hallmark of SOD1-related fALS cases; however, the molecular mechanism of SOD1 aggregation remains controversial. Here, I have used *E. coli* as a model organism and shown multiple distinct pathways of SOD1 aggregation that are dependent upon its thiol-disulfide status. Overexpression of fALS-mutant SOD1s in the cytoplasm of *E. coli* BL21 and SHuffle™, where redox environment is reducing and oxidizing, respectively, resulted in the formation of insoluble aggregates with notable differences; a disulfide bond of SOD1 was completely reduced in BL21 or abnormally formed between SOD1 molecules in SHuffle™. Depending upon intracellular redox environment, therefore, mutant SOD1 is considered to misfold/aggregate through distinct pathways, which would be relevant in description of the pathological heterogeneity of SOD1-related fALS cases.

Keywords: SOD1, ALS, aggregation, disulfide bond

INTRODUCTION

Thiol-disulfide status is critical for functioning of many proteins (Sevier and Kaiser, 2002), and Cu,Zn-superoxide dismutase (SOD1) is one of such proteins in which formation of an intramolecular disulfide bond is required for folding into its enzymatically active conformation (Furukawa et al., 2004). An enzymatic function of SOD1 is to catalyze the removal of a toxic reactive oxygen species, superoxide anion (McCord and Fridovich, 1969), and activation steps of SOD1 *in vivo* include binding of a catalytic copper ion and a structural zinc ion and also formation of an intramolecular disulfide bond. Given that SOD1 isolated from *Bacillus subtilis* (Banci et al., 2005) and *Mycobacterium tuberculosis* (Spagnolo et al., 2004) lacks a copper and zinc binding site, respectively, metal binding seems to be dispensable for SOD1. In contrast, an intramolecular disulfide bond is conserved among all SOD1 proteins identified so far, implying its essential roles in physiological functions of SOD1.

Indeed, abnormalities in a thiol-disulfide status of SOD1 have been proposed as a pathological change in a familial form of amyotrophic lateral sclerosis (fALS) that is caused by dominant mutations in SOD1 (Rosen et al., 1993). For example, in transgenic mice expressing human SOD1 with a fALS mutation (G85R), two Cys residues (Cys57 and Cys146) of SOD1, which normally form an intramolecular disulfide bond, remained reduced (Jonsson et al., 2006). Aggregation of mutant SOD1 is a major pathological change in SOD1-related fALS cases (Bruijn et al., 1998), and inclusions reproduced in diseased mice have been shown to contain disulfide-reduced SOD1 proteins (Jonsson et al., 2006; Karch et al., 2009). *In vitro* studies have also shown increased susceptibility of a disulfide bond in several fALS-mutant SOD1 proteins toward a reducing agent (Tiwari and Hayward, 2003). Furthermore, reduction of a disulfide bond significantly decreased the thermostability and thus facilitated misfolding and aggregation of SOD1 *in vitro*, supporting important roles of a conserved disulfide bond in maintaining an aggregation-resistant structure of SOD1 (Furukawa and O'Halloran, 2005; Furukawa et al., 2008).

In contrast, increased oxidative stress has been reported in fALS patients (Barber and Shaw, 2010), and SOD1 appears to be one of intracellular targets susceptible to oxidative modifications (Guareschi et al., 2012). In transgenic mice expressing human SOD1 with fALS mutations, mutant SOD1 has been shown to form insoluble oligomers cross-linked *via* intermolecular disulfide bonds (Furukawa et al., 2006). *In vitro* experiments have also revealed that aggregation of mutant SOD1 is triggered by abnormal oxidation of histidine and tryptophan residues (Rakhit et al., 2002; Zhang et al., 2003). Under such oxidative conditions, a disulfide-reduced form of SOD1 would not stably exist. Furthermore, structural destabilization of SOD1 by pathogenic mutations has been recently reported to facilitate isomerization of a conserved intramolecular disulfide bond (Cys57–Cys146) into an intermolecular disulfide crosslink (Toichi et al., 2013). Taken together, reduction of a disulfide bond may not be a prerequisite for aggregation of SOD1 *in vivo*; rather, a redox environment surrounding SOD1 would determine how mutant SOD1 is misfolded and aggregated. Indeed, most (>70%) of intracellular SOD1 exist in the reducing environment of cytoplasm (Chang et al., 1988), but a small fraction (~3%) of SOD1 is also detected in the intermembrane space (IMS) of mitochondria (Okado-Matsumoto and Fridovich, 2001), which is considerably more oxidizing than cytoplasm (Hu et al., 2008). Intracellular SOD1 is thus considered to experience a broad range of redox environment, which would affect its folding/misfolding processes.

In this study, effects of intracellular redox environment on SOD1 aggregation have been examined in *Escherichia coli* as a model organism. Overexpression of heterologous proteins in bacteria such as *E. coli* often leads to the formation of insoluble aggregates called inclusion bodies, and inclusion bodies of several proteins have been shown to possess amyloid-like properties (Carrio et al., 2005; de Groot et al., 2009; Villar-Pique and Ventura, 2012). Cytoplasm of *E. coli* has been well known as strongly reducing environment (Hwang et al., 1992), while genetically modified *E. coli*, SHuffle^{TM}, provides considerably oxidizing cytoplasm (Lobstein et al., 2012). FALS-mutant human SOD1 proteins in *E. coli* BL21 were found to exist as a disulfide-reduced state and form insoluble fibrillar aggregates. In contrast, expression of mutant SOD1 in the oxidizing cytoplasm of SHuffle^{TM} resulted in the formation of insoluble oligomers crosslinked *via* intermolecular disulfide bonds albeit with fibrillar morphologies. Depending upon the intracellular redox environment, therefore, mutant SOD1 proteins form insoluble aggregates with distinct properties, suggesting roles of organelle-specific misfolding pathways of mutant SOD1 in fALS pathomechanism.

RESULTS AND DISCUSSION

SOD1 AGGREGATES UNDER REDUCING ENVIRONMENT OF *E. coli* CYTOPLASM

Introduction of an intramolecular disulfide bond between Cys57 and Cys146 in SOD1 has been known to increase the electrophoretic mobility of SOD1 (Furukawa et al., 2004); therefore, thiol-disulfide status of SOD1 can be determined by non-reducing SDS-PAGE analysis. When overexpressed in *E. coli* BL21, wild-type human SOD1 (SOD1(WT)) was found to be in a disulfide-reduced form (SOD1^{SH}) with a small fraction of a disulfide-form (SOD1^{S-S}; **Figure 1A**). Also notably, most of SOD1^{SH} was insoluble, while SOD1^{S-S} remained soluble (**Figure 1A**). These results are consistent with a previous finding that SOD1^{SH} is highly prone to insoluble aggregation *in vitro* (Furukawa et al., 2008). Given that cytoplasm of *E. coli* provides a highly reducing environment (Hwang et al., 1992), formation of a disulfide bond in proteins will be an unfavorable process in the cytoplasm. Furthermore, metal-chelating capacity of bacterial cytoplasm has been reported to be extremely high (Outten and O'Halloran, 2001; Changela et al., 2003), where SOD1 is supposed to be in a metal-deficient apo state. Indeed, exogenous supplementation of $ZnSO_4$ in a growth media increased the soluble fraction of overexpressed SOD1$^{SH/S-S}$ (**Figure 1A**), supporting previous reports that binding of a zinc ion protects SOD1 from aggregation (Furukawa et al., 2008). In the reducing environment of cytoplasm, where metal-chelating capacity is also significant, SOD1 remain in a disulfide-reduced apo state and is prone to insoluble aggregation.

OXIDIZING ENVIRONMENT PROTECTS SOD1 FROM AGGREGATION BY DISULFIDE FORMATION

To examine effects of disulfide formation on SOD1 aggregation *in vivo*, SOD1(WT) was overexpressed in *E. coli* SHuffle^{TM}, where cytoplasmic reductive pathways are genetically diminished (Lobstein et al., 2012). More specifically, thioredoxin reductase (*trxB*) and glutathione reductase (*gor*) have been removed in *E. coli*

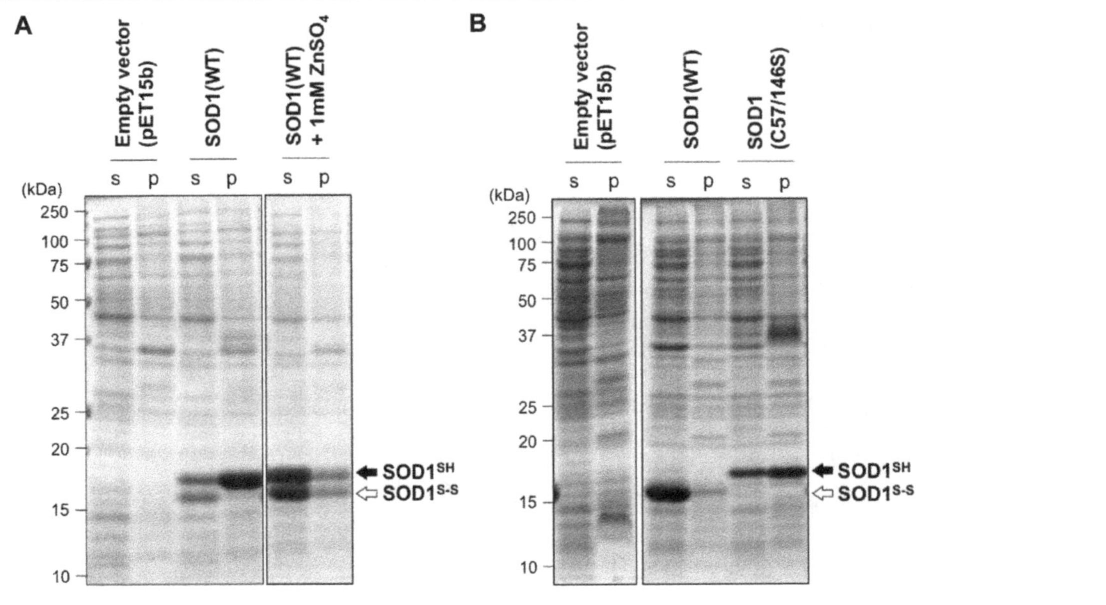

FIGURE 1 | Redox environment of *E. coli* cytoplasm influences the aggregation propensities of SOD1 by modulating its thiol-disulfide status. (A) *E. coli* BL21(DE3) or **(B)** SHuffle^{TM} was transformed with pET15b (an empty vector) or pET15b harboring human SOD1(WT) cDNA, and the protein expression was induced with IPTG (see Materials and Methods). Results obtained by addition of 1 mM $ZnSO_4$ at the induction of protein expression were also included in **(A)** (SOD1(WT) + 1 mM $ZnSO_4$). Also, expression of SOD1 with C57/146S mutations, in which an intramolecular disulfide bond cannot form, was examined in *E. coli* SHuffle^{TM} and shown in **(B)**. Cell lysates were fractionated into soluble supernatant (s) and insoluble pellets (p), treated with iodoacetamide, and then analyzed with non-reducing SDS-PAGE by using a 15% polyacrylamide gel. White (SOD1^{S-S}) and black (SOD1^{SH}) arrows at the right side of the gel image indicate positions of bands corresponding to SOD1 with and without a disulfide bond, respectively.

SHuffle^{TM}, which provides oxidizing cytoplasm and thus enables to introduce disulfide bonds in cytoplasmically expressed proteins. As shown in **Figure 1B**, SOD1(WT) overexpressed in *E. coli* SHuffle^{TM} was found to form a disulfide bond and remain soluble, showing that correct introduction of a disulfide bond in SOD1 can prevent its insoluble aggregation *in vivo*. When SOD1 with C57S/C146S mutations, in which a conserved disulfide bond (Cys57–Cys146) cannot form, was overexpressed in *E. coli* SHuffle^{TM}, significant amounts of mutant SOD1 was again found in the insoluble fraction. This result hence emphasizes a protective role of the disulfide bond against aggregation of SOD1. In eukaryotes, a copper chaperone for SOD1 (CCS) has been shown to introduce the intramolecular disulfide bond in SOD1 (Furukawa et al., 2004), while CCS-independent pathway(s) for disulfide formation in SOD1 also appears to exist (Subramaniam et al., 2002; Leitch et al., 2009). Given no CCS homologues in bacteria, the results obtained by using SHuffle^{TM} (**Figure 1B**) implies that oxidizing environment is sufficient for introducing a correct disulfide bond into wild-type SOD1 even without CCS and thereby protecting the protein from being misfolded/aggregated.

ALS MUTATIONS COMMONLY AGGRAVATE THE AGGREGATION PHENOTYPE OF SOD1 UNDER REDUCING ENVIRONMENT

To test effects of fALS-causing mutations on SOD1 aggregation *in vivo*, several types of mutant SOD1 were overexpressed in *E. coli* BL21. SOD1 with A4V mutation has been reported to be expressed in *E. coli* BL21 as insoluble pellets (Leinweber et al., 2004), and all of the other mutant SOD1s tested here were found as a disulfide-reduced form in insoluble pellets regardless of the absence (data not shown) or presence (**Figure 2**) of 1 mM $ZnSO_4$ in a growth media. This is in sharp contrast to wild-type SOD1, which was expressed as a soluble form when cultured in a growth media supplemented with zinc ions (**Figure 1A**). It has been suggested that the decreased affinity of zinc ion is a common pathogenic denominator of fALS-mutant SOD1 (Goto et al., 2000; Hayward et al., 2002); therefore, supplementation of 1 mM $ZnSO_4$ to a growth media is considered to be insufficient for metallation of mutant SOD1 in the *E. coli* cytoplasm. Also notably, significant amounts of SOD1^{S-S} were observed in a soluble fraction when the wild-type protein was expressed in *E. coli* BL21 (**Figure 1A**); however, in fALS-mutant SOD1s, formation of the disulfide bond was hardly observed (**Figure 2**). These results are consistent with previous reports showing increased susceptibility of the disulfide bond to reducing agents by pathogenic mutations (Tiwari and Hayward, 2003). Under the reducing environment with high metal-chelating capacity of *E. coli* cytoplasm, therefore, SOD1 is found to exhibit increased propensities for aggregation with fALS-causing mutations.

FALS-MUTANT SOD1 TEND TO FORM DISULFIDE-LINKED OLIGOMERS UNDER OXIDIZING ENVIRONMENT

In wild-type SOD1, the intramolecular disulfide bond was efficiently introduced under the oxidizing environment, which then protected the protein from aggregation (**Figure 1B**). In contrast, when several fALS-mutant SOD1s were expressed in the oxidizing cytoplasm of *E. coli* SHuffle^{TM}, significant amounts of SOD1 were found to remain in insoluble pellets (**Figure 3**). More specifically, a monomer and higher-order oligomers of mutant SOD1 (G37R, G41S, G85R, G93R, C111Y, and L126X) were evident in an insoluble fraction, while SOD1s with H46R and H80R mutations were obtained as soluble proteins with an intramolecular disulfide bond (**Figure 3A**). When analyzed in reducing SDS-PAGE, furthermore, those higher-order oligomer bands were collapsed and merged to the monomer band (**Figure 3B**), indicating that the oligomers were formed *via* disulfide-crosslinks. Formation of intra- or inter-molecular disulfide bond is considered to depend

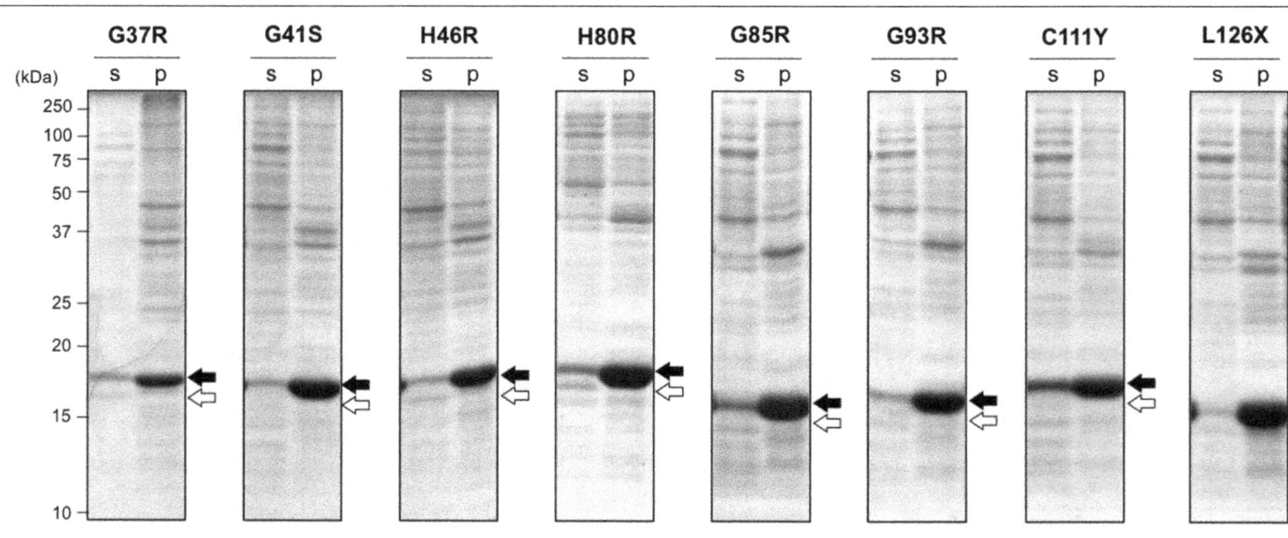

FIGURE 2 | Aggregation of disulfide-reduced SOD1 with fALS mutations in *E. coli* BL21 was not rescued by addition of $ZnSO_4$. *E. coli* BL21(DE3) was transformed with pET15b harboring human SOD1 cDNA with indicated fALS mutations, and the protein expression was induced by IPTG in the presence of 1 mM $ZnSO_4$. Cell lysates were fractionated into soluble supernatant (s) and insoluble pellets (p), treated with iodoacetamide, and then analyzed with non-reducing SDS-PAGE by using a 15% polyacrylamide gel. White (SOD1^{S-S}) and black (SOD1^{SH}) arrows at the right side of the gel image indicate positions of bands corresponding to SOD1 with and without a disulfide bond, respectively.

upon intracellular concentration of SOD1 proteins, but **Figure 3B** shows similar expression levels of SOD1 proteins in *E. coli* examined here. In those mutant SOD1s forming disulfide-linked oligomers (G37R, G41S, G85R, G93R, C111Y, but not L126X), small amounts of proteins were also detected in a soluble fraction with an intramolecular disulfide bond. Notably, SOD1 with H46R and H80R mutations have been shown to exhibit thermostability comparable to that of the wild-type protein (Rodriguez et al., 2005; Vassall et al., 2011); therefore, fALS-causing mutations that significantly destabilize a native structure of SOD1 favor the formation of disulfide-crosslinked oligomers under oxidizing environment.

MUTANT SOD1 FORMS AMYLOID-LIKE FIBRILLAR AGGREGATES IN *E. coli*

To further characterize the SOD1 aggregates formed in *E. coli*, a protocol to purify those insoluble aggregates were first established, in which insoluble fractions of *E. coli* lysates were extensively washed with 1 M NaCl, 1% Sarkosyl, and then acetone (see Materials and Methods). When purified aggregates of SOD1(G37R) were reacted with iodoacetamide to protect free thiol groups and then analyzed in non-reducing SDS-PAGE, disulfide-linked oligomers were found to be successfully isolated from *E. coli* SHuffle^{TM} (**Figure 4A**, +IA). In contrast, purified aggregates of SOD1(G37R)

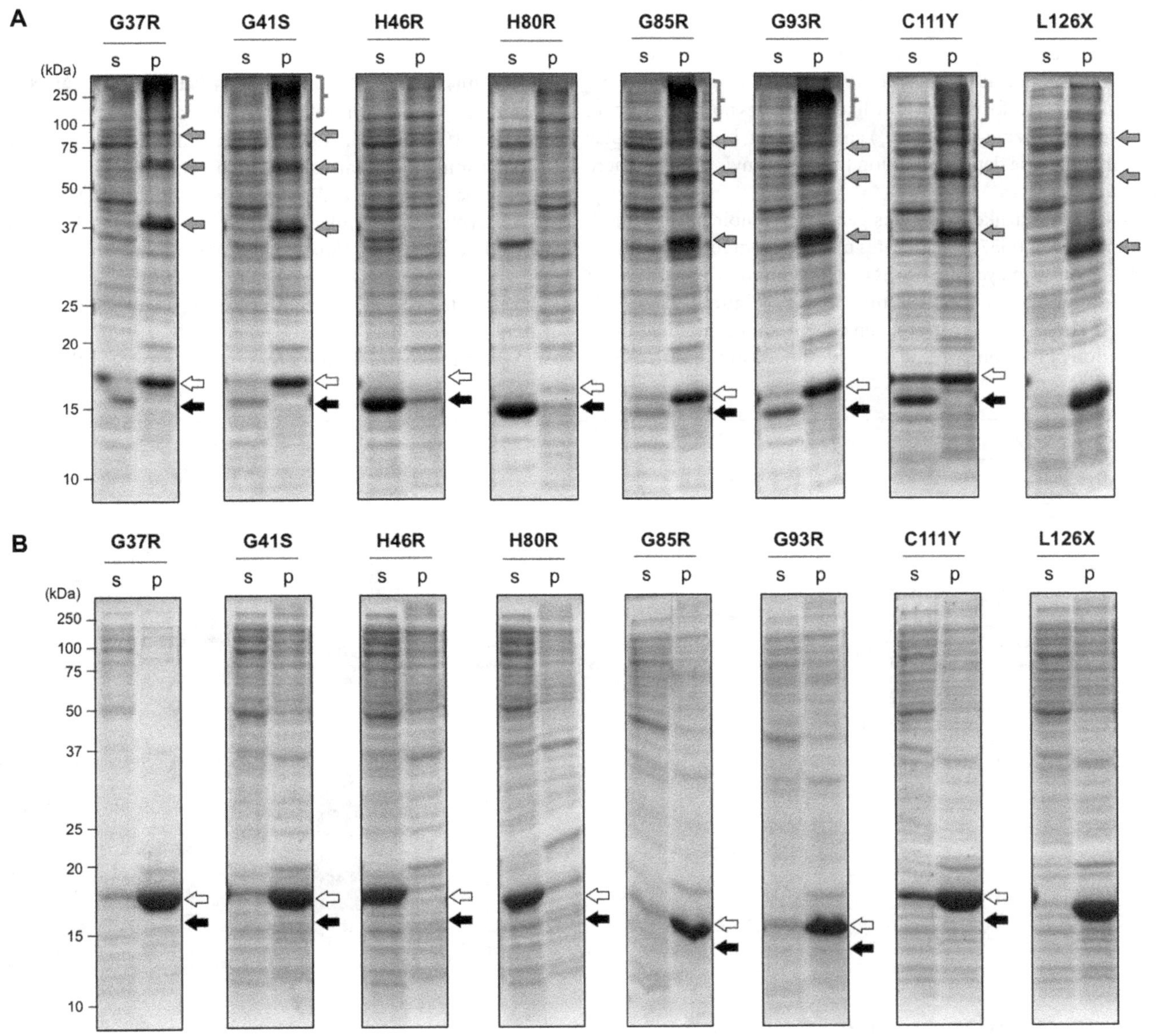

FIGURE 3 | Aggregation of mutant SOD1 in *E. coli* SHuffle^{TM} associates with the formation of inter-molecular disulfide crosslinks. *E. coli* SHuffle^{TM} was transformed with pET15b harboring human SOD1 cDNA with indicated fALS mutations, and the protein expression was induced by IPTG. Cell lysates were fractionated into soluble supernatant (s) and insoluble pellets (p), treated with iodoacetamide, and then analyzed with **(A)** non-reducing or **(B)** reducing SDS-PAGE by using a 15% polyacrylamide gel. White ($SOD1^{S-S}$) and black ($SOD1^{SH}$) arrows at the right side of the gel image indicate positions of bands corresponding to SOD1 with and without a disulfide bond, respectively. In addition, gray arrows and braces in **(A)** represent the disulfide-linked SOD1 oligomers, which disappeared in reducing SDS-PAGE **(B)**.

from *E. coli* BL21 were mainly composed of disulfide-reduced monomers with slight contamination of dimers (**Figure 4A**, +IA). Furthermore, after extensive washes, both SOD1(G37R) aggregates from BL21 and SHuffle™ produced a single band in reducing SDS-PAGE (+β-ME), supporting successful purification of the SOD1 aggregates.

Aggregates of SOD1 *in vitro* have been shown to have structural features similar to those of amyloid, which are characterized by fibrillar morphologies with β-sheet-rich structures (Furukawa et al., 2008). As shown in **Figure 4B**, both SOD1(G37R) aggregates purified from *E. coli* BL21 and SHuffle™ were found to increase the thioflavin T fluorescence but with distinct intensity. In addition, those SOD1(G37R) aggregates were found to red-shift an electronic absorption spectrum of Congo red (**Figure 4C**). These tinctorial changes of thioflavin T and Congo red have been typically observed in protein aggregates with amyloid-like properties (Klunk et al., 1999; LeVine, 1999). It is, therefore, possible that SOD1(G37R) forms amyloid-like aggregates both in reducing (BL21) and oxidizing (SHuffle™) environment, but its molecular structure might be dependent upon the redox environment where the aggregates form.

While amyloid-like aggregates generally exhibit fibrillar morphologies, SOD1(G37R) aggregates purified from insoluble inclusions in *E. coli* displayed not fibrils but amorphous, large lump-like structures under an electron microscope (**Figures 4D,E**, left panels). These structures are considered to be attained with aggregation of monomeric and disulfide-linked multimeric SOD1 proteins through SDS-sensitive interactions. When these inclusions were briefly treated with a non-specific protease, Proteinase K, however, a protease-resistant core of inclusions became exposed and was found to exhibit fibrillar morphologies with *approx.* 5.5 nm of the diameter (**Figures 4D,E**, right panels). While morphological differences of SOD1(G37R) aggregates were not clear between *E. coli* BL21 and SHuffle™, exposure of fibrillar structures by treatment with proteases have been previously reported in *E. coli* inclusions of Aβ peptide (Morell et al., 2008) and HET-s (Sabate et al., 2009), which are known to be fibrillogenic. Taken together, therefore, this study successfully reproduces fibrillar aggregation of mutant SOD1 proteins in the cytoplasm of *E. coli* and further implies that intracellular redox environment could modulate the properties of SOD1 aggregates by changing its thiol-disulfide status.

IMPLICATIONS TO PATHOLOGIES OF SOD1-RELATED fALS CASES

More than 70% of intracellular SOD1 has been detected in the cytoplasm (Chang et al., 1988), which is normally kept as reducing environment by maintaining high concentrations of reduced glutathione (Hwang et al., 1992). Indeed, mutant SOD1 proteins are abnormally accumulated in the cytoplasm as Lewy body-like hyaline inclusions (Shibata et al., 1996), and those insoluble forms of mutant SOD1 have been characterized as a disulfide-reduced state in SOD1-fALS model mice (**Figure 5**, left; Jonsson et al., 2006; Karch et al., 2009). These observations are consistent with the *in vitro* findings that inability to form the disulfide

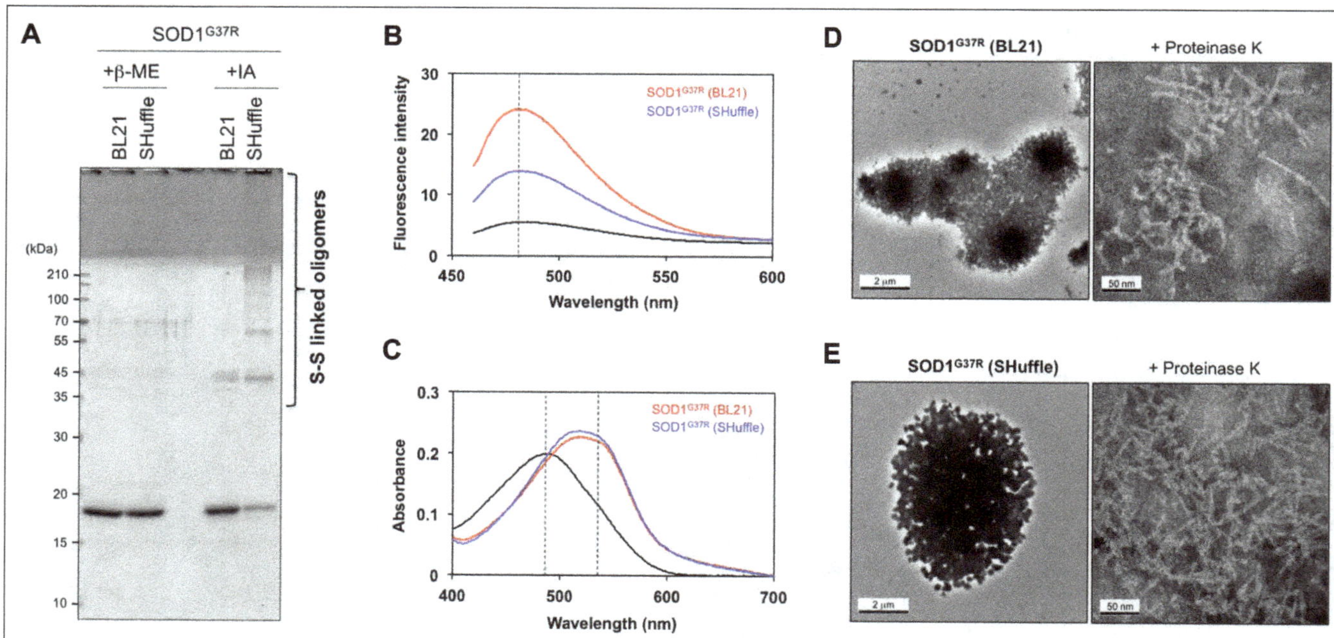

FIGURE 4 | Amyloid-like characters of SOD1 aggregates purified from insoluble inclusions in *E. coli*. **(A)** SOD1(G37R) aggregates purified from insoluble inclusions in *E. coli* were reacted with iodoacetamide for protection of free thiol groups and analyzed with reducing (+β-ME) and non-reducing (+IA) SDS-PAGE. Disulfide-crosslinked oligomers were identified in SOD1(G37R) aggregates purified from insoluble inclusions in *E. coli* SHuffle™ but not in BL21(DE3). **(B, C)** Tinctorial properties of SOD1(G37R) aggregates purified from *E. coli* BL21 and SHuffle™ (red and blue curves, respectively) were examined by **(B)** fluorescence of thioflavin T and **(C)** absorption of Congo red. Black curves represent **(B)** fluorescence spectrum of thioflavin T and **(C)** absorption spectrum of Congo red without addition of SOD1 aggregates. **(D, E)** Electron micrograms of SOD1(G37R) aggregates purified from *E. coli* **(D)** BL21 and **(E)** SHuffle™. SOD1(G37R) aggregates exhibit large, amorphous morphologies (left panels), while fibrillar structures become evident after brief treatment of aggregates with Proteinase K (right panels). A bar represents 2 μm (left panels) or 50 nm (right panels).

bond significantly increases the propensities of SOD1 for fibrillar aggregation (Furukawa et al., 2008). In reducing environment of the cytoplasm, the disulfide bond in SOD1 is introduced by a copper chaperone protein, CCS (Furukawa et al., 2004), and appears to be protected from the reductive cleavage by its burial at the dimer interface. Some fALS mutations would hence disturb the interaction with CCS and/or facilitates the monomerization of SOD1; thereby, stability of the disulfide bond becomes decreased, which then triggers the fibrillar aggregation of disulfide-reduced SOD1 in the cytoplasm (the disulfide-reduction model; Toichi et al., 2013).

In contrast to such disulfide-reduction model of SOD1 aggregation, little accumulation of cytoplasmic inclusions has been observed in some fALS model mice expressing mutant SOD1, albeit with significant mitochondrial pathologies (Nagai et al., 2001; Watanabe et al., 2001). *Approximately* 3% of total SOD1 is known to localize at the IMS of mitochondria (Okado-Matsumoto and Fridovich, 2001), where the redox potential is significantly more oxidizing than that of the cytoplasm (Hu et al., 2008). Furthermore, mitochondria of a motor neuron, which is the most damaged cell in fALS cases (Bruijn et al., 2004), have been reported to provide more oxidizing environment than those of the other types of cells (Ferri et al., 2006). Given that reduction of a disulfide bond in SOD1 is required for its transport into mitochondrial IMS (Field et al., 2003), disulfide-reduced SOD1 just after transported is considered to experience significantly oxidizing environment of motorneuronal IMS (**Figure 5**, right). Transported SOD1 polypeptide then folds into the native three-dimensional conformation, and the intramolecular disulfide bond is introduced by mitochondrial CCS. The folding process of SOD1 is, however, deterred by fALS-causing mutations (Nordlund and Oliveberg, 2006; Bruns and Kopito, 2007), which would increase the chance to form aberrant disulfide crosslinks under oxidizing environment of the mitochondrial IMS (**Figure 5**, right). Indeed, SOD1 oligomers crosslinked *via* disulfide bonds have been observed in mitochondria isolated from spinal cords of fALS-model mice expressing mutant SOD1 (Deng et al., 2006). Also in cultured motorneuronal cells, disulfide-crosslinked oligomers of mutant SOD1 have been reproduced in mitochondria but not in cytoplasm (Ferri et al., 2006). In the oxidizing environment of organelles, therefore, disulfide-reduced mutant SOD1 is highly prone to crosslinking *via* abnormal disulfide bonds, which will not occur under reducing environment of the cytosol.

So far, it has been well known that misfolding/aggregation of mutant SOD1 occurs both in cytoplasm and mitochondrial IMS; however, any possible differences in the molecular properties of SOD1 aggregates between those two cellular compartments have been hardly noticed. An intracellular folding process of protein molecules into their native conformations has been well known to be significantly affected or even controlled by chaperone proteins, but motorneurons are equipped with different sets of chaperones from those in *E. coli*; therefore, a pathological process of SOD1 aggregation in SOD1-related fALS patients, which in general gradually proceed over several decades, would not be precisely reproduced in the *E. coli* overexpression system examined here. Nonetheless, distinct forms of misfolded/aggregated SOD1, especially in terms of their thiol-disulfide status, appear to be possible that depend upon the redox environment surrounding SOD1 proteins (**Figure 5**). While it is further required to test if

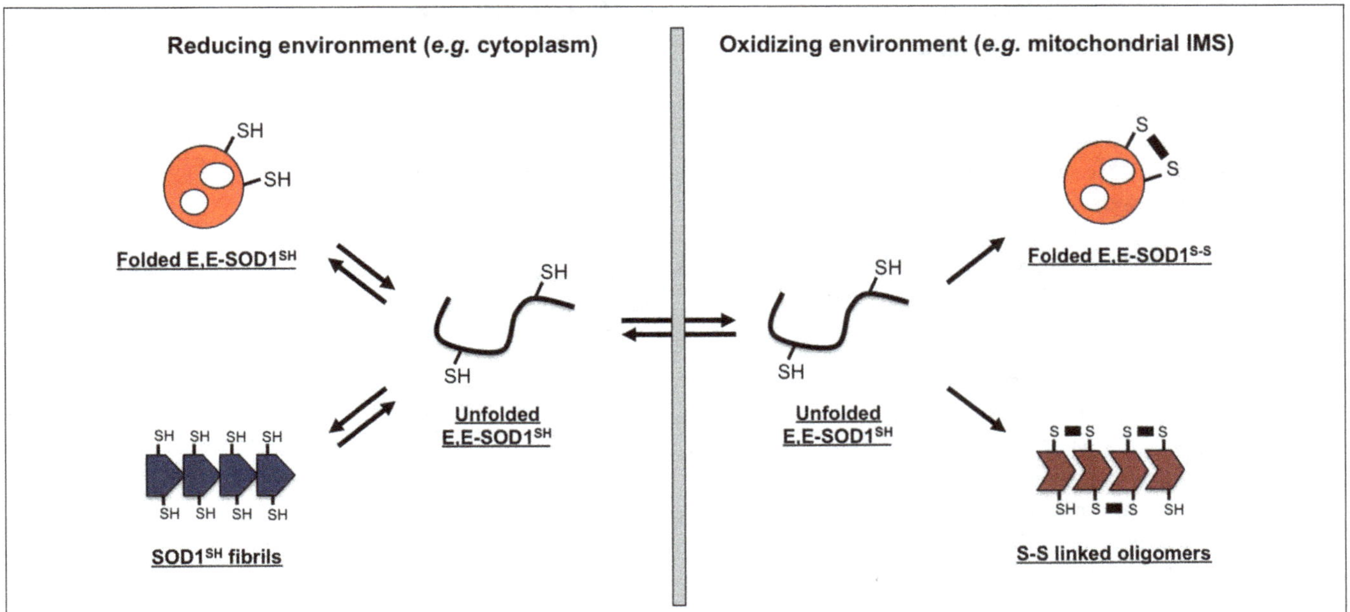

FIGURE 5 | Schematic representation of a redox-dependent SOD1 folding/misfolding model. SOD1 exists as an apo and disulfide-reduced state (E,E-SOD1^{SH}) and tends to form fibrillar aggregates (SOD1^{SH} fibrils) in reducing environment of the cytosol; in contrast, oxidizing environment stabilizes a soluble, folded state of SOD1 by introduction of an intramolecular disulfide bond (E,E-SOD1^{S-S}). Many fALS mutations are considered to destabilize the structure of E,E-SOD1^{SH}, increasing the fraction of misfolded state. In such a situation, oxidizing environment favors the formation of SOD1 oligomers cross-linked via abnormal disulfide bonds. Depending upon redox environment where SOD1 exists, several distinct forms in SOD1 aggregates are hence possible.

distinct properties of those SOD1 aggregates include toxicities to motorneurons, the redox-dependent aggregation of mutant SOD1 proteins would be one of the molecular mechanisms describing pathological heterogeneity observed in SOD1-related fALS cases.

MATERIALS AND METHODS

PLASMIDS, *E. coli* STRAINS AND PROTEIN EXPRESSION

A vector, pET15b (Novagen), was used for the construction of plasmids expressing human SOD1 without any tags; a SalI site was first introduced between BamHI and Bpu1102I sites of pET15b, and cDNA of human SOD1 was then cloned between NcoI and SalI site. Mutations were introduced by an inverse PCR method using KOD-FX-neo DNA polymerase (TOYOBO), and all constructs used in this study were confirmed by DNA sequencing. Competent cells of *E. coli*, BL21(DE3; New England Biolabs) and SHuffle^{TM} T7 Express lysY (New England Biolabs), were transformed with a plasmid. *E. coli* cells harboring a plasmid were cultured in Luria-Broth media containing 50 mg/L ampicillin (LB/Amp) by shaking at 200 rpm, and the expression of SOD1 proteins was induced with 1 mM isopropyl 1-thio-β-D-galactopyranoside at 37°C for 6 h. To test effects of Zn^{2+} ions on SOD1 aggregation, 1 mM $ZnSO_4$ was further added at the induction of protein expression.

ELECTROPHORETIC ANALYSIS OF SOD1 PROTEINS EXPRESSED IN *E. coli*

E. coli cells cultured in 5 mL LB/Amp media were collected by centrifugation (2,000 × *g*, 10 min) and lysed by ultrasonication in 100 μL of PBS with 2% Triton X-100 and 100 mM iodoacetamide. Soluble supernatant and insoluble pellets were obtained with centrifugation of cell lysates (20,000 × *g*, 10 min), and insoluble pellets were further solubilized by ultrasonication in 100 μL of PBS with 2% SDS and 100 mM iodoacetamide. The soluble supernatant and the re-solubilized insoluble pellets were incubated at 37°C for 30 min, which ensures the protection of thiol groups by modification with iodoacetamide. 0.8 (BL21) or 1.5 (SHuffle^{TM}) μL of the samples were then mixed with an SDS-PAGE sample buffer, and 10% β-mercaptoethanol was further added for reducing SDS-PAGE. The samples were boiled at 100°C for 5 min, electrophoresed on a 15% SDS-PAGE gel, and then stained with Coomassie brilliant blue.

PURIFICATION OF SOD1 AGGREGATES FROM *E. coli*

Insoluble pellets obtained by cell lysis in PBS/2% Triton X-100 were re-suspended in 1 M NaCl/H_2O with ultrasonication and centrifuged at 20,000 × *g* for 10 min to collect insoluble pellets. After washed again by 1 M NaCl, the insoluble pellets were washed three times with PBS/1% Sarkosyl and then washed with cold acetone. After dried up with SpeedVac (Savant), the pellets were re-suspended in 100 mM Na-Pi/100 mM NaCl/5 mM EDTA, pH 7.4 with ultrasonication. Purified pellets were analyzed by SDS-PAGE after being re-dissolved in PBS/2% SDS/100 mM iodoacetamide and loaded on a 15% polyacrylamide gel in the presence and absence of 10% β-mercaptoethanol (**Figure 4A**). Monomer-based concentration of SOD1 aggregates purified from inclusions was spectroscopically determined from the absorbance at 280 nm in 6 M guanidine hydrochloride using 5,500 $cm^{-1}M^{-1}$ as an extinction coefficient.

CHARACTERIZATION OF SOD1 AGGREGATES FROM *E. coli*

To test if SOD1 aggregates exhibit amyloid-like tinctorial properties, thioflavin T assay was performed. 10 μM (monomer-based) SOD1 aggregates purified from *E. coli* inclusions were mixed with 25 μM thioflavin T in 100 mM Na-Pi/100 mM NaCl/5 mM EDTA, pH 7.4, and fluorescence spectra excited at 442 nm were measured from 460 to 600 nm by using F-4500 (Hitachi). Congo red assay was also performed to test amyloid-like properties in SOD1 aggregates. 3 μM (monomer-based) SOD1 aggregates purified from *E. coli* inclusions were mixed with 5 μM Congo red in 100 mM Na-Pi/100 mM NaCl/5 mM EDTA, pH 7.4, and absorption spectra were measured by UV-2400PC (Shimadzu).

Morphologies of SOD1 aggregates formed in *E. coli* were examined by electron microscopy. Insoluble inclusions purified from *E. coli* were adsorbed on STEM100Cu grids coated by elastic carbon (Okenshoji), washed with water, and then negatively stained with 2% phosphotungstic acid. Images were obtained using an electron microscope (Tecnai^{TM} Spirit, FEI). 500 μL of *approximately* 100 μM (monomer-based) SOD1 aggregates purified from insoluble *E. coli* inclusions were mixed with 2 μL of 5 mg/mL Proteinase K and incubated at 37°C for 10 min. After ultracentrifuged at 110,000 × *g* for 15 min, insoluble pellets were washed with 500 μL of water and again ultracentrifuged. Resultant pellets were re-suspended in 100 μL of water and observed by an electron microscope as mentioned above.

ACKNOWLEDGMENTS

This work was supported by Grants-in-Aid 24111542 (to Yoshiaki Furukawa) for Scientific Research on Innovative Areas, 25291028 for Scientific Research (B) (to Yoshiaki Furukawa), and 24657093 for Challenging Exploratory Research (to Yoshiaki Furukawa) from the Ministry of Education, Culture, Sports, Science and Technology of Japan.

REFERENCES

Banci, L., Bertini, I., Calderone, V., Cramaro, F., Del Conte, R., Fantoni, A., et al. (2005). A prokaryotic superoxide dismutase paralog lacking two Cu ligands: from largely unstructured in solution to ordered in the crystal. *Proc. Natl. Acad. Sci. U.S.A.* 102, 7541–7546. doi: 10.1073/pnas.0502450102

Barber, S. C., and Shaw, P. J. (2010). Oxidative stress in ALS: key role in motor neuron injury and therapeutic target. *Free Radic. Biol. Med.* 48, 629–641. doi: 10.1016/j.freeradbiomed.2009.11.018

Bruijn, L. I., Houseweart, M. K., Kato, S., Anderson, K. L., Anderson, S. D., Ohama, E., et al. (1998). Aggregation and motor neuron toxicity of an ALS-linked SOD1 mutant independent from wild-type SOD1. *Science* 281, 1851–1854. doi: 10.1126/science.281.5384.1851

Bruijn, L. I., Miller, T. M., and Cleveland, D. W. (2004). Unraveling the mechanisms involved in motor neuron degeneration in ALS. *Annu. Rev. Neurosci.* 27, 723–749. doi: 10.1146/annurev.neuro.27.070203.144244

Bruns, C. K., and Kopito, R. R. (2007). Impaired post-translational folding of familial ALS-linked Cu, Zn superoxide dismutase mutants. *EMBO J.* 26, 855–866. doi: 10.1038/sj.emboj.7601528

Carrio, M., Gonzalez-Montalban, N., Vera, A., Villaverde, A., and Ventura, S. (2005). Amyloid-like properties of bacterial inclusion bodies. *J. Mol. Biol.* 347, 1025–1037. doi: 10.1016/j.jmb.2005.02.030

Chang, L. Y., Slot, J. W., Geuze, H. J., and Crapo, J. D. (1988). Molecular immunocytochemistry of the CuZn superoxide dismutase in rat hepatocytes. *J. Cell Biol.* 107, 2169–2179. doi: 10.1083/jcb.107.6.2169

Changela, A., Chen, K., Xue, Y., Holschen, J., Outten, C. E., O'Halloran, T. V., et al. (2003). Molecular basis of metal-ion selectivity and zeptomolar sensitivity by CueR. *Science* 301, 1383–1387. doi: 10.1126/science.1085950

de Groot, N. S., Sabate, R., and Ventura, S. (2009). Amyloids in bacterial inclusion bodies. *Trends Biochem. Sci.* 34, 408–416. doi: 10.1016/j.tibs.2009.03.009

Deng, H. X., Shi, Y., Furukawa, Y., Zhai, H., Fu, R., Liu, E., et al. (2006). Conversion to the amyotrophic lateral sclerosis phenotype is associated with intermolecular linked insoluble aggregates of SOD1 in mitochondria. *Proc. Natl. Acad. Sci. U.S.A.* 103, 7142–7147. doi: 10.1073/pnas.0602046103

Ferri, A., Cozzolino, M., Crosio, C., Nencini, M., Casciati, A., Gralla, E. B., et al. (2006). Familial ALS-superoxide dismutases associate with mitochondria and shift their redox potentials. *Proc. Natl. Acad. Sci. U.S.A.* 103, 13860–13865. doi: 10.1073/pnas.0605814103

Field, L. S., Furukawa, Y., O'Halloran, T. V., and Culotta, V. C. (2003). Factors controlling the uptake of yeast copper/zinc superoxide dismutase into mitochondria. *J. Biol. Chem.* 278, 28052–28059. doi: 10.1074/jbc.M304296200

Furukawa, Y., Fu, R., Deng, H. X., Siddique, T., and O'Halloran, T. V. (2006). Disulfide cross-linked protein represents a significant fraction of ALS-associated Cu, Zn-superoxide dismutase aggregates in spinal cords of model mice. *Proc. Natl. Acad. Sci. U.S.A.* 103, 7148–7153. doi: 10.1073/pnas.0602048103

Furukawa, Y., Kaneko, K., Yamanaka, K., O'Halloran, T. V., and Nukina, N. (2008). Complete loss of post-translational modifications triggers fibrillar aggregation of SOD1 in familial form of ALS. *J. Biol. Chem.* 283, 24167–24176. doi: 10.1074/jbc.M802083200

Furukawa, Y., and O'Halloran, T. V. (2005). Amyotrophic lateral sclerosis mutations have the greatest destabilizing effect on the apo, reduced form of SOD1, leading to unfolding and oxidative aggregation. *J. Biol. Chem.* 280, 17266–17274. doi: 10.1074/jbc.M500482200

Furukawa, Y., Torres, A. S., and O'Halloran, T. V. (2004). Oxygen-induced maturation of SOD1: a key role for disulfide formation by the copper chaperone CCS. *EMBO J.* 23, 2872–2881. doi: 10.1038/sj.emboj.7600276

Goto, J. J., Zhu, H. N., Sanchez, R. J., Nersissian, A., Gralla, E. B., Valentine, J. S., et al. (2000). Loss of in vitro metal ion binding specificity in mutant copper-zinc superoxide dismutases associated with familial amyotrophic lateral sclerosis. *J. Biol. Chem.* 275, 1007–1014. doi: 10.1074/jbc.275.2.1007

Guareschi, S., Cova, E., Cereda, C., Ceroni, M., Donetti, E., Bosco, D. A., et al. (2012). An over-oxidized form of superoxide dismutase found in sporadic amyotrophic lateral sclerosis with bulbar onset shares a toxic mechanism with mutant SOD1. *Proc. Natl. Acad. Sci. U.S.A.* 109, 5074–5079. doi: 10.1073/pnas.1115402109

Hayward, L. J., Rodriguez, J. A., Kim, J. W., Tiwari, A., Goto, J. J., Cabelli, D. E., et al. (2002). Decreased metallation and activity in subsets of mutant superoxide dismutases associated with familial amyotrophic lateral sclerosis. *J. Biol. Chem.* 277, 15923–15931. doi: 10.1074/jbc.M112087200

Hu, J., Dong, L., and Outten, C. E. (2008). The redox environment in the mitochondrial intermembrane space is maintained separately from the cytosol and matrix. *J. Biol. Chem.* 283, 29126–29134. doi: 10.1074/jbc.M803028200

Hwang, C., Sinskey, A. J., and Lodish, H. F. (1992). Oxidized redox state of glutathione in the endoplasmic reticulum. *Science* 257, 1496–1502. doi: 10.1126/science.1523409

Jonsson, P. A., Graffmo, K. S., Andersen, P. M., Brannstrom, T., Lindberg, M., Oliveberg, M., et al. (2006). Disulphide-reduced superoxide dismutase-1 in CNS of transgenic amyotrophic lateral sclerosis models. *Brain* 129, 451–464. doi: 10.1093/brain/awh704

Karch, C. M., Prudencio, M., Winkler, D. D., Hart, P. J., and Borchelt, D. R. (2009). Role of mutant SOD1 disulfide oxidation and aggregation in the pathogenesis of familial ALS. *Proc. Natl. Acad. Sci. U.S.A.* 106, 7774–7779. doi: 10.1073/pnas.0902505106

Klunk, W. E., Jacob, R. F., and Mason, R. P. (1999). Quantifying amyloid by congo red spectral shift assay. *Methods Enzymol.* 309, 285–305. doi: 10.1016/S0076-6879(99)09021-7

Leinweber, B., Barofsky, E., Barofsky, D. F., Ermilov, V., Nylin, K., and Beckman, J. S. (2004). Aggregation of ALS mutant superoxide dismutase expressed in *Escherichia coli*. *Free Radic. Biol. Med.* 36, 911–918. doi: 10.1016/j.freeradbiomed.2003.12.021

Leitch, J. M., Jensen, L. T., Bouldin, S. D., Outten, C. E., Hart, P. J., and Culotta, V. C. (2009). Activation of Cu,Zn-superoxide dismutase in the absence of oxygen and the copper chaperone CCS. *J. Biol. Chem.* 284, 21863–21871. doi: 10.1074/jbc.M109.000489

LeVine, H. III. (1999). Quantification of beta-sheet amyloid fibril structures with thioflavin T. *Methods Enzymol.* 309, 274–284. doi: 10.1016/S0076-6879(99)09020-5

Lobstein, J., Emrich, C. A., Jeans, C., Faulkner, M., Riggs, P., and Berkmen, M. (2012). SHuffle, a novel *Escherichia coli* protein expression strain capable of correctly folding disulfide bonded proteins in its cytoplasm. *Microb. Cell Fact.* 11, 56. doi: 10.1186/1475-2859-11-56

McCord, J. M., and Fridovich, I. (1969). Superoxide dismutase. An enzymic function for erythrocuprein (hemocuprein). *J. Biol. Chem.* 244, 6049–6055.

Morell, M., Bravo, R., Espargaro, A., Sisquella, X., Aviles, F. X., Fernandez-Busquets, X., et al. (2008). Inclusion bodies: specificity in their aggregation process and amyloid-like structure. *Biochim. Biophys. Acta* 1783, 1815–1825. doi: 10.1016/j.bbamcr.2008.06.007

Nagai, M., Aoki, M., Miyoshi, I., Kato, M., Pasinelli, P., Kasai, N., et al. (2001). Rats expressing human cytosolic copper-zinc superoxide dismutase transgenes with amyotrophic lateral sclerosis: associated mutations develop motor neuron disease. *J. Neurosci.* 21, 9246–9254.

Nordlund, A., and Oliveberg, M. (2006). Folding of Cu/Zn superoxide dismutase suggests structural hotspots for gain of neurotoxic function in ALS: parallels to precursors in amyloid disease. *Proc. Natl. Acad. Sci. U.S.A.* 103, 10218–10223. doi: 10.1073/pnas.0601696103

Okado-Matsumoto, A., and Fridovich, I. (2001). Subcellular distribution of superoxide dismutases (SOD) in rat liver: Cu,Zn-SOD in mitochondria. *J. Biol. Chem.* 276, 38388–38393. doi: 10.1074/jbc.M105395200

Outten, C. E., and O'Halloran, T. V. (2001). Femtomolar sensitivity of metalloregulatory proteins controlling zinc homeostasis. *Science* 292, 2488–2492. doi: 10.1126/science.1060331

Rakhit, R., Cunningham, P., Furtos-Matei, A., Dahan, S., Qi, X. F., Crow, J. P., et al. (2002). Oxidation-induced misfolding and aggregation of superoxide dismutase and its implications for amyotrophic lateral sclerosis. *J. Biol. Chem.* 277, 47551–47556. doi: 10.1074/jbc.M207356200

Rodriguez, J. A., Shaw, B. F., Durazo, A., Sohn, S. H., Doucette, P. A., Nersissian, A. M., et al. (2005). Destabilization of apoprotein is insufficient to explain Cu,Zn-superoxide dismutase-linked ALS pathogenesis. *Proc. Natl. Acad. Sci. U.S.A.* 102, 10516–10521. doi: 10.1073/pnas.0502515102

Rosen, D. R., Siddique, T., Patterson, D., Figlewicz, D. A., Sapp, P., Hentati, A., et al. (1993). Mutations in Cu/Zn superoxide dismutase gene are associated with familial amyotrophic lateral sclerosis. *Nature* 362, 59–62. doi: 10.1038/362059a0

Sabate, R., Espargaro, A., Saupe, S. J., and Ventura, S. (2009). Characterization of the amyloid bacterial inclusion bodies of the HET-s fungal prion. *Microb. Cell Fact.* 8, 56. doi: 10.1186/1475-2859-8-56

Sevier, C. S., and Kaiser, C. A. (2002). Formation and transfer of disulphide bonds in living cells. *Nat. Rev. Mol. Cell Biol.* 3, 836–847. doi: 10.1038/nrm954

Shibata, N., Hirano, A., Kobayashi, M., Siddique, T., Deng, H. X., Hung, W. Y., et al. (1996). Intense superoxide dismutase-1 immunoreactivity in intracytoplasmic hyaline inclusions of familial amyotrophic lateral sclerosis with posterior column involvement. *J. Neuropathol. Exp. Neurol.* 55, 481–490. doi: 10.1097/00005072-199604000-00011

Spagnolo, L., Toro, I., D'Orazio, M., O'Neill, P., Pedersen, J. Z., Carugo, O., et al. (2004). Unique features of the sodC-encoded superoxide dismutase from Mycobacterium tuberculosis, a fully functional copper-containing enzyme lacking zinc in the active site. *J. Biol. Chem.* 279, 33447–33455. doi: 10.1074/jbc.M404699200

Subramaniam, J. R., Lyons, W. E., Liu, J., Bartnikas, T. B., Rothstein, J., Price, D. L., et al. (2002). Mutant SOD1 causes motor neuron disease independent of copper chaperone-mediated copper loading. *Nat. Neurosci.* 5, 301–307. doi: 10.1038/nn823

Tiwari, A., and Hayward, L. J. (2003). Familial amyotrophic lateral sclerosis mutants of copper/zinc superoxide dismutase are susceptible to disulfide reduction. *J. Biol. Chem.* 278, 5984–5992. doi: 10.1074/jbc.M210419200

Toichi, K., Yamanaka, K., and Furukawa, Y. (2013). Disulfide scrambling describes the oligomer formation of superoxide dismutase (SOD1) proteins in the familial form of amyotrophic lateral sclerosis. *J. Biol. Chem.* 288, 4970–4980. doi: 10.1074/jbc.M112.414235

Vassall, K. A., Stubbs, H. R., Primmer, H. A., Tong, M. S., Sullivan, S. M., Sobering, R., et al. (2011). Decreased stability and increased formation of soluble aggregates by immature superoxide dismutase do not account for disease severity in ALS. *Proc. Natl. Acad. Sci. U.S.A.* 108, 2210–2215. doi: 10.1073/pnas.0913021108

Villar-Pique, A., and Ventura, S. (2012). Modeling amyloids in bacteria. *Microb. Cell Fact.* 11, 166. doi: 10.1186/1475-2859-11-166

Watanabe, M., Dykes-Hoberg, M., Culotta, V. C., Price, D. L., Wong, P. C., and Rothstein, J. D. (2001). Histological evidence of protein aggregation in mutant SOD1 transgenic mice and in amyotrophic lateral sclerosis neural tissues. *Neurobiol. Dis.* 8, 933–941. doi: 10.1006/nbdi.2001.0443

Zhang, H., Andrekopoulos, C., Joseph, J., Chandran, K., Karoui, H., Crow, J. P., et al. (2003). Bicarbonate-dependent peroxidase activity of human Cu, Zn-superoxide dismutase induces covalent aggregation of protein: intermediacy of tryptophan-derived oxidation products. *J. Biol. Chem.* 278, 24078–24089. doi: 10.1074/jbc.M302051200

11

Cellular and molecular mechanisms involved in the neuroprotective effects of VEGF on motoneurons

***Jerònia Lladó*[1,2]*, *Laia Tolosa*[1,2†] *and Gabriel Olmos*[1,2]**

[1] *Grup de Neurobiologia Celular, Departament de Biologia, Universitat de les Illes Balears, Palma de Mallorca, Spain*
[2] *Institut Universitari d'Investigacions en Ciències de la Salut (IUNICS), Universitat de les Illes Balears, Palma de Mallorca, Spain*

Edited by:
Ricardo Tapia, Universidad Nacional Autónoma de México, Mexico

Reviewed by:
Angel M. Pastor, Universidad de Sevilla, Spain
Carmen Ruiz De Almodovar, University of Heidelberg, Germany

****Correspondence:***
Jerònia Lladó, Grup de Neurobiologia Celular, Departament de Biologia, Universitat de les Illes Balears, Ed. Guillem Colom, Cra. de Valldemossa, km 7.5, E-07122 Palma de Mallorca, Illes Balears, Spain
e-mail: jeronia.llado@uib.es

Vascular endothelial growth factor (VEGF), originally described as a factor with a regulatory role in vascular growth and development, it is also known for its direct effects on neuronal cells. The discovery in the past decade that transgenic mice expressing reduced levels of VEGF developed late-onset motoneuron pathology, reminiscent of amyotrophic lateral sclerosis (ALS), opened a new field of research on this disease. VEGF has been shown to protect motoneurons from excitotoxic death, which is a relevant mechanism involved in motoneuron degeneration in ALS. Thus, VEGF delays motoneuron degeneration and increases survival in animal models of ALS. VEGF exerts its anti-excitotoxic effects on motoneurons through molecular mechanisms involving the VEGF receptor-2 resulting in the activation of the PI3-K/Akt signaling pathway, upregulation of GluR2 subunit of AMPA receptors, inhibition of p38MAPK, and induction of the anti-apoptotic molecule Bcl-2. In addition, VEGF acts on astrocytes to reduce astroglial activation and to induce the release of growth factors. The potential use of VEGF as a therapeutic tool in ALS is counteracted by its vascular effects and by its short effective time frame. More studies are needed to assess the optimal isoform, route of administration, and time frame for using VEGF in the treatment of ALS.

Keywords: VEGF, motoneuron, ALS, AMPA receptors, excitotoxicity, Akt

INTRODUCTION

Vascular endothelial growth factor (VEGF) was originally described as a factor with a regulatory role in vascular growth and development (reviewed by Carmeliet, 2003; Ferrara, 2004); currently, it is also known for its direct effects on a variety of neuronal cells, modulating neuronal migration, neuritic outgrowth, axon guidance and neuronal survival (reviewed by Ruiz de Almodovar et al., 2009; Mackenzie and Ruhrberg, 2012; Rosenstein et al., 2012).

The VEGFs form a family of growth factors that includes VEGF-A, VEGF-B, VEGF-C, VEGF-D, VEGF-E, and placental growth factor (Takahashi and Shibuya, 2005). The biological activity of the VEGF family is mediated through the binding to two classes of receptors. The tyrosine kinase receptors include the VEGF receptor-1 (VEGFR1, Flt-1), VEGF receptor-2 (VEGFR2, KDR, Flk-1), and VEGF receptor-3 (VEGFR3, Flt-4). The second class, the non-tyrosine kinase receptors, are the neuropilin-1 (NP-1) and neuropilin-2 (NP-2), which are also receptors for semaphorins, and function as co-receptors for the VEGFRs (reviewed by Carmeliet and Ruiz de Almodovar, 2013).

Vascular endothelial growth factor-A (hereafter referred as VEGF) is expressed in different isoforms in humans, which differ in molecular mass, solubility, receptor affinity, and most likely, in its biological function. $VEGF_{165}$ is the predominant isoform and is secreted as a 45-kDa covalently linked homodimer (reviewed by Bogaert et al., 2006). VEGF is widely expressed throughout the central nervous system. Its expression has been reported in neurons (Ogunshola et al., 2002; Schiera et al., 2007), astroglia (Ijichi et al., 1995), and microglia (Bartholdi et al., 1997). VEGF expression is low in the normal adult spinal cord (Fu et al., 2005); however, it increases in response to injury (Choi et al., 2007). VEGF binds to VEGFR1, VEGFR2, NP-1, and NP-2. VEGFR2 is expressed in many populations of neurons and some glial cells; whereas VEGFR1 is predominantly expressed by activated astrocytes and microglia following acute injury (Ogunshola et al., 2002; Choi et al., 2007; Krum et al., 2008; Ruiz de Almodovar et al., 2009). In addition, direct effects of VEGF on Schwann cells have been described (Sondell et al., 1999). NP-1 and NP-2 are expressed in different types of neurons (Kolodkin et al., 1997; Giger et al., 1998), and also in spinal cord motoneurons (Oosthuyse et al., 2001).

Vascular endothelial growth factor has pro-survival effects on some neuronal cells, protects against experimentally induced cell death (Jin et al., 2000), stimulates axonal growth, and guidance (Sondell et al., 2000; Erskine et al., 2011; Ruiz de Almodovar et al., 2011), stimulates neurogenesis (Jin et al., 2002), regulates neuronal migration (Schwarz et al., 2004; Ruiz de Almodovar et al., 2010), and promotes dendrite patterning and synaptic plasticity (Licht et al., 2010, 2011). In addition to the vascular effects of VEGF protecting motoneurons by ensuring optimal blood supply to brain and spinal cord, it functions as a neurotrophic factor for motoneurons (Oosthuyse et al., 2001; Van Den Bosch et al., 2004). VEGF protects motoneurons from insults such as oxidative stress (Li et al., 2003), hypoxia/hypoglycemia (Van Den Bosch et al., 2004), and glutamate-excitotoxicity (Tovar-Y-Romo et al., 2007; Tolosa et al., 2008; Tovar-Y-Romo and Tapia, 2010).

ROLE OF VEGF IN AMYOTROPHIC LATERAL SCLEROSIS PATHOGENESIS

The discovery in the past decade that transgenic mice with a homozygous deletion in the hypoxia response element site in the VEGF promoter (VEGF$^{\delta/\delta}$ mice) expressed reduced levels of VEGF (25–40% less) and developed late-onset motoneuron pathology reminiscent of amyotrophic lateral sclerosis (ALS), opened a new field of research on this dramatic disease. Interestingly, all the classic features of ALS including misaccumulation of neurofilaments in brainstem and spinal cord motoneurons, degeneration of motor axons, and denervation-induced muscle atrophy can be observed in these mice (Oosthuyse et al., 2001). As expected, mice engineered to overexpress VEGF had a delayed motoneuron degeneration and an increased survival when crossed to the superoxide dismutase-1 (SOD1) mouse model of ALS (Wang et al., 2007). In addition, the reduction in the levels of VEGF in the SOD1 mutant mice by crossbreeding the SOD1 mouse model of ALS with VEGF$^{\delta/\delta}$ mice worsened the disease, resulting in a decrease in survival due to more severe motoneuron degeneration and earlier onset of muscle weakness (Lambrechts et al., 2003). Interestingly, in the SOD1 mutant mice model of ALS, mutant SOD1 can disrupt the post-transcriptional regulation of VEGF, leading to decreased production of this neurotrophic factor. This effect seems to be restricted to spinal cord, and the decline in VEGF mRNA levels is apparent before onset of weakness, and is more pronounced at middle and end-stages of the disease (Lu et al., 2007). Together, these results suggest a clear relationship between VEGF expression and the familial forms of ALS linked to SOD1 mutations. It still remains unknown the role that VEGF could play in sporadic ALS. In this sense, genetic studies in humans have indicated that VEGF is a modifier of motoneuron degeneration, as a low-VEGF genotype was associated to an increased susceptibility to ALS (Lambrechts et al., 2009).

It is accepted that the major mediator of the trophic effects on spinal cord motoneurons is VEGFR2 (Tolosa et al., 2008; Tovar-Y-Romo and Tapia, 2010), and the concurrent expression of VEGF and VEGFR2 may suggest autocrine/paracrine effects on these cells (Oosthuyse et al., 2001; Ogunshola et al., 2002; Brockington et al., 2006). Interestingly, both VEGF and VEGFR2 expression is reduced in motoneurons and spinal cord of ALS patients (Brockington et al., 2006). Furthermore, the importance of VEGFR2 has been reinforced by experiments showing increased survival of SOD1 mutant mice after overexpression of VEGFR2 (Storkebaum et al., 2005). These findings support the hypothesis that reduced VEGF signaling may play a role in the pathogenesis of ALS (reviewed by Sathasivam, 2008).

Excitotoxicity is a fundamental mechanism involved in motoneuron degeneration in ALS (reviewed by Van Den Bosch et al., 2006). Defective glutamate transport, causing an abnormally increased extracellular concentration of glutamate and over activation of glutamate receptors, has been proposed as an important mechanism in the excitotoxic process in ALS (Rothstein, 2009). In this regard, a decreased expression of the GLT-1 astroglial transporter has been found in the SOD1 animal models around spinal cord motoneurons (Bendotti et al., 2001; Howland et al., 2002). Excessive calcium influx through α-amino-3-hydroxy-5-methyl-4-isoxazole propionic acid (AMPA) glutamate receptors is the final effector of motoneuron death in the excitotoxic process. Motoneurons are especially vulnerable to AMPA receptor-mediated excitotoxicity both *in vitro* and *in vivo* as they express a high number of Ca^{2+}-permeable AMPA receptors (Carriedo et al., 1996; Van Den Bosch et al., 2000). The permeability of the AMPA receptor depends upon the GluR2 subunit, which regulates the permeability to calcium: only AMPA receptors lacking GluR2 are permeable to calcium. In this regard, motoneurons express low levels of GluR2 and this renders them vulnerable to AMPA receptor-mediated excitotoxicity (Van Damme et al., 2002). Thus, selective loss of motoneurons can be induced experimentally by intrathecal or intraspinal administration of AMPA receptor agonists (Corona and Tapia, 2004; Sun et al., 2006).

In our laboratory, we used spinal cord organotypic cultures to create a model of chronic glutamate excitotoxicity in which glutamate transporters were inhibited by threohydroxyaspartate (THA) to induce motoneuron death. The exposure of these cultures to THA in the presence of VEGF significantly increased motoneuron survival (Tolosa et al., 2008). Similar results were previously obtained *in vivo* after AMPA-induced chronic excitotoxicity in rat spinal cord (Tovar-Y-Romo et al., 2007). Thus, VEGF protects motoneurons from excitotoxic death; however, it has been recently demonstrated *in vivo* that the therapeutic potential of VEGF against excitotoxicity has a short effective time frame, i.e., VEGF was effective only when administered before the onset of motor symptoms (Tovar-y-Romo and Tapia, 2012).

MECHANISMS OF VEGF PROTECTION AGAINST EXCITOTOXICITY IN ALS

Matsuzaki et al. (2001) initially identified VEGFR2 as the receptor responsible for the neuroprotective effects of VEGF against excitotoxicity in hippocampal neurons. VEGFR2 is expressed by motoneurons in humans (Brockington et al., 2006), mouse (Oosthuyse et al., 2001), and neonatal (Tolosa et al., 2008) and adult rats (Tovar-Y-Romo and Tapia, 2010), and the anti-excitotoxic effects of VEGF in these cells have also been attributed to this receptor (Bogaert et al., 2006; Tolosa et al., 2008; Tovar-Y-Romo and Tapia, 2010).

The signal transduction pathways activated by VEGF are well-characterized in endothelial cells; however, the knowledge of the signaling pathways involved in the anti-excitotoxic effects of VEGF is still incomplete. Upon ligand binding, VEGFR2 undergoes phosphorylation (Meyer et al., 1999), activating intracellular signaling pathways including phosphatidylinositol 3-kinase (PI3-K)/Akt and mitogen-activated protein kinase/extracellular signal-regulated kinase (MEK)/extracellular signal-regulated kinase (ERK). The relevance of the PI3-K/Akt pathway in the neuroprotective effects of VEGF was first proven on the motoneuron-like NSC34 cell line (Li et al., 2003) and also in SOD1 mutant rats where it was shown to counteract the loss of Akt activity preceding motoneuron degeneration (Dewil et al., 2007b). We demonstrated for the first time in spinal cord organotypic cultures that inhibition of the PI3-K/Akt pathway abolishes the anti-excitotoxic effects of VEGF on motoneurons exposed to a glutamate transporter inhibitor (Tolosa et al., 2008). These results were further confirmed *in vivo* in rats exposed to AMPA (Tovar-Y-Romo and

Tapia, 2010). These studies also suggested that the MEK/ERK was less relevant than the PI3-K/Akt signaling pathway, as MEK inhibition had a limited effect on the VEGF-mediated neuroprotection against AMPA-induced excitotoxicity (Tovar-Y-Romo and Tapia, 2010).

Activation of PI3-K by VEGF has additional neuroprotective implications as Akt phosphorylates and activates the cyclic AMP-response element binding protein (CREB), involved in the transcription of the Bcl-2 gene (Pugazhenthi et al., 2000). We demonstrated that excitotoxic conditions are associated to a decreased expression of Bcl-2 in spinal cord cultures, and that VEGF-induced neuroprotection in motoneurons could be related to the restoration, via PI3-K, of Bcl-2 levels in these cultures, and specifically in motoneurons (Tolosa et al., 2008). Bcl-2, besides its ability to block cytochrome *c* release, has been shown to increase calcium uptake and buffering capacity in mitochondria (Zhong et al., 1993), thus protecting against excitotoxicity. Additionally, it has been shown that Bcl-2 overexpression attenuates motoneuron degeneration in the SOD1 animal model (Azzouz et al., 2000).

Interestingly, it has been suggested that the PI3-K/Akt signaling pathway could be involved in GluR2 subunit assembly into AMPA receptors (Rainey-Smith et al., 2010). In this sense, VEGF has been shown, both *in vitro* and *in vivo*, to increase the expression of GluR2 subunit, thus reducing the permeability of AMPA receptors to calcium, and minimizing the vulnerability of motoneurons to AMPA-mediated excitotoxicity (Bogaert et al., 2010). Thus, a potential mechanism for VEGF protection against excitotoxicity would be through a PI3-K/Akt-mediated insertion of the GluR2 subunit of the AMPA receptor in motoneurons. Astrocytes are able to protect against excitotoxicity by inducing GluR2 expression in motoneurons. Interestingly, mutant SOD1 abolishes the ability of astrocytes to regulate GluR2 and thus, increase the susceptibility of motoneurons to excitotoxicity (Van Damme et al., 2007). It remains unknown if the VEGF-induced insertion of GluR2 could be astrocyte-mediated.

p38 mitogen-activated protein kinase (p38MAPK) belongs to a family of protein kinases activated by a range of stimuli including proinflammatory cytokines and oxidative stress (Mielke and Herdegen, 2000). As increased phosphorylation of p38MAPK has been reported in the spinal cord of SOD1 mutant mice, in motoneurons and glial cells, this kinase has been suggested to play a role in the pathogenesis of ALS (Tortarolo et al., 2003; Bendotti et al., 2004). In addition, a motoneuron specific death pathway, involving Fas, p38MAPK, and neuronal nitric oxide synthase activation has been described. Motoneurons from SOD1 mutant mice displayed increased susceptibility to activation of this pathway (Raoul et al., 2002).

Rho-mediated calcium-dependent activation of p38αMAPK has been described as a trigger of excitotoxic cell-death (Semenova et al., 2007). In this regard, it has been shown that VEGF is able to block the AMPA-induced phosphorylation of p38MAPK (Tovar-Y-Romo and Tapia, 2010), thus identifying another molecular mechanism for the anti-excitotoxic effects of VEGF. However, the sole inhibition of p38MAPK activity is not sufficient to protect motoneurons against excitotoxicity as the anti-excitotoxic effects of VEGF are also dependent on the activation of the PI3-K/Akt pathway (Tovar-Y-Romo and Tapia, 2010). In this regard, PI3-K/Akt has been reported to inhibit the phosphorylation of p38MAPK in an apoptosis signal-regulating kinase 1 (ASK1)-dependent manner (Ichijo et al., 1997; Kim et al., 2001). In agreement with that, our group has demonstrated that VEGF protects motoneurons from serum deprivation-induced cell death through PI3-K-mediated inhibition of p38MAPK phosphorylation (Tolosa et al., 2009). Moreover, the inhibition by VEGF of p38MAPK might protect motoneurons in ALS tissue exerting a dual role both through an indirect effect on glial cells (Tortarolo et al., 2003), and a direct anti-apoptotic effect on motoneurons (Dewil et al., 2007a).

ROLE OF NON-NEURONAL CELLS IN THE NEUROPROTECTIVE EFFECTS OF VEGF

Astroglia (Oosthuyse et al., 2001) and microglia (Bartholdi et al., 1997) are sources of VEGF in the spinal cord and a role for non-neuronal cells has been described in the onset and progression of the pathology in ALS (Clement et al., 2003; Barbeito et al., 2004; Sargsyan et al., 2005). It has been hypothesized that VEGF may also affect motoneurons through an indirect effect on glial cells, as both astrocytes (Krum et al., 2002) and microglia (Ryu et al., 2009) respond to VEGF stimulation. On the one hand, VEGF may affect the glial release of trophic factors, and thus, indirectly, protect motoneurons (reviewed by Bogaert et al., 2006). On the other hand, VEGF decreases the astroglial activation observed in the SOD1 mouse model of ALS, and also enhances neuromuscular junction formation (Zheng et al., 2007). Moreover, the neuroprotective effects observed with lithium in animal models of ALS could be due, in part, to an upregulation of VEGF in non-neuronal cells, as an increase in VEGF has been observed after lithium exposure in brain astrocytes and endothelial cells (Guo et al., 2009). In spite of these potential neuroprotective effects of VEGF involving non-neuronal cells, recently, it has been demonstrated that, under inflammatory conditions, astrocytic expression of VEGF is a key driver of blood–brain barrier disruption, leading to edema, excitotoxicity, and entry of inflammatory cells (Argaw et al., 2012).

Several *in vivo* and *in vitro* studies have indicated that VEGF induces adult neurogenesis (Jin et al., 2002; Cao et al., 2004). It still remains unknown if VEGF *in vivo* induces neurogenesis directly in neural stem cells or indirectly through effects on endothelial cells or other cell types (reviewed by Carmeliet and Ruiz de Almodovar, 2013). The potential of VEGF generating new neurons, together with its ability to induce axon growth could be relevant in its neuroprotective effects on ALS.

POTENTIAL USE OF VEGF AS A THERAPEUTIC TOOL IN ALS

Vascular endothelial growth factor clearly ameliorates the illness in the mutant SOD1 mice and rats (Azzouz et al., 2004; Storkebaum et al., 2005; Wang et al., 2007), supporting the hypothesis of a role for VEGF in ALS. VEGF has been administered to animals using different strategies. VEGF was administered using lentiviral vectors (intramuscularly delivered and then retrogradely transported) increasing the life expectancy of ALS mice. The treatment was more effective when initiated before disease onset (Azzouz et al., 2004).

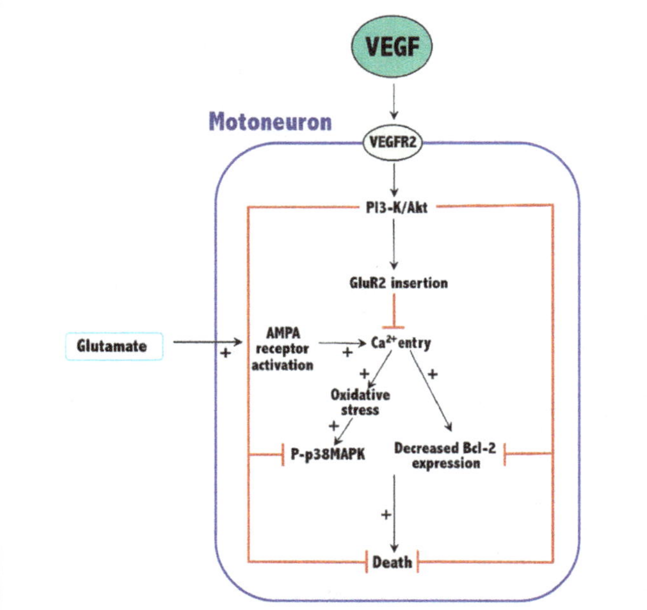

FIGURE 1 | Mechanisms involved in the neuroprotective effects of VEGF against excitotoxicity in spinal cord motoneurons. The plus symbols (+) indicate the signaling pathways that are potentiated by excitotoxicity. See Section "Conclusion" for further details.

Intravenous administration of VEGF induces vascular effects: blood vessel growth or blood–brain barrier alterations (Young et al., 2004). To avoid these problematic side-effects, continuous intracerebroventricular (i.c.v.) administration of VEGF in ALS rats was performed. VEGF at doses between 0.2 and 2 $\mu g \cdot kg^{-1} \cdot day$ was safe as it did not induce angiogenesis or inflammation. Besides, it was demonstrated that VEGF diffused from the cerebrospinal fluid to the spinal cord parenchyma, reaching motoneurons, and thus, improving motor performance and prolonging survival of SOD1 rats (Storkebaum et al., 2005). Thus, either retrograde (Azzouz et al., 2004) or paracrine (Storkebaum et al., 2005) delivery of VEGF is effective in the animal models of ALS.

Poesen et al. (2008) have demonstrated that the VEGF-B_{186} isoform is also expressed in the nervous system, has less vascular effects, and also functions as a neuroprotective factor for motoneurons. Interestingly, in contrast to VEGF-A, the presence of VEGF-B is not critical for survival or for motoneuron development in physiological conditions; however, crossing VEGF-$B^{-/-}$ mice with SOD1 mice aggravated motoneuron degeneration. The effect of VEGF-B_{186} seems to be mediated by VEGFR-1, which is also expressed by spinal cord motoneurons, indicating that they can respond to this VEGF-B isoform. In addition, as VEGFR1 is also expressed on astrocytes, an indirect effect on glia could not be ruled out. Finally, the authors demonstrated that i.c.v. delivery of VEGF-B ameliorated the disease in SOD1 rats without exhibiting side vascular effects (Poesen et al., 2008).

Taking advantage of these previous studies on animal models of ALS, ongoing clinical trials are essaying direct i.c.v. administration of VEGF in humans. Clinical trials on phase I/II investigate safety parameters in ALS patients and those on phase II/III are intended to evaluate the efficacy to increase lifespan (http://www.neuronova.com/index.php?option=com_content&task=view&id=40&Itemid=71).

CONCLUSION

Current knowledge indicates that VEGF can prevent excitotoxic motoneuron death, thus prolonging survival in an animal model of ALS. These effects are VEGFR2-mediated and involve the activation of the PI3-K/Akt signaling pathway, which results in an increased expression of both Bcl-2 and the GluR2 subunit of AMPA receptors. The overall effect of these proteins would be to reduce the excessive entry of calcium characteristic of the excitotoxic process. Thus, Bcl-2 increases the calcium uptake and the buffering capacity of mitochondria, and GluR2 assembly into AMPA receptors reduces their permeability to calcium. By reducing calcium levels into motoneurons of ALS tissue, VEGF reduces oxidative stress and p38MAPK activity, thus improving survival (**Figure 1**).

Although many of the experimental evidences of the benefits of VEGF in ALS are taken from *in vitro* or *ex vivo* experiments, the promising results obtained in animal models of familial ALS substantiate a potential use of VEGF as a therapeutic tool. However, its effectiveness may be counteracted by its vascular effects and by its expected short effective time frame (Tovar-y-Romo and Tapia, 2012). Clearly, more studies are needed to assess the optimal family member/isoform, the route of administration and the time frame for using VEGF in the treatment of ALS. In addition, a better understanding of the cellular and molecular mechanisms involved in the neuroprotective effects of VEGF will be crucial for its therapeutic development.

REFERENCES

Argaw, A. T., Asp, L., Zhang, J., Navrazhina, K., Pham, T., Mariani, J. N., et al. (2012). Astrocyte-derived VEGF-A drives blood–brain barrier disruption in CNS inflammatory dis- ease. *J. Clin. Invest.* 122, 2454–2468. doi: 10.1172/JCI60842

Azzouz, M., Hottinger, A., Paterna, J. C., Zurn, A. D., Aebischer, P., and Bueler, H. (2000). Increased motoneuron survival and improved neuromus- cular function in transgenic ALS mice after intraspinal injection of an adeno-associated virus encoding Bcl-2. *Hum. Mol. Genet.* 9, 803–811. doi: 10.1093/hmg/9.5.803

Azzouz, M., Ralph, G. S., Storke- baum, E., Walmsley, L. E., Mitro- phanous, K. A., Kingsman, S. M., et al. (2004). VEGF delivery with retrogradely transported lentivector prolongs survival in a mouse ALS model. *Nature* 429, 413–417. doi: 10.1038/nature02544

Barbeito, L. H., Pehar, M., Cassina, P., Vargas, M. R., Peluffo, H., Viera, L., et al. (2004). A role for astro- cytes in motor neuron loss in amy- otrophic lateral sclerosis. *Brain Res. Brain Res. Rev.* 47, 263–274. doi: 10.1016/j.brainresrev.2004.05.003

Bartholdi, D., Rubin, B. P., and Schwab, M. E. (1997). VEGF mRNA induction correlates with changes in the vas- cular architecture upon spinal cord damage in the rat. *Eur. J. Neurosci.* 9, 2549–2560. doi: 10.1111/j.1460- 9568.1997.tb01684.x

Bendotti, C., Atzori, C., Piva, R., Tortarolo, M., Strong, M. J., Debi- asi, S., et al. (2004). Activated p38MAPK is a novel component of the intracellular inclusions found in human amyotrophic lateral sclerosis and mutant SOD1 transgenic mice. *J. Neuropathol. Exp. Neurol.* 63, 113– 119.

Bendotti, C., Tortarolo, M., Suchak, S. K., Calvaresi, N., Carvelli, L., Bastone, A., et al. (2001). Transgenic SOD1 G93A mice develop reduced GLT- 1 in spinal cord without alterations in cerebrospinal fluid glutamate lev- els. *J. Neurochem.* 79, 737–746. doi: 10.1046/j.1471-4159.2001.00572.x

Bogaert, E., Van Damme, P., Poesen, K., Dhondt, J., Hersmus, N., Kiraly, D., et al. (2010). VEGF protects motor neurons against excitotoxicity by upregulation of GluR2. *Neu- robiol. Aging* 31, 2185–2191. doi: 10.1016/j.neurobiolaging.2008.12.007

Bogaert, E., Van Damme, P., Van Den Bosch, L., and Robberecht, W. (2006). Vascular endothelial growth factor in amyotrophic lateral sclero- sis and other neurodegenerative dis- eases. *Muscle Nerve* 34, 391–405. doi: 10.1002/mus.20609

Brockington, A., Wharton, S. B., Fer- nando, M., Gelsthorpe, C. H., Bax- ter, L., Ince, P. G., et al. (2006). Expression of vascular endothelial growth factor and its receptors in the central nervous system in amy- otrophic lateral sclerosis. *J. Neu- ropathol. Exp. Neurol.* 65, 26–36. doi: 10.1097/01.jnen.0000196134.51 217.74

Cao, L., Jiao, X., Zuzga, D. S., Liu, Y., Fong, D. M., Young, D., et al. (2004). VEGF links hippocampal activity with neurogenesis, learning and memory. *Nat. Genet.* 36, 827–835. doi: 10.1038/ng1395

Carmeliet, P. (2003). Angiogenesis in health and disease. *Nat. Med.* 9, 653–660. doi: 10.1038/nm0603-653

Carmeliet, P., and Ruiz de Almodovar, C. (2013). VEGF ligands and recep- tors: implications in neurodevelop- ment and neurodegeneration. *Cell. Mol. Life Sci.* 70, 1763–1778. doi: 10.1007/s00018-013-1283-7

Carriedo, S. G., Yin, H. Z., and Weiss, J. H. (1996). Motor neurons are selectively vulnerable to AMPA/kainate receptor-mediated injury *in vitro. J. Neurosci.* 16, 4069–4079.

Choi, J. S., Kim, H. Y., Cha, J. H., Choi, J. Y., Park, S. I., Jeong, C. H., et al. (2007). Upregulation of vascu- lar endothelial growth *factor* recep- tors Flt-1 and Flk-1 following acute spinal cord contusion in rats. *J. His- tochem. Cytochem.* 55, 821–830. doi: 10.1369/jhc.6A7139.2007

Clement, A. M., Nguyen, M. D., Roberts, E. A., Garcia, M. L., Boillee, S., Rule, M., et al. (2003). Wild-type nonneuronal cells extend survival of SOD1 mutant motor neurons in ALS mice. *Science* 302, 113–117. doi: 10.1126/science.1086071

Corona, J. C., and Tapia, R. (2004). AMPA receptor activation, but not the accumulation of endoge- nous extracellular glutamate, induces paralysis and motor neuron death in rat spinal cord *in vivo. J. Neurochem.* 89, 988–997. doi: 10.1111/j.1471- 4159.2004.02383.x

Dewil, M., Dela Cruz, V. F., Van Den Bosch, L., and Robberecht, W. (2007a). Inhibition of p38 mitogen activated protein kinase activation and mutant SOD1(G93A)- induced motor neuron death. *Neu- robiol. Dis.* 26, 332–341. doi: 10.1016/j.nbd.2006.12.023

Dewil, M., Lambrechts, D., Sciot, R., Shaw, P. J., Ince, P. G., Rob- berecht, W., et al. (2007b). Vascular endothelial growth factor counter- acts the loss of phospho-Akt preced- ing motor neurone degeneration in amyotrophic lateral sclerosis. *Neu- ropathol. Appl. Neurobiol.* 33, 499- 509. doi: 10.1111/j.1365-2990.2007. 00850.x

Erskine, L., Reijntjes, S., Pratt, T., Denti, L., Schwarz, Q., Vieira, J. M., et al. (2011). VEGF signaling through neuropilin 1 guides com- missural axon crossing at the optic chiasm. *Neuron* 70, 951–965. doi: 10.1016/j.neuron.2011.02.052

Ferrara, N. (2004). Vascular endothe- lial growth factor: basic science and clinical progress. *Endocr. Rev.* 25, 581–611. doi: 10.1210/er.2003-0027

Fu, C. Y., Hong, G. X., and Wang, F. B. (2005). Expression of vascular endothelial growth factor and its fetal liver kinase-1 receptor in spinal cord and dorsal root ganglia after neuro- tomy of sciatic nerve in rats. *Chin. J. Traumatol.* 8, 17–22.

Giger, R. J., Urquhart, E. R., Gille- spie, S. K., Levengood, D. V., Ginty, D. D., and Kolodkin, A. L. (1998). Neuropilin-2 is a receptor for semaphorin IV: insight into the structural basis of receptor function and specificity. *Neuron* 21, 1079- 1092. doi: 10.1016/S0896-6273(00) 80625-X

Guo, S., Arai, K., Stins, M. F., Chuang, D. M., and Lo, E. H. (2009). Lithium upregulates vas- cular endothelial growth factor in brain endothelial cells and astro- cytes. *Stroke* 40, 652–655. doi: 10.1161/STROKEAHA.108.524504

Howland, D. S., Liu, J., She, Y., Goad, B., Maragakis, N. J., Kim, B., et al. (2002). Focal loss of the glutamate transporter EAAT2 in a transgenic rat model of SOD1 mutant-mediated amyotrophic lateral sclerosis (ALS). *Proc. Natl. Acad. Sci. U.S.A.* 99, 1604- 1609. doi: 10.1073/pnas.032539299

Ichijo, H., Nishida, E., Irie, K., Ten Dijke, P., Saitoh, M., Moriguchi, T., et al. (1997). Induction of apopto- sis by ASK1, a mammalian MAPKKK that activates SAPK/JNK and p38 sig- naling pathways. *Science* 275, 90–94. doi: 10.1126/science.275.5296.90

Ijichi, A., Sakuma, S., and Tofilon, P. J. (1995). Hypoxia-induced vas- cular endothelial growth factor expression in normal rat astro- cyte cultures. *Glia* 14, 87–93. doi: 10.1002/glia.440140203

Jin, K., Zhu, Y., Sun, Y., Mao, X. O., Xie, L., and Greenberg, D. A. (2002). Vascular endothelial growth factor (VEGF) stimulates neurogen- esis *in vitro* and *in vivo. Proc. Natl. Acad. Sci. U.S.A.* 99, 11946–11950. doi: 10.1073/pnas.182296499

Jin, K. L., Mao, X. O., and Greenberg, D. A. (2000). Vascular endothelial growth factor: *direct* neuroprotective effect in *in vitro* ischemia. *Proc. Natl. Acad. Sci. U.S.A.* 97, 10242–10247. doi: 10.1073/pnas.97.18.10242

Kim, A. H., Khursigara, G., Sun, X., Franke, T. F., and Chao, M. V. (2001). Akt phosphorylates and negatively regulates apoptosis signal-regulating kinase 1. *Mol. Cell. Biol.* 21, 893- 901. doi: 10.1128/MCB.21.3.893-901.2001

Kolodkin, A. L., Levengood, D. V., Rowe, E. G., Tai, Y. T., Giger, R. J., and Ginty, D. D. (1997). Neu- ropilin is a semaphorin III receptor. *Cell* 90, 753–762. doi: 10.1016/S0092- 8674(00)80535-8

Krum, J. M., Mani, N., and Rosenstein, J.M. (2002). Angiogenic and astroglial responses to vascular endothelial growth factor administration in adult rat brain. *Neuroscience* 110, 589- 604. doi: 10.1016/S0306-4522(01) 00615-7

Krum, J. M., Mani, N., and Rosen- stein, J. M. (2008). Roles of the endogenous VEGF receptors flt-1 and flk-1 in astroglial and vascu- lar remodeling after brain injury. *Exp. Neurol.* 212, 108–117. doi: 10.1016/j.expneurol.2008.03.019

Lambrechts, D., Poesen, K., Fernandez- Santiago, R., Al-Chalabi, A., Del Bo, R., Van Vught, P. W., et al. (2009). Meta-analysis of vascular endothelial growth factor varia- tions in amyotrophic lateral sclero- sis: increased susceptibility in male carriers of the -2578AA genotype. *J. Med. Genet.* 46, 840–846. doi: 10.1136/jmg.2008.058222

Lambrechts, D., Storkebaum, E., Mori- moto, M., Del-Favero, J., Desmet, F., Marklund, S. L., et al. (2003). VEGF is a modifier of amyotrophic lateral sclerosis in mice and humans and protects motoneurons against ischemic death. *Nat. Genet.* 34, 383–394. doi: 10.1038/ng1211

Li, B., Xu, W., Luo, C., Gozal, D., and Liu, R. (2003). VEGF-induced activation of the PI3-K/Akt path- way reduces mutant SOD1-mediated motor neuron cell death. *Brain Res. Mol. Brain Res.* 111, 155–164. doi: 10.1016/S0169-328X(03) 00025-1

Licht, T., Eavri, R., Goshen, I., Shlo- mai, Y., Mizrahi, A., and Keshet, E. (2010). VEGF is required for dendritogenesis of newly born olfac- tory bulb interneurons. *Development* 137, 261–271. doi: 10.1242/dev. 039636

Licht, T., Goshen, I., Avital, A., Kreisel, T., Zubedat, S., Eavri, R., et al. (2011). Reversible modulations of neuronal plasticity by VEGF. *Proc. Natl. Acad. Sci. U.S.A.* 108, 5081–5086. doi: 10.1073/pnas.1007640108

Lu, L., Zheng, L., Viera, L., Suswam, E., Li, Y., Li, X., et al. (2007). Mutant Cu/Zn-superoxide dismu- tase associated with amyotrophic lateral sclerosis destabilizes vascu- lar endothelial growth factor mRNA and downregulates its expression. *J. Neurosci.* 27, 7929–7938. doi: 10.1523/JNEUROSCI.1877-07.2007

Mackenzie, F., and Ruhrberg, C. (2012). Diverse roles for VEGF-A in the nervous system. *Development* 139, 1371–1380. doi: 10.1242/dev.072348

Matsuzaki, H., Tamatani, M., Yam- aguchi, A., Namikawa, K., Kiyama, H., Vitek, M. P., et al. (2001). Vascular endothelial growth factor rescues hippocampal neurons from glutamate-induced toxicity: signal transduction cascades. *FASEB J.* 15, 1218–1220.

Meyer, M., Clauss, M., Lepple- Wienhues, A., Waltenberger, J., Augustin, H. G., Ziche, M., et al. (1999). A novel vascular endothelial growth factor encoded by Orf virus, VEGF-E, mediates angiogenesis via signalling through VEGFR-2 (KDR) but not VEGFR-1 (Flt-1) receptor tyrosine kinases. *EMBO J.* 18, 363–374. doi: 10.1093/emboj/18.2.363

Mielke, K., and Herdegen, T. (2000). JNK and p38 stresskinases – degener- ative effectors of signal-transduction- cascades in the nervous system. *Prog. Neurobiol.* 61, 45–60. doi: 10.1016/S0301-0082(99)00042-8Ogunshola, O. O., Antic, A., Donoghue,

M. J., Fan, S. Y., Kim, H., Stew- art, W. B., et al. (2002). Paracrine and autocrine functions of neuronal vascular endothelial growth factor (VEGF) in the central nervous sys- tem. *J. Biol. Chem.* 277, 11410–11415. doi: 10.1074/jbc.M111085200

Oosthuyse, B., Moons, L., Storkebaum, E., Beck, H., Nuyens, D., Brus- selmans, K., et al. (2001). Deletion of the hypoxia-response element in the vascular endothelial growth fac- tor promoter causes motor neuron degeneration. *Nat. Genet.* 28, 131- 138. doi: 10.1038/88842

Poesen, K., Lambrechts, D., Van Damme, P., Dhondt, J., Bender, F., Frank, N., et al. (2008). Novel role for vascular endothelial growth factor(VEGF) receptor-1 and its ligand VEGF-B in motor neuron degener- ation. *J. Neurosci.* 28, 10451–10459. doi: 10.1523/JNEUROSCI.1092-08. 2008

Pugazhenthi, S., Nesterova, A., Sable, C., Heidenreich, K. A., Boxer, L. M., Heasley, L. E., et al. (2000). Akt/protein kinase B up-regulates Bcl-2 expression through cAMP- response element-binding protein. *J. Biol. Chem.* 275, 10761–10766. doi: 10.1074/jbc.275.15.10761

Rainey-Smith, S. R., Andersson, D. A., Williams, R. J., and Rattray, M. (2010). Tumour necrosis fac- tor alpha induces rapid reduction in AMPA receptor-mediated calcium entry in motor neurones by increas- ing cell surface expression of the GluR2 subunit: relevance to neurode- generation. *J. Neurochem.* 113, 692– 703. doi: 10.1111/j.1471-4159.2010. 06634.x

Raoul, C., Estevez, A. G., Nishimune, H., Cleveland, D. W., Delapeyriere, O., Henderson, C. E., et al. (2002). Motoneuron death triggered by a specific pathway downstream of Fas. Potentiation by ALS-linked SOD1 mutations. *Neuron* 35, 1067–1083. doi: 10.1016/S0896-6273(02) 00905-4

Rosenstein, J. M., Krum, J. M., and Ruhrberg, C. (2012). VEGF in the nervous system. *Organogenesis* 6, 107–114. doi: 10.4161/org.6.2. 11687

Rothstein, J. D. (2009). Current hypotheses for the underlying biol- ogy of amyotrophic lateral sclerosis. *Ann. Neurol.* 65(Suppl. 1), S3–S9. doi: 10.1002/ana.21543

Ruiz de Almodovar, C., Coulon, C., Salin, P. A., Knevels, E., Chounlam- ountri, N., Poesen, K., et al. (2010). Matrix-binding vascular endothe- lial growth factor (VEGF) isoforms guide granule cell migration in the cerebellum via VEGF receptor Flk1. *J. Neurosci.* 30, 15052–15066. doi: 10.1523/JNEUROSCI.0477-10. 2010

Ruiz de Almodovar, C., Fabre, P. J., Knevels, E., Coulon, C., Segura, I., Haddick, P. C., et al. (2011). VEGF mediates commis- sural axon chemoattraction through its receptor Flk1. *Neuron* 70, 966–978. doi: 10.1016/j.neuron.2011.04. 014

Ruiz de Almodovar, C., Lambrechts, D., Mazzone, M., and Carmeliet, P. (2009). Role and therapeutic potential of VEGF in the nervous system. *Physiol. Rev.* 89, 607– 648. doi: 10.1152/physrev.00031. 2008

Ryu, J. K., Cho, T., Choi, H. B., Wang, Y. T., and Mclarnon, J. G. (2009). Microglial VEGF receptor response is an integral chemotac- tic component in Alzheimer's dis- ease pathology. *J. Neurosci.* 29, 3–13. doi: 10.1523/JNEUROSCI.2888-08. 2009

Sargsyan, S. A., Monk, P. N., and Shaw, P. J. (2005). Microglia as potential contributors to motor neuron injury in amyotrophic lateral sclerosis. *Glia* 51, 241–253. doi: 10.1002/glia. 20210

Sathasivam, S. (2008). VEGF and ALS. *Neurosci. Res.* 62, 71–77. doi: 10.1016/j.neures.2008.06.008

Schiera, G., Proia, P., Alberti, C., Mineo, M., Savettieri, G., and Di Liegro, I. (2007). Neurons produce FGF2 and VEGF and secrete them at least in part by shedding extracellular vesi- cles. *J. Cell. Mol. Med.* 11, 1384– 1394. doi: 10.1111/j.1582-4934.2007. 00100.x

Schwarz, Q., Gu, C., Fujisawa, H., Sabelko, K., Gertsenstein, M., Nagy, A., et al. (2004). Vascular endothelial growth factor controls neuronal migration and cooperates with Sema3A to pattern distinct compartments of the facial nerve. *Genes Dev.* 18, 2822–2834. doi: 10.1101/gad.322904

Semenova, M. M., Maki-Hokkonen, A. M., Cao, J., Komarovski, V., Forsberg, K. M., Koistinaho, M., et al. (2007). Rho mediates calcium- dependent activation of p38alpha and subsequent excitotoxic cell death. *Nat. Neurosci.* 10, 436–443.

Sondell, M., Lundborg, G., and Kanje, M. (1999). Vascular endothe- lial growth factor has neurotrophic activity and stimulates axonal out- growth, enhancing cell survival and Schwann cell proliferation in the peripheral nervous system. *J. Neu- rosci.* 19, 5731–5740.

Sondell, M., Sundler, F., and Kanje, M. (2000). Vascular endothelial growth factor is a neurotrophic factor which stimulates axonal outgrowth through the flk-1 receptor. *Eur. J. Neurosci.* 12, 4243–4254. doi: 10.1046/j.0953-816X.2000.01326.x

Storkebaum, E., Lambrechts, D., Dew- erchin, M., Moreno-Murciano, M. P., Appelmans, S., Oh, H., et al. (2005). Treatment of motoneuron degeneration by intracerebroventric- ular delivery of VEGF in a rat model of ALS. *Nat. Neurosci.* 8, 85–92. doi: 10.1038/nn1360

Sun, H., Kawahara, Y., Ito, K., Kanazawa, I., and Kwak, S. (2006). Slow and selective death of spinal motor neurons *in vivo* by intrathecal infusion of kainic acid: implications for AMPA receptor-mediated excitotoxicity in ALS. *J. Neurochem.* 98, 782–791. doi: 10.1111/j.1471-4159.2006. 03903.x

Takahashi, H., and Shibuya, M. (2005). The vascular endothelial growth fac- tor (VEGF)/VEGF receptor system and its role under physiological and pathological conditions. *Clin. Sci. (Lond.)* 109, 227–241. doi: 10.1042/CS20040370

Tolosa, L., Mir, M., Asensio, V. J., Olmos, G., and Llado, J. (2008). Vascu- lar endothelial growth factor protects spinal cord motoneurons against glutamate-induced excitotoxicity via phosphatidylinositol 3-kinase. *J. Neurochem.* 105, 1080–1090. doi: 10.1111/j.1471-4159.2007.05206.x

Tolosa, L., Mir, M., Olmos, G., and Llado, J. (2009). Vascular endothelial growth factor protects motoneurons from serum deprivation-induced cell death through phosphatidylinositol 3-kinase-mediated p38 mitogen- activated protein kinase inhibition. *Neuroscience* 158, 1348–1355. doi: 10.1016/j.neuroscience.2008. 10.060

Tortarolo, M., Veglianese, P., Cal- varesi, N., Botturi, A., Rossi, C., Giorgini, A., et al. (2003). Per- sistent activation of p38 mitogen- activated protein kinase in a mouse model of familial amyotrophic lateral sclerosis correlates with disease pro- gression. *Mol. Cell. Neurosci.* 23, 180–192. doi: 10.1016/S1044-7431(03) 00022-8

Tovar-Y-Romo, L. B., and Tapia, R. (2010). VEGF protects spinal motor neurons against chronic exci- totoxic degeneration *in vivo* by acti- vation of PI3-K pathway and inhi- bition of p38MAPK. *J. Neurochem.* 115, 1090–1101. doi: 10.1111/j.1471- 4159.2010.06766.x

Tovar-y-Romo, L. B., and Tapia, R. (2012). Delayed administration of VEGF rescues spinal motor neurons from death with a short effective time frame in excitotoxic experi- mental models *in vivo*. *ASN Neuro* 4, e00081. doi: 10.1042/AN2011 0057

Tovar-Y-Romo, L. B., Zepeda, A., and Tapia, R. (2007). Vascular endothelial growth factor prevents paralysis and motoneuron death in a rat model of excitotoxic spinal cord neurodegeneration. *J. Neu- ropathol. Exp. Neurol.* 66, 913– 922. doi: 10.1097/nen.0b013e31815 67c16

Van Damme, P., Bogaert, E., Dewil, M., Hersmus, N., Kiraly, D., Scheveneels, W., et al. (2007). Astrocytes reg- ulate GluR2 expression in motor neurons and their vulnerability to excitotoxicity. *Proc. Natl. Acad. Sci. U.S.A.* 104, 14825–14830. doi: 10.1073/pnas.0705046104

Van Damme, P., Van Den Bosch, L., Van Houtte, E., Callewaert, G., and Robberecht, W. (2002). GluR2- dependent properties of AMPA receptors determine the selective vul- nerability of motor neurons to exci- totoxicity. *J. Neurophysiol.* 88, 1279– 1287.

Van Den Bosch, L., Storkebaum, E., Vleminckx, V., Moons, L., Vanop- denbosch, L., Scheveneels, W., et al. (2004). Effects of vascular endothelial growth factor (VEGF) on motor neuron degeneration. *Neurobiol. Dis.* 17, 21–28. doi: 10.1016/j.nbd.2004.06.004

Van Den Bosch, L., Van Damme, P., Bogaert, E., and Robberecht, W. (2006). The role of excitotox- icity in the pathogenesis of amy- otrophic lateral sclerosis. *Biochim. Biophys. Acta* 1762, 1068–1082. doi: 10.1016/j.bbadis.2006.05.002

Van Den Bosch, L., Vandenberghe, W., Klaassen, H., Van Houtte, E., and Robberecht, W. (2000). Ca(2+)-permeable AMPA receptors and selective vulnerability of motor neurons. *J. Neurol. Sci.* 180, 29–34. doi: 10.1016/S0022-510X(00) 00414-7

Wang, Y., Mao, X. O., Xie, L., Ban- wait, S., Marti, H. H., Greenberg, D. A., et al. (2007). Vascular endothelial growth factor overexpression delays neurodegeneration and prolongs sur- vival in amyotrophic lateral sclero- sis mice. *J. Neurosci.* 27, 304–307. doi: 10.1523/JNEUROSCI.4433-06. 2007

Young, P. P., Fantz, C. R., and Sands, M. S. (2004). VEGF disrupts the neonatal blood–brain barrier and increases life span after non- ablative BMT in a murine model of congenital neurodegeneration caused by a lysosomal enzyme defi- ciency. *Exp. Neurol.* 188, 104–114. doi: 10.1016/j.expneurol.2004.03. 007

Zheng, C., Skold, M. K., Li, J., Nennesmo, I., Fadeel, B., and Henter, J. I. (2007). VEGF reduces astrogliosis and preserves neuromuscular junctions in ALS transgenic mice. *Biochem. Bio- phys. Res. Commun.* 363, 989– 993. doi: 10.1016/j.bbrc.2007.09. Y088

Zhong, L. T., Kane, D. J., and Bredesen,D. E. (1993). BCL-2 blocks glutamate toxicity in neural cell lines. *Brain Res.*

Mol. Brain Res. 19, 353–355. doi: 10.1016/0169-328X(93)90139-G

12

A seeded propagation of Cu, Zn-superoxide dismutase aggregates in amyotrophic lateral sclerosis

Mariko Ogawa and Yoshiaki Furukawa*

Laboratory for Mechanistic Chemistry of Biomolecules, Department of Chemistry, Keio University, Yokohama, Japan

Edited by:
Ricardo Tapia, Universidad Nacional Autónoma de México, Mexico

Reviewed by:
Luis B. Tovar-y-Romo, Universidad Nacional Autónoma de México, Mexico
Neil Cashman, University of British Columbia, Canada

***Correspondence:**
Yoshiaki Furukawa, Laboratory for Mechanistic Chemistry of Biomolecules, Department of Chemistry, Keio University, 3-14-1 Hiyoshi, Kohoku, Yokohama, Kanagawa 223-8522, Japan
e-mail: furukawa@chem.keio.ac.jp

Abnormal accumulation of protein inclusions in motor neurons has been known as a major pathological change in amyotrophic lateral sclerosis (ALS). Increasing numbers of proteins including mutant Cu, Zn-superoxide dismutase (SOD1) have been identified as constituents of pathological inclusions in a form of insoluble fibrillar aggregates. Notably, protein fibrillar aggregates exhibit a self-perpetuating property, which can convert a soluble native protein into insoluble fibrillar aggregates. Such "seeding reaction" of protein fibrils can accelerate the aggregation significantly and would contribute to the spread of inclusion pathologies from an affected cell to its neighboring cells in neurodegenerative diseases. In ALS, a pathological change first occurs at the site of disease onset and then propagates throughout the affected tissues in a time-dependent manner; therefore, it can be assumed that seeded aggregation may be the key factor of disease progression in ALS. In this mini review, we will briefly summarize recent studies on possible roles of a seeded aggregation of SOD1 in pathomechanism of ALS.

Keywords: SOD1, aggregation, seeding reaction, protein misfolding, amyloid

INTRODUCTION

Many proteins gain physiological functions by folding into their own unique three-dimensional structures, and any disturbance during this folding process potentially disrupts protein functions, which is considered to cause a variety of diseases (Morimoto, 2008). Among those, neurodegenerative diseases have been well characterized by abnormal accumulation of "mis"-folded proteins in brains and spinal cords of patients (Soto, 2003; Ross and Poirier, 2004). More specifically, certain misfolded proteins form insoluble, fibrillar aggregates that are rich in β-sheet structures, widely known as amyloid (Nelson et al., 2005).

In many neurodegenerative diseases, neurological symptoms appear in middle age (50 years ~), suggesting that it is a rare event for proteins to become misfolded/aggregated. In fact, protein fibrillar aggregation *in vitro* requires a significant conformational conversion of proteins to form oligomers (also known as "nucleus"), which is a rate-limiting step of the overall aggregation reaction (Harper and Lansbury, 1997). Once the nucleus forms, however, it functions as a structural template (or so called "seed") to convert native proteins into β-sheet-rich structures and then elongate the protein fibril. This mechanism, which accelerates and even triggers protein aggregation, is called the seeding reaction. While it remains controversial whether protein aggregation is the direct cause or a mere result of neurodegeneration (Winklhofer et al., 2008; Treusch et al., 2009), this seeding mechanism may explain why many neurodegenerative diseases progress rapidly after the symptoms first appear.

One notable example for a seeding reaction is the infectivity of Prion diseases, in which the spread of fibrillar aggregates of prion proteins is considered to be the main cause of neurodegeneration (Prusiner, 1982; Aguzzi and Rajendran, 2009). Fibrils of prion proteins are considered to work as infectious agents that can be transmitted between individuals. As exemplified in kuru (Gibbs et al., 1980), eating affected tissues of the disease could introduce fibrillar prion aggregates into a brain of a healthy control as seeds and thereby trigger fibrillation of prion proteins and cause neurodegeneration. While no infectivity between individuals has been reported in neurodegenerative diseases besides prion diseases so far, a seeding phenomenon appears to be common to protein fibrillar aggregates (Dobson, 1999); therefore, increasing numbers of researchers have pursued possible roles of seeding reactions in pathologies of neurodegenerative diseases (Aguzzi and Rajendran, 2009; Polymenidou and Cleveland, 2011; Soto, 2012). For example, Alzheimer's disease (AD) is characterized by fibrillar aggregation of Aβ peptides in brains (Hardy and Selkoe, 2002), and accelerated accumulation of Aβ fibrils has been confirmed in primate and rodent models that are injected with brain homogenates of an AD patient (Meyer-Luehmann et al., 2006; Ridley et al., 2006). Several other pathogenic proteins also forms fibrillar aggregates *in vitro*, which have been tested for their *in vivo* seeding activity by being transduced into cultured cells and brains of transgenic mouse model (Aguzzi and Rajendran, 2009; Polymenidou and Cleveland, 2011; Soto, 2012). A seeding reaction of protein fibrils is thus considered to play important roles in pathological progression of neurodegenerative diseases, and in this mini review, we will focus upon roles of seeded aggregation of proteins in pathologies of amyotrophic lateral sclerosis (ALS).

A SEEDED FIBRILLATION OF SUPEROXIDE DISMUTASE (SOD1) AS A PATHOLOGICAL PROPAGATION OF AMYOTROPHIC LATERAL SCLEROSIS (ALS)

ALS is a devastating motor neuron disease, mainly caused by abnormal accumulation of inclusions in the spinal cord (Bruijn et al., 2004). Notably, ALS has been known to occur as a focal process, which spreads contiguously throughout upper and lower motor neurons (Ravits and La Spada, 2009; Holmes and Diamond, 2012; Kanouchi et al., 2012). In other words, motor neuron degeneration in ALS is an orderly and actively propagating process, which appears to share characteristics of a seeded aggregation of proteins seen in Prion diseases.

Most ALS cases (~90%) are sporadic with no known genetic factors (sporadic ALS, sALS), while the remaining cases have been known to exhibit a family history (familial ALS, fALS; Robberecht and Philips, 2013). In 1993, dominant mutations in the gene encoding Cu, Zn-superoxide dismutase (SOD1) were identified as one of major genetic causes of fALS (Rosen et al., 1993), and mutant SOD1 proteins have been known to accumulate abnormally in the form of insoluble inclusions within affected spinal motor neurons of SOD1-related fALS patients (Bruijn et al., 1998). Ultrastructural analysis of SOD1-positive inclusions in fALS cases has identified their fibrillar morphologies (Kato et al., 2000); however, those inclusions were not stained by amyloid-diagnostic dye, Thioflavin S, which has made it controversial whether fibrillar aggregates of mutant SOD1 *in vivo* are rich in β-sheets (Kerman et al., 2010). Moreover, SOD1-positive inclusions have never been isolated from fALS cases, so further biochemical tests will be required to characterize pathological SOD1 aggregates.

In contrast, SOD1-positive inclusions with ALS-like symptoms were reproduced in a fALS-model mouse expressing human SOD1 with a pathogenic mutation (Turner and Talbot, 2008) and were found to be stained by Thioflavin S, supporting the formation of amyloid-like, β-sheet-rich fibrils in mouse (Wang et al., 2002; Furukawa et al., 2008). Insoluble SOD1 aggregates were also successfully isolated from the spinal cords of affected fALS-model mice, and quite notably, those SOD1 aggregates exhibited seeding activity toward fibrillation of purified SOD1 proteins *in vitro*. Chia et al. have prepared homogenates of spinal cords of transgenic mice expressing human SOD1 with G93A mutation and shown that the homogenates triggered fibrillation of wild-type as well as G93A-mutant human SOD1 proteins under *in vitro* conditions with acidic pH of solution in the presence of a chaotropic reagent, guanidine hydrochloride (Chia et al., 2010). While destabilization of SOD1 proteins under artificial conditions appears to be required for a seeded acceleration of fibrillar aggregation, inclusions containing mutant SOD1 would function as seeds and thereby contribute to propagation of pathological changes among contiguous motor neurons and then disease progression of SOD1-related fALS cases.

Fibrillogenic propensities of SOD1 proteins have been well characterized in *in vitro* studies using purified recombinant proteins. SOD1 is a cytoplasmic enzyme (Chang et al., 1988) that catalyzes the conversion of superoxide radicals to hydrogen peroxide and oxygen (McCord and Fridovich, 1969) and is activated by binding of a catalytic copper and a structural zinc ion and also by forming an intramolecular disulfide bond (Furukawa et al., 2004). Wild-type holo-SOD1 with a disulfide bond exhibits high thermostability (T_m ~ 90°C), conferring significant resistance to structural changes and aggregation (Forman and Fridovich, 1973). In contrast, when SOD1 lacks both metal ions and a disulfide bond (apo-SOD1^{SH}), its melting temperature decreases down to 43°C and become more prone to misfolding and aggregation at physiological temperature (Furukawa and O'Halloran, 2005). *In vitro* aggregates of human SOD1 polypeptide without any modifications possess amyloid-like characters with fibrillar morphologies and show a seeding activity to accelerate fibrillation of native human SOD1 proteins (Furukawa et al., 2008). More importantly, amyloid-like fibrils of human apo-SOD1^{SH} retain their seeding activity in the intracellular environment; transduction of those human SOD1 fibrils into cultured cells (mouse neuroblastoma, *Neuro2a*) has been shown to trigger the aggregation of stably-transfected human SOD1 (Furukawa et al., 2013).

fALS-causing mutations have been shown to decrease affinity for copper/zinc ions and/or stability of a disulfide bond (Hayward et al., 2002; Tiwari and Hayward, 2003; Furukawa et al., 2008). Therefore, in a reducing environment of the cytoplasm with high metal-chelating capacity, pathogenic mutations are supposed to increase intracellular fractions of fibrillation-prone apo-SOD1^{SH} (Furukawa et al., 2008). Nonetheless, it remains unclear how mutant SOD1 forms aggregates under pathological conditions. To elucidate how SOD1 aggregates form, several pathways for aggregation have been proposed in SOD1 proteins *in vitro* (Furukawa, 2012b). As reported by Munch et al. mutant SOD1 was found to form fibrillo-granular aggregates by addition of trifluoroethanol (TFE; Münch and Bertolotti, 2010), which penetrated inside neuronal cells through macropinocytosis and then acted as seeds to trigger intracellular aggregation of endogenously expressed SOD1 variants (Münch et al., 2011). Once SOD1 aggregation occurs in a cell, the aggregates can be released to the extracellular space and then transferred from cell to cell (*vide infra*). Intracellular aggregation of mutant SOD1 is thus considered to be persistent and heritable after passages, supporting prion-like propagation of aggregation phenotypes.

As mentioned above, two distinct types of SOD1 aggregates, i.e., apo-SOD1^{SH} amyloids and TFE-induced aggregates, have been found to function as seeds to trigger SOD1 aggregation intracellularly, but their structural and biochemical properties depend on how aggregation was induced (Furukawa et al., 2008; Münch and Bertolotti, 2010). Based upon previous *in vitro* studies, several distinct pathways for aggregation are possible in SOD1 (Toichi et al., 2013) and are expected to produce SOD1 aggregates with a varying degree of a seeding activity. This might describe heterologous progression and severity of diseases among SOD1-related fALS patients. Indeed, disease phenotypes of fALS cases have been known to be variable among different mutations in SOD1 (Wang et al., 2008), and furthermore, mutation-dependent structures of SOD1 fibrils closely correlate with their distinct biochemical properties (Furukawa et al., 2010). Therefore, it will be interesting to test if SOD1 fibrils with different mutations exhibit distinct activity as seeds *in vitro* and *in vivo*.

PROPAGATION OF PROTEIN MISFOLDING IN AMYOTROPHIC LATERAL SCLEROSIS (ALS)

In a seeding reaction, sheared pieces of insoluble fibrils can act as structural templates for a "phase-like transition" from soluble native conformers to generally insoluble fibrillar state, but this view now appears to be necessary for revision. Grad et al. utilized antibodies (3H1 and 10C12) that exclusively recognize misfolded SOD1 with disease-specific epitopes, which are not available in the natively folded state, and showed that misfolding of endogenous wild-type SOD1 in human cells (e.g., human embryonic kidney 293 cells (HEK293)) is induced by co-expression of a soluble misfolded form of human SOD1 with pathogenic mutations (Grad et al., 2011). In other words, soluble misfolded conformers of SOD1 are also transmissible without adopting classical, insoluble fibrillar states. Furthermore, transient expression of mutant human SOD1 in murine cells (e.g., *Neuro2a*) did not induce misfolding of endogenous mouse wild-type SOD1 (Grad et al., 2011). The difference lies in the amino acid sequence of murine and human SOD1, where the only tryptophan in human SOD1 (Trp32) is replaced by serine in murine counterpart. Indeed, misfolding of wild-type human SOD1 was observed by human SOD1 with a pathogenic (G127X) mutation but was significantly mitigated when G127X human SOD1 with W32S mutation was used (Grad et al., 2011). Trp32 in human SOD1 is highly solvent-exposed and distant from the native dimer interface, which might provide an alternative site for abnormal intermolecular interactions through hydrophobic interactions. It is interesting to note that expression of mutant TAR DNA binding protein 43 (TDP-43) and Fused in Sarcoma (FUS), pathogenic proteins also known to be found in ALS patients (Arai et al., 2006; Neumann et al., 2006; Kwiatkowski et al., 2009; Vance et al., 2009), can increase the immunoreactivity for misfolded SOD1 using a disease-specific antibody (3H1), both in patients and cultured human cells (SH-SY5Y; Pokrishevsky et al., 2012). While pathological involvement of wild-type SOD1 in ALS remains to be established, aberrant conformers of wild-type SOD1 have been reported in sporadic ALS with no genetic background (Furukawa, 2012a). Accordingly, toxic conformers of SOD1 might be produced by abnormal interactions of folded SOD1 with misfolded SOD1 or other proteins (such as TDP-43/FUS) at the site surrounding Trp32. In other words, as proposed in the template-assisted misfolding of prion proteins (Horwich and Weissman, 1997), soluble but misfolded conformers of protein molecules can be propagated through abnormal interactions among homologous proteins even without the formation of classical amyloid-like fibrils.

A CELL-TO-CELL TRANSFER OF INTRACELLULAR SUPEROXIDE DISMUTASE (SOD1)

SOD1 is known as one of major intracellular proteins, and most of SOD1 (~70%) exist in the cytoplasm (Chang et al., 1988). To confirm that seeded aggregation or misfolding of SOD1 is the key molecular mechanism of pathological propagation of SOD1-fALS, it is required to understand how intracellular misfolded/aggregated SOD1 is transferred from the cytoplasm to extracellular environment. As a relatively simple process, misfolded/aggregated SOD1 would be released to extracellular environment by death of an affected cell and then phagocytosed by the other cell. Recent studies have nonetheless suggested more sophisticated processes for a cell-to-cell transfer of SOD1 proteins (Grad et al., 2011; Münch et al., 2011). In fact, active secretion of SOD1 to extracellular space has been suggested in several different types of cultured cells (Mondola et al., 1996, 1998), and both wild-type and mutant SOD1 can be also detected in the cerebrospinal fluid of healthy controls as well as fALS patients (Zetterström et al., 2011).

In conditioned media of mouse motor neuron-like hybrid (NSC-34) cell line, impaired secretion of mutant SOD1 was associated with intracellular formation of inclusions and toxicity, suggesting secretion of mutant SOD1 as a beneficial process for cell survival (Turner et al., 2005). In contrast, Urushitani et al. have found that mutant SOD1 proteins are secreted in association with chromogranins and cause microgliosis and neuron death (Urushitani et al., 2006), leading to the idea that suppression of extracellular mutant SOD1 is a promising strategy for therapeutics of SOD1-related fALS cases. Indeed, passive as well as active immunizations targeting extracellular mutant SOD1 proteins have successfully prolonged lifespan of transgenic mice expressing mutant human SOD1 (Urushitani et al., 2007). Toxic roles of secreted SOD1 are further supported by the findings that motor neurons are killed by being co-cultured with astrocytes derived from adult neural progenitor cells isolated from post-mortem lumber spinal cord tissues from sporadic ALS as well as SOD1-related fALS (Haidet-Phillips et al., 2011). Also importantly, suppression of SOD1 in both fALS and sporadic ALS astrocytes was found to negate such toxicity of astrocytes toward motor neurons. Recently, furthermore, Basso et al. have shown the increased release of exosomes from astrocytes overexpressing fALS-causing mutant SOD1 and found that astrocyte-derived exosomes contained mutant SOD1 proteins and were transferred to the cytoplasm of spinal neurons (Basso et al., 2013).

Based upon these results, secretion of SOD1 is considered to occur through several distinct pathways and appears to be a normal physiological process. Experimental evidences are further required to show that secretory vesicles act as a messenger to generate seeding activity of SOD1. More specifically, conformational analysis of SOD1 (folded, misfolded, or fibrillized) included in those vesicles will reveal the molecular mechanism of pathological propagation in ALS through a seeding reaction.

SUMMARY

As briefly summarized above, increasing numbers of recent studies have supported the idea that misfolding/aggregation of mutant SOD1 is transmissible through a seeding mechanism inside the cell and among cells. In that sense, it is interesting to test pathological roles, if any, of SOD3, which resides at the extracellular matrix and possesses a structural domain almost homologous to SOD1 (Folz and Crapo, 1994). A SOD1-like domain of SOD3 has been shown to exhibit propensities for aggregation (Son et al., 2003), implying its involvement in the formation of seeds that can be taken up by cells. In summary, a seeded aggregation of SOD1 proteins including wild-type SOD1 will be a key event to understand progression/propagation of pathological changes in SOD1-related fALS and even sALS cases without mutations in

SOD1, and extracellular SOD1 with aberrant conformations is a promising target for therapeutics of those devastating diseases.

ACKNOWLEDGMENTS

This work was supported by Grants-in-Aid 24111542 for Scientific Research on Innovative Areas, 25291028 for Scientific Research (B), and 24657093 for Challenging Exploratory Research (to Yoshiaki Furukawa) from the Ministry of Education, Culture, Sports, Science and Technology of Japan.

REFERENCES

Aguzzi, A., and Rajendran, L. (2009). The transcellular spread of cytosolic amyloids, prions, and prionoids. *Neuron* 64, 783–790. doi: 10.1016/j.neuron.2009.12.016

Arai, T., Hasegawa, M., Akiyama, H., Ikeda, K., Nonaka, T., Mori, H., et al. (2006). TDP-43 is a component of ubiquitin-positive tau-negative inclusions in frontotemporal lobar degeneration and amyotrophic lateral sclerosis. *Biochem. Biophys. Res. Commun.* 351, 602–611. doi: 10.1016/j.bbrc.2006.10.093

Basso, M., Pozzi, S., Tortarolo, M., Fiordaliso, F., Bisighini, C., Pasetto, L., et al. (2013). Mutant copper-zinc superoxide dismutase (SOD1) induces protein secretion pathway alterations and exosome release in astrocytes: implications for disease spreading and motor neuron pathology in amyotrophic lateral sclerosis. *J. Biol. Chem.* 288, 15699–15711. doi: 10.1074/jbc.m112.425066

Bruijn, L. I., Houseweart, M. K., Kato, S., Anderson, K. L., Anderson, S. D., Ohama, E., et al. (1998). Aggregation and motor neuron toxicity of an ALS-linked SOD1 mutant independent from wild-type SOD1. *Science* 281, 1851–1854. doi: 10.1126/science.281.5384.1851

Bruijn, L. I., Miller, T. M., and Cleveland, D. W. (2004). Unraveling the mechanisms involved in motor neuron degeneration in ALS. *Annu. Rev. Neurosci.* 27, 723–749. doi: 10.1146/annurev.neuro.27.070203.144244

Chang, L. Y., Slot, J. W., Geuze, H. J., and Crapo, J. D. (1988). Molecular immunocytochemistry of the CuZn superoxide dismutase in rat hepatocytes. *J. Cell. Biol.* 107, 2169–2179. doi: 10.1083/jcb.107.6.2169

Chia, R., Tattum, M. H., Jones, S., Collinge, J., Fisher, E. M., and Jackson, G. S. (2010). Superoxide dismutase 1 and tgSOD1 mouse spinal cord seed fibrils, suggesting a propagative cell death mechanism in amyotrophic lateral sclerosis. *PLoS One* 5:e10627. doi: 10.1371/journal.pone.0010627

Dobson, C. M. (1999). Protein misfolding, evolution and disease. *Trends Biochem. Sci.* 24, 329–332. doi: 10.1016/S0968-0004(99)01445-0

Folz, R. J., and Crapo, J. D. (1994). Extracellular superoxide dismutase (SOD3): tissue-specific expression, genomic characterization, and computer-assisted sequence analysis of the human EC SOD gene. *Genomics* 22, 162–171. doi: 10.1006/geno.1994.1357

Forman, H. J., and Fridovich, I. (1973). On the stability of bovine superoxide dismutase. The effects of metals. *J. Biol. Chem.* 248, 2645–2649.

Furukawa, Y. (2012a). Pathological roles of wild-type Cu,Zn-superoxide dismutase in amyotrophic lateral sclerosis. *Neurol. Res. Int.* 2012:323261. doi: 10.1155/2012/323261

Furukawa, Y. (2012b). "Protein aggregates in pathological inclusions of amyotrophic lateral sclerosis," in *Amyotrophic Lateral Sclerosis*, ed M. H. Maurer (Rijeka, Croatia: InTech), 335–356.

Furukawa, Y., Kaneko, K., Watanabe, S., Yamanaka, K., and Nukina, N. (2013). Intracellular seeded aggregation of mutant Cu,Zn-superoxide dismutase associated with amyotrophic lateral sclerosis. *FEBS Lett.* 587, 2500–2505. doi: 10.1016/j.febslet.2013.06.046

Furukawa, Y., Kaneko, K., Yamanaka, K., and Nukina, N. (2010). Mutation-dependent polymorphism of Cu,Zn-superoxide dismutase aggregates in the familial form of amyotrophic lateral sclerosis. *J. Biol. Chem.* 285, 22221–22231. doi: 10.1074/jbc.m110.113597

Furukawa, Y., Kaneko, K., Yamanaka, K., O'Halloran, T. V., and Nukina, N. (2008). Complete loss of post-translational modifications triggers fibrillar aggregation of SOD1 in familial form of ALS. *J. Biol. Chem.* 283, 24167–24176. doi: 10.1074/jbc.m802083200

Furukawa, Y., and O'Halloran, T. V. (2005). Amyotrophic lateral sclerosis mutations have the greatest destabilizing effect on the apo, reduced form of SOD1, leading to unfolding and oxidative aggregation. *J. Biol. Chem.* 280, 17266–17274. doi: 10.1074/jbc.m500482200

Furukawa, Y., Torres, A. S., and O'Halloran, T. V. (2004). Oxygen-induced maturation of SOD1: a key role for disulfide formation by the copper chaperone CCS. *EMBO J.* 23, 2872–2881. doi: 10.1038/sj.emboj.7600276

Gibbs, C. J. Jr., Amyx, H. L., Bacote, A., Masters, C. L., and Gajdusek, D. C. (1980). Oral transmission of kuru, Creutzfeldt-Jakob disease and scrapie to nonhuman primates. *J. Infect. Dis.* 142, 205–208. doi: 10.1093/infdis/142.2.205

Grad, L. I., Guest, W. C., Yanai, A., Pokrishevsky, E., O'Neill, M. A., Gibbs, E., et al. (2011). Intermolecular transmission of superoxide dismutase 1 misfolding in living cells. *Proc. Natl. Acad. Sci. U S A* 108, 16398–16403. doi: 10.1073/pnas.1102645108

Haidet-Phillips, A. M., Hester, M. E., Miranda, C. J., Meyer, K., Braun, L., Frakes, A., et al. (2011). Astrocytes from familial and sporadic ALS patients are toxic to motor neurons. *Nat. Biotechnol.* 29, 824–828. doi: 10.1038/nbt.1957

Hardy, J., and Selkoe, D. J. (2002). The amyloid hypothesis of Alzheimer's disease: progress and problems on the road to therapeutics. *Science* 297, 353–356. doi: 10.1126/science.1072994

Harper, J. D., and Lansbury, P. T. Jr. (1997). Models of amyloid seeding in Alzheimer's disease and scrapie: mechanistic truths and physiological consequences of the time-dependent solubility of amyloid proteins. *Annu. Rev. Biochem.* 66, 385–407. doi: 10.1146/annurev.biochem.66.1.385

Hayward, L. J., Rodriguez, J. A., Kim, J. W., Tiwari, A., Goto, J. J., Cabelli, D. E., et al. (2002). Decreased metallation and activity in subsets of mutant superoxide dismutases associated with familial amyotrophic lateral sclerosis. *J. Biol. Chem.* 277, 15923–15931. doi: 10.1074/jbc.m112087200

Holmes, B. B., and Diamond, M. I. (2012). Amyotrophic lateral sclerosis and organ donation: is there risk of disease transmission? *Ann. Neurol.* 72, 832–836. doi: 10.1002/ana.23684

Horwich, A. L., and Weissman, J. S. (1997). Deadly conformations–protein misfolding in prion disease. *Cell* 89, 499–510. doi: 10.1016/s0092-8674(00)80232-9

Kanouchi, T., Ohkubo, T., and Yokota, T. (2012). Can regional spreading of amyotrophic lateral sclerosis motor symptoms be explained by prion-like propagation? *J. Neurol. Neurosurg. Psychiatry* 83, 739–745. doi: 10.1136/jnnp-2011-301826

Kato, S., Takikawa, M., Nakashima, K., Hirano, A., Cleveland, D. W., Kusaka, H., et al. (2000). New consensus research on neuropathological aspects of familial amyotrophic lateral sclerosis with superoxide dismutase 1 (SOD1) gene mutations: inclusions containing SOD1 in neurons and astrocytes. *Amyotroph. Lateral Scler. Other Motor Neuron Disord.* 1, 163–184. doi: 10.1080/14660820050515160

Kerman, A., Liu, H. N., Croul, S., Bilbao, J., Rogaeva, E., Zinman, L., et al. (2010). Amyotrophic lateral sclerosis is a non-amyloid disease in which extensive misfolding of SOD1 is unique to the familial form. *Acta Neuropathol.* 119, 335–344. doi: 10.1007/s00401-010-0646-5

Kwiatkowski, T. J. Jr., Bosco, D. A., Leclerc, A. L., Tamrazian, E., Vanderburg, C. R., Russ, C., et al. (2009). Mutations in the FUS/TLS gene on chromosome 16 cause familial amyotrophic lateral sclerosis. *Science* 323, 1205–1208. doi: 10.1126/science.1166066

McCord, J. M., and Fridovich, I. (1969). Superoxide dismutase. An enzymic function for erythrocuprein (hemocuprein). *J. Biol. Chem.* 244, 6049–6055.

Meyer-Luehmann, M., Coomaraswamy, J., Bolmont, T., Kaeser, S., Schaefer, C., Kilger, E., et al. (2006). Exogenous induction of cerebral beta-amyloidogenesis is governed by agent and host. *Science* 313, 1781–1784. doi: 10.1126/science.1131864

Mondola, P., Annella, T., Santillo, M., and Santangelo, F. (1996). Evidence for secretion of cytosolic CuZn superoxide dismutase by Hep G2 cells and human fibroblasts. *Int. J. Biochem. Cell Biol.* 28, 677–681. doi: 10.1016/1357-2725(96)00004-0

Mondola, P., Annella, T., Seru, R., Santangelo, F., Iossa, S., Gioielli, A., et al. (1998). Secretion and increase of intracellular CuZn superoxide dismutase content in human neuroblastoma SK-N-BE cells subjected to oxidative stress. *Brain Res. Bull.* 45, 517–520. doi: 10.1016/s0361-9230(97)00438-3

Morimoto, R. I. (2008). Proteotoxic stress and inducible chaperone networks in neurodegenerative disease and aging. *Genes Dev.* 22, 1427–1438. doi: 10.1101/gad.1657108

Münch, C., and Bertolotti, A. (2010). Exposure of hydrophobic surfaces initiates aggregation of diverse ALS-causing superoxide dismutase-1 mutants. *J. Mol. Biol.* 399, 512–525. doi: 10.1016/j.jmb.2010.04.019

Münch, C., O'Brien, J., and Bertolotti, A. (2011). Prion-like propagation of mutant superoxide dismutase-1 misfolding in neuronal cells. *Proc. Natl. Acad. Sci. U S A* 108, 3548–3553. doi: 10.1073/pnas.1017275108

Nelson, R., Sawaya, M. R., Balbirnie, M., Madsen, A. O., Riekel, C., Grothe, R., et al. (2005). Structure of the cross-beta spine of amyloid-like fibrils. *Nature* 435, 773–778. doi: 10.1038/nature03680

Neumann, M., Sampathu, D. M., Kwong, L. K., Truax, A. C., Micsenyi, M. C., Chou, T. T., et al. (2006). Ubiquitinated TDP-43 in frontotemporal lobar degeneration and amyotrophic lateral sclerosis. *Science* 314, 130–133. doi: 10.1126/science.1134108

Pokrishevsky, E., Grad, L. I., Yousefi, M., Wang, J., Mackenzie, I. R., and Cashman, N. R. (2012). Aberrant localization of FUS and TDP43 is associated with misfolding of SOD1 in amyotrophic lateral sclerosis. *PLoS One* 7:e35050. doi: 10.1371/journal.pone.0035050

Polymenidou, M., and Cleveland, D. W. (2011). The seeds of neurodegeneration: prion-like spreading in ALS. *Cell* 147, 498–508. doi: 10.1016/j.cell.2011.10.011

Prusiner, S. B. (1982). Novel proteinaceous infectious particles cause scrapie. *Science* 216, 136–144. doi: 10.1126/science.6801762

Ravits, J. M., and La Spada, A. R. (2009). ALS motor phenotype heterogeneity, focality, and spread: deconstructing motor neuron degeneration. *Neurology* 73, 805–811. doi: 10.1212/wnl.0b013e3181b6bbbd

Ridley, R. M., Baker, H. F., Windle, C. P., and Cummings, R. M. (2006). Very long term studies of the seeding of beta-amyloidosis in primates. *J. Neural Transm.* 113, 1243–1251. doi: 10.1007/s00702-005-0385-2

Robberecht, W., and Philips, T. (2013). The changing scene of amyotrophic lateral sclerosis. *Nat. Rev. Neurosci.* 14, 248–264. doi: 10.1038/nrn3430

Rosen, D. R., Siddique, T., Patterson, D., Figlewicz, D. A., Sapp, P., Hentati, A., et al. (1993). Mutations in Cu/Zn superoxide dismutase gene are associated with familial amyotrophic lateral sclerosis. *Nature* 362, 59–62. doi: 10.1038/364362c0

Ross, C. A., and Poirier, M. A. (2004). Protein aggregation and neurodegenerative disease. *Nat. Med.* 10(Suppl.), S10–S17. doi: 10.1038/nm1066

Son, M., Cloyd, C. D., Rothstein, J. D., Rajendran, B., and Elliott, J. L. (2003). Aggregate formation in Cu,Zn superoxide dismutase-related proteins. *J. Biol. Chem.* 278, 14331–14336. doi: 10.1074/jbc.m211698200

Soto, C. (2003). Unfolding the role of protein misfolding in neurodegenerative diseases. *Nat. Rev. Neurosci.* 4, 49–60. doi: 10.1038/nrn1007

Soto, C. (2012). Transmissible proteins: expanding the prion heresy. *Cell* 149, 968–977. doi: 10.1016/j.cell.2012.05.007

Tiwari, A., and Hayward, L. J. (2003). Familial amyotrophic lateral sclerosis mutants of copper/zinc superoxide dismutase are susceptible to disulfide reduction. *J. Biol. Chem.* 278, 5984–5992. doi: 10.1074/jbc.m210419200

Toichi, K., Yamanaka, K., and Furukawa, Y. (2013). Disulfide scrambling describes the oligomer formation of superoxide dismutase (SOD1) proteins in the familial form of amyotrophic lateral sclerosis. *J. Biol. Chem.* 288, 4970–4980. doi: 10.1074/jbc.m112.414235

Treusch, S., Cyr, D. M., and Lindquist, S. (2009). Amyloid deposits: protection against toxic protein species? *Cell Cycle* 8, 1668–1674. doi: 10.4161/cc.8.11.8503

Turner, B. J., Atkin, J. D., Farg, M. A., Zang, D. W., Rembach, A., Lopes, E. C., et al. (2005). Impaired extracellular secretion of mutant superoxide dismutase 1 associates with neurotoxicity in familial amyotrophic lateral sclerosis. *J. Neurosci.* 25, 108–117. doi: 10.1523/jneurosci.4253-04.2005

Turner, B. J., and Talbot, K. (2008). Transgenics, toxicity and therapeutics in rodent models of mutant SOD1-mediated familial ALS. *Prog. Neurobiol.* 85, 94–134. doi: 10.1016/j.pneurobio.2008.01.001

Urushitani, M., Ezzi, S. A., and Julien, J. P. (2007). Therapeutic effects of immunization with mutant superoxide dismutase in mice models of amyotrophic lateral sclerosis. *Proc. Natl. Acad. Sci. U S A* 104, 2495–2500. doi: 10.1073/pnas.0606201104

Urushitani, M., Sik, A., Sakurai, T., Nukina, N., Takahashi, R., and Julien, J. P. (2006). Chromogranin-mediated secretion of mutant superoxide dismutase proteins linked to amyotrophic lateral sclerosis. *Nat. Neurosci.* 9, 108–118. doi: 10.1038/nn1603

Vance, C., Rogelj, B., Hortobagyi, T., De Vos, K. J., Nishimura, A. L., Sreedharan, J., et al. (2009). Mutations in FUS, an RNA processing protein, cause familial amyotrophic lateral sclerosis type 6. *Science* 323, 1208–1211. doi: 10.1126/science.1165942

Wang, J., Xu, G., Gonzales, V., Coonfield, M., Fromholt, D., Copeland, N. G., et al. (2002). Fibrillar inclusions and motor neuron degeneration in transgenic mice expressing superoxide dismutase 1 with a disrupted copper-binding site. *Neurobiol. Dis.* 10, 128–138. doi: 10.1006/nbdi.2002.0498

Wang, Q., Johnson, J. L., Agar, N. Y., and Agar, J. N. (2008). Protein aggregation and protein instability govern familial amyotrophic lateral sclerosis patient survival. *PLoS Biol.* 6:e170. doi: 10.1371/journal.pbio.0060170

Winklhofer, K. F., Tatzelt, J., and Haass, C. (2008). The two faces of protein misfolding: gain- and loss-of-function in neurodegenerative diseases. *EMBO J.* 27, 336–349. doi: 10.1038/sj.emboj.7601930

Zetterström, P., Andersen, P. M., Brännström, T., and Marklund, S. L. (2011). Misfolded superoxide dismutase-1 in CSF from amyotrophic lateral sclerosis patients. *J. Neurochem.* 117, 91–99. doi: 10.1111/j.1471-4159.2011.07177.x

13

Self perceived emotional functioning of Spanish patients with amyotrophic lateral sclerosis: a longitudinal study

Jesús S. Mora[1]*, Teresa Salas[1], María L. Fajardo[2], Lourdes Iváñez[3] and Francisco Rodríguez-Santos[4]

[1] *ALS Unit, Department of Neurology, Hospital Carlos III, Madrid, Spain*
[2] *Department of Epidemiology, Consejería de Salud de Andalucía, Huelva, Spain*
[3] *Department of Epidemiology, Consejería de Salud de Andalucía, Sevilla, Spain*
[4] *Department of Clinical Psychology, School of Psychology, Universidad Autónoma, Madrid, Spain*

Edited by:
Francesco Pagnini, Catholic University of Milan, Italy

Reviewed by:
Luca Filipponi, Padua University, Italy
Xenia Savva, Ellen Langer Mindfulness Lab, USA

****Correspondence:***
Jesús S. Mora, Unidad de Esclerosis Lateral Amiotrófica, Hospital Carlos III, Sinesio Delgado 10, Madrid 28029, Spain.
e-mail: jmora.hciii@salud.madrid.org

Background: ALS is a neurodegenerative disease of the entire motor system that most frequently ends with respiratory arrest in few years. Its diagnosis and the rapid progression of the motor dysfunctions produce a continued emotional impact. Studies on this impact are helpful to plan adequate psychotherapeutic strategies. **Objective:** To assess and analyze: First: How the patients with ALS perceive their emotional health. Second: The emotional impact of their physical disabilities. Third: The physical disabilities with highest emotional impact. Fourth: The feelings with highest emotional impact. **Methods:** Up to 110 Spanish patients with ALS were assessed less than 1 year from diagnosis, then twice more at 6 month intervals, using the ALS Quality of Life Assessment Questionnaire (ALSAQ-40) validated for use in Spanish. Descriptive analysis and correlation between variables were obtained. **Results:** Worries about the future, of lack of freedom, and of being a burden were prevalent feelings. On average depression was felt only "sometimes." Only 25% of the variations in the emotional state were explained by changes in the physical state at first evaluation, and 16% at the last one. Emotional functioning correlated significantly with the physical disabilities at first and second evaluation, less so at third. Communication disabilities always had the highest impact. Depression at first evaluation and hopelessness at the next two evaluations had the highest emotional impact. Hopelessness did not correlate with any physical disability at the third evaluation. On the whole, emotional dysfunction was self perceived as intermediate (between none and worst), and remained stable at 1 year follow up, in both bulbar and spinal onset patients. **Conclusions:** Physical dysfunctions *per se* have a limited role in patients´ emotional distress. Communication disabilities, as well as feelings of depression at early stages of illness, and of hopelessness later on, had the most impact. This requires their careful therapeutic attention. On average, Spanish patients with ALS cope with their disease, overcoming depression, which is not felt often, and with just mid levels of emotional dysfunction.

Keywords: amyotrophic lateral sclerosis, ALS, quality of life, emotional functioning, ALSAQ-40, self evaluation, depression, hopelessness

INTRODUCTION

ALS causes a progressive and generally rapid degeneration of the entire motor neuron system and, as a result of the subsequent muscle denervation, atrophy and weakness of the skeletal muscles, including limbs, bulbar, and respiratory muscles. Mean survival is about 3.5 years. 50% of patients may survive 3 years, 20% 5 years, and less than 10% 10 years. Minor cognitive deficits have been documented in up to 50% of patients, but 5–13% of patients may also develop frontotemporal dementia (FTD). ALS and FTD may have genetic overlapping (Mora Pardina, 2011). At present, ALS does not have a cure, or even a treatment that patients might perceive as clinically significant. Patients experience the progression of their disease as their physical disabilities progress and extend relentless. People suffering from ALS go through a tremendous amount of continuous emotional distress, right after a shocking diagnosis. The rapid decline in skeletal muscle strength causes physical dependence up to for the basic activities of daily life (ADL), which entails complex and mixed emotional reactions. The disease affects not only the patient but also their caregivers and family members, all of whom face hard emotional challenges that interrelate with those of the patient (Salas and Lacasta, 1999; Pagnini et al., 2010a,b).

We often observe that severe physical deficits do not systematically correlate with increased levels of depression, self perception of poor quality of life (QoL), or high emotional distress (Salas and Lacasta, 1999), as others have also observed (Pagnini, 2012). Moreover, the impact the disease has on emotional well-being differs significantly between individuals, and the psychological reaction of the patients to their disease and their ability to cope has an effect on the disease's evolution (Chiò et al., 2004; Roach et al., 2009; Montel et al., 2012). Therefore, the traditional assumption of a tight correlation between rapidly progressive severe physical disabilities and emotional distress ought to be reconsidered. To study the relationship between the different physical disabilities caused by the disease and the emotional impact they may produce for the patient may contribute to better understanding and treatment of the emotional distress that ALS patients and their families endure. We understand that the way patients cope with their disease may be influenced by their cultural background; this is the first study to look at a Spanish population.

OBJECTIVE

To assess and analyze, at different times during their disease:

First: How the patients with ALS perceive their own emotional health.

Second: The emotional impact of each one of their physical disabilities.

Third: The physical disabilities with the highest emotional impact.

Fourth: The feelings with the highest emotional impact.

MATERIALS AND METHODS

MEASURING TOOL

We considered the ALS Assessment Questionnaire (ALSAQ-40) to be the most appropriate measuring tool for our objectives. The ALSAQ-40 is a specific state of health self appraisal questionnaire for ALS patients that looks at physical and emotional areas considered important by patients (Jenkinson et al., 1999; Epton et al., 2009). The ALSQ-40 has been validated for use in the Spanish language (Salas et al., 2008).

The ALSAQ-40 consists of 40 questions assessing four physical and one emotional area or dimension as self perceived by the patient. These are Physical Mobility (MOB), Independence/ADL (ADL), Eating and Drinking (EAT), Communication (COM), and Emotional Functioning (EMO). The first four dimensions assess physical deficiencies or disabilities that occur along with the disease. The fifth area evaluates the way that the patient deals emotionally with the disease. Each question or item is scored 0 to 4 according to the frequency of the symptom or feeling (never, rarely, sometimes, frequently, always). From the direct scores it is possible to obtain for each dimension an index ranging from 0 (best state of health) to 100 (worst state) which allows comparisons to be made between dimensions or over time. This ALS specific QoL measuring tool has demonstrated high validity, consistency, and reliability and appears sensitive to changes that have an impact on the overall status of patients (Jenkinson et al., 1999; Epton et al., 2009). It has been validated in different languages (Yamaguchi et al., 2004; Maessen et al., 2007; Salas et al., 2008; Palmieri et al., 2010; Pavan et al., 2010).

PATIENT SAMPLE AND METHODS

A total of 231 Spanish ALS patients were originally included in a 4-year long study. All were diagnosed with probable or definite ALS according to the El Escorial diagnostic criteria. None had clinical evidence of FTD, and all were receiving treatment with riluzol, the only approved ALS drug. They were living in different regions of Spain but they attended the ALS clinic at differing intervals. Of the total, only 110 patients whose first assessment was done no later than 12 months after diagnosis have been included in this study, in order to ensure a homogenous sample in terms of disease timeline. The evaluation of patients was longitudinal. Each patient filled out the questionnaire at three different times at 6 month intervals. Responses were always written or dictated by the patient. The questionnaire was first mailed accompanied by a request and an explanatory letter, and it was returned in clinic or by mail. The second and third evaluations were done in clinic or at home if the patient could not attend the clinic, and then mailed to us. The questionnaire could be completed in 10 min.

STATISTICAL ANALYSIS

Independent or explanatory variables were age, gender, site of onset (bulbar vs. spinal), time from onset of symptoms, time from diagnosis, and 30 functional variables, questions or items taken from the physical areas of the ALSAQ-40: Items 1–10 (MOB), 11–20 (ADL), 21–23 (EAT), and 24–30 (COM). Dependent variables were the 10 items, 31–40 (EMO) from the emotional dimension. These are:

1. I have felt lonely
2. I have been bored
3. I have felt embarrassed in social situations
4. I have felt hopeless about the future
5. I have worried that I am a burden to other people
6. I have wondered why I keep going
7. I have felt angry because of the disease
8. I have felt depressed
9. I worried about how the disease will affect me in the future
10. I have felt as if I have no freedom

The statistical analyses were descriptive, of correlation (regression analysis, Pearson's correlation), and of mean differences (t-test for independent samples), using SSPS v.15.0 for Windows, Microsoft Excel, and EPI INFO 2000.

RESULTS

DEMOGRAPHY

The sample size was 110 patients, 50 women and 60 men. 70 patients had spinal onset, 40 had bulbar onset (**Table 1**). Mean age at the first evaluation of 59 ± 14 years. Mean time between diagnosis and first assessment was 5.8 ± 4.0 months. The second evaluation was completed 5.7 ± 1.5 months after the first one by 76 patients (69.1%). The third assessment was filled out 6.5 ± 1.0 months later by 52 patients (47.3%).

SELF PERCEPTION OF EMOTIONAL HEALTH

In spite of increasing scores in the physical areas (MOB, ADL, EAT, COM) as the disease progresses, the emotional area (EMO) scores did not significantly increase (t-test for independent samples;

Table 1 | Sample distribution by gender and site of onset.

	Bulbar	Spinal	Total
Women	24 (21.8%)	26 (23.7%)	50 (45.5%)
Men	16 (14.6%)	44 (39.9%)	60 (54.5%)
Total	40 (36.4%)	70 (63.6%)	110 (100%)

Table 2). During the three evaluations, there are no significant differences in EMO between patients with bulbar and spinal onset, in spite of them having significant differences in physical functions: higher MOB scores in spinal onset patients, and higher EAT and COM scores in bulbar onset patients, as expected (**Table 2**). During the study period, mean EMO scores remain at around mid level, between best and worst. There are no significant differences in EMO scores between the first and third evaluations (1.74 points), and even less between the second and third evaluations (0.33 points; **Figure 1**).

At the first evaluation, less than 12 months after diagnosis, the feelings most often felt (that is, a score higher than 2: "*sometimes*") were worries about how the disease will affect the patient in the future (2.77), and feelings of being a burden to others (2.45), of lack of freedom (2.24), and of hopelessness (2.21). Anger at the disease (2.00) and depression (1.94) came after, but scored higher in patients who had been diagnosed less than 6 months ago (**Table 3**). At the second evaluation, about 6 months later, the feelings most often felt remain the same: worries about the future (2.66), lack of freedom (2.64), being a burden (2.53), hopelessness (2.33), and anger (2.22). Depression remained lower than 2 (1.91). At the third evaluation, 1 year after the first one, feelings of lack of freedom (2.98), worries about the future (2.73), and of being a burden (2.60) got close to a score of 3: "*frequently*." Hopelessness (2.21), anger (2.06), and depression (2.02) maintained similar scores to the first evaluation (**Table 3**).

EMOTIONAL IMPACT OF PHYSICAL DISABILITIES

To calculate how much the physical disability may be directly responsible for the emotional distress experienced by the patients,

Table 2 | Mean and SD for each area in bulbar and spinal onset.

	MOB		ADL		EAT		COM		EMO	
	Bulbar	**Spinal**	**Bulbar**	**Spinal**	**Bulbar**	**Spinal**	**Bulbar**	**Spinal**	**Bulbar**	**Spinal**
Maximun score	40	40	40	40	12	12	28	28	40	40
First evaluation	14.5 ± 11.4	19.8 ± 9.7	18.1 ± 12.9	20.6 ± 11.6	8.1 ± 3.6	1.9 ± 2.9	20.6 ± 7.5	4.6 ± 6.1	19.7 ± 13.1	17.4 ± 8.4
Second evaluation	19.3 ± 13.1	25.1 ± 11.9	23.9 ± 13.3	25.4 ± 11.6	9.4 ± 3.4	2.2 ± 3.5	23.5 ± 6.5	8.8 ± 9.3	21.0 ± 9.7	19.1 ± 10.5
Third evaluation	21.6 ± 12.9	29.4 ± 10.9	24.9 ± 12.7	30.7 ± 11.3	9.6 ± 2.4	4.3 ± 4.4	23.0 ± 5.6	11.6 ± 10.2	19.3 ± 9.4	20.3 ± 11.7

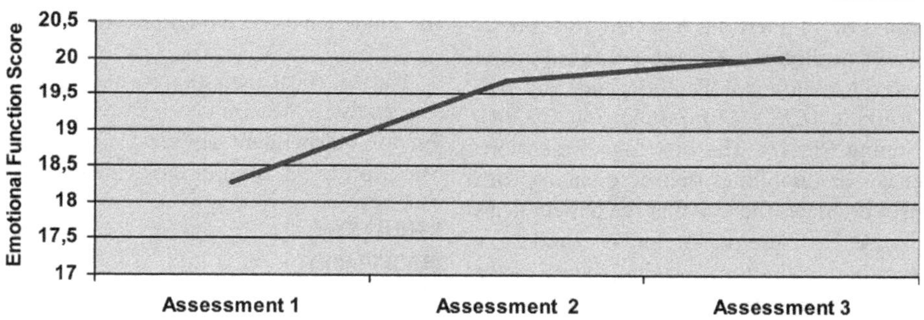

FIGURE 1 | Evolution of EMO along the three evaluations for the total sample.

Table 3 | Mean scores and SD of EMO items at the three evaluations.

EMO items*	First evaluation	Second evaluation	Third evaluation
1. I have felt lonely	0.98 ± 1.3	1.16 ± 1.5	1.10 ± 1.5
2. I have felt bored	1.30 ± 1.3	1.64 ± 1.5	1.67 ± 1.4
3. I have felt embarrassed in social situations	1.07 ± 1.3	1.10 ± 1.4	1.15 ± 1.3
4. I have felt hopelessness about the future	2.21 ± 1.2	2.33 ± 1.4	2.21 ± 1.5
5. I have worried about being a burden to other people	**2.45 ± 1.2**	**2.53 ± 1.2**	**2.60 ± 1.4**
6. I have wondered why I keep going	1.30 ± 1.4	1.49 ± 1.5	1.56 ± 1.5
7. I have felt angry because of the disease	2.00 ± 1.4	2.22 ± 1.4	2.06 ± 1.5
8. I have felt depressed	1.94 ± 1.2	1.91 ± 1.3	2.02 ± 1.4
9. I have worried about how the disease will affect me in the future	**2.77 ± 1.0**	**2.66 ± 1.3**	**2.73 ± 1.4**
10. I have felt as if I have no freedom	**2.24 ± 1.4**	**2.64 ± 1.5**	**2.98 ± 1.3**

**Items are scored as: Never = 0, Rarely = 1, Some times = 2, Frequently = 3, Always = 4.*

Bold indicates higher values that are most significant.

we carried out a dispersion diagram and calculated its linear regression. We used the EMO score as dependent variable and the sum of the scores of the physical areas (MOB, ADL, EAT, COM) as independent variables. The null hypothesis establishes that there is no relationship whatsoever between the two variables. To calculate the linear regression with 5% error and 95% confidence interval, we obtained $y = 8.298 + 0.191x$ with a correlation coefficient $R = 0.51$ and a determination coefficient of $R^2 = 0.25$. This indicates that only 25% of the variations that occur in the emotional state are explained by the changes in the physical state. The same analysis at the last evaluation produced the linear regression equation $y = 7.80 + 0.16x$, with a correlation coefficient of $R = 0.42$ and a determination coefficient of $R^2 = 16$. This shows an even smaller relationship between emotional and physical functions: only 16% of the variations that occur in the emotional state at the third evaluation, when patients experience more severe disabilities, are explained by the variations in the physical state (**Figure 2**).

PHYSICAL DISABILITIES WITH HIGHEST EMOTIONAL IMPACT

At the first evaluation there were significant correlations between EMO and COM, MOB and EAT ($p < 0.01$; bilateral, Pearson's correlation) in that order, and less significantly with ADL ($p < 0.05$; **Table 4**). At the second assessment there were significant correlations with all four physical areas ($p < 0.01$), the highest seen with COM, then with ADL (**Table 5**). At the third evaluation, the highest correlation continued being with COM ($p < 0.01$), and less so with MOB and EAT ($p < 0.05$; **Table 6**).

FEELINGS WITH HIGHEST EMOTIONAL IMPACT

Since physical dysfunctions were only partially responsible for the emotional impact, with an impact ranging from 25% at first evaluation to 16% at last evaluation, as shown in section 2, we assessed correlations between the different emotional states in EMO and the total EMO. To assess which emotions are elicited by the different physical disabilities, we calculated correlations between each EMO item and MOB, ADL, EAT, and COM (**Tables 7–9**). At the first evaluation all EMO items correlated highly with total EMO ($p < 0.01$ bilateral). The highest were items 8 on depression (Pearson $r = 0.81$), 7 on anger ($r = 0.75$), and 6 on keep going ($r = 0.74$). Item 8 on depression correlated highly ($p < 0.01$) with disabilities in MOB ($r = 0.27$) and COM ($r = 2.5$), and less so ($p < 0.05$) with ADL and EAT. All of them significantly less than with EMO ($r = 0.81$). Item 7 on anger correlated highly with MOB, COM, and ADL ($p < 0.01$) and less so with EAT ($p < 0.05$). Item 6 on keep going correlated highly with EAT, COM, and MOB. In all cases, the correlations were at much lower levels than with EMO (**Table 7**).

At the second assessment all EMO items kept a high correlation ($p < 0.01$) with total EMO. The feelings with highest correlations were items 4 on hopelessness ($r = 0.85$), 8 on depression ($r = 0.84$), and 10 on lack of freedom ($r = 0.78$). Item 4 on hopelessness and 8 on depression correlated highly with COM ($r = 0.32$) and less so with the other physical areas. Item 10 on lack of freedom correlated highly with COM, MOB, and ADL, and less so with EAT. All EMO items correlated highly with COM, except items 5 on being a burden and 9 on worries about future (**Table 8**).

At the third evaluation every EMO item maintained its high correlation with total EMO. The feelings with the highest correlations were items 4 on hopelessness ($r = 0.91$), 6 on keep going ($r = 0.84$), 2 on feeling bored ($r = 0.83$), and 8 on depression ($r = 0.80$). Item

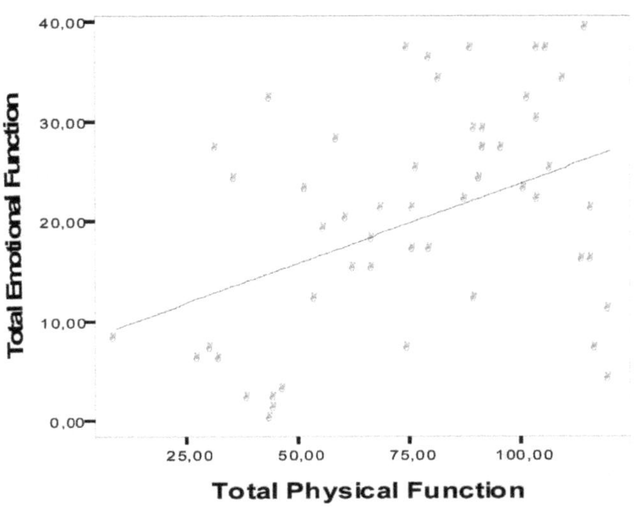

FIGURE 2 | Dispersion graph for emotional functioning and total combined physical functions at the third evaluation.

Table 4 | Correlations between areas at the first evaluation.

	ADL	EAT	COM	EMO
MOB	0.400**	0.001	−0.046	0.360**
ADL	1	0.095	0.017	0.242*
EAT		1	0.856**	0.307**
COM			1	0.398**

*$p < 0.05$ bilateral; **$p < 0.01$ bilateral.*

Table 5 | Correlation between areas at the second evaluation.

	ADL	EAT	COM	EMO
MOB	0.552**	0.022	0.165	0.331**
ADL		0.203	0.317**	0.346**
EAT		1	0.854**	0.342**
COM			1	0.444**

*$p < 0.05$ bilateral; **$p < 0.01$ bilateral.*

Table 6 | Correlation between areas at the third evaluation.

	ADL	EAT	COM	EMO
MOB	0.556**	0.278*	0.300*	0.330*
ADL	1	0.220	0.301*	0.267
EAT		1	0.845**	0.301*
COM			1	0.355**

*$p < 0.05$ bilateral; **$p < 0.01$ bilateral.*

Table 7 | Correlations between EMO items and other areas at the first evaluation.

EMO Items	MOB	ADL	EAT	COM	EMO
1. I have felt lonely	0.148	0.112	0.386**	0.399**	0.673**
2. I have felt bored	0.217*	0.183	0.249**	0.332**	0.625**
3. I have felt embarrassed in social situations	0.052	−0.011	0.433**	0.507**	0.540**
4. I have felt hopelessness about the future	0.294**	0.144	−0.049	0.017	0.670**
5. I have worried about being a burden to other people	0.265**	0.241*	0.087	0.133	0.702**
6. I have wondered why I keep going	0.274**	0.163	0.306**	0.290**	**0.740****
7. I have felt angry because of the disease	0.297**	0.272**	0.227*	0.293**	**0.751****
8. I have felt depressed	0.274**	0.214*	0.200*	0.254**	**0.812****
9. I have worried about how the disease will affect me in the future	0.198*	0.154	0.054	0.154	0.712**
10. I have felt as if I have no freedom	0.441**	0.197*	0.168	0.309**	0.688**

**p* < 0.05 bilateral; ***p* < 0.01 bilateral.
Bold indicates higher values that are most significant.

Table 8 | Correlations between EMO items and other areas at the second evaluation.

EMO Items	MOB	ADL	EAT	COM	EMO
1. I have felt lonely	0.081	0.106	0.416**	0.462**	0.620**
2. I have felt bored	0.253*	0.406**	0.351**	0.408**	0.757**
3. I have felt embarrassed in social situations	0.170	0.125	0.337**	0.371**	0.561**
4. I have felt hopelessness about the future	0.271*	0.260*	0.241*	0.324**	**0.847****
5. I have worried about being a burden to other people	0.216	0.289*	0.085	0.123	0.704**
6. I have wondered why I keep going	0.290*	0.252*	0.235*	0.295**	0.766**
7. I have felt angry because of the disease	0.290*	0.295**	0.223	0.334**	0.769**
8. I have felt depressed	0.254*	0.252*	0.181	0.326**	**0.844****
9. I have worried about how the disease will affect me in the future	0.088	0.066	0.118	0.162	0.658**
10. I have felt as if I have no freedom	0.477**	0.450**	0.256*	0.380**	**0.783****

***p* < 0.01 bilateral; **p* < 0.05 bilateral.
Bold indicates higher values that are most significant.

Table 9 | Correlations between EM items and other areas at the third evaluation.

EMO Items	MOB	ADL	EAT	COM	EM
1. I have felt lonely	0.254	0.011	0.149	0.145	0.682**
2. I have felt bored	0.319*	0.163	0.364**	0.298*	**0.826****
3. I have felt embarrassed in social situations	0.164	0.174	0.255	0.317*	0.634**
4. I have felt hopelessness about the future	0.238	0.220	0.076	0.152	**0.913****
5. I have worried about being a burden to other people	0.234	0.286*	0.138	0.219	0.698**
6. I have wondered why I keep going	0.193	0.166	0.143	0.209	**0.836****
7. I have felt angry because of the disease	0.233	0.181	0.245	0.152	0.777**
8. I have felt depressed	0.370**	0.313*	0.339*	0.494**	**0.801****
9. I have worried about how the disease will affect me in the future	0.121	0.186	0.205	0.299*	0.762**
10. I have felt as if I have no freedom	0.425**	0.377**	0.433**	0.488**	0.764**

***p* < 0.01 bilateral; **p* < 0.05 bilateral.
Bold indicates higher values that are most significant.

4 on hopelessness and item 6 on keep going did not correlate with any of the physical disabilities. Item 2 on boredom correlated highly with EAT and less so with MOB and COM. Item 8 on depression correlated highly with COM and MOB and less so with ADL. Item 10 on lack of freedom was highly correlated ($p < 0.01$) with the five areas (**Table 9**).

DISCUSSION

This study shows that as the physical deterioration of the patients with ALS increased, the self perception of the emotional distress remained more or less stable, and this happened in both spinal and bulbar onset patients, who have different timings of their physical disabilities. Emotional distress was felt, on average, as intermediate between none or worst. At the first evaluation the most frequent worries, felt more than *sometimes* but less than *frequently*, were those about the future, of losing autonomy, of being a burden, and then of despair. Less frequently felt, just *sometimes*, were depression and anger, which were more frequently felt nearer the time of diagnosis. This pattern continued at the second evaluation, with a slight increase in loss of freedom and with depression felt slightly less than *sometimes*. At the last evaluation, between 18 and 24 months after diagnosis, the pattern continues but lack of autonomy is the prevalent feeling followed by fear of the future and of being a burden, these three feelings got closer to being felt *frequently*. Depression remained stable, just being felt *sometimes*.

This pattern suggests that, for Spanish patients attending an ALS unit, the most frequent distressful thoughts are those related to fear of the future and of loss of autonomy with concerns for loved ones. Feelings of hopelessness, of depression and anger were felt less often. This might be explained by the attendance of a specialized clinic whose professionals try to fight those negative feelings with constant information on research, clinical trials, and psychological surveillance. Other explanations could be linked to the patients′ shared cultural and social background.

All four physical disabilities correlate with EMO, but it is the COM disability that has the most emotional impact as soon as it appears. This implies that dedicated care of this disability is important since it is a cause of significant distress. On the whole, physical disabilities accounted for only 25–16% of the emotional distress, and less so as the disease advances. Other varied psychosocial factors may contribute to modify the EMO (Pagnini, 2012). However, each negative feeling tested correlated highly with the global emotional dysfunction. It seems plausible that any psychosocial factor, such as advanced health care, strong familial, and social support, spirituality, or an optimistic personality, could influence the EMO of the patient by changing their patterns of feelings or emotions. Negative thoughts, not the physical disabilities *per se*, may account for an important part of the emotional distress felt by patients. We have known for a long time that emotional distress does not depend on the physical damage that one experiences but on the way that the mind processes the experience (adapted from Epicurus, 300 B.C.: "*To humans, the things do not affect us by themselves, but by the way we interpret them*").

All 10 feelings or emotional states tested correlate strongly with the global EMO, but each one has a different weight as representative of the patient's EMO at different times. Less than 1 year after diagnosis depression is the feeling with most emotional impact, followed by anger, although on average they were felt only "*some times.*" Both are highly related to the dysfunctions in COM and MOB. Once most disabilities are present, 18 months after diagnosis, feelings of hopelessness reach the same power as depression, with the COM disabilities contributing most to these feelings. Two years after diagnosis, most feelings have increased their impact, but those of hopelessness and of stopping fighting are the most representative. Worries about the future and of lack of freedom are perceived often but produce a lesser impact. Interestingly, except for lack of freedom, none of the emotional states are related to the severity of the physical dysfunctions at this stage of the disease. In this way, they are negative states of mind, not directly related to the physical disabilities, and so, subject to be treated by dedicated psychotherapy.

Many studies have tried to determine what is called the QoL of patients with ALS, and many scales have been created that try to measure it. QoL may be a confusing concept in this dreadful disease, which makes it more difficult to "measure." The methodological limitations inherent to this measurement contribute to a wide range of reported results, and statements on QoL must be considered dependent of the scale used. An excellent review has recently been published (Pagnini, 2012). QoL has been reported to be negatively correlated to suffering, a sense of burden, and hopelessness, and positively correlated to social support (Epton et al., 2009). Its relation with physical functioning was unclear to some (Ganzini et al., 1999) and it was more related to psychosocial rather than physical aspects of life, particularly in those patients with physical disabilities (Clarke et al., 2001). QoL, as assessed by the patient, has not been correlated to physical function or strength, but to psychological and existential factors, as well as to spiritual factors and support systems (Simmons et al., 2000, 2006). Hopelessness in ALS has been correlated with suffering and negatively with QoL (Ganzini et al., 1999). Hope did not correlate with physical and respiratory functions (Fanos et al., 2008). The real prevalence of depressive and anxious symptom in ALS is unclear (Norris et al., 2010; Taylor et al., 2010) although some studies found depressive symptoms common, and severe in 11–15% of the patients (McLeod and Clarck, 2007). Swallowing and breathing difficulties have been related to depressive symptoms, however the severity of the disease as such or its duration were not (Hillemaker et al., 2004). Most of these studies are in accordance with our findings.

An evaluation of 28 studies concluded that clinically significant depression is neither as prevalent nor as severe as might be expected and that patients are more likely to present with hopelessness and end-of-life concerns than clinically significant depression (Averill et al., 2007), this is consistent with our findings. Thirty ALS patients showed good psychosocial adjustment and subjective QoL, mild depressive symptoms, and no clinically relevant depression (Lulé et al., 2012). Another study rated QoL on average as satisfactory and found a moderate positive relation to physical impairment and a weak negative relation to time since diagnosis (Kubler et al., 2005). Despite marked deterioration in the patients' health, there was no change in mental well-being and QoL. Psychological well-being appeared more important in maintaining QoL than physical factors (O'Doherty et al., 2010). Few changes were observed in the QoL of 35 patients over time (Olsson et al., 2010). The general QoL changed little overtime in 60 patients (Robbins et al., 2001). Individual QoL remained stable in 42 patients and was not dependant on physical function but on family, friends/social life, health, and profession (Neudert et al., 2004). There was substantial steadiness of QoL in 31 patients over 9 months (Gauthier et al., 2007). No relationship between EMO and muscle strength or functional ability was found in 30 patients (Palmieri et al., 2010). Most of these studies are in accordance with our findings.

What emerges from our study and others is that for ALS patients, as a group, physical dysfunction *per se* is not the main contributor to emotional suffering. Emotional suffering seems more related to negative feelings linked to the new physical condition. However, emotional dysfunction, and depression at its paradigm, do not seem to be exaggerated in spite of severe physical dysfunction and remain somehow stable along most of the disease. Terminal phases need additional studies. Since we do not agree with the idea of ALS affecting only nice and suffering-resilient people, we understand that ALS patients as a group behave as any other human group who try to cope with misfortune the best they can. As in any human disaster the emotional health of each ALS patient is not completely dependent on his/her physical strength but on the strength of the coping mechanisms that he/she may build to deal with the situation These mechanisms may be individual, familial, social, or spiritual, health care provided or other. It is difficult and risky to extrapolate results obtained from groups to individual patients since the individual variables that influence the specific QoL of each person are so varied. To facilitate the work of the therapists, our study tries to understand the contribution of specific negative feelings and worries, and their subsequent emotional states, to the emotional suffering of the patients throughout their disease, and which specific physical disabilities are most related to them. Specific psychotherapeutic interventions should be implemented to help the patient to overcome them. Development of adequate protocols is needed (Pagnini et al., 2012).

ACKNOWLEDGMENTS

This work was made possible by the financial support of the Spanish ALS Research Foundation FUNDELA (*Fundación Española para el Fomento de la Investigación de la Esclerosis Lateral Amiotrófica*).

REFERENCES

Averill, A. J., Kasarskin, E. J., and Segerstrom, S. C. (2007). Psy- chological health in patients with amyotrophic lateral sclerosis. *Amy- otroph. Lateral Scler.* 8, 243–254.

Chiò, A., Gauthier, A., Montuschi, A., Calvo, A., Di Vito, N., Ghiglione, P., et al. (2004). A cross sectional study on determinants of quality of life in ALS. *J. Neurol. Neurosurg. Psychiatr.* 75, 1597–1601.

Clarke, S., Hickey, A., O'Boyle, C., and Hardiman, O. (2001). Assess- ing individual quality of life in amy- otrophic lateral sclerosis. *Qual. Life Res.* 10, 149–158.

Epton, J., Harris, R., and Jenkinson, C. (2009). Quality of life in amy- otrophic lateral sclerosis/motor neuron disease: a structured review. *Amyotroph. Lateral Scler.* 10, 15–26.

Fanos, J. H., Gelinas, D. F., Foster, R. H., Postone, N., and Miller, R. G. (2008). Hope in palliative care: from narcis- sism to self-transcendence in amy- otrophic lateral sclerosis. *J. Palliat. Med.* 11, 470–475.

Ganzini, L., Johnston, W. S., and Hoff- man, W. F. (1999). Correlates of suf- fering in amyotrophic lateral sclero- sis. *Neurology* 52, 1434–1440.

Gauthier, A., Vignola, A., Calvo, A., Cav-allo, E., Moglia, C., Sellitti, L., et al. (2007). A longitudinal study on quality of life and depression in ALS pa- tient-caregiver couples. *Neurology* 68, 923–926.

Hillemaker, T., Grassel, E., Tigges, S., Bleich, S., Neundorfer, B., Kornhu- ber, J., et al. (2004). Depression and bulbar involvement in amyotrophic lateral sclerosis. *Amyotroph. Lateral Scler.* 5, 245–249.

Jenkinson, C., Fitzpatrick, R., Brennan, C., and Swash, M. (1999). Evidence for the validity and reliability of the ALS assessment questionnaire: the ALSQ-40. *Amyotroph. Lateral Scler. Other Motor Neuron Disord.* 1, 33–40.

Kubler, A., Winter, S., Ludolph, A. C., Hautzinger, M., and Birbaumer, N. (2005). Severity of depressive symp- toms and quality of life in patients with amyotrophic lateral sclero- sis. *Neurorehabil. Neural Repair* 19, 182–193.

Lulé, D., Pauli, S., Altintas, E., Singer, U., Merk, T., Uttner, I., et al. (2012). Emotional adjustments in amyotrophic lateral sclerosis (ALS). *J. Neurol.* 259, 334–341.

Maessen, M., Post, M. W., Maillé, R., Lindeman, E., Mooij, R., Veldink, J. H., et al. (2007). Validity of the Dutch version of the amy- otrophic lateral sclerosis assessment questionnaire, ALSQ-40, ALSAQ-5. *Amyotroph. Lateral Scler.* 8, 96–100.

McLeod, J. E., and Clarck, D. M. (2007). A review of psychosocial aspects of motor neurone disease. *J. Neuro. Sci.* 258, 4–10.

Montel, S., Albertini, L., and Spitz, E. (2012). Coping strategies in rela- tion to quality of life in amyotrophic lateral sclerosis. *Muscle Nerve* 45, 131–134.

Mora Pardina, J. S. (2011). "Escle- rosis lateral amiotrófica y otras enfer- medades de la motoneurona," in *Tratado de Neurología*, ed. J. Pascual (Madrid: Luzán 5 S. A.), 1013–1048.

Neudert, C., Wasner, M., and Borasio, G. D. (2004). Individual quality of life is not correlated with healthy-related quality of life or physical func- tion in patients with amyotrophic lateral sclerosis. *J. Palliat. Med.* 7, 551–557.

Norris, L., Que, G., and Bayat, E. (2010). Psychiatric aspects of amyotrophic lateral sclerosis (ALS). *Curr. Psychi- atry Rep.* 12, 239–245.

O'Doherty, L. J., Hickey, A., and Hardi- man, O. (2010). Measuring life qual- ity, physical function and psycholog- ical well-being in neurological ill- ness. *Amyotroph. Lateral Scler.* 11, 461–468.

Olsson, A. G., Markhede, I., Strang, S., and Persson, L. I. (2010). Differ- ences in quality of life modalities give rise to needs of individual sup- port in patients with ALS and their next kin. *Palliat. Support. Care* 8, 75–82.

Pagnini, F. (2012). Psychological wellbeing and quality of life in amyotrophic lateral sclero- sis: a review. *Int. J. Psychol.* doi:10.1080/00207594.2012.691977 . [Epub ahead of print].

Pagnini, F., Rossi, G., Lunetta, C., Banfi, P., and Corbo, M. (2010a). Clinical psychology and amyotrophic lat- eral sclerosis. *Front. Psychol.* 1:33. doi:10.3389/fpsyg.2010.00033

Pagnini, F., Rossi, G., Lunetta, C., Banfi, P., Castelnuovo, G., Corbo, M., et al. (2010b). Burden, depression, and anxiety in caregivers of people with amyotrophic lateral sclerosis. *Psy- chol. Health Med.* 15, 685–693.

Pagnini, F., Simmons, Z., Corbo, M., and Molinari, E. (2012). Amyotrophic lateral sclerosis: time for research on psychological intervention?. *Amy- otroph. Lateral Scler.* 13, 416–417.

Palmieri, A., Sorarù, G., Lombardi, L., D'Ascenzo, C., Baggio, L., Ermani, M., et al. (2010). Quality of life and motor impairment in ALS: Italian validation of ALSQ. *Neurol. Res.* 32, 32–40.

Pavan, K., Marangoni, B. E., Zinezzi, M. O., Schmidt, K. B., Oliveira, B. C., Buainain, R. P., et al. (2010). Val- idation of the amyotrophic lateral sclerosis assessment questionnaire (ALSQ-40) scale in the Portuguese language. *Arq. Neuropsychiatr.* 68, 48–51.

Roach, A. R., Averill, A. J., Segerstrom, S. C., and Kasarskis, E. J. (2009). The dynamics of quality of life in ALS patients and caregivers. *Ann. Behav. Med.* 37, 197–206.

Robbins, R. A., Simmons, Z., Bremer, B. A., Walsh, S. M., and Fischer, S. (2001). Quality of life in ALS is maintained as physical function declines. *Neurology* 56, 442–444.

Salas, T., and Lacasta, M. (1999). "Asistencia psicológica," in *Esclero- sis Lateral Amiotrófica: Una Enfer- medad Tratable*, ed. J. S. Mora Par- dina (Barcelona: Prous Science), 455–469.

Salas, T., Mora, J., Esteban, J., Rodríguez, F., Díaz-Lobato, S., and Fajardo, M. (2008). Spanish adaptation of the amyotrophic lateral sclerosis questionnaire ALSQ-40 for ALS patients. *Amyotroph. Lateral Scler.* 9, 168–172.

Simmons, Z., Bremer, B. A., Robins, A., Walsh, S. M., and Fisher, (2000). Quality of life in ALS depends on factors other than strength and physical function. *Neu- rology* 55, 388–392.

Simmons, Z., Felgoise, S. H., Bremer, B. A., Walsh, S. M., Hufford, D. J., Bromber, M. B., et al. (2006). The ALSSQOL: balancing physical and nonphysical factors in assessing quality of life in ALS. *Neurology* 67, 1659–1664.

Taylor, L., Wicks, P., Leigh, P. N., and Goldstein, L. H. (2010). Prevalence of depression in amyotrophic lateral sclerosis and other motor disorders. *Eur. J. Neurol.* 17, 1047–1053.

Yamaguchi, T., Ohbu, S., Saito, M., Ito, Y., Moriwaka, F., Tashiro, K., et al. (2004). Validity and clinical applicability of the Japanese version of amy- otrophic lateral sclerosis-assessment questionnaire 40 (ALSAQ-40). *No To Shinkei* 56, 483–494.

14

Blood–CNS barrier impairment in ALS patients versus an animal model

***Svitlana Garbuzova-Davis*[1,2,3]* *and Paul R. Sanberg*[1,2,3,4]**

[1] *Department of Neurosurgery and Brain Repair, Center of Excellence for Aging and Brain Repair, Morsani College of Medicine, University of South Florida, Tampa, FL, USA*
[2] *Department of Molecular Pharmacology and Physiology, Morsani College of Medicine, University of South Florida, Tampa, FL, USA*
[3] *Department of Pathology and Cell Biology, Morsani College of Medicine, University of South Florida, Tampa, FL, USA*
[4] *Department of Psychiatry, Morsani College of Medicine, University of South Florida, Tampa, FL, USA*

Edited by:
Ricardo Tapia, Universidad Nacional Autónoma de México, Mexico

Reviewed by:
Hari S. Sharma, Uppsala University, Sweden
Yang D. Teng, Brigham and Women's Hospital and Harvard Medical School, USA

Correspondence:
Svitlana Garbuzova-Davis, Department of Neurosurgery and Brain Repair, Center of Excellence for Aging and Brain Repair, Morsani College of Medicine, University of South Florida, 12901 Bruce B. Downs Boulevard, Tampa, FL 33612, USA
e-mail: sgarbuzo@health.usf.edu

Amyotrophic lateral sclerosis (ALS) is a severe neurodegenerative disease with a complicated and poorly understood pathogenesis. Recently, alterations in the blood–Central Nervous System barrier (B-CNS-B) have been recognized as a key factor possibly aggravating motor neuron damage. The majority of findings on ALS microvascular pathology have been determined in mutant superoxide dismutase (SOD1) rodent models, identifying barrier damage during disease development which might similarly occur in familial ALS patients carrying the SOD1 mutation. However, our knowledge of B-CNS-B competence in sporadic ALS (SALS) has been limited. We recently showed structural and functional impairment in postmortem gray and white matter microvessels of medulla and spinal cord tissue from SALS patients, suggesting pervasive barrier damage. Although numerous signs of barrier impairment (endothelial cell degeneration, capillary leakage, perivascular edema, downregulation of tight junction proteins, and microhemorrhages) are indicated in both mutant SOD1 animal models of ALS and SALS patients, other pathogenic barrier alterations have as yet only been identified in SALS patients. Pericyte degeneration, perivascular collagen IV expansion, and white matter capillary abnormalities in SALS patients are significant barrier related pathologies yet to be noted in ALS SOD1 animal models. In the current review, these important differences in blood–CNS barrier damage between ALS patients and animal models, which may signify altered barrier transport mechanisms, are discussed. Understanding discrepancies in barrier condition between ALS patients and animal models may be crucial for developing effective therapies.

Keywords: amyotrophic lateral sclerosis, blood–CNS barrier, patients, animal models, microvascular pathology

INTRODUCTION

Amyotrophic lateral sclerosis (ALS) is a neurodegenerative disease affecting upper and lower motor neurons in the brain and spinal cord, damage which leads to progressive muscle atrophy, paralysis and death typically within three to five years from diagnosis (Rowland and Shneider, 2001). Most ALS cases are sporadic amyotrophic lateral sclerosis(SALS) with only 5–10% genetically linked familial amyotrophic lateral sclerosis (FALS); 20% of FALS cases show missense mutations in the Cu/Zn superoxide dismutase (SOD1) gene (Rosen et al., 1993). Clinical presentation and pathology of SALS and FALS, however, are similar. Numerous hypotheses exist regarding ALS pathogenesis (Alexianu et al., 2001; Cleveland and Rothstein, 2001; Bruijn et al., 2004; Strong et al., 2005; Pasinelli and Brown, 2006; Van Den Bosch et al., 2006; Mitchell and Borasio, 2007; Rothstein, 2009; Saleh et al., 2009; Hovden et al., 2013), but the causes of the diffuse motor neuron degeneration are still uncertain.

The blood–Central Nervous System barrier (B-CNS-B) is composed of the blood–brain barrier (BBB), blood–spinal cord barrier (BSCB), and blood–cerebrospinal fluid barrier (BCSFB) and has a crucial role in controlling CNS homeostasis by selective transport of substances to and from the systemic compartment and blocking passive diffusion of harmful blood solutes (Bradbury, 1985; Dermietzel and Krause, 1991; Pardridge, 1991, 1999; Nag, 2003; Vorbrodt and Dobrogowska, 2003; Ballabh et al., 2004). This control is possible due to the unique composition of the microvasculature – capillaries formed by endothelial cells (BBB and BSCB) and epithelial cells of the choroids plexus (BCSFB). Exchange by free diffusion is limited to molecules massing less than 450 Da; more massive substances require specific transport mechanisms. These mechanisms allow influx of required substances and efflux of cell waste (Begley and Brightman, 2003; Begley, 2004; Pardridge, 2005). Endothelial cells and their tight/adherens junctions are the primary components of the BBB and BSCB systems, while other barrier elements (pericytes, astrocytes, perivascular macrophages, and the basal lamina) also have essential roles in the tightly integrated unit maintaining the CNS environment for proper function of neuronal cells. Although major structural and functional properties are shared between the BBB and BSCB, some morphological and physiological differences have been noted in the BSCB (Bartanusz et al., 2011). Glycogen microvessel deposits, increased capillary permeability for some tracers, and decreased tight/adherence junction protein expressions were described for the BSCB in comparison to the BBB. Therefore, dysfunctional or structural impairment of any B-CNS-B component may lead to an increasingly toxic CNS environment. Microvascular endothelial dysfunction, in particular, might be implicated in the pathogenesis of various neurodegenerative diseases (Grammas et al., 2011).

Early studies in the 1980s reported altered BCSFB permeability as indicated by abnormal serum proteins and complement in the CSF of ALS patients (Leonardi et al., 1984; Annunziata and Volpi, 1985). These observations were followed by detection of blood-borne substances in the CNS tissue of ALS patients (Donnenfeld et al., 1984), suggesting BBB and BSCB leakage. Only relatively recent research has focused on microvascular competence in the brain and spinal cord, indicating impairment of BBB and BSCB integrity in animal models of ALS and in ALS patients. Compelling evidence of this B-CNS-B damage has been demonstrated at structural and functional levels in an animal model of ALS at initial stage of disease and this damage was exacerbated with disease progression (Garbuzova-Davis et al., 2007a,b; Zhong et al., 2008; Nicaise et al., 2009a,b; Miyazaki et al., 2011). Importantly, BSCB breakdown was found in SOD1 mutant mice and rats prior to motor neuron degeneration and neuroinflammation (Zhong et al., 2008; Nicaise et al., 2009a; Miyazaki et al., 2011). Evidence of BSCB impairment has also been observed in postmortem tissue from ALS patients. Loss of endothelium integrity, as shown by significant reductions of tight junction proteins and astrocyte end-feet dissociated from the endothelium, was observed in spinal cords from ALS patients (Henkel et al., 2009; Miyazaki et al., 2011). Recently, we showed structural and functional impairment in postmortem gray and white matter microvessels of medulla and spinal cord tissue from SALS patients, suggesting pervasiveness of the B-CNS-B damage (Garbuzova-Davis et al., 2012). These results strengthen the likelihood that barrier disruption contributes to disease pathogenesis (Garbuzova-Davis et al., 2008). However, B-CNS-B disruption could also trigger, as well as aggravate, motor neuron degeneration in ALS. Vascular impairment has only recently been recognized as a key factor in ALS, identifying ALS as a neurovascular disease (Garbuzova-Davis et al., 2011; Rodrigues et al., 2012). Although numerous similarities in barrier damage have been identified in mutant SOD1 animal models of ALS and ALS patients, some differences in the B-CNS-B alterations have been noted. In the current review, these discrepancies in the BBB and BSCB competence between ALS patients and animal models are discussed with an aim toward developing effective new therapies for ALS.

BBB AND BSCB IMPAIRMENT IN TRANSGENIC RODENT MODELS OF ALS

Only comparatively recent research has focused on investigations of BBB and BSCB integrity in ALS. Initially, Garbuzova-Davis et al. (2007a) demonstrated ultrastructural capillary alterations in the brainstem and spinal cord (cervical and lumbar) in both early and late stages of disease in G93A SOD1 mice. Electron microscopy analysis showed highly vacuolated and degenerated endothelial cells, mitochondrial degeneration within endothelial cells, extensive perivascular edema, and swelling of astrocyte end-feet adjacent to capillaries. Capillary rupture was also indicated by the presence of erythrocytes in the extracellular space of brainstem microvessels in early symptomatic G93A mice. These findings were later confirmed by a study from the same research group (Garbuzova-Davis et al., 2007b), showing Evans blue leakage in spinal cord capillaries of G93A mice at 13 weeks of age, indicating functional impairment of the BSCB in early stage disease. The study also demonstrated endothelial damage through downregulation of the transporter protein Glut-1 and CD146 expressions, associated with decreased laminin, a component of the basement membrane in capillaries. The alterations were mainly detected in the ventral horns of the spinal cords, areas most affected by ALS. Importantly, motor neurons demonstrated intracellular edema and cytoplasmic vacuolization, in addition to degenerated axons with myelin disruption near capillaries in the brainstem and spinal cords of G93A mice at early disease stage.

The study by Zhong et al. (2008) not only confirmed these observations on microvascular barrier damage in the spinal cord of symptomatic G93A mice, but also showed that BSCB disruption precedes neuroinflammation and might initiate disease symptoms. Western blot analysis evidenced diminished levels of zonula occludens-1 (ZO-1), occludin, and claudin-5 tight junction proteins and Glut-1 prior to disease onset in ALS mice. Although these alterations were observed, markers of endothelial activation (intercellular adhesion molecule-1, ICAM-1) and inflammation (monocyte chemoattractant protein-1, MCP-1) and cycloxygenase-2 (COX-2) were not indicated. Also prior to motor neuron loss and inflammatory changes, the investigators showed 10–15% reductions in total capillary length and 30 to 45% decreases in spinal cord blood flow of SOD1 transgenic mice. Additionally, microhemorrhages and hemosiderin deposits were found in spinal cord parenchyma, demonstrating BSCB functional impairment and disruption.

Miyazaki et al. (2011) also evaluated BSCB integrity in G93A SOD1 mice and observed progressive downregulation of occludin and platelet-endothelium cell adhesion molecule-1 (PECAM-1 or CD31) and vascular collagen IV, associated with increased activity of matrix metalloproteinase-9 (MMP-9), indicating endothelial cell and basement membrane involvement in microvascular pathological changes. All of these observations preceded motor neuron death and were in agreement with Zhong et al. (2008). However, the decline of occludin expression was moderate in the spinal cord tissues from ALS mice from 10 to 15 weeks of age and the expression of this protein significantly decreased in late symptomatic mice at 18 weeks of age. Surprisingly, the quantification of collagen IV in gray matter tissue evidenced protein up-regulation, a finding in opposition to immunohistochemical observations in the perivascular areas. These divergent results were ascribed to increased glial production of collagen IV as a consequence of disease progression and neuroinflammation, possibly reflecting an attempt by neural cells to compensate for endothelium disruption. In support of this suggestion, the authors showed higher collagen IV expression in microglia of G93A mice at 18 weeks of age vs. controls. Hence, it is still unclear whether glial cells, especially astrocytes, induce or prevent microvascular CNS barrier damage.

Another study, based on the G93A SOD1 rat model of ALS, demonstrated interesting results. Ultrastructural alterations of the capillaries such as perivascular swollen astrocyte end-feet, Evans blue leakage, reduced mRNA expression of ZO-1 and occludin, and of agrin, a basement membrane component, were observed in animals only at symptomatic stage (Nicaise et al., 2009a). Conversely, IgG and hemosiderin deposits, other indicators of capillary leakage, were detected in the brainstem and lumbar spinal cord of pre-symptomatic ALS rats. Additionally, the same group (Nicaise et al., 2009b) showed increased expression of aquaporin-4 (AQP4) mRNA and protein in the spinal cord gray matter of end-stage SOD1 rats. Immunohistochemistry revealed increased AQP4 in areas surrounding vessels and motoneuron perikaria. Electron microscopic analysis confirmed localization of this protein in association with perivascular swollen astrocytic processes. The authors suggested that the aquaporin channels may promote perivascular edema and AQR4 might be a potential marker of barrier disruption in ALS (Nicaise et al., 2010). Since elevated AQP4 was also detected near motor neurons, it is possible that dysfunctional astrocytes contribute to further motor neuron degeneration. A more recent study by Bataveljić et al. (2012) confirmed overexpression of AQP4 in the brainstem (facial and trigeminal nuclei) and motor cortex of G93A SOD1 rats at end-stage of disease. Notably, increased AQP4 immunoreactivity was observed in astrocytic processes around blood vessels in studied brain areas of ALS rats. In parallel, the authors determined decreased expression of potassium channel (Kir4.1) in the brainstem and cortex of rats by immunolabeling and Western blot analyses. The authors concluded that the functional changes in these channels could reduce astrocytes' ability to properly maintain water and potassium CNS homeostasis, not only affecting the BBB but also impeding motor neuron survival in ALS. Moreover, increased vascular permeability in the brain was determined in symptomatic G93A SOD1 rats using Gd-DTPA-enhanced MRI (Andjus et al., 2009). In addition to the BBB leakage, the authors showed marked lateral ventricle dilatation in ALS rats as "the most apparent feature of brain tissue atrophy."

Thus, the compromised BBB and BSCB are evident in the SOD1 animal model of ALS. Endothelial cell degeneration, swollen astrocyte end-feet and dissociation from the endothelium, capillary leakage, perivascular edema, downregulation of tight junction proteins, microhemorrhages, and reduction of basement membrane components are the main hallmarks of the B-CNS-B impairment. This altered vascular barrier, normally preventing entry of various blood-borne harmful substances into the CNS, could contribute to motor neuron death. Although capillary barrier damage in the CNS of both mouse and rat SOD1 models of ALS has been demonstrated prior to motor neuron loss and neuroinflammation, the specific cause of B-CNS-B breakdown has not yet been identified. It is possible that endothelial cells are more susceptible to detrimental involvement of the misfolding mutant SOD1 protein. However, the particular mechanism(s) responsible for the endothelial cell alteration observed in ALS still needs to be determined.

BBB AND BSCB IMPAIRMENT IN SPORADIC AND FAMILIAL ALS PATIENTS

The transgenic rodent models expressing mutant SOD1 have greatly contributed to the understanding of ALS pathogenesis. Relatively new research on B-CNS-B competence in ALS has largely used mutant SOD1 rodent models, but determination of barrier integrity without involvement of the mutant SOD1 protein is necessary to clarify the pathogenesis of sporadic human ALS cases. ALS is a multifactorial disease with a complexity of underlying intrinsic and extrinsic factors related to motor neuron death. Some of these detrimental factors might be directly associated with B-CNS-B impairment.

Although the B-CNS-B regulates cellular infiltration into the CNS (Engelhardt, 2008), under inflammatory conditions, extensive leukocyte migration into the CNS occurs following cytokine releases from inflammatory/immune cells (de Vries et al., 1997; Sagar et al., 2012; Sallusto et al., 2012). Leukocyte trafficking through the B-CNS-B is a multistep process mediated by adhesion molecules, classified as immunoglobulins, integrins, cadherins, or selectins. These molecules are up-regulated on the surfaces of the endothelial cells, allowing adhesion and migration of cells from the bloodstream to the CNS (Ley et al., 2007) and are often accompanied by an increased influx of serum proteins. In example, Lindsberg et al. (2010) discussed the deleterious role of the mast cell, a potent inflammatory cell, in cerebral ischemia. These cells located within the cerebral microvasculature secrete cytokines, histamine, heparin, and proteases which can degrade the basement membrane and exacerbate barrier damage, promoting edema, prolonged extravasation, and microhemorrhage and attracting new inflammatory cells. The paracellular pathway of cell migration through the capillary wall is most common, but some authors hypothesize that penetration of immune cells into the CNS can also be accomplished through the transcellular pathway with intact tight junctions (Carman and Springer, 2008).

In the CNS tissue of ALS patients, inflammation and immune cell activation have been detected and are associated with motor neuron degeneration (Donnenfeld et al., 1984; Engelhardt and Appel, 1990; Engelhardt et al., 1993, 1995; Henkel et al., 2004; Boillée et al., 2006). Early studies found IgG and C3/C4 complement deposits in the spinal cord and motor cortex tissues from ALS patients (Donnenfeld et al., 1984). Engelhardt and Appel, (1990) also detected active macrophages and IgG within the endoplasmic reticulum of motor neurons in ALS patients. Interestingly, IgG from sera of ALS patients induced death of a motor neuron cell line (VSC 4.1) *in vitro* (Engelhardt et al., 1995). These study results suggest alteration of B-CNS-B permeability and thus recent investigations have begun to focus on potential endothelial barrier damage in ALS patients.

Henkel et al. (2009) demonstrated diminished mRNA expression of occludin and ZO-1 in human lumbar spinal cord tissue from both sporadic and familial forms of ALS. Similarly, decreased immunostaining for occludin was observed in a small cohort of ALS patients (Miyazaki et al., 2011). These results agreed with the experimental findings, confirming loss of endothelial integrity, and indicating BSCB disruption that might contribute to disease pathogenesis.

A study by Garbuzova-Davis et al. (2010) showed a significant reduction in the numbers of circulating endothelial cells in the peripheral blood of ALS patients with moderate or severe disease. Increased circulating endothelial cells is considered a marker for endothelial damage (Blann et al., 2005) and has been noted in several vascular diseases, including acute myocardial infarct and acute ischemic stroke (Nadar et al., 2005; Chong et al., 2006). These unexpected results in ALS may be explained by a lack of endothelial shedding, resulting in the attachment of new endothelial cells over the damaged cells and thus a multilayer endothelium (Garbuzova-Davis et al., 2010). Indeed, electron microscopy images of ALS mouse tissue have revealed multiple layers of endothelial cells in the brain and spinal cord capillaries (Garbuzova-Davis et al., 2007a). Also, a reduction of circulating endothelial cells in peripheral blood of ALS patients with disease progression could be due to impaired re-endothelialization. The structural and functional integrity of the vascular network, normally maintained by continuous renewal of the endothelial cell layer with a low replication rate of 0.1% per day (Hunting et al., 2005), might be weakened in ALS. It is possible that insufficient production of endothelial progenitor cells by the bone marrow might be an issue. Recent reports demonstrated the functional deficiency of bone marrow mesenchymal stromal cell in ALS patients by reductions in pluripotency and secretion of various trophic factors (Koh et al., 2012) as well as by abnormal productions of MMPs and tissue inhibitors of metalloproteinases (TIMPs; Bossolasco et al., 2010).

In our recent study (Garbuzova-Davis et al., 2012), we examined structural and functional integrities of capillaries in the gray and white matter of the brainstem (medulla) and spinal cord (cervical and lumbar) in postmortem tissue from SALS patients. Study results showed capillary ultrastructural abnormalities in CNS tissues from SALS patients, similar to results from our animal studies (Garbuzova-Davis et al., 2007a). Mainly, severe intra- and extracellular edema, endothelial cell impairment as characterized by swelling and cytoplasmic vacuolization, pericyte degeneration, and degeneration of astrocyte end-feet processes surrounding capillaries were determined by electron microscopic analysis of the medulla and spinal cords. Also, separation of the endothelial cells from the basement membrane, allowing plasma to contact the basal lamina, was a significant capillary alteration noted in brain and spinal cord tissues of SALS patients. Observed capillary endothelium damage led to vascular leakage in the brain and spinal cord as determined by immunostaining for endogenous IgG, confirming previous study results on an animal model of ALS (Garbuzova-Davis et al., 2007b; Nicaise et al., 2009a). Microvascular leakage was also determined in CNS tissues from SALS patients by perivascular fibrin deposits in our electron microscopy images and was recently confirmed (Winkler et al., 2013). Winkler et al. (2013) additionally demonstrated parenchymal accumulation of the plasma-derived proteins trombin and IgG as well as erythrocyte-derived hemoglobin and iron-containing hemosiderin in the cervical gray matter from both SALS and FALS patients via immunostaining. The authors noted that these abnormal deposits in the postmortem tissues were detected only in tissues from ALS patients, but not from controls, and there were unusually widespread pathological depositions at a significant distance from capillaries. In our study (Garbuzova-Davis et al., 2012), fibrin filament deposits and IgG leakage, determined by electron microscopic and immunostaining analysis respectively, were predominantly limited to within the capillary basement membrane or were in close proximity to capillaries. Moreover, erythrocyte extravasation was not determined perivascularly or at neuropil locations in our numerous electron microscope images at different magnifications of the medulla, cervical and lumbar spinal cords from ALS patients. Microhemorrhages within CNS tissues in ALS are possible, even though not supported by MRI evaluations of microbleeds in the brain of ALS patients (Verstraete et al., 2010), so the presence of erythrocytes in CNS parenchyma observed by Winkler et al. (2013) needs further confirmation. Erythrocytes are normally restricted from entry into the CNS and these cells typically extravasate into CNS tissue due to capillary rupture as shown in multiple sclerosis (Adams, 1988), post-traumatic epilepsy (Willmore and Triggs, 1984), and cerebral ischemia (Simard et al., 2007). However, capillary rupture was not evident morphologically in the brain or spinal cords from ALS patients, even by electron microscopy imaging.

Importantly, complementary approaches have identified pericyte degeneration by electron microscopy (Garbuzova-Davis et al., 2012) and shown reduction in pericyte numbers via immunostaining (Winkler et al., 2013) in capillaries of ALS patients, deficiencies which might severely compromise the B-CNS-B. Hence, the cause(s) of pericyte deterioration in human ALS tissues should be determined.

Additionally, analysis of tight junction protein expressions in our study (Garbuzova-Davis et al., 2012) using Western immunoblot showed significant decreases of primarily ZO-1 expression in gray and white matter in all examined SALS tissues, similarly to previous studies (Henkel et al., 2009; Miyazaki et al., 2011). For occludin and claudin-5, diminished protein expressions were mostly found in ALS medulla and cervical spinal cord.

Moreover, our new findings (Garbuzova-Davis et al., 2012) showed extensive vascular basement membrane collagen IV accumulation, 2–2.5 times higher than controls, in the majority of brain and spinal cord vessels from SALS patients. Also, collagen fiber calcifications were determined in some CNS capillaries. Although similar results were noted in Alzheimer's patients (Claudio, 1996), some previous reports conflict with our study results. Decreased perivascular collagen IV was noted in postmortem ALS spinal cord tissue (Ono et al., 1998; Miyazaki et al., 2011). This discrepancy needs clarification.

Finally, our study results showed a significant increase of microvascular density in gray matter of the lumbar spinal cord from SALS patients vs. controls (Garbuzova-Davis et al., 2012) suggesting that neovascularization occurred to compensate for vascular insufficiency due to dysfunctional capillaries. Currently, we are investigating possible new vessel formation in both an ALS mouse model and ALS patients. Supporting the likelihood of ALS neovascularization, Biron et al. (2011) similarly (to our results) demonstrated increased microvascular density in brains from Alzheimer's patients, suggesting a relationship between hypervascularity, neoangiogenesis and BBB disruption. Also, ongoing angiogenesis resulted in increased vascular density in postmortem brain tissues, mainly in the hippocampus, in Alzheimer's patients (Desai et al., 2009). Recently, Desai Bradaric et al. (2012) showed the presence of newly created vessels in postmortem brain tissues such as the substantia nigra pars compacta, locus ceruleus, and putamen from subjects with Parkinson's disease and progressive supranuclear palsy. The authors suggest that these new angiogenic vessels could contribute to disease inflammatory processes by failing to restrict extravasation of immune cells and inflammatory or toxic factors from the peripheral circulation to the CNS due to the new vessels having incompletely developed BBB properties. This possibility might also be an issue for ALS.

Thus, there is compelling evidence of BBB and BSCB impairment in areas of motor neuron degeneration in ALS patients. Importantly, microvascular alterations seen in both gray and white matter of medulla, cervical, and lumbar spinal cord from SALS patients indicate pervasive B-CNS-B damage that might contribute to disease pathogenesis.

SIMILARITIES AND DIFFERENCES IN THE B-CNS-B IMPAIRMENT BETWEEN ALS PATIENTS AND ANIMAL MODELS OF ALS

Convincing findings indicate B-CNS-B alterations in both ALS patients and the SOD1 animal model of ALS and suggest these alterations as a possible factor aggravating motor neuron damage. Numerous signs of barrier damage, such as endothelial cell degeneration, capillary leakage, perivascular edema, downregulation of tight junction proteins, and microhemorrhages are common in both mutant SOD1 animal models of disease and ALS patients. To date, other pathogenic features linked to barrier alterations have so far only been identified in ALS patients. Mainly, pericyte degeneration, perivascular basement membrane collagen IV expansion, and white matter capillary abnormalities in SALS patients are significant barrier related pathologies yet to be noted in ALS SOD1 animal models. In **Table 1**, current evidence of B-CNS-B impairment in ALS is provided from animal and human studies.

Severe capillary pericyte damage (Garbuzova-Davis et al., 2012; Winkler et al., 2013) is an important finding in ALS patients. At the ultrastructural level, complete pericyte degeneration or cell fragmentation in the adjacent extracellular space was determined in numbers of gray and white matter microvessels in the medulla and cervical/lumbar spinal cord of SALS patients (Garbuzova-Davis et al., 2012). Pericytes play essential roles in maintaining B-CNS-B integrity by regulating capillary permeability, blood flow, vascular tone, and angiogenesis (Hirschi and D'Amore, 1996; Kutcher and Herman, 2009; Armulik et al., 2010; Winkler et al., 2011, 2012; Sá-Pereira et al., 2012). These functions are associated with the cells' anatomical location, in close proximity to endothelial cells and sharing a common basement membrane. Pericytes are also involved in modulation of immunological response by their phagocytic function (Balabanov and Dore-Duffy, 1998; Dalkara et al., 2011). For example, amyloid deposits within degenerating pericytes were detected in the brains of Alzheimer's patients (Dalkara et al., 2011). The authors discussed the role of pericyte dysfunction in cerebral hypoperfusion and suggest that "microvascular dysfunction due to pericyte degeneration initiates secondary neurodegenerative changes" (Dalkara et al., 2011). In ALS, Rule et al. (2010) reported reduced capillary blood flow in

Table 1 | Evidence of blood–CNS barrier impairment in ALS patients and SOD1 animal models of ALS.

	References	
Description of evidence	**Animal model of ALS**	**Human ALS**
Endothelial cell degeneration or damage	Garbuzova-Davis et al. (2007a), Nicaise et al. (2009a), Miyazaki et al. (2011)	Garbuzova-Davis et al. (2012)
Capillary leakage	Garbuzova-Davis et al. (2007b), Nicaise et al. (2009a), Andjus et al. (2009)	Garbuzova-Davis et al. (2012), Winkler et al. (2013)
Pericyte degeneration or damage		Garbuzova-Davis et al. (2012), Winkler et al. (2013)
Perivascular edema	Garbuzova-Davis et al. (2007a)	Garbuzova-Davis et al. (2012)
Astrocyte end-feet capillary damage and dissociation	Garbuzova-Davis et al. (2007a,b), Nicaise et al. (2009a), Miyazaki et al. (2011), Bataveljić et al. (2012)	Miyazaki et al. (2011), Garbuzova-Davis et al. (2012)
Altered basement membrane components	Garbuzova-Davis et al. (2007b), Nicaise et al. (2009a), Miyazaki et al. (2011)	Ono et al. (1998), Miyazaki et al. (2011), Garbuzova-Davis et al. (2012)
Microhemorrhages or perivascular hemosiderin	Garbuzova-Davis et al. (2007a), Zhong et al. (2008), Nicaise et al. (2009a)	Verstraete et al. (2010) (unsupporting), Winkler et al. (2013)
Altered blood flow or capillary lengths and diameters	Zhong et al. (2008), Miyazaki et al. (2011)	Rule et al. (2010)
Downregulation of junctional complex proteins	Zhong et al. (2008), Nicaise et al. (2009a), Miyazaki et al. (2011)	Henkel et al. (2009), Miyazaki et al. (2011), Garbuzova-Davis et al. (2012)
Altered endothelial transporter protein expression	Garbuzova-Davis et al. (2007b), Zhong et al. (2008), Milane et al. (2010), Jablonski et al. (2012)	Jablonski et al. (2012)

brains of patients correlating with disease severity, a reduction likely associated with pericyte impairment. A similar decrease in blood flow was determined in the spinal cord of G93A SOD1 mice preceding inflammation and motor neuron injury (Zhong et al., 2008). However, there were no obvious abnormalities detected in pericyte morphology in the brainstem or spinal cord capillaries via electron microscope even in late symptomatic G93A mice (Garbuzova-Davis et al., 2007a). This discrepancy between animal data and results from ALS patients should be investigated.

Another difference between human and animal studies in ALS is vascular basement membrane collagen IV abnormalities. As we noted above, our recent study (Garbuzova-Davis et al., 2012) showed extensive basement membrane collagen IV accumulation and even collagen fiber calcifications in numerous capillaries in gray and white matter brain and spinal cords from SALS patients. However, opposing reports demonstrated decreased perivascular collagen IV in postmortem ALS spinal cord tissue (Ono et al., 1998; Miyazaki et al., 2011). In a study by Miyazaki et al. (2011), reduction of immunoexpression for collagen IV was observed in the anterior horns of the spinal cord from ALS patients as well as in G93A mice during disease progression and was accompanied by MMP-9 up-regulation. The authors conclude that this vascular damage is common to humans and this ALS animal model. However, the observed collagen IV reduction might be due to the diminished capillary density described in the same study. In addition, the authors provided conflicting data with double immunofluorescence staining for collagen IV and Iba-1 (microglial marker) in the spinal anterior horn of G93A mice at 18 weeks of age showing higher collagen IV expression vs. controls along with the appearance of collagen IV-positive microglia. Microglial cells are resident cells in the CNS with macrophagic properties upon their activation and likely overexpression of collagen IV by microglia indicates uptake of this protein. Supportive evidence of the ability of microglia to express collagen IV was not provided (Miyazaki et al., 2011). Also, it is unclear if this collagen IV immunostaining was also associated with capillaries or astrocytes. Double immunostaining for collagen IV and astrocytes might be a reasonable confirming procedure. It has been shown that reactive astrocytes expressed type IV collagen after spinal cord injury in promoting glial scar formation (Liesi and Kauppila, 2002). In the same study, the authors reported that IL-1 beta and TGF beta-1 cytokines induced collagen IV expression in astrocytes *in vitro*. Since reactive astrogliosis and microglia activation are major contributors to inflammatory processes in ALS by secretion of various pro-inflammatory cytokines, particularly TNF-alpha and TGF beta-1 (Schiffer et al., 1996; Hall et al., 1998; McGeer and McGeer, 1998; Elliott, 2001; McGeer and McGeer, 2002; Consilvio et al., 2004; Henkel et al., 2004; Xie et al., 2004; Vargas and Johnson, 2010; Appel et al., 2011; Haidet-Phillips et al., 2011; Sica, 2012; Evans et al., 2013; Phatnani et al., 2013) it is possible that reactive astrocytes not only affect motor neurons but also promote a collagenous vascular basement membrane. Moreover, inflammation may initiate barrier damage by impairing endothelial cell function. Mantovani et al. (1992) showed that the inflammatory environment in ALS affected endothelial cell gene expression, altering cell function. An additional discrepancy between our and the above mentioned studies regarding basement membrane collagen deposition was discussed in detail (Garbuzova-Davis et al., 2012) and primarily focused on the potential imbalance between MMPs and TIMPs due to defective regulation of the MMP pathway by damaged endothelial cells. Also, since downregulation of other basement membrane components such as laminin (Garbuzova-Davis et al., 2007b) and argin (Nicaise et al., 2009a) has been shown in symptomatic G93A mice but not yet confirmed in ALS patients, it is possible that buildup of perivascular collagen IV occurs as a compensatory mechanism for maintenance of vascular integrity.

We strongly believe that abnormal perivascular collagen accumulation in SALS patients takes place over a long period of time. Our notion is partially supported by Ono et al. (1998) who showed widely separated and fragmented collagen bundles in the interstitial tissue surrounding capillaries in the posterior half of lateral funiculus and anterior horn of cervical spinal cord from ALS patients by ultrastructural analysis. Yet total collagen content determined for each of these spinal cord regions was lower in ALS patients than in controls with or without neurological diseases. Although these data are interesting, the existence of basement collagen abnormalities needs clarification.

Thus, the complexity of the B-CNS-B alterations in ALS is evident. Commonalities in barrier pathologies between humans and an animal model of ALS are essential for understanding involvement of the B-CNS-B in disease pathogenesis. However, the disparities in barrier competence in humans with ALS vs. animal model should be considered. Despite a growing research effort, more studies are needed to reveal specific mechanisms of barrier breakdown in ALS. The question still remains: is barrier damage an initial disease factor or a secondary element in human ALS?

CONCLUSION

ALS has been, and remains, a challenge for developing therapeutics. More than 30 drug compounds have already been tested in ALS clinical trials yet the only modestly effective treatment is riluzole (Aggarwal and Cudkowicz, 2008). Some tested substances failed to prove effective and even showed harmful effects in Phase III clinical trials: IGF-1 (insulin-like growth factor type 1; Sorenson et al., 2008), minocycline (Gordon et al., 2007), creatine (Groeneveld et al., 2003), and topiramate (Cudkowicz et al., 2003).

These disappointing results might reflect defective transport systems in damaged BBB and BSCB in ALS. Degeneration of endothelial and pericyte cells, compromising vascular barrier integrity in the brain and spinal cord in ALS patients, could be the main obstacles for effective drug delivery to the CNS. Also, it is hard to imagine proper transport of pharmaco-therapeutics across an extensively expanded vascular collagenous basement membrane. Such abnormal buildup of basement membrane collagen seems likely to alter barrier influx and efflux transport systems and, as result, motor neurons might suffer both from reduced nutritional deliveries and increased metabolite levels. Additionally, increases of P-glycoprotein (P-gp) along with the breast cancer resistance protein (BCRP) were determined in brain and spinal cord microvessels in both SOD1 animal models and ALS patients (Milane et al., 2010; Jablonski et al., 2012). Jablonski et al. (2012) conclude that the impairment of these P-gp and BCRP efflux transporters might induce pharmaco-resistance in ALS.

Numerous comprehensive reviews discuss therapeutic strategies of transport drugs across the blood–CNS barrier (Abbott and Romero, 1996; Pardridge, 2002; Misra et al., 2003; McCarty, 2005; Patel et al., 2009; Pathan et al., 2009; Gabathuler, 2010) including chemical (i.g., lipid-mediated transport), biological (i.g., specific transporters for pharmaceuticals), or particular drug carrier systems. Also, various drug delivery systems (e.g., liposomes, nanoparticles, or microspheres) and routes (e.g., intranasal, intraventricular, or intrathecal) have been proposed. However, all of these various strategies for effective drug delivery to the CNS rely on a normally functioning BBB/BSCB. In ALS, deliveries of therapeutic drugs are likely to be complicated by the pervasiveness of the B-CNS-B damage.

In conclusion, the blood–CNS barrier should be considered as a primary therapeutic target prior to development of any treatment approach for ALS.

ACKNOWLEDGMENTS

This work was supported in part by the Muscular Dystrophy Association (Grant #92452) and the USF Department of Neurosurgery and Brain Repair.

REFERENCES

Abbott, N. J., and Romero, I. A. (1996). Transporting therapeutics across the blood-brain barrier. *Mol. Med. Today* 2, 106–113. doi: 10.1016/1357-4310(96)88720-X

Adams, C. W. (1988). Perivascular iron deposition and other vascular damage in multiple sclerosis. *J. Neurol. Neurosurg. Psychiatry* 51, 260–265. doi: 10.1136/jnnp.51.2.260

Aggarwal, S., and Cudkowicz, M. (2008). ALS drug development: reflections from the past and a way forward. *Neurother. J. Am. Soc. Exp. Neurother.* 5, 516–527. doi: 10.1016/j.nurt.2008.08.002

Alexianu, M. E., Kozovska, M., and Appel, S. H. (2001). Immune reactivity in a mouse model of familial ALS correlates with disease progression. *Neurology* 57, 1282–1289. doi: 10.1212/WNL.57.7.1282

Andjus, P. R., Bataveljić, D., Vanhoutte, G., Mitrecic, D., Pizzolante, F., Djogo, N., et al. (2009). In vivo morphological changes in animal models of amyotrophic lateral sclerosis and Alzheimer's-like disease: MRI approach. *Anat. Rec. (Hoboken.)* 292, 1882–1892. doi: 10.1002/ar.20995

Annunziata, P., and Volpi, N. (1985). High levels of C3c in the cerebrospinal fluid from amyotrophic lateral sclerosis patients. *Acta Neurol. Scand.* 72, 61–64. doi: 10.1111/j.1600-0404.1985.tb01548.x

Appel, S. H., Zhao, W., Beers, D. R., and Henkel, J. S. (2011). The microglial-motoneuron dialogue in ALS. *Acta Myol.* 30, 4–8.

Armulik, A., Genové, G., Mäe, M., Nisancioglu, M. H., Wallgard, E., Niaudet, C., et al. (2010). Pericytes regulate the blood-brain barrier. *Nature* 468, 557–561. doi: 10.1038/nature09522

Balabanov, R., and Dore-Duffy, P. (1998). Role of the CNS microvascular pericyte in the blood-brain barrier. *J. Neurosci. Res.* 53, 637–644. doi: 10.1002/(SICI)1097-4547(19980915)53:6<637::AID-JNR1>3.0.CO;2-6

Ballabh, P., Braun, A., and Nedergaard, M. (2004). The blood-brain barrier: an overview: structure, regulation, and clinical implications. *Neurobiol. Dis.* 16, 1–13. doi: 10.1016/j.nbd.2003.12.016

Bartanusz, V., Jezova, D., Alajajian, B., and Digicaylioglu, M. (2011). The blood-spinal cord barrier: morphology and clinical implications. *Ann. Neurol.* 70, 194–206. doi: 10.1002/ana.22421

Bataveljić, D., Nikolić, L., Milosević, M., Todorović, N., and Andjus, P. R. (2012). Changes in the astrocytic aquaporin-4 and inwardly rectifying potassium channel expression in the brain of the amyotrophic lateral sclerosis SOD1(G93A) rat model. *Glia* 60, 1991–2003. doi: 10.1002/glia.22414

Begley, D. J. (2004). ABC transporters and the blood-brain barrier. *Curr. Pharm. Des.* 10, 1295–1312. doi: 10.2174/1381612043384844

Begley, D. J., and Brightman, M. W. (2003). Structural and functional aspects of the blood-brain barrier. *Prog. Drug Res.* 61, 39–78.

Biron, K. E., Dickstein, D. L., Gopaul, R., and Jefferies, W. A. (2011). Amyloid triggers extensive cerebral angiogenesis causing blood brain barrier permeability and hypervascularity in Alzheimer's disease. *PLoS ONE* 6:e23789. doi: 10.1371/journal.pone.0023789

Blann, A. D., Woywodt, A., Bertolini, F., Bull, T. M., Buyon, J. P., Clancy, R. M., et al. (2005). Circulating endothelial cells. Biomarker of vascular disease. *Thromb. Haemost.* 93, 228–235. doi:10.1267/THRO05020228

Boillée, S., Yamanaka, K., Lobsiger, C. S., Copeland, N. G., Jenkins, N. A., Kassiotis, G., et al. (2006). Onset and progression in inherited ALS determined by motor neurons and microglia. *Science* 312, 1389–1392. doi: 10.1126/science.1123511

Bossolasco, P., Cova, L., Calzarossa, C., Servida, F., Mencacci, N. E., Onida, F., et al. (2010). Metalloproteinase alterations in the bone marrow of ALS patients. *J. Mol. Med. (Berl.)* 88, 553–564. doi: 10.1007/s00109-009-0584-7

Bradbury, M. W. (1985). The blood-brain barrier. Transport across the cerebral endothelium. *Circ. Res.* 57, 213–222. doi: 10.1161/01.RES.57.2.213

Bruijn, L. I., Miller, T. M., and Cleveland, D. W. (2004). Unraveling the mechanisms involved in motor neuron degeneration in ALS. *Annu. Rev. Neurosci.* 27, 723–749. doi: 10.1146/annurev.neuro.27.070203.144244

Carman, C. V., and Springer, T. A. (2008). Trans-cellular migration: cell-cell contacts get intimate. *Curr. Opin. Cell Biol.* 20, 533–540. doi: 10.1016/j.ceb.2008.05.007

Chong, A. Y., Lip, G. Y. H., Freestone, B., and Blann, A. D. (2006). Increased circulating endothelial cells in acute heart failure: comparison with von Willebrand factor and soluble E-selectin. *Eur. J. Heart Fail.* 8, 167–172. doi: 10.1016/j.ejheart.2005.06.010

Claudio, L. (1996). Ultrastructural features of the blood-brain barrier in biopsy tissue from Alzheimer's disease patients. *Acta Neuropathol. (Berl.)* 91, 6–14. doi: 10.1007/s004010050386

Cleveland, D. W., and Rothstein, J. D. (2001). From Charcot to Lou Gehrig: deciphering selective motor neuron death in ALS. *Nat. Rev. Neurosci.* 2, 806–819. doi: 10.1038/35097565

Consilvio, C., Vincent, A. M., and Feldman, E. L. (2004). Neuroinflammation, COX-2, and ALS–a dual role? *Exp. Neurol.* 187, 1–10. doi: 10.1016/j.expneurol.2003.12.009

Cudkowicz, M. E., Shefner, J. M., Schoenfeld, D. A., Brown, R. H. Jr., Johnson, H., Qureshi, M., et al. (2003). A randomized, placebo-controlled trial of topiramate in amyotrophic lateral sclerosis. *Neurology* 61, 456–464. doi: 10.1212/WNL.61.4.456

Dalkara, T., Gursoy-Ozdemir, Y., and Yemisci, M. (2011). Brain microvascular pericytes in health and disease. *Acta Neuropathol. (Berl.)* 122, 1–9. doi: 10.1007/s00401-011-0847-6

Dermietzel, R., and Krause, D. (1991). Molecular anatomy of the blood-brain barrier as defined by immunocytochemistry. *Int. Rev. Cytol.* 127, 57–109.

Desai Bradaric, B., Patel, A., Schneider, J. A., Carvey, P. M., and Hendey, B. (2012). Evidence for angiogenesis in Parkinson's disease, incidental Lewy body disease, and progressive supranuclear palsy. *J. Neural Transm.* 119, 59–71. doi: 10.1007/s00702-011-0684-8

Desai, B. S., Schneider, J. A., Li, J.-L., Carvey, P. M., and Hendey, B. (2009). Evidence of angiogenic vessels in Alzheimer's disease. *J. Neural Transm.* 116, 587–597. doi: 10.1007/s00702-009-0226-9

de Vries, H. E., Kuiper, J., de Boer, A. G., Van Berkel, T. J., and Breimer, D. D. (1997). The blood-brain barrier in neuroinflammatory diseases. *Pharmacol. Rev.* 49, 143–155.

Donnenfeld, H., Kascsak, R. J., and Bartfeld, H. (1984). Deposits of IgG and C3 in the spinal cord and motor cortex of ALS patients. *J. Neuroimmunol.* 6, 51–57. doi: 10.1016/0165-5728(84)90042-0

Elliott, J. L. (2001). Cytokine upregulation in a murine model of familial amyotrophic lateral sclerosis. *Brain Res. Mol. Brain Res.* 95, 172–178. doi: 10.1016/S0169-328X(01)00242-X

Engelhardt, B. (2008). The blood-central nervous system barriers actively control immune cell entry into the central nervous system. *Curr. Pharm. Des.* 14, 1555–1565. doi: 10.2174/138161208784705432

Engelhardt, J. I., and Appel, S. H. (1990). IgG reactivity in the spinal cord and motor cortex in amyotrophic lateral sclerosis. *Arch. Neurol.* 47, 1210–1216. doi: 10.1001/archneur.1990.00530110068019

Engelhardt, J. I., Siklós, L., Kömüves, L., Smith, R. G., and Appel, S. H. (1995). Antibodies to calcium channels from ALS patients passively transferred to mice selectively increase intracellular calcium and induce ultrastructural changes in motoneurons. *Synapse* 20, 185–199. doi: 10.1002/syn.890200302

Engelhardt, J. I., Tajti, J., and Appel, S. H. (1993). Lymphocytic infiltrates in the spinal cord in amyotrophic lateral sclerosis. *Arch. Neurol.* 50, 30–36. doi: 10.1001/archneur.1993.00540010026013

Evans, M. C., Couch, Y., Sibson, N., and Turner, M. R. (2013). Inflammation and neurovascular changes in amyotrophic lateral sclerosis. *Mol. Cell. Neurosci.* 53, 34–41. doi: 10.1016/j.mcn.2012.10.008

Gabathuler, R. (2010). Approaches to transport therapeutic drugs across the blood-brain barrier to treat brain diseases. *Neurobiol. Dis.* 37, 48–57. doi: 10.1016/j.nbd.2009.07.028

Garbuzova-Davis, S., Haller, E., Saporta, S., Kolomey, I., Nicosia, S. V., and Sanberg, P. R. (2007a). Ultrastructure of blood-brain barrier and blood-spinal cord barrier in SOD1 mice modeling ALS. *Brain Res.* 1157, 126–137. doi: 10.1016/j.brainres.2007.04.044

Garbuzova-Davis, S., Saporta, S., Haller, E., Kolomey, I., Bennett, S. P., Potter, H., et al. (2007b). Evidence of compromised blood-spinal cord barrier in early and late symptomatic SOD1 mice modeling ALS. *PLoS ONE* 2:e1205. doi: 10.1371/journal.pone.0001205

Garbuzova-Davis, S., Hernandez-Ontiveros, D. G., Rodrigues, M. C. O., Haller, E., Frisina-Deyo, A., Mirtyl, S., et al. (2012). Impaired blood-brain/spinal cord barrier in ALS patients. *Brain Res.* 1469, 114–128. doi: 10.1016/j.brainres.2012.05.056

Garbuzova-Davis, S., Rodrigues, M. C. O., Hernandez-Ontiveros, D. G., Louis, M. K., Willing, A. E., Borlongan, C. V., et al. (2011). Amyotrophic lateral sclerosis: a neurovascular disease. *Brain Res.* 1398, 113–125. doi: 10.1016/j.brainres.2011.04.049

Garbuzova-Davis, S., Saporta, S., and Sanberg, P. R. (2008). Implications of blood-brain barrier disruption in ALS. *Amyotroph. Lateral Scler.* 9, 375–376. doi: 10.1080/17482960802160990

Garbuzova-Davis, S., Woods, R. L., Louis, M. K., Zesiewicz, T. A., Kuzmin-Nichols, N., Sullivan, K. L., et al. (2010). Reduction of circulating endothelial cells in peripheral blood of ALS patients. *PLoS ONE* 5:e10614. doi: 10.1371/journal.pone.0010614

Gordon, P. H., Moore, D. H., Miller, R. G., Florence, J. M., Verheijde, J. L., Doorish, C., et al. (2007). Efficacy of minocycline in patients with amyotrophic lateral sclerosis: a phase III randomised trial. *Lancet Neurol.* 6, 1045–1053. doi: 10.1016/S1474-4422(07)70270-3

Grammas, P., Martinez, J., and Miller, B. (2011). Cerebral microvascular endothelium and the pathogenesis of neurodegenerative diseases. *Expert Rev. Mol. Med.* 13, e19. doi: 10.1017/S1462399411001918

Groeneveld, G. J., Veldink, J. H., van der Tweel, I., Kalmijn, S., Beijer, C., de Visser, M., et al. (2003). A randomized sequential trial of creatine in amyotrophic lateral sclerosis. *Ann. Neurol.* 53, 437–445. doi: 10.1002/ana.10554

Haidet-Phillips, A. M., Hester, M. E., Miranda, C. J., Meyer, K., Braun, L., Frakes, A., et al. (2011). Astrocytes from familial and sporadic ALS patients are toxic to motor neurons. *Nat. Biotechnol.* 29, 824–828. doi: 10.1038/nbt.1957

Hall, E. D., Oostveen, J. A., and Gurney, M. E. (1998). Relationship of microglial and astrocytic activation to disease onset and progression in a transgenic model of familial ALS. *Glia* 23, 249–256. doi: 10.1002/(SICI)1098-1136(199807)23:3<249::AID-GLIA7>3.0.CO;2-#

Henkel, J. S., Beers, D. R., Wen, S., Bowser, R., and Appel, S. H. (2009). Decreased mRNA expression of tight junction proteins in lumbar spinal cords of patients with ALS. *Neurology* 72, 1614–1616. doi: 10.1212/WNL.0b013e3181a41228

Henkel, J. S., Engelhardt, J. I., Siklós, L., Simpson, E. P., Kim, S. H., Pan, T., et al. (2004). Presence of dendritic cells, MCP-1, and activated microglia/macrophages in amyotrophic lateral sclerosis spinal cord tissue. *Ann. Neurol.* 55, 221–235. doi: 10.1002/ana.10805

Hirschi, K. K., and D'Amore, P. A. (1996). Pericytes in the microvasculature. *Cardiovasc. Res.* 32, 687–698.

Hovden, H., Frederiksen, J. L., and Pedersen, S. W. (2013). Immune system alterations in amyotrophic lateral sclerosis. *Acta Neurol. Scand.* doi: 10.1111/ane.12125 [Epub ahead of print].

Hunting, C. B., Noort, W. A., and Zwaginga, J. J. (2005). Circulating endothelial (progenitor) cells reflect the state of the endothelium: vascular injury, repair and neovascularization. *Vox Sang.* 88, 1–9. doi: 10.1111/j.1423-0410.2005.00589.x

Jablonski, M. R., Jacob, D. A., Campos, C., Miller, D. S., Maragakis, N. J., Pasinelli, P., et al. (2012). Selective increase of two ABC drug efflux transporters at the blood-spinal cord barrier suggests induced pharmacoresistance in ALS. *Neurobiol. Dis.* 47, 194–200. doi: 10.1016/j.nbd.2012.03.040

Koh, S.-H., Baik, W., Noh, M. Y., Cho, G. W., Kim, H. Y., Kim, K. S., et al. (2012). The functional deficiency of bone marrow mesenchymal stromal cells in ALS patients is proportional to disease progression rate. *Exp. Neurol.* 233, 472–480. doi: 10.1016/j.expneurol.2011.11.021

Kutcher, M. E., and Herman, I. M. (2009). The pericyte: cellular regulator of microvascular blood flow. *Microvasc. Res.* 77, 235–246. doi: 10.1016/j.mvr.2009.01.007

Leonardi, A., Abbruzzese, G., Arata, L., Cocito, L., and Vische, M. (1984). Cerebrospinal fluid (CSF) findings in amyotrophic lateral sclerosis. *J. Neurol.* 231, 75–78. doi: 10.1007/BF00313720

Ley, K., Laudanna, C., Cybulsky, M. I., and Nourshargh, S. (2007). Getting to the site of inflammation: the leukocyte adhesion cascade updated. *Nat. Rev. Immunol.* 7, 678–689. doi: 10.1038/nri2156

Liesi, P., and Kauppila, T. (2002). Induction of type IV collagen and other basement-membrane-associated proteins after spinal cord injury of the adult rat may participate in formation of the glial scar. *Exp. Neurol.* 173, 31–45. doi: 10.1006/exnr.2001.7800

Lindsberg, P. J., Strbian, D., and Karjalainen-Lindsberg, M.-L. (2010). Mast cells as early responders in the regulation of acute blood-brain barrier changes after cerebral ischemia and hemorrhage. *J. Cereb. Blood Flow Metab.* 30, 689–702. doi: 10.1038/jcbfm.2009.282

Mantovani, A., Bussolino, F., and Dejana, E. (1992). Cytokine regulation of endothelial cell function. *Faseb J.* 6, 2591–2599.

McCarty, J. H. (2005). Cell biology of the neurovascular unit: implications for drug delivery across the blood-brain barrier. *Assay Drug Dev. Technol.* 3, 89–95. doi: 10.1089/adt.2005.3.89

McGeer, P. L., and McGeer, E. G. (1998). Glial cell reactions in neurodegenerative diseases: pathophysiology and therapeutic interventions. *Alzheimer Dis. Assoc. Disord.* 12(Suppl. 2), S1–S6. doi: 10.1097/00002093-199803001-00001

McGeer, P. L., and McGeer, E. G. (2002). Inflammatory processes in amyotrophic lateral sclerosis. *Muscle Nerve* 26, 459–470. doi: 10.1002/mus.10191

Milane, A., Fernandez, C., Dupuis, L., Buyse, M., Loeffler, J.-P., Farinotti, R., et al. (2010). P-glycoprotein expression and function are increased in an animal model of amyotrophic lateral sclerosis. *Neurosci. Lett.* 472, 166–170. doi: 10.1016/j.neulet.2010.01.078

Misra, A., Ganesh, S., Shahiwala, A., and Shah, S. P. (2003). Drug delivery to the central nervous system: a review. *J. Pharm. Pharm. Sci.* 6, 252–273.

Mitchell, J. D., and Borasio, G. D. (2007). Amyotrophic lateral sclerosis. *Lancet* 369, 2031–2041. doi: 10.1016/S0140-6736(07)60944-1

Miyazaki, K., Ohta, Y., Nagai, M., Morimoto, N., Kurata, T., Takehisa, Y., et al. (2011). Disruption of neurovascular unit prior to motor neuron degeneration in amyotrophic lateral sclerosis. *J. Neurosci. Res.* 89, 718–728. doi: 10.1002/jnr.22594

Nadar, S. K., Lip, G. Y. H., Lee, K. W., and Blann, A. D. (2005). Circulating endothelial cells in acute ischaemic stroke. *Thromb. Haemost.* 94, 707–712.

Nag, S. (ed.). (2003). "Morphology and molecular properties of cellular components of normal cerebral vessels," in *The Blood-Brain Barrier: Biology and Research Protocols* (Totowa, NJ: Humana Press Inc.), 3–36.

Nicaise, C., Mitrecic, D., Demetter, P., De Decker, R., Authelet, M., Boom, A., et al. (2009a). Impaired blood-brain and blood-spinal cord barriers in mutant SOD1-linked ALS rat. *Brain Res.* 1301, 152–162. doi: 10.1016/j.brainres.2009.09.018

Nicaise, C., Soyfoo, M. S., Authelet, M., De Decker, R., Bataveljic, D., Delporte, C., et al. (2009b). Aquaporin-4 overexpression in rat ALS model. *Anat. Rec. (Hoboken.)* 292, 207–213. doi: 10.1002/ar.20838

Nicaise, C., Soyfoo, M. S., Delporte, C., and Pochet, R. (2010). Aquaporin-4 as a potential marker of BBB disruption in ALS models. *Amyotroph. Lateral Scler.* 11, 253–254. doi: 10.3109/17482960902803457

Ono, S., Imai, T., Munakata, S., Takahashi, K., Kanda, F., Hashimoto, K., et al. (1998). Collagen abnormalities in the spinal cord from patients with amyotrophic lateral sclerosis. *J. Neurol. Sci.* 160, 140–147. doi: 10.1016/S0022-510X(98)00223-8

Pardridge, W. M. (1991). Advances in cell biology of blood-brain barrier transport. *Semin. Cell Biol.* 2, 419–426.

Pardridge, W. M. (1999). Blood-brain barrier biology and methodology. *J. Neurovirol.* 5, 556–569. doi: 10.3109/13550289909021285

Pardridge, W. M. (2002). Drug and gene targeting to the brain with molecular Trojan horses. *Nat. Rev. Drug Discov.* 1, 131–139. doi: 10.1038/nrd725

Pardridge, W. M. (2005). The blood-brain barrier: bottleneck in brain drug development. *Neurorx J. Am. Soc. Exp. Neurother.* 2, 3–14.

Pasinelli, P., and Brown, R. H. (2006). Molecular biology of amyotrophic lateral sclerosis: insights from genetics. *Nat. Rev. Neurosci.* 7, 710–723. doi: 10.1038/nrn1971

Patel, M. M., Goyal, B. R., Bhadada, S. V., Bhatt, J. S., and Amin, A. F. (2009). Getting into the brain: approaches to enhance brain drug delivery. *CNS Drugs* 23, 35–58. doi: 10.2165/0023210-200923010-00003

Pathan, S. A., Iqbal, Z., Zaidi, S. M. A., Talegaonkar, S., Vohra, D., Jain, G. K., et al. (2009). CNS drug delivery systems: novel approaches. *Recent Pat. Drug Deliv. Formul.* 3, 71–89. doi: 10.2174/187221109787158355

Phatnani, H. P., Guarnieri, P., Friedman, B. A., Carrasco, M. A., Muratet, M., O'Keeffe, S., et al. (2013). Intricate interplay between astrocytes and motor neurons in ALS. *Proc. Natl. Acad. Sci. U.S.A.* 110, E756–E765. doi: 10.1073/pnas.1222361110

Rodrigues, M. C. O., Hernandez-Ontiveros, D. G., Louis, M. K., Willing, A. E., Borlongan, C. V., Sanberg, P. R., et al. (2012). Neurovascular aspects of amyotrophic lateral sclerosis. *Int. Rev. Neurobiol.* 102, 91–106. doi: 10.1016/B978-0-12-386986-9.00004-1

Rosen, D. R., Siddique, T., Patterson, D., Figlewicz, D. A., Sapp, P., Hentati, A., et al. (1993). Mutations in Cu/Zn superoxide dismutase gene are associated with familial amyotrophic lateral sclerosis. *Nature* 362, 59–62. doi: 10.1038/362059a0

Rothstein, J. D. (2009). Current hypotheses for the underlying biology of amyotrophic lateral sclerosis. *Ann. Neurol.* 65(Suppl. 1), S3–S9. doi: 10.1002/ana.21543

Rowland, L. P., and Shneider, N. A. (2001). Amyotrophic lateral sclerosis. *N. Engl. J. Med.* 344, 1688–1700. doi: 10.1056/NEJM200105313442207

Rule, R. R., Schuff, N., Miller, R. G., and Weiner, M. W. (2010). Gray matter perfusion correlates with disease severity in ALS. *Neurology* 74, 821–827. doi: 10.1212/WNL.0b013e3181d3e2dd

Sagar, D., Foss, C., El Baz, R., Pomper, M. G., Khan, Z. K., and Jain, P. (2012). Mechanisms of dendritic cell trafficking across the blood-brain barrier. *J. Neuroimmune Pharmacol.* 7, 74–94. doi: 10.1007/s11481-011-9302-7

Saleh, I. A., Zesiewicz, T., Xie, Y., Sullivan, K. L., Miller, A. M., Kuzmin-Nichols, N., et al. (2009). Evaluation of humoral immune response in adaptive immunity in ALS patients during disease progression. *J. Neuroimmunol.* 215, 96–101. doi: 10.1016/j.jneuroim.2009.07.011

Sallusto, F., Impellizzieri, D., Basso, C., Laroni, A., Uccelli, A., Lanzavecchia, A., et al. (2012). T-cell trafficking in the central nervous system. *Immunol. Rev.* 248, 216–227. doi: 10.1111/j.1600-065X.2012.01140.x

Sá-Pereira, I., Brites, D., and Brito, M. A. (2012). Neurovascular unit: a focus on pericytes. *Mol. Neurobiol.* 45, 327–347. doi: 10.1007/s12035-012-8244-2

Schiffer, D., Cordera, S., Cavalla, P., and Migheli, A. (1996). Reactive astrogliosis of the spinal cord in amyotrophic lateral sclerosis. *J. Neurol. Sci.* 139, Suppl. 27–33. doi: 10.1016/0022-510X(96)00073-1

Sica, R. E. (2012). Is amyotrophic lateral sclerosis a primary astrocytic disease? *Med. Hypotheses* 79, 819–822. doi: 10.1016/j.mehy.2012.08.036

Simard, J. M., Kent, T. A., Chen, M., Tarasov, K. V., and Gerzanich, V. (2007). Brain oedema in focal ischaemia: molecular pathophysiology and theoretical implications. *Lancet Neurol.* 6, 258–268. doi: 10.1016/S1474-4422(07)70055-8

Sorenson, E. J., Windbank, A. J., Mandrekar, J. N., Bamlet, W. R., Appel, S. H., Armon, C., et al. (2008). Subcutaneous IGF-1 is not beneficial in 2-year ALS trial. *Neurology* 71, 1770–1775. doi: 10.1212/01.wnl.0000335970.78664.36

Strong, M. J., Kesavapany, S., and Pant, H. C. (2005). The pathobiology of amyotrophic lateral sclerosis: a proteinopathy? *J. Neuropathol. Exp. Neurol.* 64, 649–664. doi: 10.1097/01.jnen.0000173889.71434.ea

Van Den Bosch, L., Van Damme, P., Bogaert, E., and Robberecht, W. (2006). The role of excitotoxicity in the pathogenesis of amyotrophic lateral sclerosis. *Biochim. Biophys. Acta* 1762, 1068–1082. doi: 10.1016/j.bbadis.2006.05.002

Vargas, M. R., and Johnson, J. A. (2010). Astrogliosis in amyotrophic lateral sclerosis: role and therapeutic potential of astrocytes. *Neurother. J. Am. Soc. Exp. Neurother.* 7, 471–481. doi: 10.1016/j.nurt.2010.05.012

Verstraete, E., Biessels, G.-J., van Den Heuvel, M. P., Visser, F., Luijten, P. R., and van Den Berg, L. H. (2010). No evidence of microbleeds in ALS patients at 7 Tesla MRI. *Amyotroph. Lateral Scler.* 11, 555–557. doi: 10.3109/17482968.2010.513053

Vorbrodt, A. W., and Dobrogowska, D. H. (2003). Molecular anatomy of intercellular junctions in brain endothelial and epithelial barriers: electron microscopist's view. *Brain Res. Brain Res. Rev.* 42, 221–242. doi: 10.1016/S0165-0173(03)00177-2

Willmore, L. J., and Triggs, W. J. (1984). Effect of phenytoin and corticosteroids on seizures and lipid peroxidation in experimental posttraumatic epilepsy. *J. Neurosurg.* 60, 467–472. doi: 10.3171/jns.1984.60.3.0467

Winkler, E. A., Bell, R. D., and Zlokovic, B. V. (2011). Central nervous system pericytes in health and disease. *Nat. Neurosci.* 14, 1398–1405. doi: 10.1038/nn.2946

Winkler, E. A., Sengillo, J. D., Bell, R. D., Wang, J., and Zlokovic, B. V. (2012). Blood-spinal cord barrier pericyte reductions contribute to increased capillary permeability. *J. Cereb. Blood Flow Metab.* 32, 1841–1852. doi: 10.1038/jcbfm.2012.113

Winkler, E. A., Sengillo, J. D., Sullivan, J. S., Henkel, J. S., Appel, S. H., and Zlokovic, B. V. (2013). Blood-spinal cord barrier breakdown and pericyte reductions in amyotrophic lateral sclerosis. *Acta Neuropathol. (Berl.)* 125, 111–120. doi: 10.1007/s00401-012-1039-8

Xie, Y., Weydt, P., Howland, D. S., Kliot, M., and Möller, T. (2004). Inflammatory mediators and growth factors in the spinal cord of G93A SOD1 rats. *Neuroreport* 15, 2513–2516. doi: 10.1097/00001756-200411150-00016

Zhong, Z., Deane, R., Ali, Z., Parisi, M., Shapovalov, Y., O'Banion, M. K., et al. (2008). ALS-causing SOD1 mutants generate vascular changes prior to motor neuron degeneration. *Nat. Neurosci.* 11, 420–422.doi: 10.1038/nn2073

15

Trophic factors as modulators of motor neuron physiology and survival: implications for ALS therapy

Luis B. Tovar-y-Romo, Uri Nimrod Ramírez-Jarquín, Rafael Lazo-Gómez and Ricardo Tapia*

División de Neurociencias, Instituto de Fisiología Celular, Universidad Nacional Autónoma de México, Mexico City, Mexico

Edited by:
Yosef Yarom, Hebrew University of Jerusalem, Israel

Reviewed by:
Daniel Kaganovich, Hebrew University of Jerusalem, Israel
Ping Liu, University of Connecticut Health Center, USA

Correspondence:
Ricardo Tapia, División de Neurociencias, Instituto de Fisiología Celular, Universidad Nacional Autónoma de México, 04510 Mexico City, Distrito Federal, Mexico
e-mail: rtapia@ifc.unam.mx

Motor neuron physiology and development depend on a continuous and tightly regulated trophic support from a variety of cellular sources. Trophic factors guide the generation and positioning of motor neurons during every stage of the developmental process. As well, they are involved in axon guidance and synapse formation. Even in the adult spinal cord an uninterrupted trophic input is required to maintain neuronal functioning and protection from noxious stimuli. Among the trophic factors that have been demonstrated to participate in motor neuron physiology are vascular endothelial growth factor (VEGF), glial-derived neurotrophic factor (GDNF), ciliary neurotrophic factor (CNTF) and insulin-like growth factor 1 (IGF-1). Upon binding to membrane receptors expressed in motor neurons or neighboring glia, these trophic factors activate intracellular signaling pathways that promote cell survival and have protective action on motor neurons, in both *in vivo* and *in vitro* models of neuronal degeneration. For these reasons these factors have been considered a promising therapeutic method for amyotrophic lateral sclerosis (ALS) and other neurodegenerative diseases, although their efficacy in human clinical trials have not yet shown the expected protection. In this minireview we summarize experimental data on the role of these trophic factors in motor neuron function and survival, as well as their mechanisms of action. We also briefly discuss the potential therapeutic use of the trophic factors and why these therapies may have not been yet successful in the clinical use.

Keywords: amyotrophic lateral sclerosis, spinal cord neurodegeneration, motor neurons, neurotrophic factors, VEGF

INTRODUCTION

Neuronal development and survival depend on a balanced and tightly regulated support from trophic factors. Such factors are capable of regulating several important physiological processes, such as neuronal differentiation, maintenance of synapses, neuronal survival through the inhibition of apoptosis, neurogenesis and axonal outgrowth (Korsching, 1993; Boonman and Isacson, 1999; Hou et al., 2008). In addition, they provide an environmental niche suitable for neuronal survival (Mudò et al., 2009). Trophic support is essential for neurons in the spinal cord and is conferred from many different cellular sources including astrocytes, microglia, neurons and endothelial cells (Ikeda et al., 2001; Béchade et al., 2002; Dugas et al., 2008; Su et al., 2009; Hawryluk et al., 2012). Therefore, trophic support is considered a promising therapeutic strategy for neurodegenerative diseases (Kotzbauer and Holtzman, 2006), and it plays an important role in cellular therapy aimed at the reinnervation of lost neuromuscular synapses (Casella et al., 2010).

Amyotrophic lateral sclerosis (ALS) is caused by the selective and progressive loss of spinal, bulbar and cortical motor neurons that lead to irreversible paralysis, speech, swallowing and respiratory malfunctions and eventually death of the affected individuals in a rapid disease course. ALS is mostly sporadic with 90% of the cases occurring without a family history of the disease. However, in the recent years it has become evident that many sporadic cases carry alterations in proteins that have been found mutated in familial cases that might, at least, increase the probability for developing ALS (Deng et al., 2010). Many of these mutations involve alterations in the TAR DNA-binding protein 43 (TDP43) and Fused in sarcoma (FUS) genes that bind RNA molecules (Gordon, 2013; Sreedharan and Brown, 2013), whereas most familial cases with a dominant autosomal inheritance pattern are caused by mutations in superoxide dismutase 1 (SOD1; Rosen et al., 1993). Transgenic mice expressing a mutant form of the human SOD1 are the most widely used model for *in vivo* studies of ALS (Gurney et al., 1994). Trophic factors have been thought as therapeutic targets for ALS, aiming at restoring lost neuromuscular synapses and rescuing motor neurons from toxicity.

There is a series of well characterized trophic factors for the CNS, such as brain-derived neurotrophic factor (BDNF), insulin-like growth factor 1 (IGF-1), ciliary neurotrophic factor (CNTF), glial-derived neurotrophic factor (GDNF), nerve growth factor (NGF), growth hormone and vascular endothelial growth factor (VEGF). Many of these have been tested for neuroprotective potential in different experimental models of ALS. In fact, viral vectors encoding growth factors are among the most effective ways to delay the progression of degenerative processes and prolong survival in ALS mice (Wang et al.,

2002; Kaspar et al., 2003; Azzouz et al., 2004; Dodge et al., 2008).

TROPHIC FACTORS DURING MOTOR NEURON DEVELOPMENT

Motor neuron development is differentially affected by specific trophic factor shortage, and loss of particular trophic signaling alters the development of different subpopulations of motor neurons in heterogeneous ways. The absence of GDNF alters the location of developing motor neurons that innervate the limbs in the spinal cord (Haase et al., 2002; Kramer et al., 2006) and selectively affects the innervation of intrafusal muscle spindles (Gould et al., 2008). Interestingly, the overexpression of this factor in muscle during development causes a hyperinnervation of neuromuscular junctions (Nguyen et al., 1998). In contrast, BDNF may not be as important for motor neurons, because although the lack of this trophic factor severely affects the normal development of sensory neurons, motor neurons are able to develop without major alterations (Ernfors et al., 1994a; Jones et al., 1994). Furthermore, distinct motor neuron subpopulations show different sensitivities to the lack of neurotrophins. For example, the absence of neurotrophin-3 produces a complete loss of spinal motor neurons while facial motor neurons are spared (Ernfors et al., 1994b; Gould et al., 2008), and the absence of CNTF produces no alterations for motor neuron development at the spinal or cranial levels (DeChiara et al., 1995), although the loss of its receptor CNTFRα generates severe motor neuron deficits and mice lacking this receptor die perinatally (DeChiara et al., 1995). A possible alternate ligand for this receptor is the dimer formed by cardiotrophin-like cytokine/cytokine-like factor 1, whose deletions have been shown to cause a significant reduction in the number of motor neurons (Forger et al., 2003). The absence of other factors such as cardiotrophin-1 has also been reported to produce a significant loss of motor neurons (Oppenheim et al., 2001; Forger et al., 2003), and the loss of IGF-1 causes significant reduction in the number of trigeminal and facial motor neurons (Vicario-Abejón et al., 2004). Finally, while the lack of VEGF is lethal, a deletion of the hypoxia response element in the promoter region of the VEGF gene causes a decrease in the expression of this factor that leads to an adult-onset progressive loss of motor neurons in mice (Oosthuyse et al., 2001). After this fortuitous discovery, it was reported that certain VEGF haploytpes (-2578C/A, -1154G/A and -634G/C) conferred an increased susceptibility to ALS in humans, but later on in a meta-analysis conducted with more than 7000 subjects from at least eight different populations no association between these haplotypes and ALS was found (Lambrechts et al., 2009). Moreover, no mutations in the hypoxia response element of the VEGF promoter (Gros-Louis et al., 2003), or in the VEGF receptor 2 (Brockington et al., 2007) were found in ALS patients.

Neurotrophic factors are not only important during development, but they also regulate motor neuron maintenance and survival even long after neurons have become fully differentiated. As well, they might be able to trigger the activation of endogenous regenerative processes. Aside from the synthesis of trophic factors in the local spinal microenvironment, synaptic targets of motor neurons also play important roles in the trophic feedback. As a matter of fact, this is an essential event for the development of the CNS during which originating neurons receive trophic input from their target tissues that enables them to surpass an endogenous-codified programmed cell death (Oppenheim, 1991). In the case of motor neurons these effects are mostly mediated by skeletal muscle-derived factors (Oppenheim et al., 1988; Grieshammer et al., 1998; Kablar and Rudnicki, 1999).

TROPHIC FACTOR EFFECTS ON MOTOR NEURON SURVIVAL

Among all the trophic factors tested in experimental ALS models, VEGF has been shown to be one of the most potent motor neuron protectors. VEGF remarkably retards the progression of the disease and the loss of motor neurons in familial (Azzouz et al., 2004; Zheng et al., 2004; Storkebaum et al., 2005; Wang et al., 2007), as well as in sporadic (Tovar-Y-Romo et al., 2007; Tovar-Y-Romo and Tapia, 2010, 2012) experimental models of motor neurodegeneration.

Activation of VEGF receptor 2 triggers the phosphorylation of intracellular pathways driven by phosphatidyl-inositol-3-kinase (PI3-K), phospholipase C-γ, and mitogen-activated protein kinase (MEK) that promote the inhibition of pro-apoptotic factors like Bad (Yu et al., 2005) and caspases 9 (Cardone et al., 1998) and 3 (Góra-Kupilas and Joško, 2005; Kilic et al., 2006). The activation of these intracellular signaling pathways has been extensively studied in the CNS (Zachary, 2005). VEGF-dependent activation of PI3-K/Akt is sufficient to prevent motor neuronal death in familial models of ALS *in vitro* (Li et al., 2003; Koh et al., 2005; Tolosa et al., 2008) and in experimental *in vitro* models of excitotoxic neuronal death (Matsuzaki et al., 2001). Furthermore, the activation of PI3-K/Akt is required for motor neuron survival and axonal regeneration after spinal cord injury (Namikawa et al., 2000). We have demonstrated that the signaling mediated by PI3-K is critically involved in the protective effect of VEGF against AMPA-induced excitotoxic spinal neurodegeneration *in vivo* (Tovar-Y-Romo and Tapia, 2010).

VEGF also mediates neuroprotection through the inhibition of stress activated protein kinases like p38 mitogen-activated protein kinase. Increased levels of phosphorylated p38 have been found in motor neurons and glia in the familial mouse model of ALS (Tortarolo et al., 2003; Holasek et al., 2005; Veglianese et al., 2006; Dewil et al., 2007), even at the pre-symptomatic stage (Tortarolo et al., 2003), and p38 is also an important factor in a cell death pathway specific for motor neurons (Raoul et al., 2006). Interestingly, the inhibition of p38 prevents motor neuron death in an *in vitro* familial model of ALS (Dewil et al., 2007), and we and others have proven that VEGF can suppress p38 activation in both familial (Tolosa et al., 2009) and excitotoxic (Tovar-Y-Romo and Tapia, 2010) models of spinal cord neurodegeneration.

An increased expression of the VEGF-inducing factor Hypoxia induced factor 1 (HIF-1α) in the spinal cord may occur due to relative hypoxic conditions that exist in the spinal microenvironment, although motor neurons seem to be unable to fully respond to increased downstream effectors such as VEGF (Sato et al., 2012). One possible explanation for this and for the decrease of VEGF levels found in human patients (Devos et al., 2004) might be that inducing factors such as HIF-1α are prevented from translocating to the nucleus even though their concentrations are increased in the cytoplasm (Nagara et al., 2013). This failure to mount the complete response of VEGF synthesis during hypoxia is not cell type specific and it has been demonstrated to occur in monocytes from ALS patients (Moreau et al., 2011).

In contrast to the good protection potential of VEGF, other factors like BDNF failed to protect in different experimental paradigms. BDNF is synthesized by activated microglia in the first stages of the disease when the glial response mainly exerts anti-inflammatory and protective effects, but its production is lost when microglia turns toxic at later stages (Liao et al., 2012). In addition, BDNF does not protect motor neurons from excitotoxicity in experimental models *in vitro* (Fryer et al., 2000) and *in vivo* (Tovar-Y-Romo and Tapia, 2012). This could be possibly due to the sequestration of the ligand by a truncated isoform of the high affinity receptor that is known to be expressed in motor neurons, because removing this truncated receptor significantly delays the disease onset in the mouse familial model (Yanpallewar et al., 2012). In spite of this, BDNF may be a risk factor for neurons by increasing their sensitivity to excitotoxicity (Fryer et al., 2000), or through the activation of NADPH oxidase (Kim et al., 2002), an enzyme involved in motor neuron pathology by damaging the survival pathways activated by trophic factors (Wu et al., 2006). Other growth factors have also been shown to be beneficial although to a lesser extent.

The expression of GDNF by astrocytes is up-regulated after spinal cord ischemia and this might be a mechanism of protection for motor neurons against excitotoxic death (Tokumine et al., 2003). GDNF exerts its neuroprotective effects preferentially on neuronal somas rather than on nerve endings at the neuromuscular synapse when it is administered directly in the spinal cord (Suzuki et al., 2007). Conversely, when it is administered directly in the muscle, GDNF preserves the muscle-nerve synapse and promotes motor neuron function and survival in a familial model of ALS (Suzuki et al., 2008), implying that the protective effects exerted by GDNF are rather limited by the proximity to the trophic source. Nonetheless, GDNF can be retrogradely transported along motor neuronal axons (Leitner et al., 1999), which allows the opportunity to explore a delivery route that will impact both somas and nerve endings. Interestingly, human ALS patients show an up-regulation of GDNF in muscle (Grundström et al., 1999), and the overexpression of GDNF in muscle but not in astrocytes extends lifespan in ALS mice (Mohajeri et al., 1999). Combined growth factor therapy might be an alternative that is worth exploring, as suggested by a recent report in the rat transgenic ALS model showing that VEGF and GDNF administered through an implant of human mesenchymal stem cells exert a synergistic protection in preserving nerve muscular synapses (Krakora et al., 2013).

In the case of CNTF, although the blockade of its expression has been reported to result in the loss of motor neurons and the development of motor symptoms (Masu et al., 1993), these effects are relatively mild when compared to those induced by the loss of other factors like VEGF. Interestingly, ALS patients have a selective decrease of CNTF expression in the CNS regions affected by the disease (Anand et al., 1995). Conversely, serum levels of CNTF are generally elevated in ALS patients, especially among those with the lumbar-onset form of the disease (Laaksovirta et al., 2008).

TROPHIC FACTORS AS THERAPY FOR AMYOTROPHIC LATERAL SCLEROSIS (ALS)

Clinical trials administering trophic factors to ALS patients have not been successful yet. Subcutaneous injections of CNTF, which was effective in the mutant mice models of motor neuron disease *pmn/pmn* (Sendtner et al., 1992) and wobbler (Mitsumoto et al., 1994), did not affect the progression of disease in humans, but caused minor adverse side effects (ALS CNTF Treatment Study Group, 1996). Similarly, disease progression was not modified in ALS patients treated with subcutaneous administration of BDNF (The BDNF Study Group, 1999). Two randomized double-blind placebo-controlled clinical trials administering recombinant human IGF showed little (Lai et al., 1997) or no effect (Borasio et al., 1998) on disease progression, even when IGF-1 was found to be protective in the transgenic rodent model of ALS (Kaspar et al., 2003; Dodge et al., 2008). A combined meta-analysis of both trials showed slight retardation in the disease progression in the group treated with IGF-1, although the results are not conclusive (Beauverd et al., 2012). Interestingly, it has been recently reported that skeletal muscle fiber production of IGF-1 is impaired in ALS patients (Lunetta et al., 2012), so that the modest effects found in some of the patients enrolled in the clinical trials might have been due to a compensation of impaired IGF-1 production by the exogenous administration of the factor. Finally, even when according to one report (Morselli et al., 2006) the majority of ALS patients showed deficiencies in growth hormone secretion, in a recent clinical trial the administration of this hormone to ALS patients did not produce any benefit as compared to patients that received placebo (Saccà et al., 2012).

The time of administration after symptom onset in a trophic factor-based therapy is critical. Trophic factors have a short time frame for protection of motor neurons once the noxious process is triggered and this is probably due to the rate at which motor neurons die during the time course of the disease. Histological studies of human spinal cord showed a large variability between the degree of motor neuron loss and muscle weakness (Stephens et al., 2006), and transgenic familial amyotrophic lateral sclerosis (FALS) mice bearing human (Dal Canto and Gurney, 1995; Bruijn et al., 1997) or murine (Morrison et al., 1998) mutant SOD1 do not present a significant loss of motor neurons prior to the onset of symptoms, and the neuronal loss occurs at a very fast rate over a period of 10 days. In our model of chronic spinal cord excitotoxicity we found that the onset of motor deficits, characterized by limping of the rear limbs, occurs before the loss of motor neurons, suggesting that the time at which the cellular death process starts but prior to clear neuronal degeneration constitutes a therapeutic frame within which growth factor administration could result effective (Tovar-Y-Romo et al., 2007; Tovar-Y-Romo and Tapia, 2012). In fact, in the FALS murine models the administration of VEGF (Azzouz et al., 2004; Storkebaum et al., 2005) or IGF-1 (Kaspar et al., 2003; Dodge et al., 2008) well before the beginning of symptoms confers a significantly better protection, observed by a delay in the progression of symptoms and increased lifespan, as compared to that produced when administered at the symptoms onset. A similar result was obtained in rats subjected to spinal AMPA-induced excitotoxicity, in which a delayed administration of VEGF clearly protected but only when administered before the beginning of motor deficit symptoms (Tovar-Y-Romo and Tapia, 2012). This difference possibly means that growth factors are helpful at preventing the accumulating toxicity that arises from neurodegenerative processes that begin before motor neuron death or symptoms onset (Dal Canto and Gurney, 1995; Bendotti et al., 2001). Unfortunately, obtaining a correct diagnosis of ALS is a complicated and slow process due to the many parameters needed to meet diagnosis criteria (Shook and Pioro, 2009; Bedlack, 2010), so that the earliest intervention with trophic factors once a patient is diagnosed may be already too late.

Administration routes for trophic factor therapy are also important. This is of special interest when considering that in the actual human disease cellular alterations take place along the entire spinal cord, which might be a target particularly difficult to reach. Therefore, assessing different ways to deliver trophic factors is worth trying. Intracerebroventricular (ICV) administration of VEGF has been proven efficient in the rat transgenic model of FALS (Storkebaum et al., 2005) and in our acute model of spinal cord excitotoxicity (Tovar-Y-Romo and Tapia, 2012). ICV administration has the capability to cover the entire spinal cord although it most probably creates a concentration gradient (Storkebaum et al., 2005). The continuous perfusion of trophic factors in the spinal cord by intrathecal infusions or into the brain by ICV injections overcome the blockade that the blood brain barrier represents for the delivery of these molecules. In fact, intrathecal injections have been tried in ALS patients for the delivery of IGF-1, with modest results (Nagano et al., 2005). Clinical trials for VEGF are now underway to assess the safety and tolerability of VEGF (Siciliano et al., 2010).

Other important aspects to consider in growth factor therapies are the stability of the molecule, the half-life of the proteins, the need for sustained delivery and exposure, the dose, their ability to cross the blood brain barrier, and the unwanted side effects on non-targeted cells (Suzuki and Svendsen, 2008). Nonetheless, the neuroprotective potential that growth factor represent overweighs the obstacles that need to be overcome in order to achieve a successful therapy.

CONCLUSIONS

Because trophic support is an essential component for neuronal maintenance and survival, supplying motor neurons subjected to stressful or noxious stimuli with molecular factors that help them counteract cellular death processes, growth factors represent a therapeutic tool that is undoubtedly worth exploring for ALS. However, we still need to understand a great deal of the molecular pathways that cause growth factor shortage during the course of disease and the cellular and molecular mechanisms that limit the responses elicited by these factors when they are supplied exogenously. As well, we still need to identify proper therapeutic regimens and treatment approaches to be able to translate the findings we have made in experimental models into useful therapeutic procedures.

ACKNOWLEDGMENTS

This work was supported by Dirección General de Asuntos del Personal Académico, UNAM (Project IN201013) and Consejo Nacional de Ciencia y Tecnología (CONACYT), México (Project 128229). Uri Nimrod Ramírez-Jarquín and Rafael Lazo-Gómez are recipients of a CONACyT scholarship.

REFERENCES

ALS CNTF Treatment Study Group. (1996). A double-blind placebo-controlled clinical trial of subcutaneous recombinant human ciliary neurotrophic factor (rHCNTF) in amyotrophic lateral sclerosis. ALS CNTF Treatment Study Group. *Neurology* 46, 1244–1249. doi: 10.1212/wnl.46.5.1244

Anand, P., Parrett, A., Martin, J., Zeman, S., Foley, P., Swash, M., et al. (1995). Regional changes of ciliary neurotrophic factor and nerve growth factor levels in post mortem spinal cord and cerebral cortex from patients with motor disease. *Nat. Med.* 1, 168–172. doi: 10.1038/nm0295-168

Azzouz, M., Ralph, G. S., Storkebaum, E., Walmsley, L. E., Mitrophanous, K. A., Kingsman, S. M., et al. (2004). VEGF delivery with retrogradely transported lentivector prolongs survival in a mouse ALS model. *Nature* 429, 413–417. doi: 10.1038/nature02544

Béchade, C., Mallecourt, C., Sedel, F., Vyas, S., and Triller, A. (2002). Motoneuron-derived neurotrophin-3 is a survival factor for PAX2-expressing spinal interneurons. *J. Neurosci.* 22, 8779–8784.

Bedlack, R. S. (2010). Amyotrophic lateral sclerosis: current practice and future treatments. *Curr. Opin. Neurol.* 23, 524–529. doi: 10.1097/wco.0b013e32833c7ac2

Beauverd, M., Mitchell, J. D., Wokke, J. H., and Borasio, G. D. (2012). Recombinant human insulin-like growth factor I (rhIGF-I) for the treatment of amyotrophic lateral sclerosis/motor neuron disease. *Cochrane Database Syst. Rev.* 11:CD002064. doi: 10.1002/14651858.CD002064.pub3

Bendotti, C., Calvaresi, N., Chiveri, L., Prelle, A., Moggio, M., Braga, M., et al. (2001). Early vacuolization and mitochondrial damage in motor neurons of FALS mice are not associated with apoptosis or with changes in cytochrome oxidase histochemical reactivity. *J. Neurol. Sci.* 191, 25–33. doi: 10.1016/s0022-510x(01)00627-x

Boonman, Z., and Isacson, O. (1999). Apoptosis in neuronal development and transplantation: role of caspases and trophic factors. *Exp. Neurol.* 156, 1–15. doi: 10.1006/exnr.1999.7056

Borasio, G. D., Robberecht, W., Leigh, P. N., Emile, J., Guiloff, R. J., Jerusalem, F., et al. (1998). A placebo-controlled trial of insulin-like growth factor-I in amyotrophic lateral sclerosis. European ALS/IGF-I Study Group. *Neurology* 51, 583–586. doi: 10.1212/wnl.51.2.583

Brockington, A., Wokke, B., Nixon, H., Hartley, J., and Shaw, P. J. (2007). Screening of the transcriptional regulatory regions of vascular endothelial growth factor receptor 2 (VEGFR2) in amyotrophic lateral sclerosis. *BMC Med. Genet.* 8:23. doi: 10.1186/1471-2350-8-23

Bruijn, L. I., Becher, M. W., Lee, M. K., Anderson, K. L., Jenkins, N. A., Copeland, N. G., et al. (1997). ALS-linked SOD1 mutant G85R mediates damage to astrocytes and promotes rapidly progressive disease with SOD1-containing inclusions. *Neuron* 18, 327–338. doi: 10.1016/s0896-6273(00)80272-x

Cardone, M. H., Roy, N., Stennicke, H. R., Salvesen, G. S., Franke, T. F., Stanbridge, E., et al. (1998). Regulation of cell death protease caspase-9 by phosphorylation. *Science* 282, 1318–1321. doi: 10.1126/science.282.5392.1318

Casella, G. T., Almeida, V. W., Grumbles, R. M., Liu, Y., and Thomas, C. K. (2010). Neurotrophic factors improve muscle reinnervation from embryonic neurons. *Muscle Nerve* 42, 788–797. doi: 10.1002/mus.21757

Dal Canto, M. C., and Gurney, M. E. (1995). Neuropathological changes in two lines of mice carrying a transgene for mutant human Cu,Zn SOD and in mice overexpressing wild type human SOD: a model of familial amyotrophic lateral sclerosis (FALS). *Brain Res.* 676, 25–40. doi: 10.1016/0006-8993(95)00063-V

DeChiara, T. M., Vejsada, R., Poueymirou, W. T., Acheson, A., Suri, C., Conover, J. C., et al. (1995). Mice lacking the CNTF receptor, unlike mice lacking CNTF, exhibit profound motor neuron deficits at birth. *Cell* 83, 313–322. doi: 10.1016/0092-8674(95)90172-8

Deng, H. X., Zhai, H., Bigio, E. H., Yan, J., Fecto, F., Ajroud, K., et al. (2010). FUS-immunoreactive inclusions are a common feature in sporadic and non-SOD1 familial amyotrophic lateral sclerosis. *Ann. Neurol.* 67, 739–748. doi: 10.1002/ana.22051

Devos, D., Moreau, C., Lassalle, P., Perez, T., De Seze, J., Brunaud-Danel, V., et al. (2004). Low levels of the vascular endothelial growth factor in CSF from early ALS patients. *Neurology* 62, 2127–2129. doi: 10.1212/01.wnl.0000129913.44351.a3

Dewil, M., Dela Cruz, V. F., Van Den Bosch, L., and Robberecht, W. (2007). Inhibition of p38 mitogen activated protein kinase activation and mutant SOD1(G93A)-induced motor neuron death. *Neurobiol. Dis.* 26, 332–341. doi: 10.1016/j.nbd.2006.12.023

Dodge, J. C., Haidet, A. M., Yang, W., Passini, M. A., Hester, M., Clarke, J., et al. (2008). Delivery of AAV-IGF-1 to the CNS extends survival in ALS mice through modification of aberrant glial cell activity. *Mol. Ther.* 16, 1056–1064. doi: 10.1038/mt.2008.60

Dugas, J. C., Mandemakers, W., Rogers, M., Ibrahim, A., Daneman, R., and Barres, B. A. (2008). A novel purification method for CNS projection neurons leads to the identification of brain vascular cells as a source of trophic support for corticospinal motor neurons. *J. Neurosci.* 28, 8294–8305. doi: 10.1523/jneurosci.2010-08.2008

Ernfors, P., Lee, K. F., and Jaenisch, R. (1994a). Mice lacking brain-derived neurotrophic factor develop with sensory deficits. *Nature* 368, 147–150. doi: 10.1038/368147a0

Ernfors, P., Lee, K. F., Kucera, J., and Jaenisch, R. (1994b). Lack of neurotrophin-3 leads to deficiencies in the peripheral nervous system and loss of limb proprioceptive afferents. *Cell* 77, 503–512. doi: 10.1016/0092-8674(94)90213-5

Forger, N. G., Prevette, D., Delapeyriere, O., De Bovis, B., Wang, S., Bartlett, P., et al. (2003). Cardiotrophin-like cytokine/cytokine-like factor 1 is an essential trophic factor for lumbar and facial motoneurons in vivo. *J. Neurosci.* 23, 8854–8858.

Fryer, H. J., Wolf, D. H., Knox, R. J., Strittmatter, S. M., Pennica, D., O'leary, R. M., et al. (2000). Brain-derived neurotrophic factor induces excitotoxic sensitivity in cultured embryonic rat spinal motor neurons through activation of the phosphatidylinositol 3-kinase pathway. *J. Neurochem.* 74, 582–595. doi: 10.1046/j.1471-4159.2000.740582.x

Góra-Kupilas, K., and Joško, J. (2005). The neuroprotective function of vascular endothelial growth factor (VEGF). *Folia Neuropathol.* 43, 31–39.

Gordon, P. H. (2013). Amyotrophic lateral sclerosis: an update for 2013 clinical features, pathophysiology, management and therapeutic trials. *Aging Dis.* 4, 295–310. doi: 10.14336/ad.2013.0400295

Gould, T. W., Yonemura, S., Oppenheim, R. W., Ohmori, S., and Enomoto, H. (2008). The neurotrophic effects of glial cell line-derived neurotrophic factor on spinal motoneurons are restricted to fusimotor subtypes. *J. Neurosci.* 28, 2131–2146. doi: 10.1523/jneurosci.5185-07.2008

Grieshammer, U., Lewandoski, M., Prevette, D., Oppenheim, R. W., and Martin, G. R. (1998). Muscle-specific cell ablation conditional upon Cre-mediated DNA recombination in transgenic mice leads to massive spinal and cranial motoneuron loss. *Dev. Biol.* 197, 234–247. doi: 10.1006/dbio.1997.8859

Gros-Louis, F., Laurent, S., Lopes, A. A., Khoris, J., Meininger, V., Camu, W., et al. (2003). Absence of mutations in the hypoxia response element of VEGF in ALS. *Muscle Nerve* 28, 774–775. doi: 10.1002/mus.10498

Grundström, E., Askmark, H., Lindeberg, J., Nygren, I., Ebendal, T., and Aquilonius, S. M. (1999). Increased expression of glial cell line-derived neurotrophic factor mRNA in muscle biopsies from patients with amyotrophic lateral sclerosis. *J. Neurol. Sci.* 162, 169–173. doi: 10.1016/s0022-510x(98)00333-5

Gurney, M. E., Pu, H., Chiu, A. Y., Dal Canto, M. C., Polchow, C. Y., Alexander, D. D., et al. (1994). Motor neuron degeneration in mice that express a human Cu,Zn superoxide dismutase mutation. *Science* 264, 1772–1775. doi: 10.1126/science.8209258

Haase, G., Dessaud, E., Garces, A., De Bovis, B., Birling, M., Filippi, P., et al. (2002). GDNF acts through PEA3 to regulate cell body positioning and muscle innervation of specific motor neuron pools. *Neuron* 35, 893–905. doi: 10.1016/s0896-6273(02)00864-4

Hawryluk, G. W., Mothe, A., Wang, J., Wang, S., Tator, C., and Fehlings, M. G. (2012). An in vivo characterization of trophic factor production following neural precursor cell or bone marrow stromal cell transplantation for spinal cord injury. *Stem Cells Dev.* 21, 2222–2238. doi: 10.1089/scd.2011.0596

Holasek, S. S., Wengenack, T. M., Kandimalla, K. K., Montano, C., Gregor, D. M., Curran, G. L., et al. (2005). Activation of the stress-activated MAP kinase, p38, but not JNK in cortical motor neurons during early presymptomatic stages of amyotrophic lateral sclerosis in transgenic mice. *Brain Res.* 1045, 185–198. doi: 10.1016/j.brainres.2005.03.037

Hou, S. T., Jiang, S. X., and Smith, R. A. (2008). Permissive and repulsive cues and signalling pathways of axonal outgrowth and regeneration. *Int. Rev. Cell Mol. Biol.* 267, 125–181. doi: 10.1016/s1937-6448(08)00603-5

Ikeda, O., Murakami, M., Ino, H., Yamazaki, M., Nemoto, T., Koda, M., et al. (2001). Acute up-regulation of brain-derived neurotrophic factor expression resulting from experimentally induced injury in the rat spinal cord. *Acta Neuropathol.* 102, 239–245.

Jones, K. R., Farinas, I., Backus, C., and Reichardt, L. F. (1994). Targeted disruption of the BDNF gene perturbs brain and sensory neuron development but not motor neuron development. *Cell* 76, 989–999. doi: 10.1016/0092-8674(94)90377-8

Kablar, B., and Rudnicki, M. A. (1999). Development in the absence of skeletal muscle results in the sequential ablation of motor neurons from the spinal cord to the brain. *Dev. Biol.* 208, 93–109. doi: 10.1006/dbio.1998.9184

Kaspar, B. K., Llado, J., Sherkat, N., Rothstein, J. D., and Gage, F. H. (2003). Retrograde viral delivery of IGF-1 prolongs survival in a mouse ALS model. *Science* 301, 839–842. doi: 10.1126/science.1086137

Kilic, U., Kilic, E., Jarve, A., Guo, Z., Spudich, A., Bieber, K., et al. (2006). Human vascular endothelial growth factor protects axotomized retinal ganglion cells in vivo by activating ERK-1/2 and Akt pathways. *J. Neurosci.* 26, 12439–12446. doi: 10.1523/jneurosci.0434-06.2006

Kim, S. H., Won, S. J., Sohn, S., Kwon, H. J., Lee, J. Y., Park, J. H., et al. (2002). Brain-derived neurotrophic factor can act as a pronecrotic factor through transcriptional and translational activation of NADPH oxidase. *J. Cell Biol.* 159, 821–831. doi: 10.1083/jcb.200112131

Koh, S. H., Roh, H., Lee, S. M., Kim, H. J., Kim, M., Lee, K. W., et al. (2005). Phosphatidylinositol 3-kinase activator reduces motor neuronal cell death induced by G93A or A4V mutant SOD1 gene. *Toxicology* 213, 45–55. doi: 10.1016/j.tox.2005.05.009

Korsching, S. (1993). The neurotrophic factor concept: a reexamination. *J. Neurosci.* 13, 2739–2748.

Kotzbauer, P. T., and Holtzman, D. M. (2006). Expectations and challenges in the therapeutic use of neurotrophic factors. *Ann. Neurol.* 59, 444–447. doi: 10.1002/ana.20794

Krakora, D., Mulcrone, P., Meyer, M., Lewis, C., Bernau, K., Gowing, G., et al. (2013). Synergistic effects of GDNF and VEGF on lifespan and disease progression in a familial als rat model. *Mol. Ther.* 21, 1602–1610. doi: 10.1038/mt.2013.108

Kramer, E. R., Knott, L., Su, F., Dessaud, E., Krull, C. E., Helmbacher, F., et al. (2006). Cooperation between GDNF/Ret and ephrinA/EphA4 signals for motor-axon pathway selection in the limb. *Neuron* 50, 35–47. doi: 10.1016/j.neuron.2006.02.020

Laaksovirta, H., Soinila, S., Hukkanen, V., Roytta, M., and Soilu-Hanninen, M. (2008). Serum level of CNTF is elevated in patients with amyotrophic lateral sclerosis and correlates with site of disease onset. *Eur. J. Neurol.* 15, 355–359. doi: 10.1111/j.1468-1331.2008.02080.x

Lai, E. C., Felice, K. J., Festoff, B. W., Gawel, M. J., Gelinas, D. F., Kratz, R., et al. (1997). Effect of recombinant human insulin-like growth factor-I on progression of ALS. A placebo-controlled study. The North America ALS/IGF-I Study Group. *Neurology* 49, 1621–1630. doi: 10.1212/wnl.49.6.1621

Lambrechts, D., Poesen, K., Fernandez-Santiago, R., Al-Chalabi, A., Del Bo, R., Van Vught, P. W., et al. (2009). Meta-analysis of vascular endothelial growth factor variations in amyotrophic lateral sclerosis: increased susceptibility in male carriers of the -2578AA genotype. *J. Med. Genet.* 46, 840–846. doi: 10.1136/jmg.2008.058222

Leitner, M. L., Molliver, D. C., Osborne, P. A., Vejsada, R., Golden, J. P., Lampe, P. A., et al. (1999). Analysis of the retrograde transport of glial cell line-derived neurotrophic factor (GDNF), neurturin, and persephin suggests that in vivo signaling for the GDNF family is GFRalpha coreceptor-specific. *J. Neurosci.* 19, 9322–9331.

Li, B., Xu, W., Luo, C., Gozal, D., and Liu, R. (2003). VEGF-induced activation of the PI3-K/Akt pathway reduces mutant SOD1-mediated motor neuron cell death. *Brain Res. Mol. Brain Res.* 111, 155–164. doi: 10.1016/s0169-328x(03)00025-1

Liao, B., Zhao, W., Beers, D. R., Henkel, J. S., and Appel, S. H. (2012). Transformation from a neuroprotective to a neurotoxic microglial phenotype in a mouse model of ALS. *Exp. Neurol.* 237, 147–152. doi: 10.1016/j.expneurol.2012.06.011

Lunetta, C., Serafini, M., Prelle, A., Magni, P., Dozio, E., Ruscica, M., et al. (2012). Impaired expression of insulin-like growth factor-1 system in skeletal muscle of amyotrophic lateral sclerosis patients. *Muscle Nerve* 45, 200–208. doi: 10.1002/mus.22288

Masu, Y., Wolf, E., Holtmann, B., Sendtner, M., Brem, G., and Thoenen, H. (1993). Disruption of the CNTF gene results in motor neuron degeneration. *Nature* 365, 27–32. doi: 10.1038/365027a0

Matsuzaki, H., Tamatani, M., Yamaguchi, A., Namikawa, K., Kiyama, H., Vitek, M. P., et al. (2001). Vascular endothelial growth factor rescues hippocampal neurons from glutamate-induced toxicity: signal transduction cascades. *FASEB J.* 15, 1218–1220. doi: 10.1096/fj.00-0495fje

Mitsumoto, H., Ikeda, K., Holmlund, T., Greene, T., Cedarbaum, J. M., Wong, V., et al. (1994). The effects of ciliary neurotrophic factor on motor dysfunction in wobbler mouse motor neuron disease. *Ann. Neurol.* 36, 142–148. doi: 10.1002/ana.410360205

Mohajeri, M. H., Figlewicz, D. A., and Bohn, M. C. (1999). Intramuscular grafts of myoblasts genetically modified to secrete glial cell line-derived neurotrophic factor prevent motoneuron loss and disease progression in a mouse model of familial amyotrophic lateral sclerosis. *Hum. Gene Ther.* 10, 1853–1866. doi: 10.1089/10430349950017536

Moreau, C., Gosset, P., Kluza, J., Brunaud-Danel, V., Lassalle, P., Marchetti, P., et al. (2011). Deregulation of the hypoxia inducible factor-1alpha pathway in monocytes from sporadic amyotrophic lateral sclerosis patients. *Neuroscience* 172, 110–117. doi: 10.1016/j.neuroscience.2010.10.040

Morrison, B. M., Janssen, W. G., Gordon, J. W., and Morrison, J. H. (1998). Time course of neuropathology in the spinal cord of G86R superoxide dismutase transgenic mice. *J. Comp. Neurol.* 391, 64–77. doi: 10.1002/(sici)1096-9861(19980202)391:1<64::aid-cne6>3.0.co;2-p

Morselli, L. L., Bongioanni, P., Genovesi, M., Licitra, R., Rossi, B., Murri, L., et al. (2006). Growth hormone secretion is impaired in amyotrophic lateral sclerosis. *Clin. Endocrinol. (Oxf)* 65, 385–388. doi: 10.1111/j.1365-2265.2006.02609.x

Mudò, G., Bonomo, A., Di Liberto, V., Frinchi, M., Fuxe, K., and Belluardo, N. (2009). The FGF-2/FGFRs neurotrophic system promotes neurogenesis in the adult brain. *J. Neural Transm.* 116, 995–1005. doi: 10.1007/s00702-009-0207-z

Nagano, I., Shiote, M., Murakami, T., Kamada, H., Hamakawa, Y., Matsubara, E., et al. (2005). Beneficial effects of intrathecal IGF-1 administration in patients with amyotrophic lateral sclerosis. *Neurol. Res.* 27, 768–772. doi: 10.1179/016164105x39860

Nagara, Y., Tateishi, T., Yamasaki, R., Hayashi, S., Kawamura, M., Kikuchi, H., et al. (2013). Impaired cytoplasmic-nuclear transport of hypoxia-inducible factor-1alpha in amyotrophic lateral sclerosis. *Brain Pathol.* 23, 534–546. doi: 10.1111/bpa.12040

Namikawa, K., Honma, M., Abe, K., Takeda, M., Mansur, K., Obata, T., et al. (2000). Akt/protein kinase B prevents injury-induced motoneuron death and accelerates axonal regeneration. *J. Neurosci.* 20, 2875–2886.

Nguyen, Q. T., Parsadanian, A. S., Snider, W. D., and Lichtman, J. W. (1998). Hyperinnervation of neuromuscular junctions caused by GDNF overexpression in muscle. *Science* 279, 1725–1729. doi: 10.1126/science.279.5357.1725

Oosthuyse, B., Moons, L., Storkebaum, E., Beck, H., Nuyens, D., Brusselmans, K., et al. (2001). Deletion of the hypoxia-response element in the vascular endothelial growth factor promoter causes motor neuron degeneration. *Nat. Genet.* 28, 131–138. doi: 10.1038/88842

Oppenheim, R. W. (1991). Cell death during development of the nervous system. *Annu. Rev. Neurosci.* 14, 453–501. doi: 10.1146/annurev.neuro.14.1.453

Oppenheim, R. W., Haverkamp, L. J., Prevette, D., Mcmanaman, J. L., and Appel, S. H. (1988). Reduction of naturally occurring motoneuron death in vivo by a target-derived neurotrophic factor. *Science* 240, 919–922. doi: 10.1126/science.3363373

Oppenheim, R. W., Wiese, S., Prevette, D., Armanini, M., Wang, S., Houenou, L. J., et al. (2001). Cardiotrophin-1, a muscle-derived cytokine, is required for the survival of subpopulations of developing motoneurons. *J. Neurosci.* 21, 1283–1291.

Raoul, C., Buhler, E., Sadeghi, C., Jacquier, A., Aebischer, P., Pettmann, B., et al. (2006). Chronic activation in presymptomatic amyotrophic lateral sclerosis (ALS) mice of a feedback loop involving Fas, Daxx, and FasL. *Proc. Natl. Acad. Sci. U S A* 103, 6007–6012. doi: 10.1073/pnas.0508774103

Rosen, D. R., Siddique, T., Patterson, D., Figlewicz, D. A., Sapp, P., Hentati, A., et al. (1993). Mutations in Cu/Zn superoxide dismutase gene are associated with familial amyotrophic lateral sclerosis. *Nature* 362, 59–62. doi: 10.1038/362059a0

Saccà, F., Quarantelli, M., Rinaldi, C., Tucci, T., Piro, R., Perrotta, G., et al. (2012). A randomized controlled clinical trial of growth hormone in amyotrophic lateral sclerosis: clinical, neuroimaging, and hormonal results. *J. Neurol.* 259, 132–138. doi: 10.1007/s00415-011-6146-2

Sato, K., Morimoto, N., Kurata, T., Mimoto, T., Miyazaki, K., Ikeda, Y., et al. (2012). Impaired response of hypoxic sensor protein HIF-1alpha and its downstream proteins in the spinal motor neurons of ALS model mice. *Brain Res.* 1473, 55–62. doi: 10.1016/j.brainres.2012.07.040

Sendtner, M., Schmalbruch, H., Stockli, K. A., Carroll, P., Kreutzberg, G. W., and Thoenen, H. (1992). Ciliary neurotrophic factor prevents degeneration of motor neurons in mouse mutant progressive motor neuronopathy. *Nature* 358, 502–504. doi: 10.1038/358502a0

Shook, S. J., and Pioro, E. P. (2009). Racing against the clock: recognizing, differentiating, diagnosing and referring the amyotrophic lateral sclerosis patient. *Ann. Neurol.* 65(Suppl. 1), S10–S16. doi: 10.1002/ana.21545

Siciliano, G., Carlesi, C., Pasquali, L., Piazza, S., Pietracupa, S., Fornai, F., et al. (2010). Clinical trials for neuroprotection in ALS. *CNS Neurol. Disord. Drug Targets* 9, 305–313. doi: 10.2174/187152710791292648

Sreedharan, J., and Brown, R. H. Jr. (2013). Amyotrophic lateral sclerosis: problems and prospects. *Ann. Neurol.* 74, 309–316. doi: 10.1002/ana.24012

Stephens, B., Guiloff, R. J., Navarrete, R., Newman, P., Nikhar, N., and Lewis, P. (2006). Widespread loss of neuronal populations in the spinal ventral horn in sporadic motor neuron disease. A morphometric study. *J. Neurol. Sci.* 244, 41–58. doi: 10.1016/j.jns.2005.12.003

Storkebaum, E., Lambrechts, D., Dewerchin, M., Moreno-Murciano, M. P., Appelmans, S., Oh, H., et al. (2005). Treatment of motoneuron degeneration by intracerebroventricular delivery of VEGF in a rat model of ALS. *Nat. Neurosci.* 8, 85–92. doi: 10.1038/nn1360

Su, H., Zhang, W., Guo, J., Guo, A., Yuan, Q., and Wu, W. (2009). Neural progenitor cells enhance the survival and axonal regeneration of injured motoneurons after transplantation into the avulsed ventral horn of adult rats. *J. Neurotrauma* 26, 67–80. doi: 10.1089/neu.2008.0656

Suzuki, M., and Svendsen, C. N. (2008). Combining growth factor and stem cell therapy for amyotrophic lateral sclerosis. *Trends Neurosci.* 31, 192–198. doi: 10.1016/j.tins.2008.01.006

Suzuki, M., Mchugh, J., Tork, C., Shelley, B., Hayes, A., Bellantuono, I., et al. (2008). Direct muscle delivery of GDNF with human mesenchymal stem cells improves motor neuron survival and function in a rat model of familial ALS. *Mol. Ther.* 16, 2002–2010. doi: 10.1038/mt.2008.197

Suzuki, M., Mchugh, J., Tork, C., Shelley, B., Klein, S. M., Aebischer, P., et al. (2007). GDNF secreting human neural progenitor cells protect dying motor neurons, but not their projection to muscle, in a rat model of familial ALS. *PLoS One* 2:e689. doi: 10.1371/journal.pone.0000689

The BDNF Study Group. (1999). A controlled trial of recombinant methionyl human BDNF in ALS: the BDNF study group (phase III). *Neurology* 52, 1427–1433. doi: 10.1212/WNL.52.7.1427

Tokumine, J., Sugahara, K., Kakinohana, O., and Marsala, M. (2003). The spinal GDNF level is increased after transient spinal cord ischemia in the rat. *Acta Neurochir. Suppl.* 86, 231–234. doi: 10.1007/978-3-7091-0651-8_50

Tolosa, L., Mir, M., Asensio, V. J., Olmos, G., and Llado, J. (2008). Vascular endothelial growth factor protects spinal cord motoneurons against glutamate-induced excitotoxicity via phosphatidylinositol 3-kinase. *J. Neurochem.* 105, 1080–1090. doi: 10.1111/j.1471-4159.2007.05206.x

Tolosa, L., Mir, M., Olmos, G., and Llado, J. (2009). Vascular endothelial growth factor protects motoneurons from serum deprivation-induced cell death through phosphatidylinositol 3-kinase-mediated p38 mitogen-activated protein kinase inhibition. *Neuroscience* 158, 1348–1355. doi: 10.1016/j.neuroscience.2008.10.060

Tortarolo, M., Veglianese, P., Calvaresi, N., Botturi, A., Rossi, C., Giorgini, A., et al. (2003). Persistent activation of p38 mitogen-activated protein kinase in a mouse model of familial amyotrophic lateral sclerosis correlates with disease progression. *Mol. Cell. Neurosci.* 23, 180–192. doi: 10.1016/s1044-7431(03)00022-8

Tovar-Y-Romo, L. B., and Tapia, R. (2010). VEGF protects spinal motor neurons against chronic excitotoxic degeneration in vivo by activation of PI3-K pathway and inhibition of p38MAPK. *J. Neurochem.* 115, 1090–1101. doi: 10.1111/j.1471-4159.2010.06766.x

Tovar-Y-Romo, L. B., and Tapia, R. (2012). Delayed administration of VEGF rescues spinal motor neurons from death with a short effective time frame in excitotoxic experimental models in vivo. *ASN Neuro* 4, 121–129. doi: 10.1042/an20110057

Tovar-Y-Romo, L. B., Zepeda, A., and Tapia, R. (2007). Vascular endothelial growth factor prevents paralysis and motoneuron death in a rat model of excitotoxic spinal cord neurodegeneration. *J. Neuropathol. Exp. Neurol.* 66, 913–922. doi: 10.1097/nen.0b013e3181567c16

Veglianese, P., Lo Coco, D., Bao Cutrona, M., Magnoni, R., Pennacchini, D., Pozzi, B., et al. (2006). Activation of the p38MAPK cascade is associated with upregulation of TNF alpha receptors in the spinal motor neurons of mouse models of familial ALS. *Mol. Cell. Neurosci.* 31, 218–231. doi: 10.1016/j.mcn.2005.09.009

Vicario-Abejón, C., Fernández-Moreno, C., Pichel, J. G., and De Pablo, F. (2004). Mice lacking IGF-I and LIF have motoneuron deficits in brain stem nuclei. *Neuroreport* 15, 2769–2772.

Wang, L. J., Lu, Y. Y., Muramatsu, S., Ikeguchi, K., Fujimoto, K., Okada, T., et al. (2002). Neuroprotective effects of glial cell line-derived neurotrophic factor mediated by an adeno-associated virus vector in a transgenic animal model of amyotrophic lateral sclerosis. *J. Neurosci.* 22, 6920–6928.

Wang, Y., Mao, X. O., Xie, L., Banwait, S., Marti, H. H., Greenberg, D. A., et al. (2007). Vascular endothelial growth factor overexpression delays neurodegeneration and prolongs survival in amyotrophic lateral sclerosis mice. *J. Neurosci.* 27, 304–307. doi: 10.1523/jneurosci.4433-06.2007

Wu, D. C., Re, D. B., Nagai, M., Ischiropoulos, H., and Przedborski, S. (2006). The inflammatory NADPH oxidase enzyme modulates motor neuron degeneration in amyotrophic lateral sclerosis mice. *Proc. Natl. Acad. Sci. U S A* 103, 12132–12137. doi: 10.1073/pnas.0603670103

Yanpallewar, S. U., Barrick, C. A., Buckley, H., Becker, J., and Tessarollo, L. (2012). Deletion of the BDNF truncated receptor TrkB.T1 delays disease onset in a mouse model of amyotrophic lateral sclerosis. *PLoS One* 7:e39946. doi: 10.1371/journal.pone.0039946

Yu, F., Sugawara, T., Maier, C. M., Hsieh, L. B., and Chan, P. H. (2005). Akt/Bad signaling and motor neuron survival after spinal cord injury. *Neurobiol. Dis.* 20, 491–499. doi: 10.1016/j.nbd.2005.04.004

Zachary, I. (2005). Neuroprotective role of vascular endothelial growth factor: signalling mechanisms, biological function and therapeutic potential. *Neurosignals* 14, 207–221. doi: 10.1159/000088637

Zheng, C., Nennesmo, I., Fadeel, B., and Henter, J. I. (2004). Vascular endothelial growth factor prolongs survival in a transgenic mouse model of ALS. *Ann. Neurol.* 56, 564–567. doi: 10.1002/ana.20223

16

Mitochondrial DNMT3A and DNA methylation in skeletal muscle and CNS of transgenic mouse models of ALS

Margaret Wong[1†], Barry Gertz[1,2†], Barry A. Chestnut[1,2] and Lee J. Martin[1,2,3]*

[1] *Department of Pathology, Division of Neuropathology, Johns Hopkins University School of Medicine, Baltimore, MD, USA*
[2] *Department of Pathology, Pathobiology Graduate Program, Johns Hopkins University School of Medicine, Baltimore, MD, USA*
[3] *Department of Neuroscience, Johns Hopkins University School of Medicine, Baltimore, MD, USA*

Edited by:
Ricardo Tapia, Universidad Nacional Autónoma de México, Mexico

Reviewed by:
P. Hemachandra Reddy, Oregen Health and Science University, USA
Alexander K. Murashov, East Carolina University, USA
Shirley M. Taylor, Virginia Commonwealth University, USA

****Correspondence:***
Lee J. Martin, Department of Pathology, Johns Hopkins University School of Medicine, 558 Ross Building, 720 Rutland Avenue, Baltimore, MD 21205-2196, USA
e-mail: martinl@jhmi.edu

† Co-first authors.

Cytosine methylation is an epigenetic modification of DNA catalyzed by DNA methyltransferases. Cytosine methylation of mitochondrial DNA (mtDNA) is believed to have relative underrepresentation; however, possible tissue and cell differences in mtDNA methylation and relationships to neurodegenerative disease have not been examined. We show by immunoblotting that DNA methyltransferase 3A (Dnmt3a) isoform is present in pure mitochondria of adult mouse CNS, skeletal muscle, and testes, and adult human cerebral cortex. Dnmt1 was not detected in adult mouse CNS or skeletal muscle mitochondria but appeared bound to the outer mitochondrial membrane. Immunofluorescence confirmed the mitochondrial localization of Dnmt3a and showed 5-methylcytosine (5mC) immunoreactivity in mitochondria of neurons and skeletal muscle myofibers. DNA pyrosequencing of two loci (D-loop and 16S rRNA gene) and twelve cytosine-phosphate-guanine (CpG) sites in mtDNA directly showed a tissue differential presence of 5mC. Because mitochondria have been implicated in the pathogenesis of amyotrophic lateral sclerosis (ALS), but the disease mechanisms are uncertain, we evaluated mitochondrial Dnmt3a and 5mC levels in human *superoxide dismutase-1* (SOD1) transgenic mouse models of ALS. Mitochondrial Dnmt3a protein levels were reduced significantly in skeletal muscle and spinal cord at presymptomatic or early disease. Immunofluorescence showed that 5mC immunoreactivity was present in mitochondria of neurons and skeletal myofibers, and 5mC immunoreactivity became aggregated in motor neurons of ALS mice. DNA pyrosequencing revealed significant abnormalities in 16S rRNA gene methylation in ALS mice. Immunofluorescence showed that 5mC immunoreactivity can be sequestered into autophagosomes and that mitophagy was increased and mitochondrial content was decreased in skeletal muscle in ALS mice. This study reveals a tissue-preferential mitochondrial localization of Dnmt3a and presence of cytosine methylation in mtDNA of nervous tissue and skeletal muscle and demonstrates that mtDNA methylation patterns and mitochondrial Dnmt3a levels are abnormal in skeletal muscle and spinal cord of presymptomatic ALS mice, and these abnormalities occur in parallel with loss of myofiber mitochondria.

Keywords: ALS, DNA pyrosequencing, Dnmt1, Dnmt3a, mitochondrial DNA, 5-methylcytosine, mitochondria, motor neuron

INTRODUCTION

Methylation of DNA on carbon five of cytosine (5-methylcytosine, 5mC) in cytosine-phosphate-guanine (CpG) dinucleotides is an epigenetic modification of DNA used by cells to regulate nuclear gene expression (Jones and Takai, 2001; Bird, 2002; Brenner and Fuks, 2006). Cytosine methylation signals through 5mC-binding proteins to remodel chromatin and downregulate gene expression. Cytosine methylation is mediated by a family of DNA methyltransferase (Dnmt) enzymes (Cheng, 1995). Dnmt1 is the most abundant isoform in proliferating cells and displays a preference for hemimethylated substrates and is targeted to replication forks, acting to maintain DNA methylation patterns during cell replication (Robertson, 2001), and to DNA repair sites (Mortusewicz et al., 2005). Recently, mutations in the *Dnmt1* gene have been identified as a cause of hereditary sensory and autonomic neuropathy type 1 (Klein et al., 2011) and autosomal dominant cerebellar ataxia, deafness, and narcolepsy (Winkelmann et al., 2012). Dnmt2 (also called tRNA methyltransferase-1) transfers methyl groups to RNA instead of DNA (Schaefer and Lyko, 2010; Motorin and Helm, 2011). DNA methyltransferase 3A (Dnmt3a) and Dnmt3b function as *de novo* methyltransferases because they methylate hemimethylated DNA and also completely unmethylated DNA (Okano et al., 1999; Xie et al., 1999). Dnmt3L functions as an essential regulatory cofactor for Dnmt3a (Jia et al., 2007). Nuclear DNA methylation attracts attention because it has been implicated in normal cell and tissue development and differentiation (Geiman and Muegge, 2010) and in human diseases, including cancer (Calvanese et al.,

2009), Rett syndrome (Amir et al., 1999), and, more recently, neurodegenerative diseases (Chestnut et al., 2011; Klein et al., 2011; Winkelmann et al., 2012; Martin and Wong, 2013).

Studies of mitochondrial DNA (mtDNA) cytosine methylation and the Dnmts that regulate mtDNA methylation are not as common as studies of nuclear DNA methylation; moreover, many mitochondrial-based mechanisms of disease have been implicated in amyotrophic lateral sclerosis (ALS) (Beal, 2005; Martin, 2010, 2012; Reddy and Reddy, 2011; Panov et al., 2012; Santa-Cruz et al., 2012), but mtDNA methylation and mitochondrial Dnmts have not been studied in ALS. Earlier work tends to minimize the occurrence and importance of mtDNA cytosine methylation. Some studies of cultured cells have found mtDNA cytosine methylation in mouse fibroblastoid cells (Pollack et al., 1984) and human fibroblasts (Shmookler Reis and Goldstein, 1983). In the latter study, ~2–5% of CCGG sites were fully methylated. Other studies have found underrepresented or no mtDNA cytosine methylation (Maekawa et al., 2004). However, the earlier studies that failed to observe mtDNA cytosine methylation were done on mitochondria isolated from blood. More recently, it has been reported that Dnmt1 localizes to mitochondria in cultured mouse embryonic fibroblasts and human colon carcinoma cells (Shock et al., 2011) and that Dnmt3a localizes to mouse brain and spinal cord mitochondria (Chestnut et al., 2011). Studies have yet to examine comparatively mtDNA methylation in different adult tissue types *in vivo* to test the hypothesis that there is tissue specificity for mtDNA cytosine methylation. Moreover, the physiological significance and potential pathophysiological relevance of mtDNA methylation in ALS merit exploration in light of findings that Dnmt3 is localized to neuronal mitochondria and appears to be upregulated in human ALS neurons and mouse spinal motor neurons during their degeneration (Chestnut et al., 2011).

In the current study, we demonstrate that Dnmt3a and 5mC are in mitochondria of adult mouse and human tissue types that are mostly excitable tissues (nervous and muscle) and that tissue Dnmt3a levels are reduced and 5mC immunoreactivity accumulates in skeletal muscle myofibers and spinal cord motor neurons in mouse models of ALS. We also show directly by pyrosequencing that mtDNA from these tissues contains 5mC and that the levels of 5mC in the 16S rRNA gene are increased in transgenic mouse models of ALS.

MATERIALS AND METHODS

MICE

Wildtype and human *superoxide dismutase-1* (hSOD1) transgenic (tg) mice were used with approval from the institutional Animal Care and Use Committee. For studies of normal DNMT3a and 5mC localizations and distributions, non-tg adult C57BL/6 and SV129 mice ($n = 20$–25) were used at 2–6 months of age. Several different tg mouse lines were used. One line was hemizygous for a low copy number of hSOD1-G37R mutant allele driven by the endogenous human promoter (line 29) derived from a founder B6.Cg-Tg SOD1-G37R 29Dpr/J (stock # 008229, The Jackson Laboratory, Bar Harbor, MA). Another tg mouse line (hSOD1-wildtype) expressed normal wildtype human *SOD1* gene (B6SJL-TgN[SOD1] 2Gur, stock #002297, The Jackson Laboratory) at high levels (copy number ~25) driven by the endogenous human promoter. These two tg lines thus expressed hSOD1 ubiquitously in many tissues (Gurney et al., 1994; Martin et al., 2007, 2009; Gertz et al., 2012). We also used tg mice with skeletal muscle-restricted expression of hSOD1-G37R, -G93A, and -wildtype variants (designated as hSOD1^{mus}) which have been described previously (Wong and Martin, 2010). All the lines of hSOD1 tg mice were studied at presymptomatic or early to middle stages of disease. Control mice were age-matched, non-tg littermates. Mouse genotypes were identified by PCR. Mitochondrial fractions were prepared from 5–10 mice/genotype.

PREPARATION OF CRUDE MITOCHONDRIAL FRACTIONS FROM SKELETAL MUSCLE AND HEART

Tissue mitochondrial preparations were isolated from fresh tissues with no prior freezing or fixation. For fresh tissue harvesting, mice were deeply anesthetized and decapitated; organs and tissues were immediately removed, weighed, and placed in ice-cold phosphate-buffered saline (PBS). Muscle crude mitochondrial fractions were obtained using a modification (**Figure 1**) of a described method (Bhattacharya et al., 1991). The tissue was finely minced using a razor. The pieces were resuspended in 10 ml/g digestion buffer (100 mM sucrose, 10 mM EDTA, 100 mM Tris-HCl, 46 mM KCl, pH 7.4) with 0.1 mg/ml nagarse (Sigma-Aldrich) and were digested at room temperature for 10–20 min. The digest was placed in an equal volume of homogenization buffer consisting of digestion buffer with 5 mg/ml BSA and complete protease inhibitor (Roche Diagnostics). The tissue pieces were allowed to settle, the buffer was aspirated, and the tissue was resuspended in an equal volume of homogenization buffer. The tissue was homogenized using a PT 3100 Polytron (Kinematica) at 20,000 rpm on ice. The homogenate was centrifuged at 500 g for 10 min and the resulting supernatant was removed to a fresh tube. The supernatant was then centrifuged at 12,000 g for 20 min. The resulting pellet was the crude mitochondrial fraction.

PREPARATION OF CRUDE MITOCHONDRIAL FRACTION FROM TISSUES OTHER THAN STRIATED MUSCLE

Crude mitochondrial fractions of organs were obtained using a described method (Okado-Matsumoto and Fridovich, 2001) with slight modifications (**Figure 1**). Brain, spinal cord, liver, kidney, colon, and spleen were homogenized in nycodenz homogenization buffer (210 mM mannitol, 70 mM sucrose, 10 mM Tris, 1 mM EDTA, and protease inhibitor, pH 7.5) at a 1:5 (w/v) ratio using a PT 3100 Polytron at 20,000 rpm on ice. The homogenate was centrifuged at 1300 g for 10 min and resultant supernatant removed to a fresh tube. The supernatant was then centrifuged at 17,000 g for 10 min. The resulting pellet was the crude mitochondrial fraction.

GENERATION OF PURE MITOCHONDRIAL FRACTION

A highly enriched mitochondrial fraction was obtained by nycodenz (Axis-Shield) discontinuous gradient centrifugation (Okado-Matsumoto and Fridovich, 2001). Gradients were prepared by diluting 50% nycodenz solution (5 mM Tris, 3 mM KCl, 0.3 mM EDTA, 25 g nycodenz, pH 7.5, prepared in 50 ml of

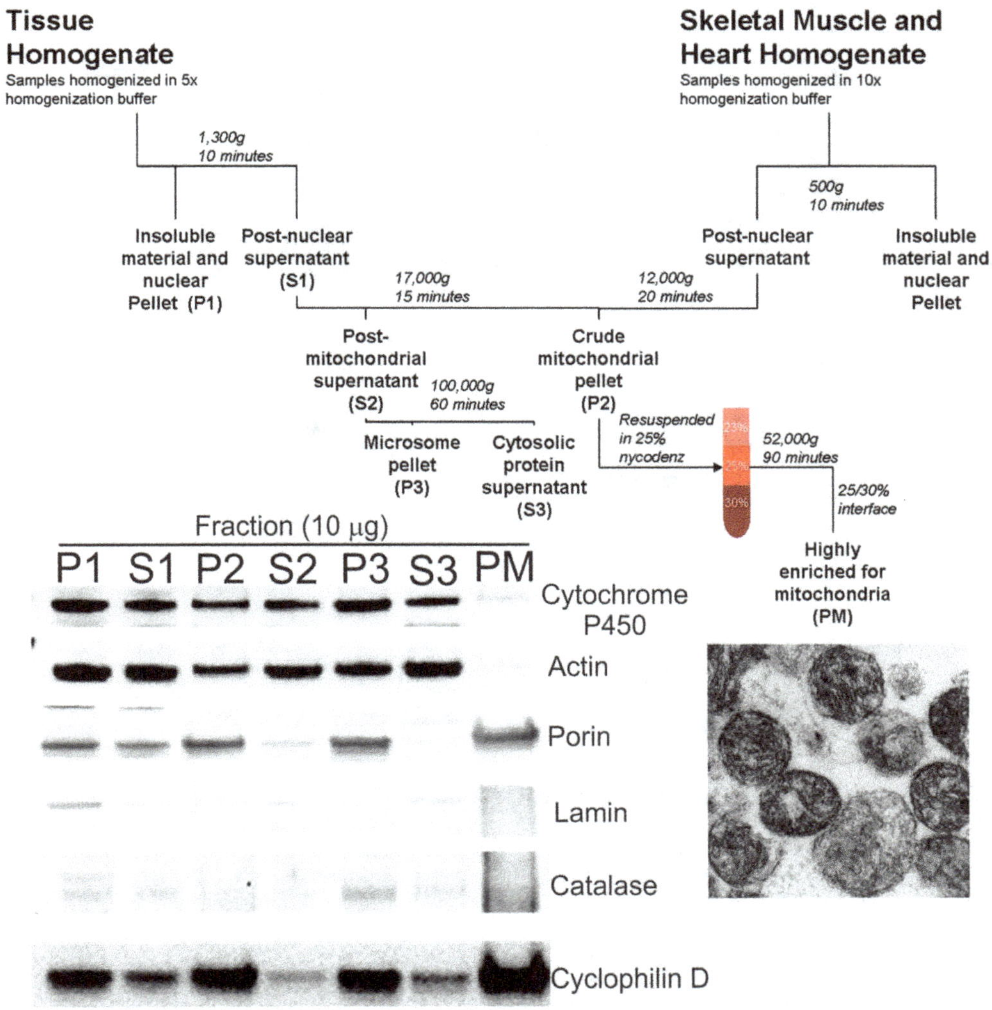

FIGURE 1 | Schematic diagram of tissue fractionation and experimental verification of mitochondrial enrichment and purity. Tissues were homogenized in appropriate buffer using a PT3100 polytron. After centrifugation to remove tissue and cellular debris, a crude mitochondrial pellet was obtained (fraction P2). The pellet was resuspended in 25% nycodenz and a highly pure mitochondrial fraction (fraction PM) was obtained by discontinuous gradient centrifugation. Bottom left panel: Immunoblotting of the various fractions confirms the pure mitochondria (PM) fraction to be highly enriched for mitochondria (porin and CyPD), with very little or no contamination by cytoplasmic (actin), microsomal (cytochrome P450), nuclear (lamin), and peroxisomal/lysosomal (catalase) compartments. Bottom right panel: Electron microscopy on PM fractions confirmed visually the very high enrichment of mitochondria.

double-distilled water) with the appropriate volume of dilution buffer (0.75 g NaCl, 5 mM Tris, 3 mM KCl, 0.3 mM EDTA, pH 7.5, prepared in 100 ml of double-distilled water) to obtain an iso-osmotic solution. The crude mitochondrial fractions were resuspended in 3 ml 25% nycodenz buffer, layered onto 2.5 ml 30% nycodenz buffer, and overlaid with 2.5 ml 23% nycodenz buffer. Samples were centrifuged at 52,000 g for 90 min in a swinging bucket rotor (Sorval TH641). The pure mitochondria (PM) fraction was isolated from the 25%/30% interface. This fraction was highly enriched in mitochondria (**Figure 1**, blot inset) as demonstrated by the absence of markers for nucleus (lamin), endoplasmic reticulum/microsomes (cytochrome P450 reductase), peroxisomes (catalase), and cytosol (actin), and the enrichment in mitochondrial markers, including porin (voltage-dependent anion channel, VDAC), cyclophilin D, and complex V (**Figures 1, 2A–C,G**). Aliquots of freshly prepared PM samples were fixed in 2% glutaraldehyde, embedded in plastic, and thin-sectioned for electron microscopy (EM) to further validate the mitochondrial purification using this approach (**Figure 1**).

To confirm that Dnmt protein was localized within mitochondria rather than being bound to the surface of mitochondria, proteinase K digestion of freshly isolated intact mitochondria was performed. PBS-resuspended mitochondria were incubated in 5 mg/ml agarose-conjugated proteinase K (Sigma) for 30 min at 37°C, and then centrifuged and washed in PBS for several cycles to remove proteinase K.

IMMUNOBLOTTING

Tissue subcellular fractions were separated by SDS-PAGE on 4–12% NuPage gels (Invitrogen) under denaturing and reducing

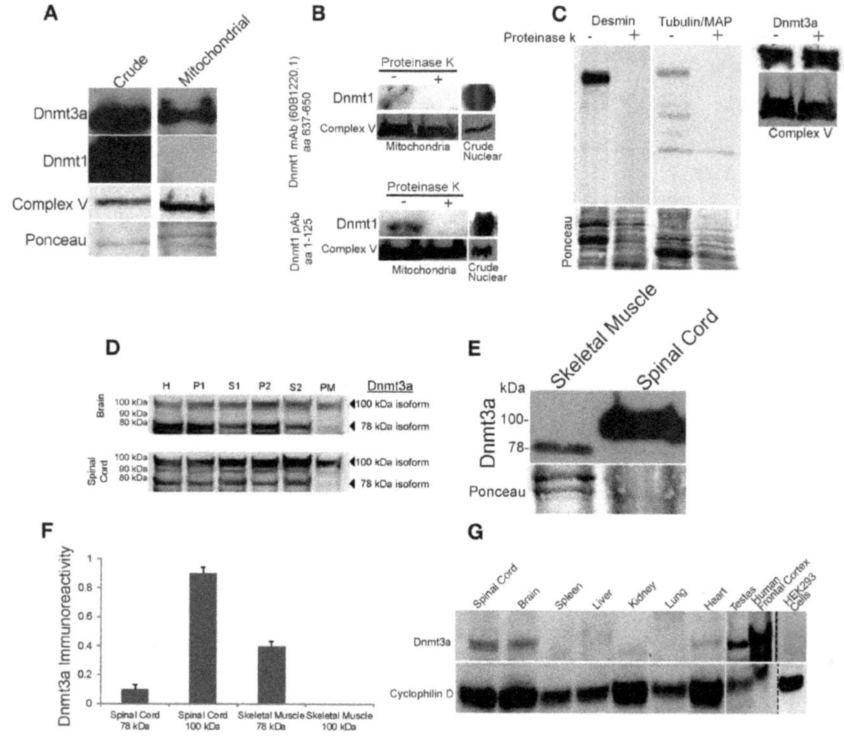

FIGURE 2 | Dnmt3a is present in skeletal muscle and CNS mitochondria of adult mouse and human. (A) Western blots showing that Dnmt3a, but not Dnmt1, is present in adult mouse skeletal muscle mitochondria. Dnmt1 was present in crude tissue fractions but was undetectable in pure mitochondrial fractions even with prolonged overexposures as shown. Western blot for the mitochondrial marker complex V is used to verify mitochondrial enrichment of the fraction. Ponceau S-stained membrane is used to show protein loading. **(B)** Experiments that establish that Dnmt1 is bound to the outer surface of mitochondria. Freshly isolated intact skeletal muscle mitochondria were treated (+) with agarose-conjugated proteinase K to digest surface-bound proteins or were not treated with proteinase K (−). Mitochondria were lysed and proteins were fractionated by SDS-PAGE and western blotted for Dnmt1 using two different antibodies that detect different amino acid (aa) domains of the protein. Protein loading was revealed by reprobing the blots for complex V. Crude nuclear fractions were used as a positive control. **(C)** Experiments that establish that Dnmt3a is within mitochondria and not merely bound to the outer surface of mitochondria. Freshly isolated intact skeletal muscle mitochondria were treated with agarose-conjugated proteinase K to digest surface-bound proteins. The efficacy of digestion is shown by the loss of desmin and tubulin/MAP immunoreactivities in the treated samples, but Dnmt3a immunoreactivity was not attenuated by proteinase K digestion. Protein loading is shown by Ponceau S staining of membranes. Mitochondrial enrichment is shown by complex V immunoreactivity. **(D)** Adult mouse brain and spinal cord were homogenized, fractionated and immunoblotted with antibody to Dnmt3a. Lanes were loaded with equivalent amounts of protein from the crude homogenate (H) and different fractions, including nuclear-enriched and insoluble material (P1), post-nuclear supernatant (S1), crude mitochondria (P2), post-mitochondrial supernatant (S2), and pure mitochondria (PM). See **Figure 1** for the validation of this fractionation method. The 100 kDa form of Dnmt3a was present in all fractions, including the pure mitochondria, while the 78 kDa form was present in all fractions except the mitochondria. **(E)** Western blot comparing the levels of Dnmt3a and isoform specificity in skeletal muscle (100 μg protein) and spinal cord (50 μg protein). Dnmt3a expression is greater in spinal cord compared to skeletal muscle. The 78 kDa isoform predominates in skeletal muscle while the 100 kDa isoform predominates in spinal cord. **(F)** Graph showing the relative levels of Dnmt3a isoform immunoreactivity determined by immunobloting of pure mitochondria isolated from adult mouse skeletal muscle and spinal cord. Values are mean ± SD. The 100 kDa isoform was not detected in skeletal muscle even after long exposures. **(G)** Immunoblot for Dnmt3a in pure mitochondria (PM) fractions from different types of adult mouse tissues, human brain, and a human cell line. The 100 kDa isoform of Dnmt3a was present in mouse spinal cord, brain, heart, testes, and human brain cerebral cortex. Dnmt3a immunoreactivity was low or undetectable in mouse spleen, liver, kidney, and lung and in human embryonic kidney cells. Western blot for the mitochondrial marker cyclophilin D is used to show protein loading.

conditions. Gels were transferred to a nitrocellulose membrane using the Xcell surelock system (Invitrogen). The membranes were stained with Ponceau S (Sigma) to determine transfer efficiency, destained, blocked with 1% BSA/0.05% Tween 20/TBS and incubated with primary antibodies: rabbit polyclonal anti-cytochrome P450 reductase (Stressgen) at 1:1000; mouse monoclonal anti-actin (Chemicon) at 1:1000; mouse monoclonal anti-porin (Mitosciences) at 1:3000; rabbit polyclonal anti-lamin (Millipore) at 1:500; sheep polyclonal anti-catalase (Biodesign International) at 1:2000; mouse anti-cyclophilin D (Mitosciences) at 1:3000; mouse monoclonal anti-complex V (Molecular Probes Invitrogen) at 1:10,000; rabbit polyclonal and mouse monoclonal anti-Dnmt3a (Cell Signaling, Abgent, and Alexis) at 1:100–1:500, rabbit polyclonal and mouse monoclonal anti-Dnmt1 (Bethyl, Novus, and Alexis) at 1:500–1:5000, and rabbit polyclonal antibody to Dnmt3b (Abcam) at 1:250. The details of the Dnmt antibodies used are shown in **Table 1.** To confirm the efficacy of proteinase K digestion of putative mitochondrial

Table 1 | Antibodies to Dnmt isoforms screened in this study.

Dnmt target	Antibody clonality	Immunogen	Company and product	Comment
Dnmt1	Mouse monoclonal 60B1220.1	Synthetic peptide corresponding to aa 637–650 (central region)	Alexis (Enzo) ALX-804-369	Good for mouse skeletal muscle and CNS westerns
Dnmt1	Rabbit polyclonal	Synthetic peptide corresponding to aa 1–125 (N-terminus)	Novus Biologicals NB100-264	Good for mouse skeletal muscle and CNS westerns
Dnmt1	Rabbit polyclonal	Synthetic peptide corresponding to ~ aa 574–846 (encoded by exon 25)	Bethyl Laboratories BL961	Suitable for mouse tissue westerns
Dnmt3a	Mouse monoclonal 64B1446	Mouse recombinant Dnmt3a (C-terminal epitope aa 705–908)	Alexis (Enzo) ALX-804-370	Good for mouse skeletal muscle and CNS westerns and immunohistochemistry
Dnmt3a	Rabbit polyclonal	N-terminus of human Dnmt3a	Cell Signaling Technology 2160	Suitable for mouse skeletal muscle and CNS westerns and immunohistochemistry
Dnmt3a	Rabbit polyclonal	Synthetic peptide corresponding to aa 400–500 of human Dnmt3a	ABGENT AP1034a	Suitable for mouse skeletal muscle and CNS westerns
Dnmt3b	Mouse monoclonal 52A1018	Mouse recombinant Dnmt3b	Abcam Ab13604	No detection of Dnmt3b in skeletal muscle mitochondria

surface-tethered proteins, treated skeletal muscle mitochondria were probed with antibodies to tubulin/microtubule associated proteins (1:1000, Sigma) and desmin (1:5000, Sigma). Antibody to LC3A (Cell Signaling) was used as a mitochondrial autophagy marker. Blots were washed, incubated with secondary antibody (1:10,000–1:50,000), and developed using ECL (Pierce Supersignal West Pico). The membranes were imaged using a CCD camera and BioRad Quantity One software or were developed using X-ray film. Immunoreactivity was quantified using ImageJ.

IMMUNOFLUORESCENCE

Age-matched non-tg and hSOD1^{mus}-G37R, -G93A, and -wildtype tg mice (12–15 months of age) received an anesthetic overdose and were perfused transcardially with 4% paraformaldehyde. The group sizes were 3–4 mice per genotype. Spinal cord, skeletal muscle, and testes were removed and cryoprotected in 20% glycerol and then frozen and cut (40 μm) on a sliding microtome. Sections were permeabilized in 0.4–1% Triton-X100/PBS, blocked in 10% normal donkey serum or goat serum/0.1% Triton/PBS, and incubated in primary antibody to mitochondrial markers SOD2 (1:100, Assay Design) or complex V (1:500, Invitrogen Molecular Probes), 5mC (1:100, Calbiochem), Dnmt3a (1:100–500, Alexis or Abgent), or the autophagy marker LC3A (1:100, Cell Signaling). The sections were then rinsed, incubated in secondary antibody (1:400–800) conjugated to AlexaFluor-488 or -594, Hoechst dye counterstained (for nuclear visualization), and imaged on a Zeiss LSM 510 Meta confocal microscope or Zeiss Axiophot epifluorescence microscope.

mtDNA ISOLATION AND mtDNA PYROSEQUENCING

The PM fraction was used to isolate mtDNA using a Qiaprep Spin Miniprep kit (Qiagen) or conventional phenol-chloroform extraction, RNase digestion, and ethanol precipitation. mtDNA concentration and relative purity was determined by measuring A260 and A280 and calculating the A260/A280 ratio.

Mouse mtDNA was sequenced using Pyromark Q24 (Qiagen). DNA (2 μg) was bisulfite treated using an Epitek Bisulfite kit (Qiagen). Purified converted DNA (10 ng) was then PCR amplified, and 25 μl of product sequenced on the Pyromark Q24 (primers and conditions supplied by Qiagen using the Pyromark software): Locus 1 (D-loop), forward primer 5′-GGGTTTATTAAATTTGGGGGTAGTT-3′, biotinylated reverse primer 5′- ATAC CAAATA CATAACACCACAAT-3′, sequencing primer 5′- ATTTGGTTTTTACTTTAGGG T-3′; Locus 2 (16S rRNA gene), forward primer 5′- TGTTGGATTAGGATA TTTTAATGGTGTAG-3′, biotinylated reverse primer 5′- CAC CACCCTAATAACCTTCTCTA-3′, sequencing primer 5′- ATT TTAATGGTGTAGAAGT-3′; run conditions: 95°C 15 min, 45× (95°C 30 s, 58°C 30 s, 72°C 30 s), 72°C 5 min. The data was validated by internal controls and presented as percent 5mC/cytosine ± standard deviation ($n = 3$, in duplicate) with high agreement in duplicate measures.

EM

Age-matched non-tg and hSOD1^{mus}-G37R, -G93A, and -wildtype tg mice (15–17 months of age) received an anesthetic overdose and were perfused transcardially with 2% paraformaldehyde/2% glutaraldehyde. The group sizes were two mice per genotype. Tissue samples of left and right biceps femoris were acquired from each mouse and process and embedded in plastic for conventional transmission EM as described (Martin et al., 1994). Tissue samples were cut in the transverse plane at 0.5 μm for high-resolution light microscopy and then thin sections were cut and collected on copper grids for EM. These sections were viewed and imaged using a Phillips CM12 electron microscope. Digital electron micrographs from each mouse genotype were used to determine subsarcolemmal mitochondrial layer thickness and intermyofibrillar mitochondrial density in at least five images per mouse.

HUMAN CNS TISSUE

Rapid autopsy neurologic disease-free control human brain ($n = 4$) cerebral cortical samples were obtained through the Human Brain Resource Center at Johns Hopkins. These fresh samples of frontal cortex were used to isolate mitochondria for western blot studies of Dnmts.

STATISTICAL ANALYSIS

Western blot densitometry measurements, cytosine methylation pyrosequencing measurements, and myofiber mitochondrial density measurements were used to determine group means and variances and comparisons among groups were analyzed using a one-way analysis of variance and a Newman-Keuls *post-hoc* test or a Student's *t*-test.

RESULTS

DNMT3A LOCALIZES TO MITOCHONDRIA

We analyzed several tissue types for the presence of Dnmts in mitochondria. A flow diagram for the mitochondrial purification preparation is shown (**Figure 1**, top), and the method was validated by western blotting (**Figure 1**, lower left). The fraction designated as PM was highly enriched for mitochondria, as determined by the enrichment of porin and cyclophilin D, and was essentially free of contamination from other subcellular organelles such as the endoplasmic reticulum (cytochrome p450), cytosol (actin), nucleus (lamin), and microsomes (catalase) (**Figure 1**, lower left). EM was used to show by direct visualization that the PM fraction had a high content of mitochondria (**Figure 1**, lower right).

We examined adult mouse skeletal muscle mitochondria for Dnmts (**Figure 2A**). The purity of the mitochondrial samples was confirmed by the enrichment of complex V (**Figure 2A**). Dnmt3a had a robust presence in skeletal muscle mitochondrial fractions (**Figure 2A**) and was detected with several different antibodies to Dnmt3a that recognize N-terminal, central, and C-terminal domains of the protein (**Table 1**). Dnmt1 was usually not detected in skeletal muscle PM fractions (**Figure 2A**), even after prolonged exposures and use of 3 different primary antibodies recognizing different domains of the protein (**Table 1**). In some mitochondrial preparations of skeletal muscle, Dnmt1 was detected at very low levels (**Figure 2B**) but was not present in fractions of intact mitochondria digested with agarose-bound proteinase K (**Figures 2A,B**). In contrast, Dnmt1 was highly concentrated in crude nucleus-enriched P1 fractions (**Figure 1**, Top) of the same tissue homogenates (**Figures 2A,B**). Dnmt3b was not detected in skeletal muscle mitochondria (data not shown).

To determine whether Dnmt3a is present within mitochondria or bound to the surface of mitochondria, fresh intact mitochondria were digested with agarose-bound proteinase K (**Figure 2C**). Tubulin, microtubule-associated proteins, and desmin are known to be tethered to the surface of striated muscle mitochondria (Capetanaki et al., 2007), and tubulin is known to specifically dock to VDAC (Carré et al., 2002). Proteinase K digestion removed completely or nearly completely mitochondrial-bound cytoskeletal proteins but did not alter the robust detection of Dnmt3a in PM (**Figure 2C**). This finding demonstrates that Dnmt3a is present within skeletal muscle mitochondria.

To confirm previous observations indicating a mitochondrial presence of Dnmt3a in nervous tissue (Chestnut et al., 2011), we tracked by subcellular fractionation the presence of Dnmt3a in mouse brain and spinal cord tissue (**Figure 2D**). Dnmt3a was present in nucleus-containing fractions (**Figure 2D**, lanes H and P1) and cytosol-containing fractions (**Figure 2D**, lanes H, S1, P2, and S2). Several isoforms of Dnmt3a have been reported (Chen et al., 2002).We detected both the 78 and 100 kDa isoforms of Dnmt3a in the different fractions of brain and spinal cord (**Figure 2D**). Brain and spinal cord PM fractions contained Dnmt3a (**Figure 2D**), as detected with three different antibodies to the N-terminal or central regions of Dnmt3a (**Table 1**). The 100 kDa isoform of Dnmt3a was concentrated in PM relative to total homogenate (**Figure 2D**). We were unable to detect Dnmt1 immunoreactivity in PM of brain and spinal cord using three different antibodies, consistent with previous data (Chestnut et al., 2011).

Western blotting for Dnmt3a in adult mouse skeletal muscle and spinal cord in a side-by-side comparison revealed tissue differences in isoform distribution (**Figure 2E**). In skeletal muscle, the 78 kDa isoform predominates over the 100 kDa isoform (**Figure 2F**), but in spinal cord the 100 kDa isoform predominates (**Figure 2E**) and accounts for nearly 100% of the total amount of this isoform in spinal cord mitochondria (**Figure 2F**).

We next tested the hypothesis that mitochondrial Dnmt3a is tissue specific. We examined by immunoblotting the presence of Dnmt3a in highly PM isolated from several adult mouse tissues, including spleen, liver, kidney, lung, heart, and testes (**Figure 2G**). The mitochondrial fractions of brain, spinal, heart, and testes contained the 100 kDa isoform of Dnmt3a (**Figure 2G**). Mitochondrial Dnmt3a protein levels were very low or undetectable in spleen, liver, kidney, and lung. The faintly detectable mitochondrial Dnmt3a in spleen, kidney, and lung appeared as the 78 kDa isoform (**Figure 2G**). To determine if the mitochondrial presence of Dnmt3a was mouse-specific, we prepared PM from human cerebral cortex (frontal cortex) and cultured human embryonic kidney (HEK) 293 cells (**Figure 2G**). Dnmt3a was detected robustly in mitochondria of the human brain but not in HEK293 cells (**Figure 2G**). Thus, the mitochondrial localization of Dnmt3a occurs primarily in the mitochondria of excitable tissues in human and mouse.

MITOCHONDRIAL DNMT3A LEVELS ARE REDUCED IN SKELETAL MUSCLE AND SPINAL CORD OF tg MOUSE MODELS OF ALS

Abnormalities in Dnmt protein levels and DNA methylation have been observed in human ALS CNS tissues and in mouse and cell models of motor neuron degeneration (Chestnut et al., 2011). Moreover, in human ALS skeletal muscle, marked mitochondrial abnormalities are found (Wiedemann et al., 1998; Vielhaber et al., 2000; Krasnianski et al., 2005; Echaniz-Laguna et al., 2006; Corti et al., 2009), and it has been proposed that skeletal muscle disease is a driving part of the disease process in ALS (Dupuis et al., 2006; Dobrowolny et al., 2008; Wong and Martin, 2010). We examined the levels of Dnmt3a in skeletal muscle mitochondria in hSOD1 tg mouse models of ALS at presymptomatic or early symptomatic stages of disease. Compared to non-tg age matched littermates, presymptomatic tg mice expressing mutant hSOD1-G37R non-conditionally in most tissues showed reduced levels of Dnmt3a in skeletal muscle mitochondria (**Figures 3A,B**). Tg early symptomatic mice with skeletal muscle-restricted expression of G37R mutant (hSOD1^{mus}-G37R) and G93A mutant (hSOD1^{mus}-G93A) also had a severe loss of skeletal muscle mitochondrial Dnmt3a (**Figures 3A,B**). Mitochondrial Dnmt3a protein levels were reduced modestly in hSOD1^{mus}-wildtype tg mice but were not changed significantly in tg mice with non-conditional expression hSOD1-wildtype allele (**Figures 3A,B**). Spinal cords of hSOD1^{mus}-G37R, -G93A, and -wildtype tg male mice at early stages of disease also had marked reduction in mitochondrial Dnmt3a (**Figures 3C,D**). The loss of Dnmt3a was selective for the mitochondrial compartment because Dnmt3a levels in crude homogenates of skeletal muscle and spinal cord were unchanged in tg mice (**Figure 3E**).

CELLULAR LOCALIZATION OF DNMT3A AND 5mC IN SPINAL CORD AND SKELETAL MUSCLE AND ABERRANT PATTERNS OF IMMUNOREACTIVITY IN hSOD1^{mus} tg MICE

Our biochemical finding that Dnmt3a is present in excitable tissue mitochondria required direct confirmation of a mitochondrial Dnmt3a localization *in situ* and an assessment of whether Dnmt3a in mitochondria overlaps with a reporter molecule for DNA methylation. We also assessed whether abnormalities in Dnmt3a and 5mC are found in tg mouse models of ALS since abnormalities has been found in human ALS (Chestnut et al., 2011). We used a highly specific monoclonal antibody to detect 5mC (Kang et al., 2006). We have done additional characterization of the 5mC antibody (Chestnut et al., 2011). By immunofluorescence, we visualized Dnmt3a and 5mC localization within spinal cord of 2–4 months old non-tg mice (**Figure 4A**). Extranuclear Dnmt3a and 5mC immunoreactivities colocalized. While Dnmt3a immunoreactivity was present diffusely in the cytoplasm, there were distinct punctate structures positive for Dnmt3a. These cytoplasmic puncta invariably were 5mC-positive (**Figure 4A**, arrows), indicating that these structures contain methylated DNA. Consistent with expectations, 5mC immunoreactivity was also detected in the nucleus of neurons (**Figures 4B,C**, red).

As the only extranuclear cellular structures known to contain DNA are mitochondria, we examined spinal cord for the presence of 5mC within mitochondria. Using immunofluorescence for SOD2, a mitochondrial marker that shows robust punctate labeling in the cytoplasm (Martin et al., 2007), we determined that mitochondria contain 5mC (**Figure 4B**). Not all SOD2-positive structures were also positive for 5mC (**Figure 4B**, arrows). The dual positive structures often appeared larger than the SOD2-only positive mitochondria.

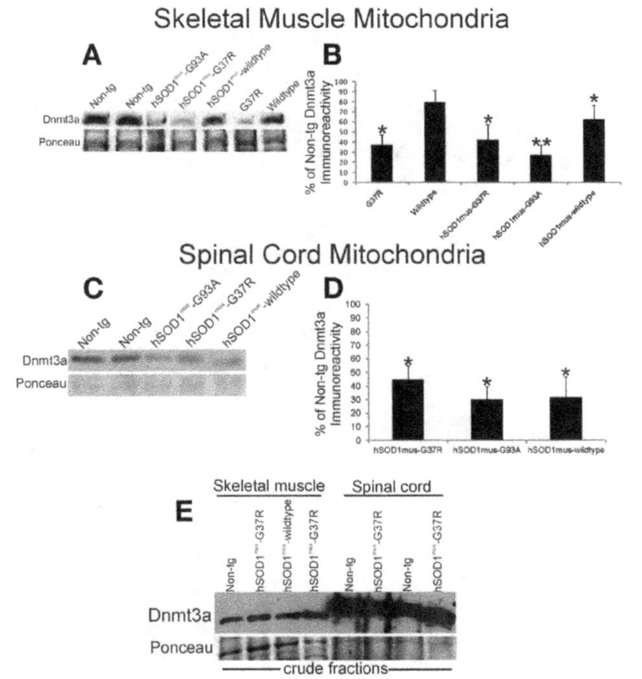

FIGURE 3 | Dnmt3a levels are reduced in hSOD1 tg mouse models of ALS. (A) Western blot for Dnmt3a in leg skeletal muscle mitochondria (100 μg/lane) in non-conditional tg mice expressing hSOD1-G37R or hSOD1-wildtype constructs and conditional (muscle-restricted) tg mice expressing hSOD1^{mus}-G37R, -G93A, or -wildtype constructs compared to age-matched non-tg littermates. Ponceau S staining of membrane shows protein loading. **(B)** Graph showing the relative levels of Dnmt3a immunoreactivity determined by immunoblotting of pure mitochondria isolated from hSOD1 tg mouse leg skeletal muscle. Values are mean ± SD. Significant differences from non-tg control are indicated by single ($p < 0.05$) or double ($p < 0.01$) asterisks. **(C)** Western blot for Dnmt3a in spinal cord mitochondria fractions (50 μg/lane) in conditional (muscle-restricted) tg mice expressing hSOD1^{mus}-G37R, -G93A, or -wildtype constructs compared to age-matched non-tg littermates. Ponceau S staining of membrane shows protein loading. **(D)** Graph showing the relative levels of Dnmt3a immunoreactivity in hSOD1^{mus} tg mouse spinal cord. Values are mean ± SD. Significant differences from non-tg control are indicated by an asterisk ($p < 0.05$). The results have been replicated in at least 3 different experiments. **(E)** Western blot for Dnmt3a in crude fractions of skeletal muscle and spinal cord of conditional (muscle-restricted) tg mice expressing hSOD1^{mus}-G37R or -wildtype constructs compared to age-matched non-tg littermates. Ponceau S staining of membrane shows protein loading.

Some of the discreet cytoplasmic puncta that contained 5mC appeared similar to autophagosomes (Martin et al., 1994; Kabeya et al., 2000) or granules based on size and shape (**Figure 4A**). The larger 5mC-positive bodies were not positive for the mitochondrial marker SOD2, while the smaller 5mC-positive bodies did stain for SOD2 (**Figure 4B**), possibly indicating degradation of mitochondria or mitochondrial marker. We next examined the immunolocalization of 5mC and LC3A (**Figure 4C**). LC3A is a marker for autophagosomes (Kabeya et al., 2000) that is known to function in mitophagy (Wang and Klionsky, 2011). 5mC-containing, SOD2-negative bodies were positive for LC3A

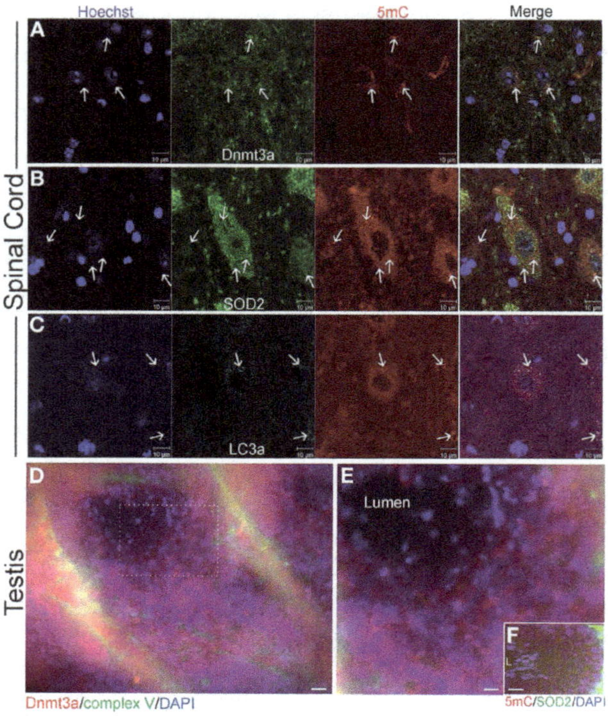

FIGURE 4 | Cellular localizations of Dnmt3a and 5-methylcytosine (5mC) in wildtype young adult mouse spinal cord and testes. (A) In 6–8 weeks old non-tg mice, Dnmt3a is present in the nucleus and in the cytoplasm of neurons in spinal cord. Extranuclear cytoplasmic Dnmt3a immunoreactivity (green) is localized diffusely and in discrete bodies (arrows). These discrete bodies also contain 5mC (red, arrows). Hoechst staining was used to identify cell nuclei. **(B)** Cytoplasmic 5mC is localized to mitochondria in neurons. Some mitochondria, identified by SOD2 immunoreactivity (green, arrows), in spinal cord colocalize with 5mC immunoreactivity (red, arrows). Many mitochondria also do not contain 5mC. The SOD2- and 5mC-positive bodies tend to be larger than normal mitochondria (white arrows). **(C)** 5mC is present in autophagosomes. Mouse spinal cord sections were immunostained for an autophagosome marker LC3A (green) and 5mC (red). Extranuclear 5mC immunoreactivity has a high colocalization with LC3A in autophagosomes (arrows). **(D,E)** Immunofluorescent localization of Dnmt3a (red) and complex V (green) in mouse testis. Cell nuclei are blue. Dnmt3a immunoreactivity (red) is enriched in cells in the seminiferous tubules of testes. The boxed area in D is represented at higher magnification in E which shows that Dnmt3a immunoreactivity (red) partly colocalizes (seen as yellow-orange) with mitochondria (green). Scale bars: 30 μm **(D)**; 15 μm **(E)**. **(F)** Immunofluorescence for 5mC (red) and SOD2 (green) in mouse testes. Cell nuclei are blue. 5mC immunoreactivity (red) partly colocalizes (seen as yellow-orange) with mitochondria (green). Mature spermatozoa with scant mitochondria are seen at left in seminiferous tubule lumen (L). Scale bar = 30 μm.

(**Figure 4C**). The prominent colocalization of 5mC and LC3A in the cytoplasm of spinal motor neurons suggests a relationship between cytosine methylation of mtDNA and mitophagy signaling.

In the mouse tissue screening for Dnmt3a protein levels we saw that testes also contained relatively high levels of Dnmt3a (**Figure 2G**). In seminiferous tubules, Dnmt3a and 5mC were discretely localized to mitochondria of spermatocytes (**Figures 4D,E**). Interestingly, immunofluorescent signal for mitochondria, Dnmt3a, and 5mC dissipated with maturation of spermatocytes to spermatozoa within the seminiferous tubule lumen (**Figures 4D,E**) consistent with a predominant pre-fertilization elimination of paternal mitochondria and mtDNA in sperm cells during their maturation, rather than a post-fertilization mechanism (Luo et al., 2013).

Immunofluorescent assessments of Dnmt3a and 5mC were done on skeletal muscle and spinal cord sections of $hSOD1^{mus}$ tg mice to confirm biochemical findings and to put our homogenate-based observations into a cellular localization framework. In non-tg control mice, Dnmt3a colocalized with complex V robustly in subsarcolemmal mitochondria and also in intermyofibrillar mitochondria (**Figure 5A**), while Dnmt3a and complex V immunoreactivity was severely attenuated in $hSOD1^{mus}$-G37R skeletal muscle myofibers (**Figure 5B**). In subsarcolemmal mitochondria adjacent to myonuclei, Dnmt3a was not colocalized with 5mC in non-tg controls (**Figure 5C**), but in $hSOD1^{mus}$ tg mice, Dnmt3a and 5mC were prominently colocalized in apparent subsarcolemmal mitochondria (**Figure 4D**). 5mC immunoreativity was also seen in subsets of myofiber nuclei (**Figures 5C,D**, green). In lumbar spinal cord motor neurons of 15–17 months old non-tg mice, Dnmt3a was normally colocalized with complex V in about a third of the mitochondria in motor neuron cell bodies (**Figure 5E**) and, similarly, about a third of the Dnmt3-positive cytoplasmic particles colocalized with 5mC (**Figure 5G**). In $hSOD1^{mus}$ tg mice, complex V immunoreactivity was enriched in remaining lumbar motor neurons and Dnmt3 immunoreactivity appeared as aggregates associated with some mitochondria (**Figure 5F**). The Dnmt3a-5mC colocalization in remaining mitochondria in motor neurons of $hSOD1^{mus}$ tg mice also revealed large numerous cytoplasmic aggregates containing 5mC (**Figure 5H**) consistent with findings in degenerating motor neurons (Chestnut et al., 2011).

DIRECT DEMONSTRATION OF 5mC IN mtDNA

We directly identified 5mC in purified mtDNA by DNA pyrosequencing (Marsh, 2007) (**Figures 6A,B**). Two different loci of the mitochondrial genome (D-loop and 16S rRNA gene) were interrogated in bisulfite-treated mtDNA isolated from mouse brain, liver, and testes (**Figure 6A**). Cytosine methylation was determined at five nucleotide sites in locus 1 and at seven nucleotide sites in locus 2 (**Figures 6A,B**). Locus 1 in the D-loop had CpG regions with 5mC content ranging from 9% (brain, position 4) to 2% (liver, position 2) (**Figure 6C**). Most of the mtDNA CpG sites in locus 1 of brain and testes had 5mC content at ~4–6% (**Figure 6C**). Liver mtDNA was generally at 4% 5mC content at locus 1 (**Figure 6C**). In contrast, locus 2 in the 16S rRNA gene had several CpG regions with 5mC content ranging from 7.5 to 18% in brain and testes mtDNA and testes (**Figure 6D**). Locus 2 CpG position 4 showed the highest 5mC content (**Figures 6B,D**). Liver mtDNA generally had ~5% 5mC content at locus 2, with the exception of CpG position 4 where it was about 10% (**Figure 6D**).

ALS MICE HAVE ABERRANT mtDNA 5mC SIGNATURES

Cytosine methylation in mtDNA was assayed in skeletal muscle and spinal cord of different hSOD1 tg mouse models of ALS (**Figures 7, 8**). Tg mice with non-conditional expression of

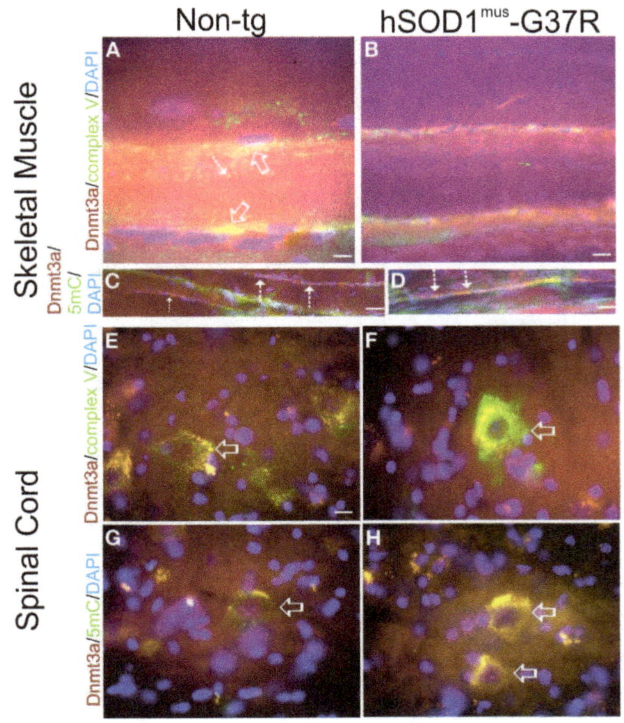

FIGURE 5 | Immunofluorescent localizations of Dnmt3a, mitochondria, and 5-methylcytosine (5mC) in hSOD1^{mus} tg mouse skeletal muscle and spinal cord. (A,B) In non-tg mouse skeletal muscle (biceps femoris), Dnmt3a (red) immunoreactivity can be found diffusely in the sarcoplasm and associated with mitochondria (colocalization is seen as yellow) identified by complex V immunoreactivity (green). Dnmt3a/complex V colocalization occur prominently in subsarcolemmal mitochondria in non-tg mice (A, open arrows) and in interfibrillar mitochondria **(A**, hatched arrow**)**. In hSOD1^{mus} mouse hindleg skeletal muscle, Dnmt3a (red) immunoreactivity and mitochondrial complex V immunoreactivity (green) are markedly attenuated. Scale bars = 9 μm **(A)**, 15 μm **(B)**. **(C,D)**. Myofiber perinuclear colocalization of Dnmt3a and 5mC is intensified in hSOD1^{mus} tg mice. In non-tg mouse skeletal muscle (biceps femoris), Dnmt3a (red) immunoreactivity can be found clustered around peripheral myonuclei **(C**, hatched arrows**)** and generally has little colocalization with 5mC. In hSOD1^{mus}mouse skeletal muscle Dnmt3a (red) and 5mC (green) immunoreactivities have prominent perinuclear colocalizations **(D**, hatched arrows, yellow-orange**)**. Scale bars = 20 μm **(C,D)**. **(E,F)** In ~17 months old non-tg mice, Dnmt3a immunoreactivity (red) is present in the nucleus and, more prominently, in the cytoplasm of spinal cord motor neurons **(E,G**, open arrows**)**. Cytoplasmic Dnmt3a immunoreactivity (red) is localized in discreet particles in motor neurons **(E,G**, arrows**)**. Many of these cytoplasmic particles colocalize (seen as yellow) with complex V immunoreactivity **(E**, green**)**, and thus are mitochondria, and with 5mC **(G**, green, arrow**)** and thus contain methylated mtDNA. Scale bar in **(E) (**same for **F–H)** = 6 μm. In age-matched hSOD1^{mus} tg mice, remaining spinal motor neurons **(F**, open arrow**)** show intensified mitochondrial immunoreactivity for complex V (green) and the Dnmt3a immunoreactivity largely is colocalized with complex V **(F)** and 5mC **(H)** and is aggregated in the cytoplasm.

mutant-G37R and wildtype variants of hSOD1 were analyzed at 8–10 months of age (**Figure 7**). Generally, 5mC content was lower in the D loop (locus 1) than in the 16S rRNA gene (locus 2) in control mice. Within the D-loop, the CpG at site 2 had the lowest % methylation, and sites 3 and 4 had the highest cytosine methylation in skeletal muscle and spinal cord (**Figure 7**). No significant differences in cytosine methylation of the D-loop were seen in tg mice expressing mutant-G37R and wildtype variants of hSOD1 compared to non-tg mice. In the 16S rRNA gene (locus 2), the CpG at site 4 had the highest % methylation of all the sites sequenced (**Figure 7**). Cytosine methylation was significantly increased at sites 1, 3, 4, 5, 6, and 7 in the 16S rRNA gene of spinal cord in tg mice with non-conditional expression of mutant-G37R (**Figure 7**), but no differences were detected in cytosine methylation in the 16S rRNA gene of skeletal muscle (**Figure 7**). Tg mice (16–20 months old) with skeletal muscle-restricted expression of mutant-G37R and -G93A and wildtype variants of hSOD1 (**Figure 8**) showed patterns of mtDNA cytosine methylation that were different compared to non-conditional hSOD1 tg mice. Cytosine methylation in D-loop site 2 of spinal cord was significantly reduced in hSOD1^{mus}-G37R (**Figure 8**), but other sites assayed for in the D-loop of spinal cord and skeletal muscle were unchanged (**Figure 8**). In contrast, cytosine methylation in all sites of the 16S rRNA gene of spinal cord was significantly lower in hSOD1^{mus}-wildtype mice compared to non-tg mice (**Figure 8**), but G37R^{mus} and G93A^{mus} mice did not differ from control.

hSOD1^{mus} tg MICE DEVELOP MITOCHONDRIAL ABNORMALITIES IN SKELETAL MUSCLE AND SPINAL CORD

The loss of mitochondrial Dnmt3a seen in tg mouse models of ALS could be related to changes in mitochondrial content. Indeed, skeletal muscle complex V was reduced significantly in hSOD1^{mus}-G37R, -G93A, and -wildtype tg mice at middle stages of disease compared to age-matched non-tg mice (**Figure 9A**). The reduced levels of complex V in skeletal muscle were mirrored by increases in the autophagy marker LC3A (**Figure 9B**). In contrast, complex V levels in spinal cord were significantly elevated in hSOD1^{mus} tg mice (**Figure 9C**), consistent with previous histologic observations showing increased numbers of mitochondria in motor neurons of these mice (Wong and Martin, 2010).

Mitochondrial distributions and numbers in skeletal muscle were examined using high-resolution light and transmission electron microscopic evaluation of plastic sections. Non-tg control mice were rich in subsarcolemmal and interfibrillar mitochondria (**Figures 10A,C**). hSOD1^{mus}tg mice showed a loss of subsarcolemmal and interfibrillar mitochondria (**Figures 10B,D,E**). In putative type I fibers of non-tg mice the subsarcolemmal mitochondrial layer thickness was ~4 μm (**Figures 10C,E**), but in hSOD1^{mus}-G37R, -G93A, and -wildtype tg mice, the subsarcolemmal mitochondrial layer was significantly attenuated (**Figure 10E**). Putative type II fibers in hSOD1^{mus} tg mouse skeletal muscle displayed a significantly reduced density of interfibrillar mitochondria (**Figure 10F**) compared to age-matched non-tg mice. EM additionally revealed evidence for subsarcolemmal and interfibrillar mitophagy (**Figure 10D**, upper inset), as well as intramitochondrial rod-like inclusions (**Figure 10D**, lower inset) indicative of mitochondrial myopathy (Schlattner et al., 2006).

DISCUSSION

We demonstrate that the DNA methylating enzyme Dnmt3a is present in mitochondria of mouse CNS, striated muscle, and

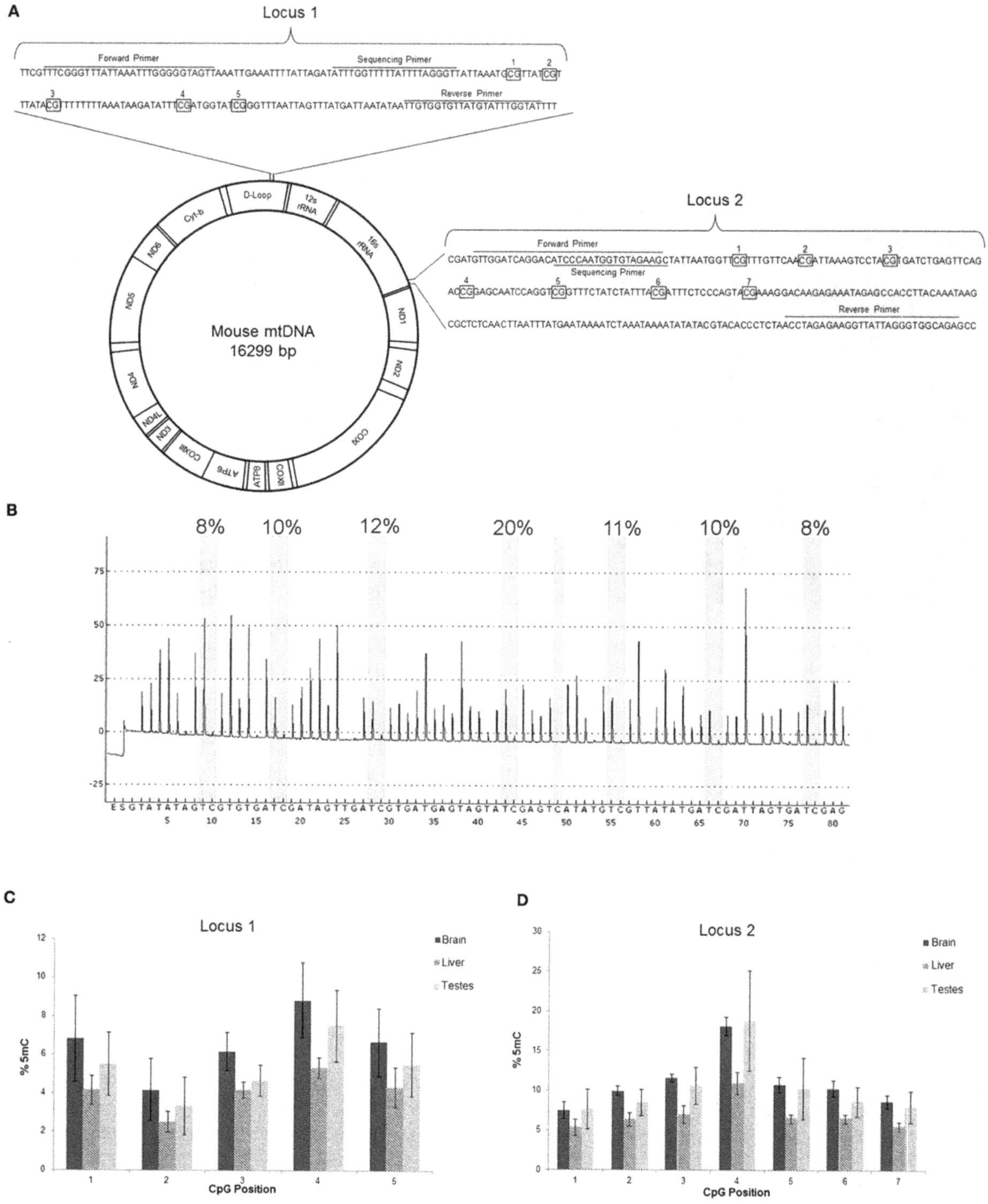

FIGURE 6 | mtDNA contains 5-methylcytosine (5mC). (A) Schematic of mouse mtDNA (Bibb et al., 1981) with depictions of the two locations assayed for 5mC. The first locus is in the D-loop, involved in mtDNA replication, and the second locus in the 16s rRNA encoding region. The primer locations are shown in sequences (wildtype or converted shown) with the CpG regions examined that are boxed and numbered. **(B)** Representative pyrogram from pyrosequencing of mouse brain mtDNA locus 2. The Y-axis is relative intensity (in arbitrary units) and the X-axis is the dispensation sequence showing the order of nucleotide addition to the reaction (E, enzyme; S, substrate). The seven thick shaded bars indicate the CpG positions with the degree of methylation (shown at top of bar) calculated from the ratio of the peak heights of C and T. The single narrow bar shows a bisulfite treatment control point where the peak only at the T dispensation and not at the C dispensation confirms full conversion by the bisulfite treatment. **(C,D)** Pyosequencing data of the two regions of mtDNA from mouse brain, liver, and testes. Numbers on the x-axis correspond to the CpG numbering in the sequence in **(A)**, and the y-axis is mtDNA 5mC content. In locus 1 the 5mC content was highest in brain mtDNA. In locus 2 the 5mC content in mtDNA was highest in the brain and testes, especially at position 4. Of the 3 tissues, liver had the lowest mtDNA 5mC content.

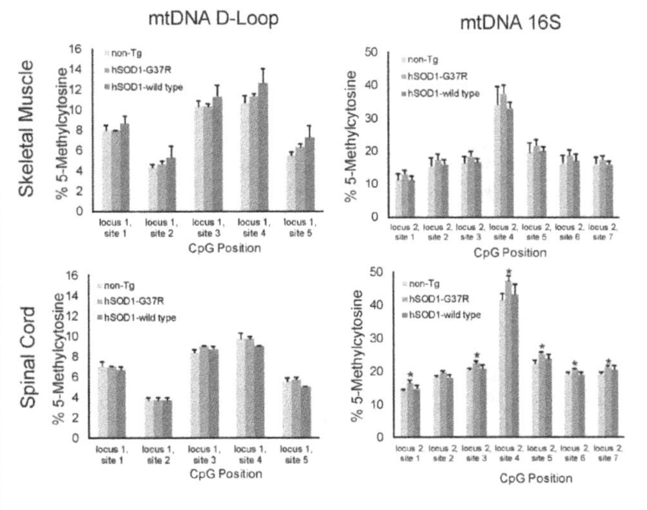

FIGURE 7 | 5-methylcytosine (5mC) content in two loci of skeletal muscle mtDNA in non-conditional transgenic mouse models of ALS. Graphs show the %5mC content at 5 CpG sites in the D-loop (**left**) and at 7 CpG sites in the 16S rRNA gene in the skeletal muscle (**top**) and spinal cord (**bottom**) of tg mice with expression of G37R or wildtype hSOD1 variants. Tg and non-tg control mice were 8–10 months of age. Values are mean ± SEM derived from mtDNA isolated from three different mice per genotype. Asterisks denote significant increase in hSOD1-G37R mice compared to non-tg control ($p < 0.05$).

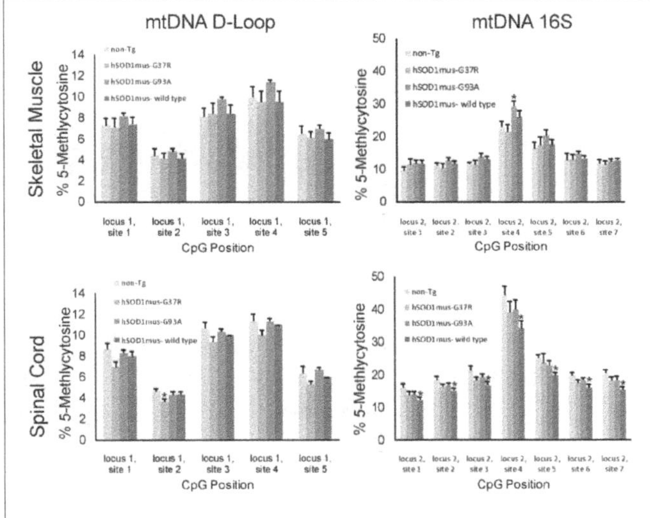

FIGURE 8 | 5-methylcytosine (5mC) content in two loci of skeletal muscle mtDNA in conditional transgenic mouse models of ALS. Graphs show the %5mC content at 5 CpG sites in the D-loop (**left**) and at 7 CpG sites in the16S rRNA gene in the skeletal muscle (**top**) and spinal cord (**bottom**) of tg mice with skeletal muscel-restricted expression of G37R, G93A, or wildtype hSOD1 variants. Tg and non-tg control mice were 16–20 months of age. Values are mean ± SEM derived from mtDNA isolated from three different mice per genotype. Asterisks denote significant differences in tg mice compared to non-tg control mice ($p < 0.05$).

testes. We also find Dnmt3a in human cerebral cortex mitochondria. Furthermore, the mtDNA of these tissues contains 5mC as shown directly by DNA pyrosequencing. Dnmt3a protein levels are reduced significantly at early disease in skeletal muscle and spinal cord of tg mouse models of ALS, and these mice also show aberrant patterns in 5mC immunoreactivity in skeletal muscle and spinal motor neurons. Some 5mC-positive structures are sequestered into autophagosomes. The skeletal muscle of presymptomatic tg mouse models of ALS shows accumulation of autophagy marker, loss of subsarcolemmal and intermyofibrillar mitochondria, and ultrastructural evidence for mitophagy. We conclude that mitochondrial localization of Dnmt3a and cytosine methylation of mtDNA are tissue-preferential, mostly confined to excitable tissues, and that regulatory mechanisms for epigenetic modification mtDNA, or non-catalytic functions of mitochondrial Dnmt3a, in skeletal muscle and spinal cord are aberrant in mouse ALS.

DNA methylating enzymes are thought traditionally to localize and function in the cell nucleus where they catalyze cytosine methylation leading to chromatin remodeling (Cheng, 1995; Jones and Takai, 2001; Bird, 2002; Brenner and Fuks, 2006). Here, we show that Dnmt3a is present the mitochondria of adult mouse excitable tissues such as brain, spinal cord, heart, and skeletal muscle. Mitochondrial Dnmt3a was also present in testes. In contrast, Dnmt3a is low or undetectable in spleen, liver, kidney, and lung. We detected mitochondrial Dnmt3a with several different antibodies to Dnmt3a that recognize different epitopes. The finding was not an artifact of subcellular contamination because the mitochondrial preparation was assessed for purity by immunoblotting and EM. Moreover, the Dnmt3a was present within mitochondria rather than being docked to the surface of mitochondria, as was the case for the mitochondrial association of Dnmt1. We also observed that different Dnmt3a isoforms were enriched preferentially in different mouse tissues. Skeletal muscle expressed primarily the 78 kDa Dnmt3a isoform, whereas, nervous tissue expressed primarily the 100 kDa Dnmt3a isoform. Dnmt3a was found also in mitochondria purified from adult human cerebral cortex. Dnmt3b was not detected in mouse skeletal muscle mitochondria (data not shown). We confirmed the mitochondrial expression of Dnmt3a by immunolocalization. Dnmt3a was found to colocalize with mitochondrial markers in spinal cord, skeletal muscle and testes. Another group has shown the presence of a Dnmt isoform associated with mitochondria, but the mitochondria were prepared from cell cultures and only one antibody to Dnmt1 and one antibody putatively to Dnmt3a was used (Shock et al., 2011). Dnmt1, but not Dnmt3a, was found associated with mitochondria from cultured mouse embryonic fibroblasts and human colon carcinoma cells (Shock et al., 2011), but mitochondrial surface-associated Dnmt1 was not ruled out by protease digestion of outer membrane-bound proteins as done here. We did not detect Dnmt1 in mouse skeletal muscle mitochondria using an antibody specifically directed to the N-terminus of Dnmt1. A commercial antibody (Abcam) to amino acids 1–10 of the N-terminus of Dnmt1 was reportedly used in this previous study (Shock et al., 2011), but this antibody was not in inventory for our use. With antibodies to N-terminal and central regions of Dnmt1, we identified here a proteinase K-sensitive Dnmt1 in some mitochondrial preparations, indicating surface-associated Dnmt1. Dnmt1 is associated with imprinting mechanisms involved in maintaining methylation patterns during cell division (Robertson, 2001), likely to be occurring in cultured cycling cells, while Dnmt3a has *de novo* methylating

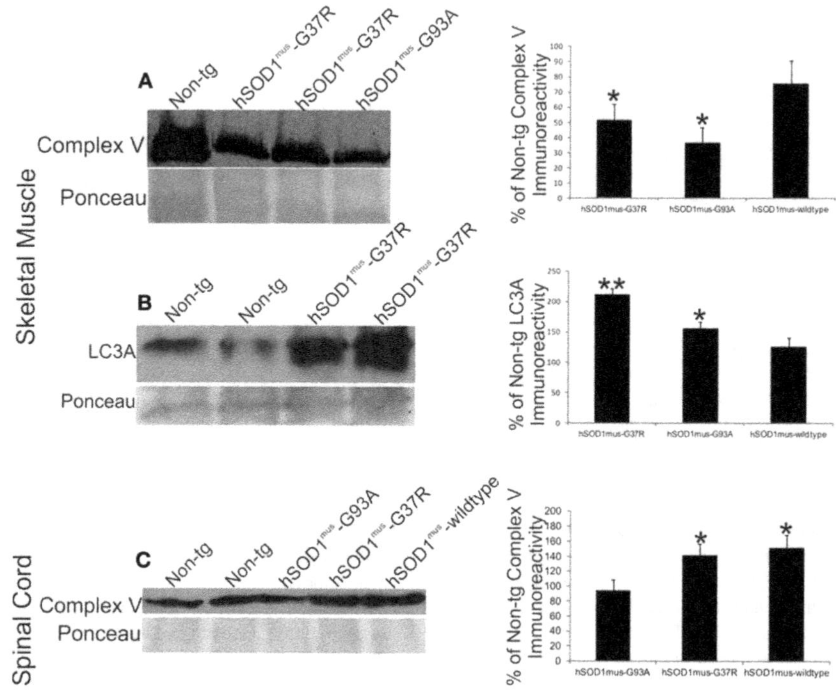

FIGURE 9 | hSOD1^{mus} tg mouse model of ALS has mitochondrial abnormalities in skeletal muscle and spinal cord. (A) Western blot for complex V in skeletal muscle crude extracts (100 μg/lane) of early symptomatic tg mice expressing skeletal muscle-restricted hSOD1^{mus}-G37R or hSOD1^{mus}-wildtype. Ponceau S-stained membrane shows protein loading. Graph (at right) shows the quantification of complex V immunoreactivity in early symptomatic hSOD1^{mus}-G37R, hSOD1^{mus}-G93A, or hSOD1^{mus}-wildtype tg mice. Values (as % of control) are mean ± SD. Asterisk denotes significant differences ($p < 0.01$) from non-tg control. **(B)** Western blot for autophagy marker LC3A in skeletal muscle crude extracts (100 μg/lane) early symptomatic tg mice expressing skeletal muscle-restricted hSOD1^{mus}-G37R or hSOD1^{mus}-wildtype. Ponceau S-stained membrane shows protein loading. Graph (at right) shows the quantification of LC3A immunoreactivity in early symptomatic hSOD1^{mus}-G37R, hSOD1^{mus}-G93A, or hSOD1^{mus}-wildtype tg mice. Values (as % of control) are mean ± SD. Significant differences from non-tg control are indicated by single ($p < 0.05$) or double ($p < 0.01$) asterisks. **(C)** Western blot for complex V in spinal cord crude extracts (50 μg/lane) of early symptomatic tg mice expressing skeletal muscle-restricted hSOD1^{mus}-G37R or hSOD1^{mus}-wildtype. Ponceau S-stained membrane shows protein loading. Graph (at right) shows the quantification of complex V immunoreactivity in spinal cord of early symptomatic hSOD1^{mus}-G37R, hSOD1^{mus}-G93A, or hSOD1^{mus}-wildtype tg mice. Values (as % of control) are mean ± SD. Asterisk denotes significant differences ($p < 0.05$) from non-tg control.

activity (Okano et al., 1999). We conclude that the major mitochondrial Dnmt in adult mouse and human excitable tissues *in vivo* is Dnmt3a.

Our finding that Dnmt3a is within mitochondria of excitable tissue led to measurements of mtDNA methylation in these tissues. We demonstrated directly the presence of 5mC in mtDNA by DNA pyrosequencing (Marsh, 2007). Because DNA pyrosequencing cannot distinguish between 5mC and 5-hydroxymethylcytosine, our pryosequencing data represents a measurement of 5mC and 5-hydroxymethylcytosine in mtDNA. A recent study has also demonstrated the presence of 5mC and 5-hydroxymethylcytosine in mtDNA of cultured mouse embryonic fibroblasts and human colon carcinoma cells using qPCR and Gla1 restriction enzyme digestion (Shock et al., 2011). While it is possible the mtDNA methylation is involved in regulating gene expression (Shock et al., 2011), as in the nucleus, the proteins involved in chromatin remodeling, such as histones, are not present in mitochondria (Spelbrink, 2010). This suggests the intriguing possibility that cytosine methylation through Dnmt3a is a major epigenetic mechanism involved in mitochondrial gene regulation without partnership with histone acetylation. Alternatively, the mtDNA methylation may serve some purpose other than gene regulation.

Our immunolocalization experiments on mouse skeletal muscle, spinal cord, and testes revealed that some 5mC-positive structures in the cytoplasm of myofibers, spinal motor neurons, and maturing spermatozoa were mitochondria because the 5mC colocalized with SOD2 or complex V and Dnmt3a. This observation confirms a previous report of mitochondrial 5mC localization using other mitochondrial makers (Chestnut et al., 2011). However, some cytoplasmic 5mC-positive structures were not positive for mitochondrial markers and had a morphology different from mitochondria because they were larger than typical mitochondria and sometimes appeared aggregated. We thus sought to determine possible relationships between methylated mtDNA and mitophagy and found that 5mC colocalized with the autophagosome marker LC3A (Klionsky and Emr, 2000). Our findings in mouse testes suggest that enhanced mtDNA methylation and mitophagy in maturing spermatoza in seminiferous tubules could be a mechanism to reduce the major burden of paternal mtDNA transmission prior to postfertilization autophagy (Al Rawi et al., 2011). Autophagy has also been

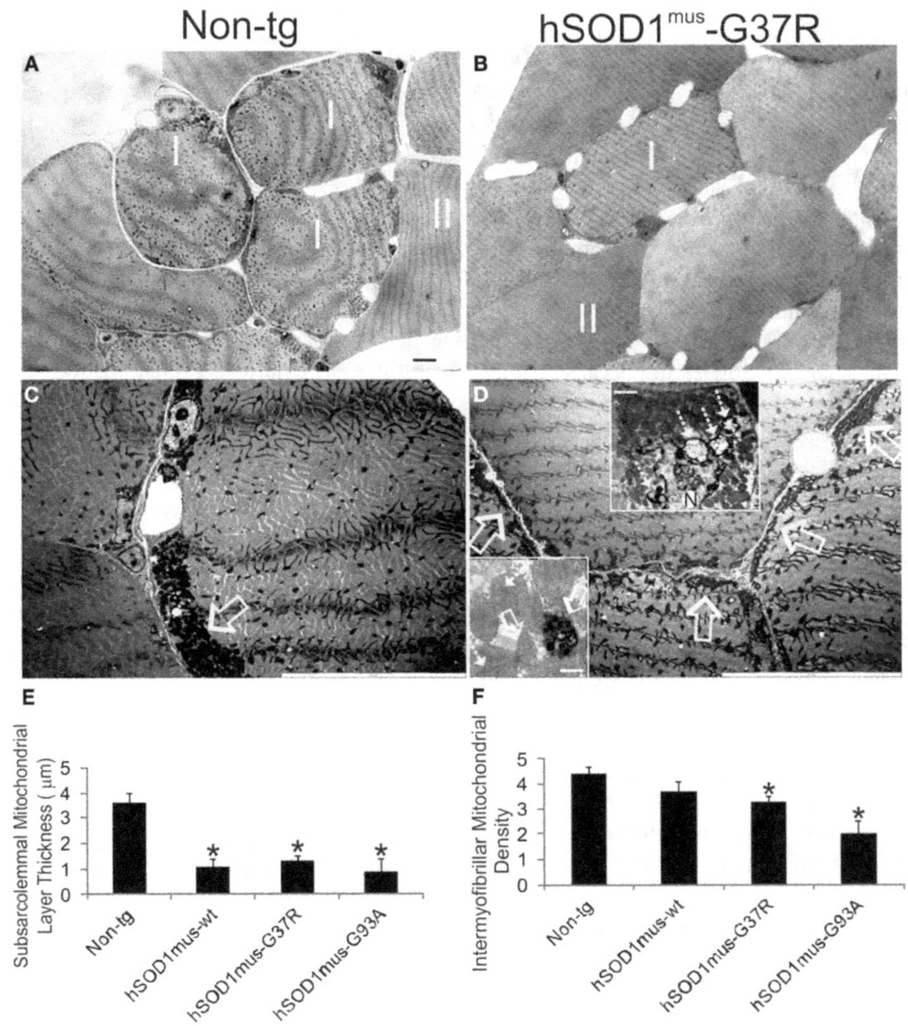

FIGURE 10 | hSOD1^{mus} tg mouse model of ALS shows loss of mitochondria in skeletal muscle. (A,B) Toluidine blue-stained plastic sections (0.5 μm thick) of biceps femoris muscle from 15 month-old non-tg and hSOD1^{mus}-G37R tg mice. In non-tg mice, type I and type II fibers have distinct appearances as evidenced by the surrounding capillary number and subsarcolemmal and interfibrillar mitochondria density. In tg mice, type I fibers are less prominent with apparent loss of subsarcolemmal and interfibrillar mitochondria. Scale bar (in **A**, same for **B**) = 8 μm. **(C,D)** Electron micrographs showing a high density of subsarcolemmal mitochondria in non-tg mice (**C**, open arrows) and prominent attenuation of the subsarcolemmal layer in hSOD1^{mus} tg mice (**D**, open arrows). Upper inset **(D)** shows prominent mitophagy of subsarcolemmal mitochondria (hatched arrows) by a myonucleus (N) in hSOD1^{mus}-G37R tg mouse skeletal muscle. Scale bar = 1.3 μm. Lower inset **(D)** shows degenerating mitochondria with round inclusions (open white arrows) or rod inclusions (hatched white arrows) from hSOD1^{mus}-G93A tg mouse skeletal muscle. Scale bar = 0.5 μm. **(E)** Graph of the thickness of type I fiber subsarcolemmal mitochondrial layers in age-matched (~17 months) non-tg and hSOD1^{mus} tg mice. Values are mean ± SD. Asterisk denotes significant differences ($p < 0.01$) from non-tg control. **(F)** Graph of type II fiber interfibrillar mitochondrial densities in age-matched (~17 months) non-tg and hSOD1^{mus} tg mice. Values are mean ± SD. Asterisk denotes significant differences ($p < 0.01$) from non-tg control.

associated with nervous system and muscle disease (Batlevi and La Spada, 2011). In hSOD1 tg mice with muscle-specific expression, large 5mC-positive aggregates were observed in the cytoplasm of subsets of spinal motor neurons. Similar observations have been shown in adult mouse spinal motor neurons undergoing axotomy-induced apoptosis (Chestnut et al., 2011). The presence of Dnmt3a and 5mC within a subset of mitochondria, many of which are associated with autophagosomes, suggests an upstream epigenetic mechanism for mitophagy in the regulation of normal and pathological mitochondrial dynamics.

We have found that epigenetic mechanisms involving DNA methylation can drive motor neuron apoptosis in cell culture and *in vivo* and that aberrant regulation of DNA methylation is part of the pathobiology of human ALS (Chestnut et al., 2011). Abnormalities in the levels and localizations of Dnmt1, Dnmt3a, and 5mC have been found in human ALS spinal cord and motor cortex (Chestnut et al., 2011), and mitochondrial abnormalities in skeletal muscle, liver, spinal motor neurons, and motor cortex have been reported in human ALS (Sasaki and Iwata, 1999; Menzies et al., 2002). However, causal disease mechanisms are difficult to pinpoint using human postmortem tissue. We therefore evaluated Dnmt3a and mtDNA methylation in several tg mouse models of ALS expressing mutant and wildtype hSOD1 either non-conditionally with global tissue expression (Gurney et al., 1994; Martin et al., 2007, 2009; Gertz et al., 2012) or conditionally with muscle-restricted expression (Wong and Martin, 2010). In skeletal muscle, mitochondrial Dnmt3a levels were markedly reduced in most hSOD1 tg mouse lines at stages of disease ranging from presymptomatic to mid-symptomatic. The loss of Dnmt3a and mitochondria in skeletal muscle was corroborated microscopically by immunohistochemistry. Interestingly, spinal cord Dnmt3a was reduced in tg mice with muscle-specific expression of hSOD1. This change is interesting because conditional ablation of Dnmt3a specifically in nervous tissue causes an age-related ALS-like phenotype in mice involving neuromuscular junction dismantling, motor neuron loss, and shortened lifespan (Nguyen et al., 2007). The localizations of 5mC immunoreactivity in skeletal muscle and spinal cord were also different in non-conditional and muscle-specific hSOD1 tg mice compared to age-matched control mice. Skeletal muscle disease in ALS mice thus appears to trigger retrograde transynaptic changes in epigenetic DNA methylation machinery in spinal cord mitochondria.

Abnormalities in mtDNA cytosine methylation were detected by pyrosequencing in mouse models of ALS. The cytosines interrogated were in the D-loop and 16S ribosomal RNA gene (**Figure 6A**). The 16S ribosomal RNA gene was more vulnerable than the D-loop to anomalous cytosine methylation. In the 16S ribosomal RNA gene, six cytosine sites showed increased methylation in spinal cord of hSOD1-G37R mice, and one cytosine site showed increased methylation in skeletal muscle of $hSOD1^{mus}$-G93A mice. While five cytosines in the D-loop showed differential levels of methylation, their methylation was similar in control and ALS mice. While the D-loop is generally thought to be a major regulator of mitochondrial genome transcription, it is now known that non-promoter CpG methylation within gene bodies can regulate gene expression in the nuclear genome (Maunakea et al., 2010). We have no direct explanation for the apparent mismatches between mitochondrial Dnmt3a protein levels which decrease and 5mC which increase. Recent studies have found that Dnmt3a has demethylase activity that is stimulated by Ca^{2+} ions (Chen et al., 2013), so the increased cytosine methylation could be construed as being consistent with the loss of Dnmt3a in mitochondria.

A mechanism for the loss of skeletal muscle mitochondria appears to be mitophagy, as evidenced by the ultrastructure of degenerating mitochondrial profiles and the marked upregulation of LC3A seen by western blotting. Because numerous copies of mtDNA reside in single mitochondrion, Dnmt3a protein levels may be more reflective of skeletal muscle mitochondrial numbers, and extensively methylated mtDNA may be more stable than Dnmt3a protein in mitochondria undergoing mitophagy. Recent evidence supports this possibility because some mtDNA can escape autophagy and participate in local inflammatory mechanisms (Oka et al., 2012). Tissue inflammation is a prominent component of the pathobiology of mouse models of ALS (Martin et al., 2007; Chen et al., 2010; Drechsel et al., 2012) and human ALS (McGeer and McGeer, 2002; Corcia et al., 2013).

AUTHOR CONTRIBUTIONS

Conceived and designed the experiments: Margaret Wong, Barry Gertz, Barry A. Chestnut, Lee J. Martin. Performed experiments: Margaret Wong, Barry Gertz, Lee J. Martin. Analyzed the data: Margaret Wong, Barry Gertz, Lee J. Martin. Wrote paper: Margaret Wong, Barry Gertz, Lee J. Martin.

ACKNOWLEDGMENTS

The authors thank Antoinette Price and Yan Pan for technical assistance. The authors are particularly grateful to Ed Roberts for his outstanding work on the EM. This work was supported by grants from the U.S. Public Health Service, National Institutes of Health, National Institute on Aging (AG016282) and National Institute of Neurological Disorders and Stroke (NS034100, NS065895, and NS052098).

REFERENCES

Al Rawi, S., Louvet-Vallée, S., Djeddi, A., Sachse, M., Culetto, E., Hajjar, C., et al. (2011). Postfertilization autophagy of sperm organelles prevents paternal mitochondrial DNA transmission. *Science* 344, 1144–1147. doi: 10.1126/science.1211878

Amir, R. E., Van den Yeyver, I. B., Wan, M., Tran, C. Q., Francke, U., and Zoghbi, H. Y. (1999). Rett syndrome is caused by mutations in X-linked MECP2, encoding methyl-CpG-binding protein 2. *Nat. Genet.* 23, 185–188. doi: 10.1038/13810

Batlevi, Y., and La Spada, A. R. (2011). Mitochondrial autophagy in neural function, neurodegenerative disease, neuron cell death, and aging. *Neurobiol. Dis.* 43, 46–51. doi: 10.1016/j.nbd.2010.09.009

Beal, M. F. (2005). Mitochondria take center stage in aging and neurodegeneration. *Ann. Neurol.* 58, 495–505. doi: 10.1002/ana.20624

Bhattacharya, S. K., Thakar, J. H., Johnson, P. L., and Shanklin, D. R. (1991). Isolation of skeletal muscle mitochondria from hamsters using ionic medium containing ethylediaminetetraacetic acid and nagarse. *Anal. Biochem.* 192, 344–349. doi: 10.1016/0003-2697(91)90546-6

Bibb, M. J., Van Etten, R. A., Wright, C. T., Walberg, M. W., and Clayton, D. A. (1981). Sequence and gene organization of mouse mitochondrial DNA. *Cell* 26, 167–80. doi: 10.1016/0092-8674(81)90300-7

Bird, A. (2002). DNA methylation patterns and epigenetic memory. *Genes Dev.* 16, 6–21. doi: 10.1101/gad.947102

Brenner, C., and Fuks, F. (2006). DNA methyltransferases: Facts, clues, mysteries. *Curr. Top. Microbiol. Immunol.* 301, 45–66. doi: 10.1007/3-540-31390-7_3

Calvanese, V., Lara, E., Kahn, A., and Fraga, M. F. (2009). The role of epigenetics in aging and age-related diseases. *Ageing Res. Rev.* 8, 268–276. doi: 10.1016/j.arr.2009.03.004

Capetanaki, Y., Bloch, R. J., Kouloumenta, A., Mavroidis, M., and Psarras, S. (2007). Muscle intermediate filaments and their links to membranes and membranous organelles. *Exp. Cell Res.* 313, 2063–2076. doi: 10.1016/j.yexcr.2007.03.033

Carré, M., André, N., Carles, G., Borghi, H., Brichese, L., Briand, C., et al. (2002). Tubulin is an inherent component of mitochondrial membranes that interacts with the voltage-dependent anion channel. *J. Biol. Chem.* 277, 33664–33669. doi: 10.1074/jbc.M203834200

Chen, C.-C., Wang, H.-Y., and Shen, C.-K. J. (2013). DNA 5-methylcytosine demethylation activities of the mammalian DNA methytransferases. *J. Biol. Chem.* 288, 9084–9091. doi: 10.1074/jbc.M112.445585

Chen, K., Northington, F. J., and Martin, L. J. (2010). Inducible nitric oxide synthase is present in motor neuron mitochondria and Schwann cells and contributes to disease mechanisms in ALS mice. *Brain Struct. Funct.* 214, 210–234. doi: 10.1007/s00429-009-0226-4

Chen, T., Ueda, Y., Xie, S., and Li, E. (2002). A novel Dnmt3a isoform product produced from an alternative promoter localizes to euchromatin and its expression correlates with active *de novo* methylation. *J. Biol. Chem.* 277, 38746–38754. doi: 10.1074/jbc.M205312200

Cheng, X. (1995). Structure and function of DNA methyltransferases. *Annu. Rev. Biophys. Biomol. Struct.* 24, 293–318. doi: 10.1146/annurev.bb.24.060195.001453

Chestnut, B. A., Chang, Q., Lesuisse, C., Wong, M., and Martin, L. J. (2011). Epigenetic regulation of motor neuron degeneration through DNA methylation. *J. Neurosci.* 31, 16619–16636. doi: 10.1523/JNEUROSCI.1639-11.2011

Corcia, P., Tauber, C., Vercoullie, J., Arlicot, N., Prunier, C., Praline, J., et al. (2013). Molecular imaging of microglial activation in amyotrophic lateral sclerosis. *PLoS ONE* 7:e52941. doi: 10.1371/journal.pone.0052941

Corti, S., Donadoni, C., Ronchi, D., Bordoni, A., Fortunato, F., Santoro, D., et al. (2009). Amyotrophic lateral sclerosis linked to a novel *SOD1* mutation with muscle mitochondrial dysfunction. *J. Neurol. Sci.* 276, 170–174. doi: 10.1016/j.jns.2008.09.030

Dobrowolny, G., Aucello, M., Rizzuto, E., Beccaficao, S., Mammucari, C., Bonconpagni, S., et al. (2008). Skeletal muscle is a primary target of SOD1^{G93A}-mediated toxicity. *Cell Metab.* 8, 425–436. doi: 10.1016/j.cmet.2008.09.002

Drechsel, D. A., Estevez, A. G., Barbeito, L., and Beckman, J. S. (2012). Nitric oxide-mediated oxidative damage and the rogressive demise of motor neurons in ALS. *Neurotox. Res.* 22, 251–264. doi: 10.1007/s12640-012-9322-y

Dupuis, L., Gonzalez de Aguilar, J. L., Echaniz-Laguna, A., and Loeffler, J.-P. (2006). Mitochondrial dysfunction in amyotrophic lateral sclerosis also affects skeletal muscle. *Muscle Nerve* 34, 253–254. doi: 10.1002/mus.20566

Echaniz-Laguna, A., Zoll, J., Ponsot, E., N'Guessan, B., Tranchant, C., Loeffler, J.-P., et al. (2006). Muscular mitochondrial function in amyotrophic lateral sclerosis is progressively altered as the disease develops: a temporal study in man. *Exp. Neurol.* 198, 25–30. doi: 10.1016/j.expneurol.2005.07.020

Geiman, T. M., and Muegge, K. (2010). DNA methylation in early development. *Mol. Reprod. Dev.* 77, 105–113. doi: 10.1002/mrd.21118

Gertz, B., Wong, M., and Martin, L. J. (2012). Nuclear localization of human SOD1 and mutant SOD1-specific disruption of survival motor neuron protein complex in transgenic amyotrophic lateral sclerosis mice. *J. Neuropathol. Exp. Neurol.* 71, 162–177. doi: 10.1097/NEN.0b013e318244b635

Gurney, M. E., Pu, H., Chiu, A. Y., Dal Canto, M. C., Polchow, C. Y., Alexander, D. D., et al. (1994). Motor neuron degeneration in mice that express a human Cu,Zn superoxide dismutase mutation. *Science* 264, 1772–1775. doi: 10.1126/science.8209258

Jia, D., Jurkowska, R. Z., Zhang, X., Jeltsch, A., and Cheng, X. (2007). Structure of Dnmt3a bound to Dnmt3L suggests a model for *de novo* DNA methylation. *Nature* 449, 248–251. doi: 10.1038/nature06146

Jones, P. A., and Takai, D. (2001). The role of DNA methylation in mammalian epigenetics. *Science* 293, 1068–1070. doi: 10.1126/science.1063852

Kabeya, Y., Mizushima, N., Ueno, T., Yamamoto, A., Kirisako, E., Noda, T., et al. (2000). LC3, a mammalian homologue of yeast Apg8p, is localized in autophagosome membranes after processing. *EMBO J.* 19, 5720–5728. doi: 10.1093/emboj/19.21.5720

Kang, J. S., Wanibuchi, H., Morimura, K., Totsuka, Y., Yoshimura, I., and Fukushima, S. (2006). Existence of a no effect level foe MeIQx hepatocarcinogenicity on a background of thioacetaminde-induced liver damage in rats. *Cancer Sci.* 97, 453–458. doi: 10.1111/j.1349-7006.2006.00201.x

Klein, C. J., Botuyan, M.-V., Wu, Y., Ward, C. J., Nicholson, G. A., Hammans, S., et al. (2011). Mutations in *DNMT1* cause hereditary sensory neuropathy with dementia and hearing loss. *Nat. Gen.* 43, 595–600. doi: 10.1038/ng.830

Klionsky, D. J., and Emr, S. D. (2000). Autophagy as a regulated pathway of cellular degradation. *Science* 290, 1717–1721. doi: 10.1126/science.290.5497.1717

Krasnianski, A., Deschauer, M., Neudecker, S., Gellerich, F. N., Müller, T., Schoser, B. G., et al. (2005). Mitochondrial changes in skeletal muscle in amyotrophic lateral sclerosis and other neurogenic atrophies. *Brain* 128, 1870–1876. doi: 10.1093/brain/awh540

Luo, S.-M., Ge, Z.-J., Wang, Z.-W., Jiang, Z.-Z., Wang, Z.-B., Ouyang, Y.-C., et al. (2013). Unique insights into maternal mitochondrial inheritance in mice. *Proc. Natl. Acad. Sci. U.S.A.* 110, 13038–13043. doi: 10.1073/pnas.1303231110

Maekawa, M., Taniguchi, T., Higashi, H., Sugimura, H., Sugano, K., and Kanno, T. (2004). Methylation of mitochondrial DNA is not a useful marker for cancer detection. *Clin. Chem.* 50, 1480–1481. doi: 10.1373/clinchem.2004.035139

Marsh, S. (2007). Pyrosequencing applications. *Methods Mol. Biol.* 373, 15–24.

Martin, L. J. (2010). Mitochondrial and cell death mechanisms in neurodegenerative diseases. *Pharmaceuticals* 3, 839–915. doi: 10.3390/ph3040839

Martin, L. J. (2012). Biology of mitochondria in neurodegenerative diseases. *Prog. Mol. Biol. Trans. Sci.* 107, 355–415. doi: 10.1016/B978-0-12-385883-2.00005-9

Martin, L. J., Gertz, B., Pan, Y., Price, A. C., Molkentin, J. D., and Chang, Q. (2009). The mitochondrial permeability transition pore in motor neurons: involvement in the pathobiology of ALS mice. *Exp. Neurol.* 218, 33–346. doi: 10.1016/j.expneurol.2009.02.015

Martin, L. J., Liu, Z., Chen, K., Price, A. C., Pan, Y., Swaby, J. A., et al. (2007). Motor neuron degeneration in amyotrophic lateral sclerosis mutant superoxide dismutase-1 transgenic mice: mechanisms of mitochondriopathy and cell death. *J. Comp. Neurol.* 500, 20–46. doi: 10.1002/cne.21160

Martin, L. J., Pardo, C., Cork, L. C., and Price, D. L. (1994). Synaptic pathology and glial responses to neuronal injury precede the formation of senile plaques and amyloid deposits in the aging cerebral cortex. *Am. J. Pathol.*145,1358-1381.

Martin, L. J., and Wong, M. (2013). Aberrant regulation of DNA methylation in amyotrophic lateral sclerosis: a new target of disease mechanism. *Neurotherapeutics* 10, 722–733. doi: 10.1007/s13311-013-0205-6

Maunakea, A. K., Nagarajan, R. P., Bilenky, M., Ballinger, T. J., D'Souza, C., Fouse, S. D., et al. (2010). Conserved role of intragenic DNA methylation in regulating alternative promoters. *Nature* 466, 253–260. doi: 10.1038/nature09165

McGeer, P. L., and McGeer, E. G. (2002). Inflammatory processes in amyotrophic lateral sclerosis. *Muscle Nerve* 26, 459–470. doi: 10.1002/mus.10191

Menzies, F. M., Ince, P. G., and Shaw, P. J. (2002). Mitochondrial involvement in amyotrophic lateral sclerosis. *Neurochem. Intl.* 40, 543–551. doi: 10.1016/S0197-0186(01)00125-5

Mortusewicz, O., Schermelleh, L., Walter, J., Cardoso, M. C., and Leonhardt, H. (2005). Recruitment of DNA methyltransferase I to DNA repair sites. *Proc. Natl. Acad. Sci. U.S.A.* 102, 8905–8909. doi: 10.1073/pnas.0501034102

Motorin, Y., and Helm, M. (2011). RNA nucleotide methylation. *WIREs RNA* 2, 611–631. doi: 10.1002/wrna.79

Nguyen, S., Meletis, K., Fu, D., Jhaveri, S., and Jaenisch, R. (2007). Ablation of *de novo* DNA methyltransferase Dnmt3a in the nervous system leads to neuromuscular defects and shortened lifespan. *Devel. Dyn.* 236, 1663–1676. doi: 10.1002/dvdy.21176

Oka, T., Hikoso, S., Yamaguchi, O., Taneike, M., Takeda, T., Tamai, T., et al. (2012). Mitochondrial DNA that escapes from autophagy causes inflammation and heart failure. *Nature* 485, 251–255. doi: 10.1038/nature10992

Okado-Matsumoto, A., and Fridovich, I. (2001). Subcellular distribution of superoxide dismutases (SOD) in rat liver: Cu,Zn-SOD in mitochondria *J. Biol. Chem.* 276, 38388–38393. doi: 10.1074/jbc.M105395200

Okano, M., Bell, D. W., Haber, D. A., and Li, E. (1999). DNA methyltransferases Dnmt3a and Dnmt3b are essential for *de novo* methylation and mammalian development. *Cell* 99, 247–257. doi: 10.1016/S0092-8674(00)81656-6

Panov, A., Steuerwald, N., Vavilin, V., Dambinova, S., and Bonkovsky, H. L. (2012). "Role of neuronal mitochondrial metabolic phenotype in pathogenesis of ALS," in *Amyotrophic Lateral Sclerosis,* ed M. Maurer (InTech), 225–248. ISBN: 978-953-307-806-9. doi: 10.5772/30418

Pollack, Y., Kasir, J., Shemer, R., Metzger, S., and Szyf, M. (1984). Methylation pattern of mouse mitochondrial DNA. *Nucleic Acid Res.* 12, 4811–4824. doi: 10.1093/nar/12.12.4811

Reddy, P. H., and Reddy, T. P. (2011). Mitochondria as a therapeutic target for aging and neurodegenerative diseases. *Curr. Alzheimer Res.* 8, 398–409. doi: 10.2174/156720511795745401

Robertson, K. D. (2001). DNA methylation, methyltransferases, and cancer. *Oncogene* 20, 3139–3155. doi: 10.1038/sj.onc.1204341

Santa-Cruz, L. D., Ramírez-Jarquín, U. N., and Tapia, R. (2012). "Role of mitochondrial dysfunction in motor neuron degeneration in ALS," *Amyotrophic Lateral Sclerosis,* ed M. Maurer (InTech), 197–224. ISBN: 978-953-307-806-9. doi: 10.5772/31290

Sasaki, S., and Iwata, M. (1999). Ultrastructural changes of synapses of Betz cell in patients with amyotrophic lateral sclerosis. *Neurosci. Lett.* 268, 29–32. doi: 10.1016/S0304-3940(99)00374-2

Schaefer, M., and Lyko, F. (2010). Solving the Dnmt2 enigma. *Chromosoma* 119, 35–40. doi: 10.1007/s00412-009-0240-6

Schlattner, U., Tokarska-Schlattner, M., and Wallimann, T. (2006). Mitochondrial creatine kinase in human health and disease. *Biochim. Biophy. Acta* 1762, 164–180. doi: 10.1016/j.bbadis.2005.09.004

Shmookler Reis, R. J., and Goldstein, S. (1983). Mitochondrial DNA in mortal and immortal cells: genome number, integrity, and methylation. *J. Biol. Chem.* 258, 9078–9085.

Shock, L. S., Thakkar, P. V., Peterson, E. J., Moran, R. G., and Taylor, S. M. (2011). DNA methyltransferase 1, cytosine methylation, and cytosine hydroxymethylation in mammalian mitochondria. *Proc. Natl. Acad. Sci. U.S.A.* 108, 3630–3635. doi: 10.1073/pnas.1012311108

Spelbrink, J. N. (2010). Functional organization of mammalian mitochondrial DNA in nucleoids: history, recent developments, and future challenges. *IUBMB Life* 62, 19–32. doi: 10.1002/iub.282

Vielhaber, S., Kunz, D., Winkler, K., Wiedemann, F. R., Kirches, E., Feistner, H., et al. (2000). Mitochondrial DNA abnormalities in skeletal muscle of patients with sporadic amyotrophic lateral sclerosis. *Brain* 123, 1339–1348. doi: 10.1093/brain/123.7.1339

Wang, K., and Klionsky, D. J. (2011). Mitochondria removal by authophagy. *Autophagy* 7, 297–300. doi: 10.4161/auto.7.3.14502

Wiedemann, F. R., Winkler, K., Kuznetsov, A. V., Bartels, C., Vielhaber, S., Feistner, H., et al. (1998). Impairment of mitochondrial function in skeletal muscle of patients with amyotrophic lateral sclerosis. *J. Neurol. Sci.* 156, 65–72. doi: 10.1016/S0022-510X(98)00008-2

Winkelmann, J., Lin, L., Schormair, B., Kornum, B. R., Faraco, J., Plazzi, G., et al. (2012). Mutations in DNMT1 cause autosomal dominant cerebellar ataxia, deafness and narcolepsy. *Hum. Mol. Genet.* 21, 2205–2210. doi: 10.1093/hmg/dds035

Wong, M., and Martin, L. J. (2010). Skeletal muscle-restricted expression of human SOD1 causes motor neuron degeneration in transgenic mice. *Hum. Mol. Genet.* 9, 2284–2302. doi: 10.1093/hmg/ddq106

Xie, S., Wang, Z., Okano, M., Nogami, M., Li, Y., He, W. W., et al. (1999). Cloning, expression and chromosome locations of the human DNMT3 gene family. *Gene* 236, 87–95. doi: 10.1016/S0378-1119(99)00252-8

Efficacy of hypnosis-based treatment in amyotrophic lateral sclerosis: a pilot study

Arianna Palmieri[1]*, Johann Roland Kleinbub[1], Vincenzo Calvo[1], Gianni Sorarù[2], Irene Grasso[2], Irene Messina[1] and Marco Sambin[1]

[1] Department of Philosophy, Sociology, Pedagogy and Applied Psychology, University of Padova, Padova, Italy
[2] Department of Neurosciences, University of Padova, Padova, Italy

Edited by:
Francesco Pagnini, Catholic University of Milan, Italy

Reviewed by:
Francesco Pagnini, Catholic University of Milan, Italy
Maria Nives Sala, Univerità degli Studi di Torino, Italy

***Correspondence:**
Arianna Palmieri, Department of Philosophy, Sociology, Pedagogy and Applied Psychology, University of Padova, via Venezia 8, Padova 35100, Italy.
e-mail: arianna.palmieri@unipd.it

Background: Amyotrophic lateral sclerosis (ALS) and its devastating neurodegenerative consequences have an inevitably psychological impact on patients and their caregivers: however, although it would be strongly needed, there is a lack of research on the efficacy of psychological intervention. Our aim was to investigate the effect of hypnosis-based intervention on psychological and perceived physical wellbeing in patients and the indirect effect on caregivers. **Methods:** We recruited eight ALS volunteers patients as a pilot sample for an hypnosis intervention and self-hypnosis training protocol lasting 1 month. Anxiety and depression level was measured in patients and caregivers at pre and post treatment phase. Quality of life and perceived physical symptoms changes were also investigated in patients. **Results:** One month pre-post treatment improvement in depression, anxiety, and quality of life was clearly clinically observed and confirmed by psychometric analyses on questionnaire data. Moreover, decreases in physical symptoms such as pain, sleep disorders, emotional lability, and fasciculations were reported by our patients. Improvements in caregiver psychological wellbeing, likely as a consequence of patients psychological and perceived physical symptomatology improvement, were also observed. **Conclusion:** To the best of our knowledge, even if at a preliminary level, this is the first report on efficacy psychological intervention protocol on ALS patients. The findings provide initial support for using hypnosis and self-hypnosis training to manage some ALS physical consequences and mainly to cope its dramatic psychological implications for patients and, indirectly, for their caregivers.

Keywords: amyotrophic lateral sclerosis, hypnotherapy, self-hypnosis, psychological intervention

INTRODUCTION

Amyotrophic Lateral Sclerosis (ALS) is classically characterized by progressive loss of upper and lower motor neurons, causing weakness and hypotrophy of upper and lower limbs, dysphagia and dysarthria, and respiratory failure, which is the most common cause of death. Frequently, patients require intubation and mechanical ventilation and, in a large proportion, receive tracheostomy, leading to inevitably, overwhelming locked-in syndrome (Vianello et al., 2011). Secondary symptoms that affects patient quality of life are also pain (Pagnini et al., 2011a; Chiò et al., 2012; Pagnini, 2012), sleep disorders (Blackhall, 2012), emotional lability (Palmieri et al., 2009), and fasciculations (Rana et al., 2009; De Carvalho and Swash, 2012). Although pharmacology and physiotherapy research efforts, effective treatments for ALS have remained elusive (Beghi et al., 2011). Not surprisingly, a very active community of researchers is dedicated to deepen the devastating psychological impact of ALS in patients and caregivers. Depression and anxiety are two reactions typically described in response of the disease, mainly in the first stage, in which are accompanied by anger, hopelessness, and suicidal ideation (Palmieri et al., 2010a; Pagnini, 2012). Patient psychic status has been found directly related to caregiver's one (Palmieri et al., 2009; Pagnini et al., 2010a, 2011b). Analogously, caregiver psychological status has a deep impact on patient (Chiò et al., 2005). Although psychological wellbeing is crucial also in determining a better prognosis in ALS (McDonald et al., 1994), there is an absence of research on efficacy of psychological intervention in ALS. That is what was recently highlighted by Pagnini et al. (2012), in a relevant short communication published in ALS leading journal, eloquently entitled: "ALS: time for research on psychological intervention?" The communication arises the importance to carry out exploratory investigation on the impact and the suitability of psychological treatments for ALS patients. Given the devastating physical involvement of the disease, which affects also speech ability and eventually may result in the locked-in syndrome, a mind-body treatment technique, such as hypnosis, mindfulness meditation, or biofeedback (techniques included among complementary therapies in neurology; Wahbeh et al., 2008), could represent the eligible psychological forms of intervention. In particular, probably no other contemporary therapeutic intervention has a longer and corroborated clinical/scientific history than that of hypnosis. Our purpose was to explore, in the form of a pilot study, the applicability and efficacy of a hypnosis-based treatment in a small sample of ALS patients. Since the potential treatment benefit obtained from individual active participation (Bandura, 1997), a self-hypnosis training, other than ericksonian hypnosis classical intervention, was proposed to patients. Our primary hypothesis was that the treatment and the training may determine relevant reductions in the two primary psychological reactions to the disease, i.e., anxiety and depression, and, in general, in quality of life. In addition, we aimed to explore if the participation to the hypnosis training could produce significant improvements in the perception of the above-mentioned physical secondary symptomatology (i.e., pain, sleep disorders, emotional lability, and fasciculations). Finally, we hypothesized an eventual reduction of caregivers' anxiety and depression, as indirect consequence of patients psychological improvement.

MATERIALS AND METHODS

PARTICIPANTS AND PROCEDURE

Eight consecutive patients with a diagnosis of probable or definite ALS (in accordance with the Revised El Escorial Criteria; Brooks et al., 2000) presenting to the Motor Neuron Disease Center of Padova University Hospital and their respective caregivers (seven spouses, one daughter) were recruited as volunteers for the pilot study. Patients underwent complete neurological and neuropsychological examination within a week before the first treatment session. Our sample was composed by four males and four females, with mean age of 55 years (SD = 7.14); ALSFRS-r (Cedarbaum et al., 1999) mean score was 35 (SD = 7.1), ranging from 21 to 42; four had bulbar onset, and one of them was completely enable to speak; two were completely enable to move upper limbs. Patient neuropsychological profiles did not revealed any alteration if compared to normative data. Further demographic and clinical characteristics of participants are reported in **Table 1**. The intervention protocol consisted of four weekly domiciliary sessions of hypnosis-based intervention, administered by a psychologist extensively trained in ericksonian hypnotic method and analgesic hypnosis. All sessions were based on a standardized, general induction followed by individual suggestion modified for the patient according to his/her psychological status and physical symptoms. Hypnotic suggestions were constituted by guided visual imagery oriented with an emphasis on developing physical symptomatology controls, such as muscle pain or emotional lability, sense of resilience, self-consciousness, and illness acceptance. After the hypnosis session, which lasted about 45 min, patient was supported by the aiding of the hypnotherapist to try again in recreating hypnotic status with self-hypnosis technique. The general induction, common for all treatment phases and for all patients, was recorded in a CD audio and was left to each patient who was encouraged to practice at least one time every day. Such procedure is inspired by Jensen et al. (2009, 2011) hypnosis-based protocol, successfully applied on multiple sclerosis patients. Sessions included also a brief clinical interview with patient and/or caregiver (separately) collected by a psychotherapist with 10-years experience with ALS. The interview aimed to investigate the subjective perception of the hypnosis treatment efficacy both on psychological and physical perspective, the frequency of application and the eventual difficulties. Each entirely domiciliary session lasted about 2 h. Immediately before the first and after the last treatment, patients and caregivers psychological variables were collected by means of standardized, Italian-validated *ad hoc* questionnaires, as described in the next paragraph. Patient impressions on physical symptomatology were also systematically recorded. The study protocol was approved by the Ethical Committee of the University of Padova and carried out in accordance with the principles of the Declaration Helsinki as revised in 1983. All the participants signed a consent statement after being informed about the study's purpose and methods.

MEASURES

The Hospital Anxiety and Depression Scale (HADS; Zigmond and Snaith, 1983), a measure largely used to identify caseness of anxiety disorders and depression among non-psychiatric patients (Bjelland et al., 2002), easy to administer and well accepted, was employed for patients and their caregivers. It is divided into an Anxiety subscale (HADS-A) and a Depression subscale (HADS-D) both containing seven intermingled items on a 4-point Likert scale (ranging 0–3).

Patients also underwent the Amyotrophic Lateral Sclerosis Specific Quality of Life – revised (ALSSQOL-r; Simmons et al., 2006; Pagnini et al., 2010b), a 46-items on a 11-point Likert scale (ranging 0–10) derived from interviews with ALS patients. The ALSSQOL-r is composed by six subscale including negative

Table 1 | Participants demographic and clinical characteristics.

Patient	Age	Gender	Time since diagnosis (months)	Onset	ALSFRS-r	FVC (%)	Caregivers age (years); gender
I	64	*F*	24	Bulbar	42	82	(32); *F**
II	55	*M*	15	Limb	38	82	(50); *F*
III	59	*F*	10	Limb	40	86	(57); *M*
IV	54	*M*	26	Limb	21	56	(50); *F*
V	43	*M*	18	Limb	39	92	(40); *F*
VI	53	*M*	40	Limb	30	75	(53); *F*
VII	55	*F*	24	Bulbar	39	91	(56); *M*
VIII	66	*F*	10	Limb	31	72	(69); *M*

ALS-FRS-r, amyotrophic lateral sclerosis functional rating scale-revised; FVC, forced vital capacity.

**Daughter; in the other cases, caregiver was the spouse.*

emotion (13 items), interaction with people and their environment (11 items), intimacy (seven items), religiousness and spirituality (four items), physical symptoms (six items), and bulbar functioning (five-items).

The five-items ALS Assessment Questionnaire (ALSAQ-5), a further, brief specific quality of life measure derived from the broader ALSAQ-40 (Jenkinson and Fitzpatrick, 2001; Palmieri et al., 2010b), was also administered to patients. Items are composed on a five-point Likert scale (ranging 1–5). Such measure was introduced, in addition to the more exhaustive, even if different in content, ALSSQOL-r, in the perspective of eventual 3 and 6 months follow-up, in order to obviate eventual drop out in quality of life measurement (such phenomenon could be due to progressive physical impairment that can frustrate responding questionnaire with many items).

Global satisfaction with hypnotic-based intervention score in terms of perceived efficacy was assessed asking patients to rate, after treatment, how satisfied they were with the treatment they received on a 1–5 Likert scale (from one as totally unsatisfied to five as extremely satisfied). Subjective perception of secondary symptoms affecting patient everyday life that could receive benefit from hypnosis-based treatment, namely pain, sleep disorders, emotional lability, and fasciculations, were qualitatively investigated before and after the treatment (for an example, in the time lapse immediately preceding the beginning of the treatment were asked to the patients: "Did you suffer physical pain (e.g., cramps)?" And, if yes, after the treatment was asked them: "Did you notice any improvement during the training period?"). To not overfatigue the patients with wide many items standardized measurements, we opted, at this preliminary level, to investigate such physical perceived changes with a simple open-answers interview, avoiding dimension-specific questionnaires for peculiar physical dysfunctions. Due to severity of motor impairment, not every patient would be able to fulfill self-report questionnaires responses. Therefore, to obviate eventual heterogeneity in the data collection, a trained psychologist administered all questionnaires in an eterodirected way.

DATA ANALYSIS

Pre-post differences in scores for each subscale of the questionnaires (HADS, ALSSQOL, ALSAQ-5) were analyzed for significance through Wilcoxon Signed Rank Tests at the 0.05 level, and the Cliff's delta (∂) statistic was used to assess effect size. Cliff's delta (Cliff, 1993) was chosen as a more robust alternative to the common Cohen's *d* in conditions were non-parametric statistics are advisable, such as small sample sizes where it is not safe to assume a normal distribution (Hess and Kromrey, 2004). An high effect size is considered $\partial \geq |0{,}474|$, a medium effect size is $\partial = |0{,}33|$ and a low effect size is $\partial < |0{,}147|$ (Cohen, 1988). Analysis were performed with R software, version 2.15.1.

RESULTS

Patients declared to have successfully practiced self-hypnosis at least once every day in the great majority of the days during month treatment. The HADS scores showed that before the treatment two out of eight patients suffered from "mild" depression while the remaining six fell in the normality range; after the treatment all eight patients fell in the normality range for depression. Before the treatment, three patients out of eight suffered from "mild" anxiety, one suffered from "severe" anxiety, and the remaining four patients fell into the normality range. After the treatment, two out of eight patients suffered from "mild" anxiety while the six remaining had a normal score (of note, one was previously ranged as "moderate" and one was previously ranged as "severe"). Pre and post analysis of the HADS scores showed significant reduction in the anxiety subscale, with very high effect sizes (where an high effect size is considered $\partial \geq |0{,}474|$) both for patients ($W = 36, p = 0.008; \partial = -1$) and caregivers ($W = 21, p = 0.031; \partial = -0.75$); moreover, the HADS depression subscale showed a significant reduction in score with high effect size ($W = 28, p = 0.016; \partial = -0.875$) for the patients group only. Significant pre-post differences were also observed in the ALSSQOL-r average total score ($W = 1, p = 0.016; \partial = 0.75$), negative emotion subscale ($W = 0, p = 0.008; \partial = 1$), and religiosity/spirituality subscale ($W = 1, p = 0.031; \partial = 0.625$). The interaction ($W = 5, p = 0.078; \partial = 0.75$) and physical symptoms ($W = 0, p = 0.125; \partial = 0.75$) subscales' pre-post differences were not found significant, but still showed a large effect size, whereas the bulbar and intimacy subscales showed only a medium to small effect size. ALSAQ-5 questionnaire did not show any significant difference before and after the treatment ($W = 16, p = 0.219; \partial = 0.25$). Patient and caregiver questionnaires mean and standard deviation score, and pre to post treatment comparison in terms of statistical indices are shown in **Table 2**.

Regarding physical symptoms, both the two patients who were suffering from sleep disorders, four out of seven patients suffering from muscular pain and cramps, four out of five patients who were suffering fasciculations and each of the four patients suffering from emotional lability declared that their symptoms improved during the training period. A question on the perceived usefulness of the training, ranging from 0: "not useful at all" to 5: "very useful," showed an average score of 4.25 (SD = 0.71).

DISCUSSION

In contrast with the prolific scientific literature addressed to investigate the psychological impact of ALS on affected patients (Felgoise et al., 2010; Palmieri et al., 2010a; Lulé et al., 2012; Pagnini, 2012), the need to outline research on efficacy of psychological intervention has recently emerged (Pagnini et al., 2012). The current pilot study represents a preliminary response to such a relevant issue. Our psychological treatment, on a small patient sample size, was focused on hypnosis-based domiciliary intervention (hypnosis intervention and self-hypnosis training) and was designed to address three related goals: to assess the effect of such intervention on both reducing psychological suffering in ALS patients and giving relief from physical symptoms of the disease and consequently contributing to a positive psychological impact on caregivers. Our findings provided a clearly encouraging, although initial, support for using hypnosis to manage psychological and some physical consequences of ALS. In particular, results showed ALS patient improvements in depressive, anxiety symptomatology, and in general quality of life after 1 month treatment. Moreover, relevant pre to post treatment improvements in pain, disorders, emotional lability, and fasciculations were reported and

Table 2 | Patient pre and post treatment psychological measures.

Patient outcome variables (questionnaire scores)	Pre treatment mean (SD)	Post treatment mean (SD)	*P* (Wilcoxon W index)	Pre-post effect size (Cliff's delta)
HADS anxiety	8.12 (4.58)	4.5 (4.44)	**0.008**** (36)	−1
HADS depression	4.87 (2)	3 (2.33)	**0.016*** (28)	−0.87
ALSSAQOL-r negative emotions	7.38 (1.21)	8.44 (0.60)	**0.008**** (0)	−1
ALSSAQOL-r interaction	7.49 (1.21)	8.21 (1.17)	0.078 (5)	0.75
ALSSAQOL-r intimacy	6.21 (2.17)	6.28 (2.25)	0.437 (6.5)	0.25
ALSSAQOL-r religiousness	8.10 (2.34)	7.12 (1.76)	**0.031*** (1)	0.62
ALSSAQOL-r physical symptoms	7.06 (1.96)	7.71 (1.53)	0.125 (0)	0.75
ALSSAQOL-r bulbar functioning	6.82 (0.96)	6.95 (1.01)	0.250 (2)	0.37
ALSSAQOL-r total score	6.95 (0.99)	7.68 (0.89)	**0.016*** (1)	0.75
ALSAQ-5	45 (17.52)	41.87 (20.86)	0.219 (16)	0.25
CAREGIVER OUTCOME VARIABLES (QUESTIONNAIRE SCORES)				
HADS anxiety	8 (4.66)	6.12 (3.88)	**0.031*** (21)	−0.75
HADS depression	4.62 (4.78)	3.25 (5.33)	0.22 (22)	−0.37

HADS, hospital anxiety and depression scale; ALSSQOL-r, amyotrophic lateral sclerosis specific quality of life – revised; ALSAQ-5, 5-items amyotrophic lateral sclerosis assessment questionnaire.
*Significant results are in bold; *p < 0.05; **p < 0.01.*

attributed by patients to hypnosis-based intervention and self-hypnosis training. A satisfaction level from good to extreme was finally reported by patients involved in our study, confirming the appreciation and the applicability of the treatment. Caregiver depression and anxiety levels were observed to decrease during 1 month patient treatment, and such positive trend was attributed by them to patient gained psychological wellbeing.

Before the beginning of the treatment, two of our patients were classified as affected by "mild" depression and half of them as affected by "mild" to "severe" level of anxiety. Moreover, at the end of the treatment, the great majority of patients qualitatively showed, from a clinical point of view, a clear amelioration in such aspects, and the global psychometric analyses, calculated on HADS questionnaire scores, confirmed such clinical evidence. These findings on patient psychopathological remission, even if should be considered with caution at this preliminary stage of investigation, are undoubtedly of great interest for clinicians. As an example, depression and anxiety appear to be strongly related in the disease: Atassi et al. (2011) found that anxiety level resulted the unique ALS related symptom that can predict the occurrence of depression. Prevalence of depression in ALS has been reported as highly variable, depending by specific interview methods and assessment tools of investigation (Taylor et al., 2010), and could reach levels as high as 75% (Wicks et al., 2007). The nature of the wide difference in estimation of mood states in ALS is conceivably due also by the fact that the existential despair some patient feel in the face of their illness may be poorly described by the word of "depression." Their experience of overwhelming sense of demoralization, hopelessness, anger, and loss of meaning in the face of their mortality is something different of feel just depressed (Blackhall, 2012).

Our study highlighted also positive psychological changes in patients' quality of life after the training. Both specific ALS measures of the quality of life employed in the study, namely the ALSSAQOL (Simmons et al., 2006) and the ALSAQ-5 (Jenkinson and Fitzpatrick, 2001; Palmieri et al., 2010b), showed a clear improvement when comparing pre to post treatment mean scores. In particular, the ALSSAQOL "negative emotion" and "spiritually/religiousness" subscales reached the psychometric significance in terms of pre to post treatment improvements, while "interaction" and "physical symptoms" subscales appeared to be marginally significant. In the palliative care field, improving or maintain global quality of life is considered the crucial challenge in patients whose disease is not responsive to curative treatment as ALS. World Health Organization (WHO) scientific panel clearly established that the main objective of palliative care is achievement of the best quality of life for patients and their families until death (Doyle et al., 2003).

Interestingly, qualitative positive results have been emerged also in the disease secondary symptomatology, as it is perceived by patients. All of them declared to have perceived an improvement, from mild to extreme depending on cases, in pain, sleep disorders emotional lability, or fasciculation syndrome, whereas there was an occurrence before treatment. Since ALS devastating impact on motor system and dysphagic/dysartric, respiratory dysfunctioning, the impression is that secondary symptoms patient suffering have been underestimated by scientific attentional focus. However, recent clinical/epidemiological investigation highlighted such relevant disease consequences for patients. In particular, Chiò et al. (2012), in a wide epidemiological study, show that pain (e.g., muscle spasms, contractures, spasticity, abnormal stresses on the musculoskeletal system imposed by weak musculature) is frequent in all stages of ALS, but it often goes underrecognized and undertreated, recommending research efforts toward the appropriate ALS pain treatment. Our intervention protocol could be interpreted as addressed in such direction as well. The arena in which the hypnosis has probably proved its efficacy most adequately is, indeed, that of hypnotically induced analgesia, providing reduction of both chronic (e.g., cancer) and acute (e.g., painful medical procedure) pain (Freeman et al., 1999). As for ALS sleep disorders (resulting from factors such as reduced mobility, muscle cramps and anxiety, restless legs, and increased myoclonic activity), it may produce daytime symptoms and impairment activities of daily living and can be further affected by an increased incidence of depression (Hetta and Jansson, 1997). In emotional lability and fasciculation syndrome, respectively underestimated source of deep embarrassment (Palmieri et al., 2009) and physical discomfort (Rana et al., 2009), as well for pain and sleep disorders, seems to play a psychological etiopathogenetic non-neglectable role (Palmieri et al., 2009; Rana et al., 2009). As a final confirmation of the treatment approval, in the overall judgment of satisfaction we asked to the patients, all of them declared a good from extreme satisfaction.

Relevant improvement in terms of depression and anxiety reduction, measured with the same patient assessment tools, was reported by caregivers. When asked, the great majority of them stated they were satisfied of hypnotic treatment and self-hypnosis training patient positive outcome, and that the improvement on patient psychological functioning, according to them, has lead to a probable effect on their own mood tone as well. The impact of patient suffering on family caregivers is a further understudied but important topic. Associations of patient distress with caregiver negative affect has recently been shown by some authors (Chiò et al., 2005; Gauthier et al., 2007; Boerner and Mock, 2012). On the other hand, patient's loss of physical functions was positively related with caregiver burden, anxiety, and somatic expression of depression (Pagnini et al., 2010a).

Our findings on treatment efficacy, in their globality, could appear surprising, but it should be mentioned the number of Authors who have recently enhanced the potentiality of hypnosis-based treatment, and, in general, mind-body techniques, leading to a rapid improvement on anxiety, and depression especially when they are reactive to a medical condition (Shih et al., 2009; Willemsen et al., 2010; Plaskota et al., 2012). Specifically, in the realm of neurological disorders, hypnosis has been reported as an effective adjunctive treatment for organic brain damage (Sullivan et al., 1974), Parkinson disease (Wain et al., 1990), stroke (Holroyd and Hill, 1989), peripheral nerve lesions (Pajntar et al., 1980), cases of organic paralysis (Lucas et al., 1981), various type of dystonia (De Benedittis, 1996), multiple sclerosis (Jensen et al., 2009, 2011), migraine (Ezra et al., 2012), and fibromialgy (Bernardy et al., 2011).

Although our results show promising and exciting insights, the study suffers of a number of limitations, including the typical ones that naturally characterize pilot studies. Primary among them, the small sample size have limited our ability to detect whole treatment effect from a psychometric point of view. A further criticism is the lack of a different treatment condition (e.g., a different mind-body intervention or psychopharmacological treatment) that controls for the effects of time, placebo condition, and expectancy effect. Lastly, additional measurement at pre treatment level in order to investigate psychological traits such as personality profile, attachment style and hypnotic absorption, dissociation, and suggestion ability could have been undoubtedly important variables to be compared with the treatment efficacy (Primavera and Patterson, 1991). Moreover it will be relevant to consider the frequency of self-hypnosis and verify its role in the efficacy of this kind of treatment with ALS patients.

In conclusion, our general aim was to lay some foundations to develop, in a future perspective, a protocol of eligible psychological interventions for ALS, "useful for a meaningful improvement in quality of life or reduction in psychological distress in patients and their caregivers" (Pagnini et al., 2012) and suitable to be proposed to patients with a such peculiar condition, involving bulbar dysfunctions and that can eventually lead to a locked-in syndrome. Despite the pilot study limitations, the findings provide clear support for the potential efficacy of hypnosis-based intervention to cope with devastating consequences of ALS. Further longitudinal researches using larger sample to help determine the reliability of the current findings are warranted.

ACKNOWLEDGMENTS

We are grateful for their help to Francesca Colombo, Carla D'Ascenzo, Giorgia Querin, Marica Scremin, Maria Sorce, without whom this study would not have been realizable.

REFERENCES

Atassi, N., Cook, A., Pineda, C. M. E., Yerramilli-Rao, P., Pulley, D., and Cudkowicz, M. (2011). Depres- sion in amyotrophic lateral scle- rosis. *Amyotroph. Lateral Scler.* 12, 109–112.

Bandura, A. (1997). *Self Efficacy: The Exercise of Control.* New York: WH Freeman and Company.

Beghi, E., Chiò, A., Couratier, P., Este- ban, J., Hardiman, O., Logroscino, G., et al. (2011). The epidemiology and treatment of ALS: focus on the heterogeneity of the disease and crit- ical appraisal of therapeutic trials. *Amyotroph. Lateral Scler.* 12, 1–10.

Bernardy, K., Fuber, N., Klose, P., and Hauser, W. (2011). Efficacy of hypnosis/guided imagery in fibromyal- gia syndrome–a systematic review and meta-analysis of controlled tri- als. *BMC Musculoskeletal Disord.* 12, 133.

Bjelland, I., Dahl, A. A., Haug, T. T., and Neckelmann, D. (2002). The validity of the hospital anxiety and depression scale: an updated liter- ature review. *J. Psychosom. Res.* 52, 69–77.

Blackhall, L. J. (2012). Amyotrophic lateral sclerosis and palliative care: where we are, and the road ahead. *Muscle Nerve* 45, 311–318.

Boerner, K., and Mock, S. E. (2012). Impact of patient suf- fering on caregiver well-being: the case of amyotrophic lateral sclerosis patients and their caregivers. *Psychol. Health Med.* 17, 457–466.

Brooks, B. R., Miller, R. G., Swash, M., and Munsat, T. L. (2000). El escorial revisited: revised criteria for the diagnosis of amyotrophic lateral sclerosis. *Amyotroph. Lateral Scler.* 1, 293–299.

Cedarbaum, J. M., Stambler, N., Malta, E., Fuller, C., Hilt, D., Thurmond, B., et al. (1999). The ALSFRS-R: a revised ALS functional rating scale that incorporates assessments of res- piratory function. *J. Neurol. Sci.* 169, 13–21.

Chiò, A., Canosa, A., Gallo, S., Moglia, C., Ilardi, A., Cammarosano, S., et al. (2012). Pain in amyotrophic lat- eral sclerosis: a population-based controlled study. *Eur. J. Neurol.* 19, 551–555.

Chiò, A., Gauthier, A., Calvo, A., Ghiglione, P., and Mutani, R. (2005). Caregiver burden and patients' per- ception of being a burden in ALS. *Neurology* 64, 1780–1782.

Cliff, N. (1993). Dominance statistics: ordinal analyses to answer ordinal questions. *Psychol. Bull.* 114, 494–509.

Cohen, J. (1988). Statistical power analysis for the behavioral sciences. Hillsdale: Lawrence Erlbaum Asso- ciates.

De Benedittis, G. (1996). Hypnosis and spasmodic torticollis – Report of four cases: a brief communica- tion. *Int. J. Clin. Exp. Hypn.* 44, 292–306.

De Carvalho, M., and Swash, M. (2012). Fasciculation potentials: still mysterious. *Clin. Neurophysiol.* 123, 227–228.

Doyle, D., Hanks, G., and Macdon- ald, N. (2003). "Introduction," in *Oxford Textbook of Pallia- tive Medicine,* eds D. Doyle, G. Hanks and N. Macdonald, 3rd Edn (Oxford: Oxford University Press).

Ezra, Y., Gotkine, M., Goldman, S., Ada- han, H. M., and Ben-Hur, T. (2012). Hypnotic relaxation vs amitripty- line for tension-type headache: let the patient choose. *Headache* 52, 785–791.

Felgoise, S. H., Chakraborty, B. H., Bond, E., Rodriguez, J., Bremer, B. A., Walsh, S. M., et al. (2010). Psycho- logical morbidity in ALS: the impor- tance of psychological assessment beyond depression alone. *Amy- otroph. Lateral Scler.* 11, 351–358.

Freeman, T. B., Vawter, D. E., Leaver- ton, P. E., Godbold, J. H., Hauser, R. A., Goetz, C. G., et al. (1999). Use of placebo surgery in controlled trials of a cellular-based therapy for Parkinson's disease. *N. Engl. J. Med.* 341, 988-992.

Gauthier, A., Vignola, A., Calvo, A., Cav- allo, E., Moglia, C., Sellitti, L., et al. (2007). A longitudinal study on quality of life and depression in ALS patient-caregiver couples. *Neurology* 68, 923-926.

Hess, M. R., and Kromrey, J. D. (2004). "Robust confidence intervals for effect sizes: a comparative study of Cohen's d and Cliff's delta under non-normality and heterogeneous variances," in *Annual Meeting of the American Educational Research Asso- ciation*, San Diego.

Hetta, J., and Jansson, I. (1997). Sleep in patients with amyotrophic lat- eral sclerosis. *J. Neurol.* 244 (Suppl), S7–S9.

Holroyd, J., and Hill, A. (1989). Pushing the limits of recovery: hypnotherapy with a stroke patient. *Int. J. Clin. Exp. Hypn.* 37, 120–128.

Jenkinson, C., and Fitzpatrick, R. (2001). Reduced item set for the amyotrophic lateral sclerosis assess- ment questionnaire: development and validation of the ALSAQ-5. *J. Neurol. Neurosurg. Psychiatr.* 70, 70–73.

Jensen, M. P., Barber, J., Romano, J. M., Molton, I. R., Raichle, K. A., Osborne, T. L., et al. (2009). A comparison of self-hypnosis ver- sus progressive muscle relaxation in patients with multiple sclerosis and chronic pain. *Int. J. Clin. Exp. Hypn.* 57, 198–221.

Jensen, M. P., Ehde, D. M., Gertz, K. J., Stoelb, B. L., Dillworth, T. M., Hirsh, A. T., et al. (2011). Effects of self-hypnosis training and cognitive restructuring on daily pain intensity and catastrophizing in individuals with multiple sclerosis and chronic pain. *Int. J. Clin. Exp. Hypn.* 59, 45–63.

Lucas, D., Stratis, D. J., and Deniz, S. (1981). From the clinic: hypno- sis in conjunction with corrective therapy in a quadriplegic patient: a case report. *Am. Correct. Ther. J.* 35, 116–120.

Lulé, D., Pauli, S., Altintas, E., Singer, U., Merk, T., Uttner, I., et al. (2012). Emotional adjustment in amyotrophic lateral sclerosis (ALS). *J. Neurol.* 259, 334–341.

McDonald, E. R., Wiedenfeld, S. A., Hil-lel, A., Carpenter, C. L., and Wal- ter, R. A. (1994). Survival in amy- otrophic lateral sclerosis: the role of psychological factors. *Arch. Neurol.* 51, 17–23.

Pagnini, F. (2012). Psychological wellbeing and quality of life in amyotrophic lateral sclero- sis: a review. *Int. J. Psychol.* doi:10.1080/00207594.2012.691977

Pagnini, F., Lunetta, C., Banfi, P., Rossi, G., Fossati, F., Marconi, A., et al. (2011a). Pain in amy- otrophic lateral sclerosis: a psycho- logical perspective. *Neurol. Sci.* 33, 1–4.

Pagnini, F., Lunetta, C., Rossi, G., Banfi, P., Gorni, K., Cellotto, N., et al. (2011b). Existential well-being and spirituality of individuals with amy- otrophic lateral sclerosis is related to psychological well-being of their caregivers. *Amyotroph. Lateral Scler.* 12, 105–108.

Pagnini, F., Rossi, G., Lunetta, C., Banfi, P., Castelnuovo, G., Corbo, M., et al. (2010a). Burden, depres- sion, and anxiety in caregivers of people with amyotrophic lateral sclerosis. *Psychol. Health Med.* 15, 685–693.

Pagnini, F., Simmons, Z., Felgoise, S., Lunetta, C., and Corbo, M. (2010b). "Italian validation of Amyotrophic Lateral Sclerosis Specific Quality of Life – Revised (ALSSQOL-R): a comparison between US and Italian samples," in *21th International Sym- posium on ALS/MND*, Orlando.

Pagnini, F., Simmons, Z., Corbo, M., and Molinari, E. (2012). Amy- otrophic lateral sclerosis: time for research on psychological interven- tion? *Amyotroph. Lateral Scler.* 13, 416–417.

Pajntar, M., Jeglic, A., Stefancic, M., and Vodovnik, L. (1980). Improve- ments of motor response by means of hypnosis in patients with periph- eral nerve lesions. *Int. J. Clin. Exp. Hypn.* 28, 16–26.

Palmieri, A., Abrahams, S., Sorarù, G., Mattiuzzi, L., D'ascenzo, C., Pego- raro, E., et al. (2009). Emotional Lability in MND: relationship to cognition and psychopathology and impact on caregivers. *J. Neurol. Sci.* 278, 16–20.

Palmieri, A., Sorarù, G., Albertini, E., Semenza, C., Vottero-Ris, F., D'ascenzo, C., et al. (2010a). Psy- chopathological features and suici- dal ideation in amyotrophic lateral sclerosis patients. *Neurol. Sci.* 31, 735–740.

Palmieri, A., Sorarú, G., Lombardi, L., D'ascenzo, C., Baggio, L., Ermani, M., et al. (2010b). Quality of life and motor impairment in ALS: Italian validation of ALSAQ. *Neurol. Res.* 32, 32–40.

Plaskota, M., Lucas, C., Pizzoferro, K., Saini, T., Evans, R., and Cook, K. (2012). A hypnotherapy interven- tion for the treatment of anxiety in patients with cancer receiving pal- liative care. *Int. J. Palliat. Nurs.* 18, 69–75.

Primavera, J. P., and Patterson, S. (1991). A tape-recorded test of hypnotic susceptibility for screening headache patients: a feasibility study of the Harvard group scale of hypnotic suscep- tibility, form A. *Headache* 31, 619–621.

Rana, S., Schramke, C., Sangha, A., and Karpinski, A. (2009). Compar- ison of psychosocial factors between patients with benign fasciculations and those with amyotrophic lateral sclerosis. *Ann. Indian Acad. Neurol.* 12, 108–110.

Shih, M., Yang, Y. H., and Koo, M. (2009). A meta-analysis of hypnosis in the treatment of depressive symp- toms: a brief communication. *Int. J. Clin. Exp. Hypn.* 57, 431–442.

Simmons, Z., Felgoise, S. H., Bremer, B. A., Walsh, S. M., Hufford, D. J., Bromberg, M. B., et al. (2006). The ALSSQOL: balancing physical and nonphysical factors in assessing quality of life in ALS. *Neurology* 67, 1659–1664.

Sullivan, D. S., Johnson, A., and Bratkovitch, J. (1974). Reduction of behavioral deficit in organic brain damage by use of hypnosis. *J. Clin. Psychol.* 30, 96–98.

Taylor, L., Wicks, P., Leigh, P. N., and Goldstein, L. H. (2010). Prevalence of depression in amyotrophic lateral sclerosis and other motor disorders. *Eur. J. Neurol.* 17, 1047–1053.

Vianello, A., Arcaro, G., Palmieri, A., Ermani, M., Braccioni, F., Gallan, F., et al. (2011). Survival and quality of life after tracheostomy for acute respiratory failure in patients with amyotrophic lateral sclerosis. *J. Crit. Care* 26, 329.

Wahbeh, H., Elsas, S. M., and Oken, B. S. (2008). Mind-body interventions: applications in neurology. *Neurology* 70, 2321–2328.

Wain, H. J., Amen, D., and Jabbari, B. (1990). The effects of hypno- sis on a Parkinsonian tremor: case report with polygraph/EEG record- ings. *Am. J. Clin. Hypn.* 33, 94–98.

Wicks, P., Abrahams, S., Masi, D., Hejda-Forde, S., Leigh, P. N., and Goldstein, L. H. (2007). Prevalence of depres- sion in a 12-month consecutive sam- ple of patients with ALS. *Eur. J. Neurol.* 14, 993–1001.

Willemsen, R., Haentjens, P., Roseeuw, D., and Vanderlinden, J. (2010). Hypnosis in refractory alopecia areata significantly improves depres- sion, anxiety, and life quality but not hair regrowth. *J. Am. Acad. Derma- tol.* 62, 517–518.

Zigmond, A. S., and Snaith, R. P. (1983). The hospital anxiety and depres- sion scale. *Acta Psychiatr. Scand.* 67, 361–370.

18

Differential effects on KCC2 expression and spasticity of ALS and traumatic injuries to motoneurons

Laura Mòdol†, Renzo Mancuso†, Albert Alé, Isaac Francos-Quijorna and Xavier Navarro*

Department of Cell Biology, Physiology, and Immunology, Centro de Investigación Biomédica en Red sobre Enfermedades Neurodegenerativas, Institute of Neurosciences, Universitat Autònoma de Barcelona, Bellaterra, Spain

Edited by:
Ricardo Tapia, Universidad Nacional Autónoma de México, Mexico

Reviewed by:
Laurent Vinay, CNRS and Aix-Marseille Université, France
Brigitte Pettmann, Institut National de la Santé et de la Recherche Médicale, France

***Correspondence:**
Xavier Navarro, Unitat de Fisiologia Mèdica, Facultad de Medicina, Edifici M, Universitat Autònoma de Barcelona, E-08193 Bellaterra, Spain
e-mail: xavier.navarro@uab.cat

† These authors have contributed equally to this work.

Amyotrophic lateral sclerosis (ALS) is a neurodegenerative disease manifested by progressive muscle atrophy and paralysis due to the loss of upper and lower motoneurons (MN). Spasticity appears in ALS patients leading to further disabling consequences. Loss of the inhibitory tone induced by downregulation of the potassium chloride cotransporter 2 (KCC2) in MN has been proposed to importantly contribute to the spastic behavior after spinal cord injury (SCI). The aim of the present study was to test whether the alterations in the expression of KCC2 are linked to the appearance of spasticity in the SOD^{G93A} ALS murine model. We compared SOD^{G93A} mice to wild type mice subjected to SCI to mimic the spinal MN disconnection from motor descending pathways, and to sciatic nerve lesion to mimic the loss of MN connectivity to muscle. Electrophysiological results show that loss of motor function is observed at presymptomatic stage (8 weeks) in SOD^{G93A} mice but hyperreflexia and spasticity do not appear until a late stage (16 weeks). However, KCC2 was not downregulated despite MN suffered disconnection both from muscles and upper MNs. Further experiments revealed decreased gephyrin expression, as a general marker of inhibitory systems, accompanied by a reduction in the number of Renshaw interneurons. Moreover, 5-HT fibers were increased in the ventral horn of the lumbar spinal cord at late stage of disease progression in $SOD1^{G93A}$ mice. Taken together, the present results indicate that spasticity appears late in the ALS model, and may be mediated by a decrease in inhibitory interneurons and an increase of 5-HT transmission, while the absence of down-regulation of KCC2 could rather indicate an inability of MNs to respond to insults.

Keywords: motoneuron disease, spasticity, hypereflexia, KCC2 transporter, $SOD1^{G93A}$ mice

INTRODUCTION

Amyotrophic lateral sclerosis (ALS) is an adult onset neurodegenerative disorder that clinically manifests by progressive muscle atrophy and paralysis (Wijesekera and Leigh, 2009) due to the loss of upper and lower motoneurons (MN). The 90% of ALS cases are sporadic with unknown etiology whereas the remaining 10% are inherited forms, caused by genetic mutations. Among these, mutations in the gene encoding for the enzyme Cu/Zn superoxide dismutase 1 (SOD1) have been reported in about 20% of the patients (Rosen, 1993). Several transgenic animal models of ALS have been developed during the last decades. The most widely used is a transgenic mouse that over-expresses the human mutated form of the *sod1* gene with a glycine to alanine conversion at the 93rd codon (Ripps et al., 1995). This model recapitulates most relevant clinical and histopathological features of both familial and sporadic forms of the human disease (Ripps et al., 1995). Moreover, it has been recently reported that alterations of SOD1 protein are also present in sporadic ALS cases, increasing the interest of this model (Bosco et al., 2010).

Spasticity is a secondary complication of different upper MN syndromes characterized by a velocity-dependent increase in muscle tone resulting from hyperexcitability of the stretch reflex (Lance, 1980). This phenomenon is present in ALS patients and leads to important disabling complications that compromise their manual dexterity and gait (Wijesekera and Leigh, 2009; Kiernan et al., 2011). It has been hypothesized that spasticity may occur due to the loss of upper MN and/or alterations of intraspinal motor circuitry (Schütz, 2005; Chang and Martin, 2009, 2011; Dentel et al., 2013). The appearance of spasticity has also been described in the SOD1 ALS murine model (Dentel et al., 2013). In fact, despite the remaining hindlimb muscle innervation at the end stage of the disease could be enough to allow movement, the animals appear paralyzed due to spastic paresis (Mancuso et al., 2011).

Recent studies have demonstrated the relevance of MN increased excitability for the appearance of spasticity after traumatic injuries to the spinal cord (Lu et al., 2008; Boulenguez et al., 2010; Kakinohana et al., 2012; Bos et al., 2013). Rather than be mediated by an increase in excitatory transmission, these studies postulated that the loss of the inhibitory tone below the lesion is mediated by downregulation of the potassium chloride cotransporter 2 (KCC2) in spinal MNs (Boulenguez et al., 2010; Bos et al., 2013). Modulation of the inhibitory amino acids (GABA and glycine) response is determined by changes in the intracellular chloride concentration $[Cl_i^-]$. KCC2 is the main chloride extruder expressed in adult neurons, being responsible for the maintenance of the low $[Cl_i^-]$ (Ganguly et al., 2001; Rivera et al., 2002; Wang et al., 2002; Payne et al., 2003; Stein et al., 2004;

Bray and Mynlieff, 2009). At birth, when GABA and glycine responses are excitatory (Ben-Ari et al., 2007), KCC2 is barely detectable but increases progressively during the early post-natal days of the murine life (Rivera et al., 1999; Wang et al., 2002; Payne et al., 2003). Although excitatory actions of GABA and glycine during early development are relevant for the establishment of circuitry in the spinal cord and the development of motor functional patterns (Stil et al., 2011), the increased excitability induced by KCC2 down regulation in the adult spinal cord after trauma has also been linked to alterations of locomotor pattern, chronic pain and spasticity (Boulenguez et al., 2010; Bos et al., 2013).

In the present experiment, we tested whether changes in the expression of KCC2 in the SOD^{G93A} ALS model are of relevance for the appearance of spasticity at late stages of the disease process. For assessing the potential contributing mechanisms we compared the changes in KCC2 induced by SCI and by peripheral nerve lesions in wild type mice.

MATERIAL AND METHODS

TRANSGENIC SOD1^{G93A} MICE

Transgenic mice with the G93A human SOD1 mutation [B6SJL-Tg(SOD1-G93A)1Gur] were obtained from the Jackson Laboratory (Bar Harbor, ME, USA), and maintained at the Animal Service of the Universidad de Zaragoza. Hemizygotes B6SJL SOD1^{G93A} males were obtained by crossing with B6SJL females from the CBATEG (Bellaterra, Spain). The offspring was identified by PCR amplification of DNA extracted from the tail tissue. All experimental procedures were approved by the Ethics Committee of the Universitat Autònoma de Barcelona, where the animal experiments were performed, and followed the guidelines of the European Commission on Animal Care and the Canadian Council on Animal Care.

SURGICAL PROCEDURES

Adult (8–10 weeks old) female wild type C57BL/6 mice (Charles River) were anesthetized by i.p. injection of ketamine (10 mg/kg; Imalgene) and xylazine (1 mg/kg; Rompun). For the nerve crush, the sciatic nerve was exposed at the mid-thigh and subjected to a crush during 30 s for three times in succession with a Dumont no. 5 forceps. For SCI a laminectomy at the 11th thoracic vertebra was performed. The exposed spinal cord was contused using the Infinite Horizon Impactor device (Precision Scientific Instrumentation), using a force of 50 kdynes and with tissue displacement ranging between 500 and 700 μm. After injury, the skin was sutured and animals were left to recover on a hot pad and returned to their home cages with free access to food and water.

FUNCTIONAL ASSESSMENT

Locomotors recovery was evaluated in an open-field test using the nine-point Basso Mouse Scale (BMS) (Basso et al., 2006; Klopstein et al., 2012), which was specifically developed for locomotors testing after spinal cord contusion injuries in mice. The BMS analysis of hindlimb movements and coordination was performed by two independent researchers and the consensus score was taken. The final score is presented as mean ± s.e.m.

NERVE CONDUCTION TESTS

The sciatic nerve was stimulated percutaneously by means of single pulses of 0.02 ms duration (Grass S88) delivered through a pair of needle electrodes placed at the sciatic notch. The compound muscle action potential (CMAP, M wave) and the reflex H wave were recorded from the tibial anterior (TA) and the plantar (interpose) muscles with microneedle electrodes (Valero-Cabré and Navarro, 2001; Mancuso et al., 2011). For evaluation of the motor central pathways, motor evoked potentials (MEP) were recorded from the same muscles in response to transcranial electrical stimulation of the motor cortex by single rectangular pulses of 0.1 ms duration, delivered through needle electrodes inserted subcutaneously, the cathode over the skull overlaying the sensorimotor cortex and the anode at the nose (García-Alías et al., 2003; Mancuso et al., 2011). All potentials were amplified and displayed on a digital oscilloscope (Tektronix 450S) at settings appropriate to measure the amplitude from baseline to the maximal negative peak. To ensure reproducibility, the recording needles were placed under microscope to secure the same placement on all animals guided by anatomical landmarks. During the tests, the mice body temperature was kept constant by means of a thermostated heating pad.

HISTOLOGY

SOD^{G93A} mice at 8, 12 and 16 weeks of age, and sciatic nerve crushed (at 7 days post injury, dpi) and spinal cord injured (at 28 dpi) wild type mice were included in the histological analysis (4–5 mice per group). Animals were transcardially perused with 4% paraformaldehyde in PBS and the lumbar segment of the spinal cord was harvested, post-fixed overnight, and cryopreserved in 30% sucrose. Transverse 40-μm thick sections were serially cut with a cry tome (Lexica) between L2 and L5 segmental levels. Spinal cord slices were sequentially collected free-floating in Olmos medium.

For immunohistochemistry, sections were blocked with PBS-Triton 0.3%-normal donkey serum 5% and incubated overnight at 4°C with primary antibodies: rabbit anti-KCC2 (KCC2, 1:500, Millipore), mouse anti-neurofilament non-phosphorylated heavy chain (SMI-32, 1:1000, Covance), mouse anti-activating transcription factor 3 (ATF3, 1:500, Abeam), rabbit anti-ionized calcium binding adaptor molecule 1 (Ibal, 1:1000, Wako), rabbit anti-serotonin (5-HT, 1:5000, Sigma) or rabbit anti-calbindin (1:200, Chemicon). After washes, sections were incubated for 1 h at room temperature with Alexi 488 or Alexi 594 conjugated secondary antibody (1:200; Life Science). For co-localization, spinal NMS were labeled with NeuroTrace 500/525 Green Fluorescent Nissl (1:200, Life Science).

To quantify microglial immunoreactivity, microphotographs of the ventral horn gray matter were taken at ×400 and, after defining the threshold for background correction, the integrated density of Ibal labeling was measured using ImageJ software (Mancuso et al., 2012). The integrated density is the area above the threshold for the mean density minus the background.

PROTEIN EXTRACTION AND WESTERN BLOT

For protein extraction, another subset of mice ($n = 3$–4) of the same experimental groups, i.e., SOD^{G93A} mice at 8, 12 or 16 weeks of age, mice with sciatic nerve crush and mice with SCI, were anesthetized and decapitated. The lumbar spinal cord was removed and divided into quarters to isolate the ventral quadrants. In animals that received a sciatic nerve crush, only the ventral horn of the lesioned side was used for protein extraction. Samples were prepared for protein extraction and homogenized in modified RIPA buffer (50 mom Tris–HCl pH 7.5, 1% Triton X-100, 0.5% sodium deoxycholate, 0.2% SDS, 100 mM NaCl, 1 mM EDTA) adding 10 µl/ml of Protease Inhibitor cocktail (Sigma) and PhosphoSTOP phosphatase inhibitor cocktail (Roche). After clearance, protein concentration was measured by Lowry assay (Bio-Rad, Dc protein assay).

Western blots were performed by loading 20 µg of protein of each sample in SDS-poliacrylamide gels. The transfer buffer was 25 mM trizma-base, 192 mM glycine, 20% (v/v) methanol, pH 8.4. The membranes were blocked with 5% BSA in PBS plus 0.1% Tween-20 for 1 h, and then incubated with primary antibodies at 4°C overnight. The primary antibodies used were: mouse anti-GAPDH (1:20000, Millipore), rabbit anti-phospho-^{Ser940} KCC2 (1:1000, Phosphosolutions), rabbit anti-KCC2 (1:500, Millipore), mouse anti-gephyrin (1:1000, BD Bioscience) and anti-GAD65/67 (1:1000, Abcam). Horseradish peroxidase–coupled secondary antibody (1:5000, Vector) incubation was performed for 1 h at room temperature. The membranes were visualized using enhanced chemiluminiscence method and the images were collected and analyzed with a Gene Genome apparatus and Gene Snap and Gene Tools software (Signee), respectively.

STATISTICAL ANALYSIS

Data are expressed as mean ± s.e.m. Electrophysiological test results were statistically analyzed using repeated measurements and One-Way ANOVA, applying Turkey *post-hoc* test when necessary. For immunobloting and histological data we used Mann-Whitney (for two groups comparison) or Kruskal-Wallis tests (for multiple groups comparison) followed by Dunn's *post-hoc* test (Prism 6 software; Graphpad). The level of significance was set at $p < 0.05$.

RESULTS

SOD1^{G93A} ANIMALS SHOW HYPERREFLEXIA AND SPASTICITY AT LATE STAGES OF DISEASE PROGRESSION

We first evaluated peripheral motor nerve conduction to assess the progressive muscle denervation by stimulating the sciatic nerve and recording in TA and plantar muscles (Mancuso et al., 2011). Results revealed a different pattern of muscle denervation in the two tested muscles; the plantar muscle CMAP showed a fast drop in amplitude at 12 weeks of age, whereas the TA CMAP progressively decreased in amplitude from 8 weeks of age (**Figure 1A**). The monosynaptic spinal reflex activity was assessed by the H/M ratio (Mancuso et al., 2011). Results evidenced a significant increase of the H/M ratio in both tested muscles ($p < 0.01$) at the end stage of the disease (16 weeks), coincident with the spastic condition (**Figure 1A**). **Figure 1B** shows representative recordings to illustrate the increased H/M ratio in the plantar muscle of 16 weeks aged SOD1^{G93A} mice. Finally, we assessed central motor conduction by means of MEPs to evaluate the state of the spinal motor descending pathways. Results showed a significant reduction of MEPs amplitude from 12 weeks of age both in TA and plantar muscles (**Figure 1A**).

SPINAL CORD INJURY CAUSES LOCOMOTOR IMPAIRMENT AND HYPERREFLEXIA

We evaluated the locomotor function of wild type mice after SCI by means of the BMS score (Basso et al., 2006; Klopstein et al., 2012). Results revealed that injured mice achieved less than 3 over the 9 points scale at 28 days, evidencing the inability to support their own weight (**Figure 1C**). Then, we assessed central motor conduction preservation and hyperreflexia of the animals at 28 dpi. Results showed a significant reduction of MEPs and an increased H/M ratio, coincident with the spastic behavior in the animals' hindlimbs (**Figure 1C**).

KCC2 EXPRESSION IS NOT ALTERED IN LUMBAR SPINAL MNs OF SOD1^{G93A} ANIMALS

We did not observe changes in the KCC2 oligomer/monomer ratio (**Figures 2A,B**) in SOD1^{G93A} mice at 8, 12, or 16 weeks of age compared to wild type mice. Accordingly, no significant changes in the phosphorylated form were observed in SOD1^{G93A} mice (**Figures 2A,B**). We then characterized the localization of KCC2 by immunohistochemistry in lumbar MNs of SOD1^{G93A} mice along disease progression. Confocal images showed no changes in subcellular localization of KCC2 at 8, 12 and 16 weeks of age (**Figure 2C**). In fact, co-labeling of KCC2 and SMI-32 confirmed that KCC2 remained in the MNs plasma membrane at late stages of the disease, as no co-localization of both markers was observed in the samples of SOD1^{G93A} mice, even in degenerating MNs (**Figure 3**). Taken together, these findings indicate that KCC2 expression and localization in the MN plasma membrane remains unchanged during ALS disease progression.

REDUCED ACTIVE FORM OF KCC2 IN LUMBAR SPINAL MNs AFTER SCI

We first examined KCC2 expression by western blotting in the lumbar ventral spinal cord of animals with SCI at 28 dpi. Compared to naïve animals, we observed a slight reduction of total KCC2 after SCI (around 20%), although the difference did not reach statistical significance ($p = 0.06$, data not shown). This tendency is in agreement with previously reported results by. Boulenguez et al. (2010) after SCI in the rat. To check the activation state of the KCC2, we also performed western blotting for the phosphorylated form of the KCC2 (pKCC2) with a specific antibody against phopho-Ser^{940}. In contrast to total KCC2 expression, the phosphorylated form was decreased after SCI compared to control samples ($p < 0.05$; **Figures 4A,B**). Since it has been previously described that KCC2 oligomer/monomer ratio is increased at maturity and correlates with KCC2 activation (Blaesse et al., 2006; Boulenguez et al., 2010; Bos et al., 2013), we also analyzed the ratio between the oligomeric and monomeric states of the KCC2. The results showed a significant reduction of the oligomer/monomer ratio (**Figures 4A,B**; $p < 0.05$), confirming the above results on the reduction of the pKCC2 expression.

Confocal immunohistochemical images confirmed KCC2 staining into the MNs cytoplasm. This labeling pattern contrasted

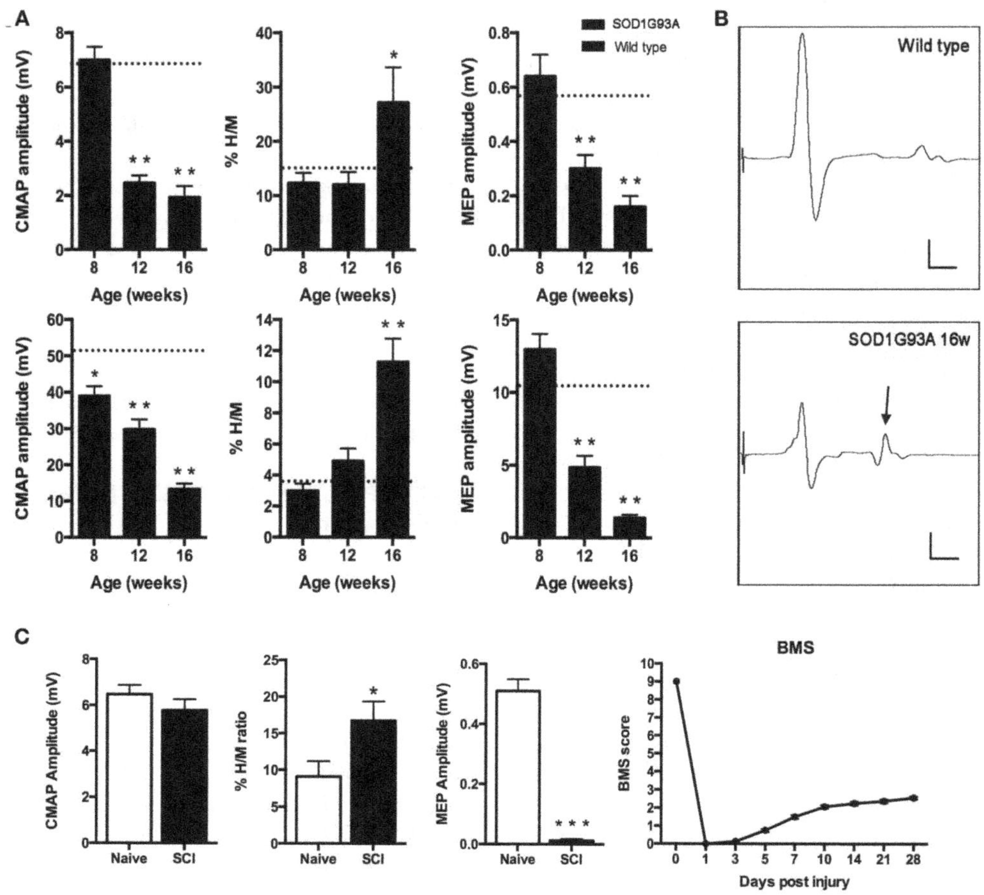

FIGURE 1 | (A,B) Peripheral and central motor conduction along disease progression in SOD1^{G93A} mice. **(A)** Plantar (upper) and tibialis anterior (lower) compound muscle action potential (CMAP) amplitude, %H/M ratio and motor evoked potentials (MEP) amplitudes of SOD1^{G93A} animals at 8, 12, and 16 weeks of age. Values are represented as mean ± s.e.m. Dashed line represents wild type mean value for each parameter. $^{*}p < 0.05$; $^{**}p < 0.01$ vs. wild type littermates. **(B)** Representative recordings of plantar muscle CMAPs. Note the relative increase of the H wave (arrow) reflecting hyperreflexia. Scale bars: 2 mV; 2 ms. **(C)** Functional assessment of SCI animals. Compound muscle action potential (CMAP) amplitude of the plantar muscle. Hyperreflexia evaluated by means of the %H/M ratio recorded in the plantar muscle after sciatic nerve stimulation. $^{*}p < 0.05$ vs. naïve mice. The lack of differences indicates that the increased %H/M ratio is not due to CMAP alterations. Motor evoked potentials (MEP) amplitude. BMS score as a measure of the locomotor capacity of the animals in the open field walking test. Note that at 28 dpi the score remains below 3, indicating that animals cannot support their own weight.

to the uniform band surrounding MNs in naïve animals (**Figure 4C**). Together, these results indicate that the translocation of KCC2 to the plasma membrane of MN is reduced after SCI.

REDUCED ACTIVE FORM OF KCC2 IS OBSERVED IN LUMBAR SPINAL MNs AFTER SCIATIC NERVE CRUSH

In order to mimic the muscle denervation that occurs early in the ALS progression, we performed a sciatic nerve crush to analyze early changes of KCC2 after MN axotomy. Results of western blotting showed a significant decrease of the KCC2 oligomer/monomer ratio and of the phosphorylated active form of KCC2 in the injured side of the spinal cord in contrast to naïve animals (**Figures 4A,B**, $p < 0.01$). Immunohistochemical labeling confirmed that after sciatic nerve crush KCC2 was internalized into the MNs cytoplasm in the injured side forming intracellular clusters. In contrast, KCC2 localization in intact animals, showed a well-defined line surrounding MNs indicating a preferably membrane location of KCC2 in non-injured conditions (**Figure 4C**).

ABSENCE OF DOWN-REGULATION KCC2 RESPONSE TO AXONAL INSULT IN ALS MNs

We then studied the KCC2 response in injured MNs, identified by labeling the activation transcription factor 3 (ATF3) as a marked of axonal damage (Tsujino et al., 2000), to assess whether KCC2 behave similarly between ALS and axotomized MNs. After sciatic nerve crush, KCC2 cytoplasmic inclusions were found into injured ATF3-positive MNs. On the contrary, the same analysis performed on SOD1^{G93A} ventral spinal cord revealed that KCC2 localization remained normal even if MNs expressed ATF3 (**Figure 5**). These results suggest an altered response regarding KCC2 expression of ALS MNs after muscle denervation.

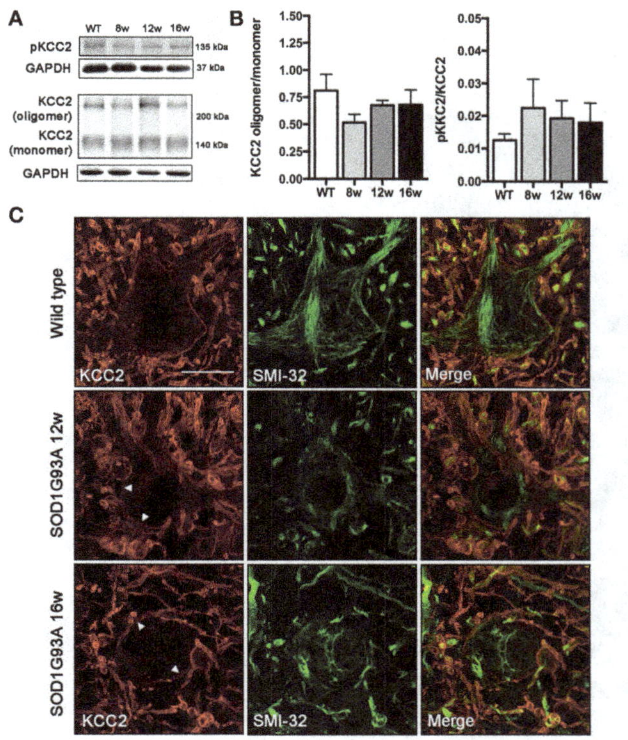

FIGURE 2 | Analysis of KCC2 and phopho-KCC2 expression in the ventral spinal cord of SOD1^{G93A} mice at 8, 12, and 16 weeks of age. (A) Representative blots of phopho-KCC2 and total KCC2 (on both monomeric and oligomeric states). **(B)** KCC2 western blots quantifications. Graphs represent the ratio between the oligomeric KCC2 (functional state) vs. monomeric KCC2 and the phopho-KCC2 (active form) vs. monomeric KCC2. Note the lack of significant differences between SOD1^{G93A} at any age and wild type littermates. Data are represented as mean ± s.e.m. **(C)** Confocal images of wild type and SOD1^{G93A} L4 spinal MNs confirmed the maintenance of membrane-bound (active) KCC2 in transgenic animals along disease progression, even in abnormal MNs at 16 weeks of age. Arrowheads show the membrane bound KCC2 in SOD1^{G93A} L4 spinal MNs. Scale bar 20 μm.

MICROGLIAL REACTIVITY IS INCREASED IN SOD1^{G93A} AND AFTER SCIATIC NERVE CRUSH AND SCI

It has been reported that microglial cells play a central role in the pathway that leads to KCC2 dephosphorylation (Coull et al., 2005; Ferrini et al., 2013). Thus, we evaluated the microglial activation by immunohistochemistry in SOD1^{G93A} , sciatic nerve crush and SCI animals. We focused on the L4-L5 lamina IX in order to analyze the reaction of the microglial cells adjacent to MNs. Results revealed a progressive increase of microglial immunoreactivity in SOD1^{G93A} mice from 8 to 16 weeks of age. On the other hand, SCI and sciatic nerve crush mice also showed an increase in Iba1 reactivity after the lesion at 28 and 7 dpi, respectively. SOD1^{G93A} mice at 16 weeks of age showed similar levels of Iba1 immunoreactivity to those observed in nerve crush and SCI mice, when compared to their respective controls (wild type and naïve) (**Figure 6**).

INCREASED SEROTONIN PROJECTIONS IN SOD1^{G93A} LUMBAR SPINAL CORD

Serotonin (5-hydroxytryptamine, 5-HT) has been postulated as an important factor that contributes to MN excitability by promoting slight depolarization of their membrane potential through increased persistent inward currents (Heckman et al., 2003). 5-HT has been also related to KCC2 phosphorylation and binding to the cell membrane and the consequent decrease in spasticity after SCI (Bos et al., 2013). For this reason, we assessed the 5-HT projections that arrive to L4-L5 spinal MNs. Immunohistochemical analysis revealed an important increase of 5-HT projections in 16 weeks old SOD1^{G93A} lumbar spinal cord (**Figure 7**, $p < 0.05$).

REDUCED INHIBITION AND RENSHAW CELLS DEGENERATION IN SOD1^{G93A} LUMBAR SPINAL CORD

Once revealed that KCC2 expression and localization is not altered along ALS progression, we studied the inhibitory circuits in the lumbar spinal cord of 16 weeks aged SOD1 animals to evaluate its potential involvement on hyperreflexia. We analyzed gephyrin as a general marker of inhibitory glycine and GABA systems. Results showed a significant decrease of gephyrin expression in SOD1^{G93A} mice compared to non-transgenic littermates (**Figures 8A,B**). We also labeled the Renshaw cells in lamina VII of the L4 spinal cord, since these cells are glycinergic and importantly contribute to the inhibition of MNs. As described previously (Chang et al., 2009), we found a significant decrease in the number of calbindin positive cells in 16 weeks aged SOD1^{G93A} when compared to WT littermates (**Figure 8C**, $p < 0.05$). The findings suggest that inhibition is reduced in SOD1^{G93A} lumbar spinal cord due to alterations of the glycinergic system.

DISCUSSION

The results of the present work demonstrate that KCC2 is downregulated after peripheral and central nerve injuries. However, although KCC2 downregulation has been demonstrated to be a key factor in the appearance of hyperreflexia and spasticity after such injuries, we did not found changes in the KCC2 dephosphorylation that could explain the appearance of spastic behavior at the late stage (16 weeks of age) of the ALS murine model. On the other hand, our results suggest that the increased spinal excitability and the appearance of spasticity in ALS may be a consequence of two abnormalities: the loss of inhibitory tone due to loss of Renshaw glycinergic interneurons, and the increased 5-HT projections present in the ventral horn that would directly contribute to increasing MN excitability.

FACTORS CONTRIBUTING TO SPASTICITY IN SOD1^{G93A} MICE

Spasticity is present in ALS patients and leads to disabling complications in hand function and gait (Wijesekera and Leigh, 2009; Kiernan et al., 2011). Several works have investigated the mechanisms underlying spasticity after traumatic SCI. A relevant finding of these studies is that KCC2 loss of function is an important hallmark of MN increased excitability and thus, of spasticity after SCI (Boulenguez et al., 2010; Bos et al., 2013). The KCC2 is a potassium-chloride cotransporter, responsible for the low intracellular chloride concentration that allows GABA and glycine inhibitory synaptic responses in the adulthood (Rivera et al., 1999; Ganguly et al., 2001; Wang et al., 2002; Payne et al., 2003; Stein et al., 2004; Bray and Mynlieff, 2009). Phosphorylation of S940 in the intracellular C-terminal domain of the KCC2 has

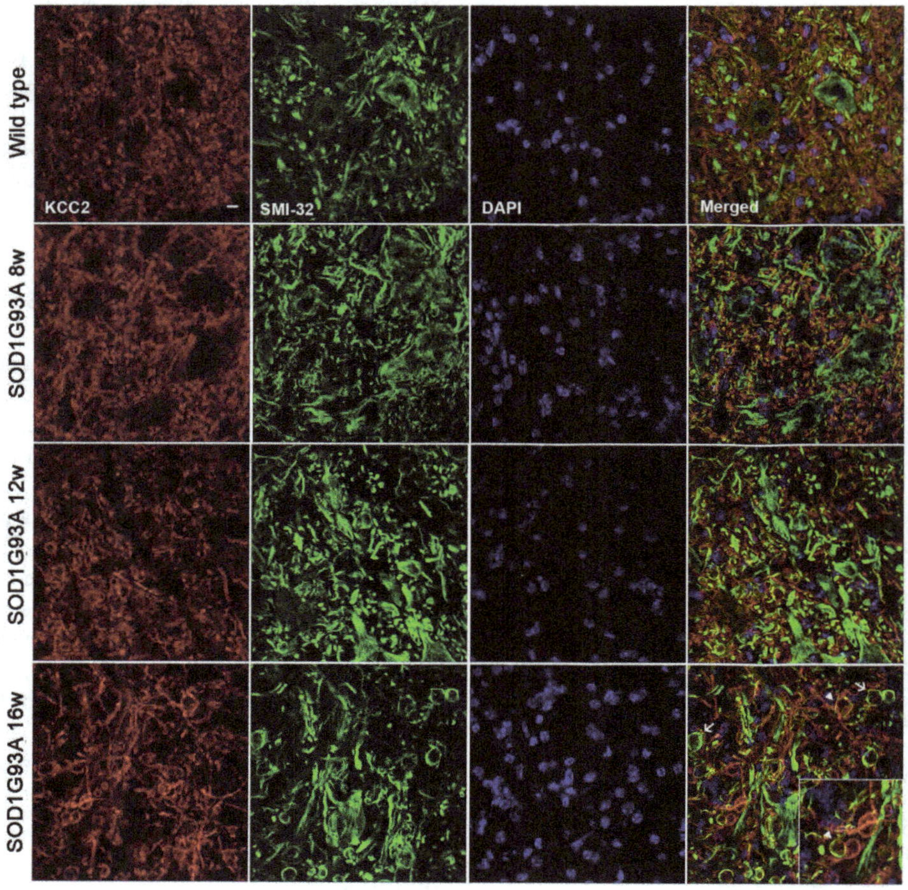

FIGURE 3 | Confocal images of L4 ventral spinal cord of wild type and SOD1^{G93A} mice at 8, 12, and 16 weeks of age. Note the progressive increase in number and volume of abnormal swollen structures (arrow) along the disease progression in SOD1^{G93A} animals. The KCC2 remained localized in the cell membrane even in these swallows (arrowheads). Scale bar 10 μm.

been demonstrated to be responsible for the stabilization of KCC2 on the neuronal cell surface, increasing its functional expression (Li et al., 2007; Lee et al., 2007, 2010). The expression and function of KCC2 is reduced after neural injuries, participating in the lowered strength of inhibitory transmission (Coull et al., 2003). The most prevalent mechanism underlying KCC2 regulation has been postulated to be mediated by brain-derived neurotrophic factor (BDNF) released through microglial signaling (Ulmann et al., 2008; Ferrini and De Koninck, 2013). Indeed, microglia react to alterations of the extracellular milieu with a protective and defensive role secreting specific messengers (including BDNF), that in turn sculpt neuronal circuit excitability (Ferrini and De Koninck, 2013). Although, this mechanism has been commonly described in the dorsal horn of the spinal cord, other studies also described the microglia-BDNF-TrkB-KCC2 signaling in the spinal motor system (Ferrini et al., 2013). In agreement, we found that the decrease of KCC2 phosphorylation after central or peripheral nerve injuries in the ventral horn of the spinal cord was also accompanied by increased microglial reactivity. Although this phenomenon has been reported to contribute to spasticity after SCI (Boulenguez et al., 2010; Bos et al., 2013), here we demonstrate that KCC2 is not altered in SOD1^{G93A} mice MN, and unlikely contributing to the hyperreflexia and spasticity that occurs in SOD1^{G93A} animals. Our results revealed that, opposite to what occurs after SCI, KCC2 remained localized in the cell membrane of MN, even in animals of 16 weeks of age when hyperreflexia and spasticity are clearly present. Fuchs et al. (2010) previously reported a down regulation of KCC2 mRNA in spinal MNs of SOD1^{G93A} mice. They found a slight reduction of mRNA signal in only a few large MNs of 80 days old animals (11 weeks of age), despite that almost 50% of lumbar MNs are not functionally connected to muscle at this time (as evidenced by the CMAP reduction). When they analyzed KCC2 mRNA at 120 days (17 weeks of age) they found a significant reduction of mRNA signal area per neuron, although some of the MNs could be in a degenerative state. KCC2 immunoreactivity was reduced in the neuropil surrounding MNs, similar to what we observed (see **Figure 3**), whereas some MNs bodies had increased KCC2 labeling in the cytoplasm (Fuchs et al., 2010). These findings suggest that KCC2 disregulation is slight and does not occur until very advanced stages in SOD1^{G93A} mice, quite later than the muscle denervation process.

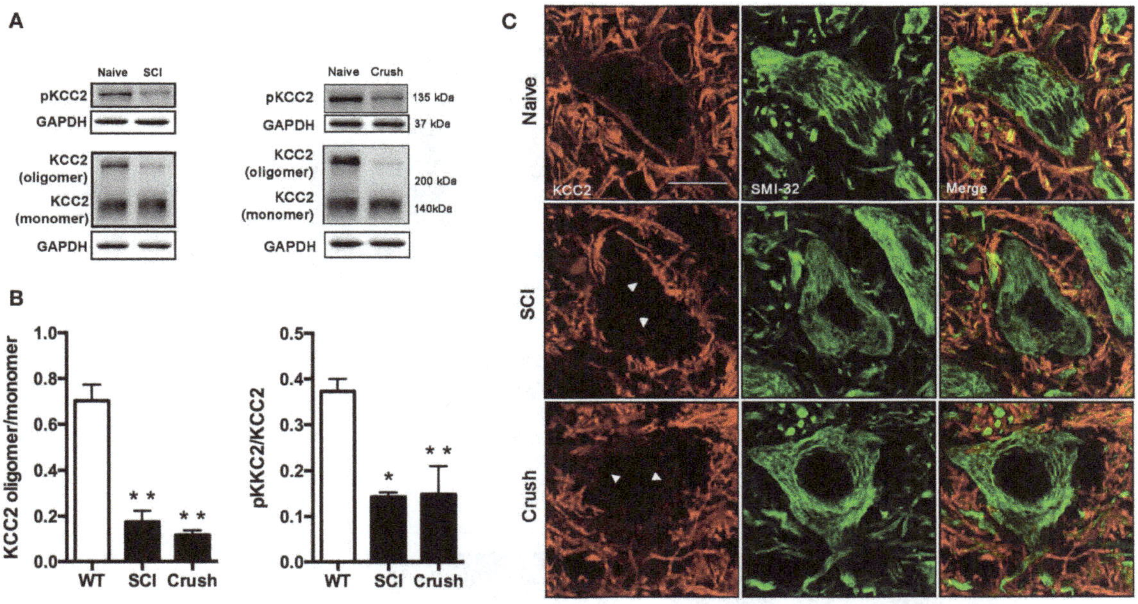

FIGURE 4 | Analysis of KCC2 and phopho-KCC2 expression in the ventral spinal cord of SCI and sciatic nerve injured mice. (A) Representative blots of phopho-KCC2 and total KCC2 (on both monomeric and oligomeric states) in SCI and crush mice. **(B)** KCC2 western blots quantifications. Graphs represent the ratio between the oligomeric KCC2 (functional state) vs. monomeric KCC2 and the phopho-KCC2 (active form) vs. monomeric KCC2. Both analyses revealed a decrease in the active form of the KCC2 in SCI (28 days after injury) and in sciatic nerve crush (7 days after injury). Data are represented as mean ± s.e.m.; $^{*}p < 0.05$, $^{**}p < 0.01$ vs. naïve animals. **(C)** Confocal images of L4 spinal MNs revealed the presence of membrane-bound (active) KCC2 in naïve but not in SCI and sciatic nerve injured animals. Arrowheads point internalized KCC2 aggregates. Scale bar 20 μm.

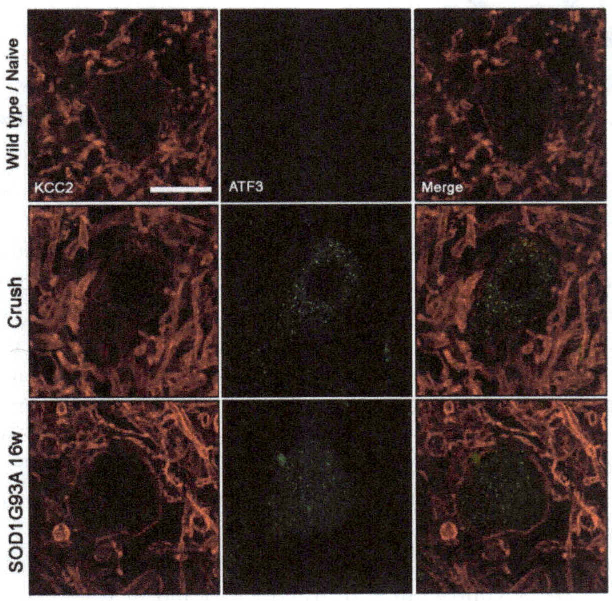

FIGURE 5 | KCC2 expression and localization in ATF3 labeled MN in wild type/naïve, sciatic nerve injured and 12 weeks old SOD1^{G93A} mice. Note that membrane-bound KCC2 is reduced in ATF3-positive injured neurons after nerve crush, but it remains in the membrane in ATF3-positive SOD1^{G93A} MNs. Scale bar 20 μm.

Mechanisms underlying spasticity have been mostly studied in experimental models of SCI. It is considered that SCI associated spasticity arises from several mechanisms, one of the most important being alterations of 5-HT inputs to spinal MNs. 5-HT descending axons from brainstem nuclei densely innervate spinal MNs, maintaining their excitability through increased persistent calcium current (Heckman et al., 2003). Although damage of serotonergic axons caused by a SCI leads to a transient hypoexcitability of spinal MNs, after a few weeks, MNs compensate for the loss of serotonin inputs through the overexpression of 5-HT receptors. These synaptic modifications promote hyperexcitability and consequent spasticity (Murray et al., 2010, 2011). In accordance, a recent study showed that the heterogeneity of 5-HT receptors is an important feature of hyperexcitability in MNs after SCI. Bos et al. (2013) reported that activation of 5-HT2B and 5-HT2C receptors induced a depolarizing shift in MNs. However, activation of 5-HT2A participated in the activation and restoration of KCC2 expression. Our results reveal that MNs of SOD1^{G93A} mice receive an increased amount of 5-HT projections at 16 weeks of age. Moreover, in contrast to the localized presence of 5-HT projections around MNs in WT animals, in SOD1^{G93A} mice they became spread over lamina IX in the ventral horn of the spinal cord. As a result, 5-HT labeling was found increased and could partially explain the hyperreflexia and spasticity observed at the late stage of the disease, but also the maintenance of KCC2 in the MN membrane. Further studies assessing the differential

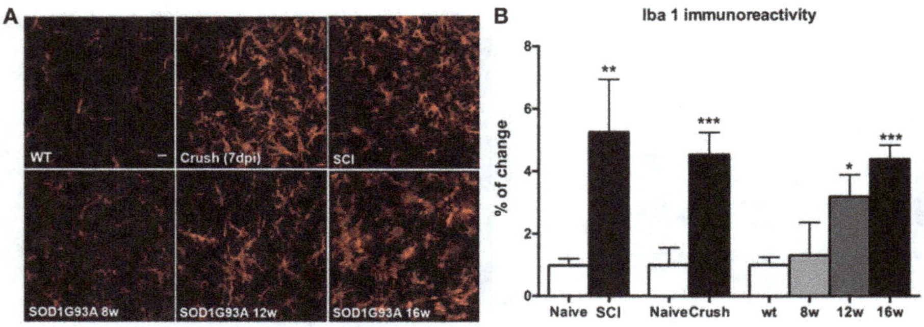

FIGURE 6 | Comparison of microglial (Iba-1 labeled) immunoreactivity in SOD1^{G93A}, SCI and sciatic nerve injured mice. (A) Representative confocal images of the ventral part of the lumbar spinal cord of wild type/naïve, SOD1^{G93A} at 8, 12, and 16 weeks of age, SCI and sciatic nerve crush injured animals. Scale bar 10 μm. **(B)** Iba-1 immunoreactivity quantification revealed a progressive increase of microglial reactivity during disease progression in SOD1^{G93A} mice. At late stages (16 weeks of age), Iba-1 immunoreactivity level is similar to that observed in SCI and sciatic nerve injured animals. Values are mean ± s.e.m. $^*p < 0.05$, $^{**}p < 0.01$, $^{***}p < 0.001$ vs. respective wild type/naïve animals.

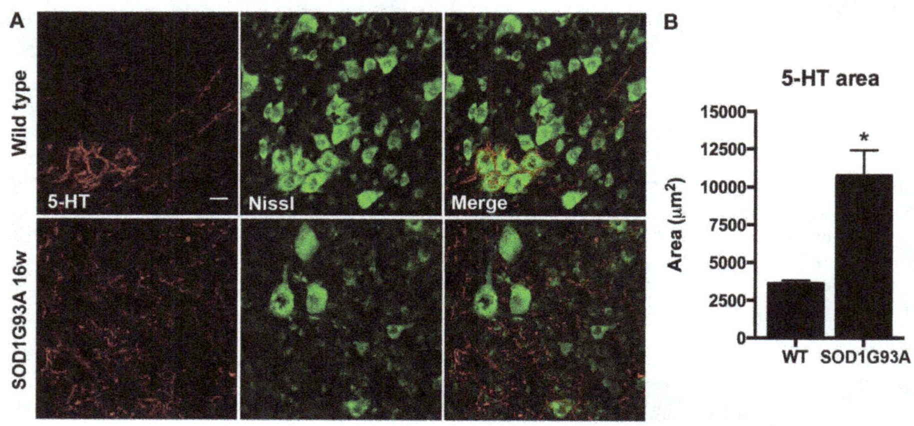

FIGURE 7 | Serotonin (5-HT) projections to MN pools in the lumbar spinal cord of 16 weeks old SOD1^{G93A} mice and wild type littermates. (A) Respresentative confocal images show increased 5-HT projections in SOD1^{G93A} compared to wild type mice. Scale bar 20 μm. **(B)** Quantification of the immunolabeling shows a 2 fold increase of 5-HT labeled area in SOD1^{G93A} animals at 16 weeks of age. Values are mean ± s.e.m. $^*p < 0.05$ vs. wild type.

expression of 5-HT receptors in SOD1^{G93A} mice would be of interest for understanding their interaction with the KCC2 role in ALS.

We further assessed the inhibitory state of the lumbar spinal cord by measuring gephyrin expression. Gephyrin is a structural component of the postsynaptic protein network of both glycine and GABA inhibitory synapses in the spinal cord (Bohlhalter et al., 1994). Our results show a significant reduction of gephyrin expression in 16 weeks old SOD1^{G93A} animals, evidencing decreased inhibition in the ventral spinal cord. Since gephyrin participates in glycine receptor clustering but not in GABAergic synapses formation (Lévi et al., 2004), we further investigated the glycinergic Renshaw cells at late stages in SOD1 mice. Renshaw cells are spinal interneurons located in the ventral horn gray matter that mediate recurrent inhibition to spinal MNs (Katz and Pierrot-Deseilligny, 1999; Alvarez and Fyffe, 2007). These cells have been related to spasticity (Mazzocchio and Rossi, 1997) and, recently, postulated as contributors to spasticity in ALS (Mazzocchio and Rossi, 2010). In fact, our results revealed a significant decrease in the number of calbindin labeled Renshaw cells in the lumbar spinal cord of SOD1 mice at 16 weeks of age. The loss of inhibitory interneurons could partially explain the abnormally increased spinal excitability found in SOD1^{G93A} animals at late stages. Indeed, Chang and Martin have reported an early presymptomatic loss of glycinergic synaptic buttons onto MNs (Chang and Martin, 2009) and the abnormal properties of glycinergic channels in dissociated G93A MNs (Chang and Martin, 2011).

Taken together, our results suggest two distinct mechanisms that may be contributing to hyperreflexia and increased spinal excitability in the SOD1 mouse model. On the one hand, increased lumbar 5-HT may enhance MN excitability through the activation of 5-HT2B and 5-HT2C receptors and, on the other hand, the loss of Renshaw cell leads to a reduction in inhibitory inputs onto MNs. Both phenomena may explain the disabling spastic paresis observed in SOD1^{G93A} animals at the late stage. These exogenous influences may add to the mild MN

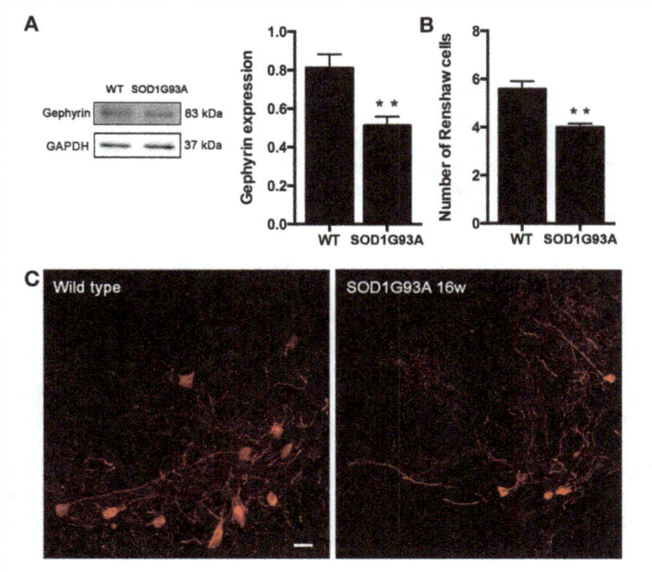

FIGURE 8 | Evaluation of inhibitory intraspinal circuits in SOD1^{G93A} mice at 16 weeks of age. (A) Representative blots and quantification of gephyrin expression in the ventral part of the lumbar spinal cord. Results revealed that gephyrin expression in 16 weeks old SOD1 mice was reduced when compared to wild type mice. **(B)** Number of Renshaw cells in the ventral horn of L4 spinal cord of wild type and SOD1^{G93A} animals at 16 weeks of age. Values are mean ± s.e.m. $^{**}p < 0.01$ vs. wild type animals. **(C)** Representative confocal images of Renshaw cells in the L4 spinal cord of wild type and 16 weeks old SOD1^{G93A} animals. Scale bar 10 μm.

depolarization state described in this ALS murine model (Boërio et al., 2010).

DIFFERENTIAL MN RESPONSE BETWEEN SOD1^{G93A} AND NERVE CRUSHED MNs

Once demonstrated the lack of KCC2 downregulation in SOD1^{G93A} MNs when compared to SCI, we explored whether the KCC2 response could be an intrinsic feature of ALS MNs. To test this hypothesis, we compared the differences in KCC2 expression between ALS and axotomized wild type MNs. Our results demonstrate for the first time that KCC2 down regulation also occurs in spinal MNs after peripheral nerve injury, as showed by the decrease in the active pKCC2 after sciatic nerve crush. Immunohistochemical evaluation also revealed that MNs labeled for ATF3, a typical marker of axonal injury (Tsujino et al., 2000; Navarro et al., 2007), presented an evident translocation of KCC2 from the plasma membrane to cytoplasmic aggregates. This fact indicates that injured MNs were actively down regulating KCC2 from their cell membrane. After lesion of peripheral axons, differential regulation of protein expression occurs and plays a role in transitioning the neuron from a transmission mode to a regenerative, growth mode (Fu and Gordon, 1997; Pieraut et al., 2007, 2011). One example of the plastic changes that occur after axotomy, are the excitatory responses to GABA and glycine induced by the loss of KCC2 in the neuronal cell membrane. This shift in the balance between excitatory and inhibitory influences that renders injured networks hyperexcitable has been implicated in the pathogenesis of neuropathic pain in dorsal horn neurons (Coull et al., 2003; Cramer et al., 2008; Hasbargen et al., 2010; Janssen et al., 2011, 2012).

Our results in SOD1^{G93A} mice revealed that KCC2 remained in its active phosphorylated form and located in the cell membrane even in MNs that highly expressed ATF3, evidencing a recent process of target muscle disconnection (Vlug et al., 2005; Saxena et al., 2009). After axotomy, KCC2 loss of function would contribute to an increase of spinal synaptic excitability and hyperreflexia (Valero-Cabré and Navarro, 2001), as a feature of the plastic changes that may play a role on nerve regeneration and functional recovery. The lack of such changes in ALS MNs could suggest an inability of these cells to initiate some cellular events in response to muscle disconnection that would allow for axonal regeneration and re-establishment of new neuromuscular junctions. The abnormal response to insults would be also manifested by a progressive increase of neurofilament aggregates (Julien, 1997) surrounded by active and phosphorylated KCC2 with age in SOD1^{G93A} MNs. This observation could explain the fact that we did not observe any changes in the KCC2 activity by analyzing the WB result when comparing with wild type animals. Nevertheless, despite the active KCC2 downregulation could be likely due to muscle disconnection *per se*, it cannot be discarded that such changes are produced by transynaptic effects of the injured primary sensory afferents, explaining the differences we observed between ALS and nerve crushed mice. Thus, further experiments are needed to understand which mechanisms underline the reduction of KCC2 activity.

In summary, the present results demonstrate that there is not downregulation of KCC2 expression from the plasma membrane of ALS MNs, even at advanced stage of the disease, when they have suffered deafferentation from upper MNs and axonal damage and muscle disconnection. This is in contrast to what we found after either SCI or peripheral nerve injury, which induced a rapid decrease of KCC2 phosphorylation in MNs. Such a KCC2 change has been previously described in spinal MNs linked to the development of spasticity (Boulenguez et al., 2010), and in dorsal horn neurons related to the appearance of neuropathic pain (Janssen et al., 2012). The fact that KCC2 is not downregulated along the lifespan of SOD1 mice could indicate that ALS MNs do not react as axotomized normal MNs after muscle denervation.

REFERENCES

Alvarez, F. J., and Fyffe, R. E. W. (2007). The continuing case for the Renshaw cell. *J. Physiol.* 584, 31–45. doi: 10.1113/jphysiol.2007.136200

Basso, D. M., Fisher, L. C., Anderson, A. J., Jakeman, L. B., McTigue, D. M., and Popovich, P. G. (2006). Basso mouse scale for locomotion detects differences in recovery after spinal cord injury in five five common mouse strains. *J. Neurotrauma* 23, 635–659. doi: 10.1089/neu.2006.23.635

Ben-Ari, Y., Gaiarsa, J.-L., Tyzio, R., and Khazipov, R. (2007). GABA: a pioneer transmitter that excites immature neurons and generates primitive oscillations. *Physiol. Rev.* 87, 1215–1284. doi: 10.1152/physrev.00017.2006

Blaesse, P., Guillemin, I., Schindler, J., Schweizer, M., Delpire, E., Khiroug, L., et al. (2006). Oligomerization of KCC2 correlates with development of inhibitory neurotransmission. *J. Neurosci.* 26, 10407–10419. doi: 10.1523/JNEUROSCI.3257-06.2006

Boërio, D., Kalmar, B., Greensmith, L., and Bostock, H. (2010). Excitability properties of mouse motor axons in the mutant SOD1(G93A) model of amyotrophic lateral sclerosis. *Muscle Nerve.* 41, 774–784. doi: 10.1002/mus.21579

Bohlhalter, S., Möhler, H., and Fritschy, J. M. (1994). Inhibitory neurotransmission in rat spinal cord: co-localization of glycine- and GABAA-receptors at GABAergic synaptic contacts demonstrated by triple immunofluorescence staining. *Brain Res.* 642, 59–69. doi: 10.1016/0006-8993(94)90905-9

Bos, R., Sadlaoud, K., Boulenguez, P., Buttigieg, D., Liabeuf, S., Brocard, C., et al. (2013). Activation of 5-HT2A receptors upregulates the function of the neuronal K-Cl cotransporter KCC2. *Proc. Natl. Acad. Sci. U.S.A.* 110, 348–353. doi: 10.1073/pnas.1213680110

Bosco, D. A., Morfini, G., Karabacak, N. M., Song, Y., Gros-Louis, F., Pasinelli, P., et al. (2010). Wild-type and mutant SOD1 share an aberrant conformation and a common pathogenic pathway in ALS. *Nat. Neurosci.* 13, 1396–1403. doi: 10.1038/nn.2660

Boulenguez, P., Liabeuf, S., Bos, R., Bras, H., Jean-Xavier, C., Brocard, C., et al. (2010). Down-regulation of the potassium-chloride cotransporter KCC2 contributes to spasticity after spinal cord injury. *Nat. Med.* 16, 302–307. doi: 10.1038/nm.2107

Bray, J. G., and Mynlieff, M. (2009). Influx of calcium through L−type calcium channels in early postnatal regulation of chloride transporters in the rat hippocampus. *Dev. Neurobiol.* 69, 885–896. doi: 10.1002/dneu.20749

Chang, Q., and Martin, L. J. (2009). Glycinergic innervation of motoneurons is deficient in amyotrophic lateral sclerosis mice: a quantitative confocal analysis. *Am. J. Pathol.* 174, 574–585. doi: 10.2353/ajpath.2009.080557

Chang, Q., and Martin, L. J. (2011). Glycine receptor channels in spinal motoneurons are abnormal in a transgenic mouse model of amyotrophic lateral sclerosis. *J. Neurosci.* 31, 2815–2827. doi: 10.1523/JNEUROSCI.2475-10.2011

Coull, J. A. M., Beggs, S., Boudreau, D., Boivin, D., Tsuda, M., Inoue, K., et al. (2005). BDNF from microglia causes the shift in neuronal anion gradient underlying neuropathic pain. *Nature* 438, 1017–1021. doi: 10.1038/nature04223

Coull, J. A. M., Boudreau, D., Bachand, K., Prescott, S. A., Nault, F., Sik, A., et al. (2003). Trans-synaptic shift in anion gradient in spinal lamina I neurons as a mechanism of neuropathic pain. *Nature* 424, 938–942. doi: 10.1038/nature01868

Cramer, S. W., Baggott, C., Cain, J., Tilghman, J., Allcock, B., Miranpuri, G., et al. (2008). The role of cation-dependent chloride transporters in neuropathic pain following spinal cord injury. *Mol. Pain.* 4, 36. doi: 10.1186/1744-8069-4-36

Dentel, C., Palamiuc, L., Henriques, A., Lannes, B., Spreux-Varoquaux, O., Gutknecht, L., et al. (2013). Degeneration of serotonergic neurons in amyotrophic lateral sclerosis: a link to spasticity. *Brain* 136, 483–493. doi: 10.1093/brain/aws274

Ferrini, F., and De Koninck, Y. (2013). Microglia control neuronal network excitability via BDNF signalling. *Neural Plast.* 2013, 429815. doi: 10.1155/2013/429815

Ferrini, F., Trang, T., Mattioli, T. A. M., Laffray, S., Del'Guidice, T., Lorenzo, L.-E., et al. (2013). Morphine hyperalgesia gated through microglia-mediated disruption of neuronal Cl^- homeostasis. *Nat. Neurosci.* 16, 183–192. doi: 10.1038/nn.3295

Fu, S. Y., and Gordon, T. (1997). The cellular and molecular basis of peripheral nerve regeneration. *Mol. Neurobiol.* 14, 67–116. doi: 10.1007/BF02740621

Fuchs, A., Ringer, C., Bilkei-Gorzo, A., Weihe, E., Roeper, J., and Schütz, B. (2010). Downregulation of the potassium chloride cotransporter KCC2 in vulnerable motoneurons in the SOD1-G93A mouse model of amyotrophic lateral sclerosis. *J. Neuropathol. Exp. Neurol.* 69, 1057–1070. doi: 10.1097/NEN.0b013e3181f4dcef

Ganguly, K., Schinder, A. F., Wong, S. T., and Poo, M. (2001). GABA itself promotes the developmental switch of neuronal GABAergic responses from excitation to inhibition. *Cell* 105, 521–532. doi: 10.1016/S0092-8674(01)00341-5

García-Alías, G., Verdú, E., Forés, J., López-Vales, R., and Navarro, X. (2003). Functional and electrophysiological characterization of photochemical graded spinal cord injury in the rat. *J. Neurotrauma* 20, 501–510. doi: 10.1089/089771503765355568

Hasbargen, T., Ahmed, M. M., Miranpuri, G., Li, L., Kahle, K. T., Resnick, D., et al. (2010). Role of NKCC1 and KCC2 in the development of chronic neuropathic pain following spinal cord injury. *Ann. N.Y Acad. Sci.* 1198, 168–172. doi: 10.1111/j.1749-6632.2010.05462.x

Heckman, C. J., Lee, R. H., and Brownstone, R. M. (2003). Hyperexcitable dendrites in motoneurons and their neuromodulatory control during motor behavior. *Trends Neurosci.* 26, 688–895. doi: 10.1016/j.tins.2003.10.002

Janssen, S. P., Gerard, S., Raijmakers, M. E., Truin, M., Van Kleef, M., and Joosten, E. A. (2012). Decreased intracellular GABA levels contribute to spinal cord stimulation-induced analgesia in rats suffering from painful peripheral neuropathy: the role of KCC2 and GABA(A) receptor-mediated inhibition. *Neurochem. Int.* 60, 21–30. doi: 10.1016/j.neuint.2011.11.006

Janssen, S. P., Truin, M., Van Kleef, M., and Joosten, E. A. (2011). Differential GABAergic disinhibition during the development of painful peripheral neuropathy. *Neuroscience* 184, 183–194. doi: 10.1016/j.neuroscience.2011.03.060

Julien, J. P. (1997). Neurofilaments and motor neuron disease. *Trends Cell Biol.* 7, 243–249. doi: 10.1016/S0962-8924(97)01049-0

Kakinohana, O., Scadeng, M., Corleto, J. A., Sevc, J., Lukacova, N., and Marsala, M. (2012). Development of AMPA receptor and GABA B receptor-sensitive spinal hyper-reflexia after spinal air embolism in rat: a systematic neurological, electrophysiological and qualitative histopathological study. *Exp. Neurol.* 237, 26–35. doi: 10.1016/j.expneurol.2012.06.004

Katz, R., and Pierrot-Deseilligny, E. (1999). Recurrent inhibition in humans. *Prog. Neurobiol.* 57, 325–355. doi: 10.1016/S0301-0082(98)00056-2

Kiernan, M. C., Vucic, S., Cheah, B. C., Turner, M. R., Eisen, A., Hardiman, O., et al. (2011). Amyotrophic lateral sclerosis. *Lancet* 377, 942–955. doi: 10.1016/S0140-6736(10)61156-7

Klopstein, A., Santos-Nogueira, E., Francos-Quijorna, I., Redensek, A., David, S., Navarro, X., et al. (2012). Beneficial effects of B-crystallin in spinal cord contusion injury. *J. Neurosci.* 32, 14478–14488. doi: 10.1523/JNEUROSCI.0923-12.2012

Lance, J. W. (1980). The control of muscle tone, reflexes, and movement: Robert Wartenberg lecture. *Neurology* 30, 1303–1313. doi: 10.1212/WNL.30.12.1303

Lee, H. H. C., Jurd, R., and Moss, S. J. (2010). Tyrosine phosphorylation regulates the membrane trafficking of the potassium chloride co-transporter KCC2. *Mol. Cell. Neurosci.* 45, 173–179. doi: 10.1016/j.mcn.2010.06.008

Lee, H. H. C., Walker, J. A., Williams, J. R., Goodier, R. J., Payne, J. A., and Moss, S. J. (2007). Direct protein kinase C-dependent phosphorylation regulates the cell surface stability and activity of the potassium chloride cotransporter KCC2. *J. Biol. Chem.* 282, 29777–29784. doi: 10.1074/jbc.M705053200

Lévi, S., Logan, S. M., Tovar, K. R., and Craig, A. M. (2004). Gephyrin is critical for glycine receptor clustering but not for the formation of functional GABAergic synapses in hippocampal neurons. *J. Neurosci.* 24, 207–217. doi: 10.1523/JNEUROSCI.1661-03.2004

Li, H., Khirug, S., Cai, C., Ludwig, A., Blaesse, P., Kolikova, J., et al. (2007). KCC2 interacts with the dendritic cytoskeleton to promote spine development. *Neuron* 56, 1019–1033. doi: 10.1016/j.neuron.2007.10.039

Lu, Y., Zheng, J., Xiong, L., Zimmermann, M., and Yang, J. (2008). Spinal cord injury-induced attenuation of GABAergic inhibition in spinal dorsal horn circuits is associated with down-regulation of the chloride transporter KCC2 in rat. *J. Physiol.* 586, 5701–5715. doi: 10.1113/jphysiol.2008.152348

Mancuso, R., Oliván, S., Rando, A., Casas, C., Osta, R., and Navarro, X. (2012). Sigma-1R agonist improves motor function and motoneuron survival in ALS mice. *Neurotherapeutics* 9, 814–826. doi: 10.1007/s13311-012-0140-y

Mancuso, R., Santos-Nogueira, E., Osta, R., and Navarro, X. (2011). Electrophysiological analysis of a murine model of motoneuron disease. *Clin. Neurophysiol.* 122, 1660–1670. doi: 10.1016/j.clinph.2011.01.045

Mazzocchio, R., and Rossi, A. (1997). Involvement of spinal recurrent inhibition in spasticity. Further insight into the regulation of Renshaw cell activity. *Brain.* 120, 991–1003. doi: 10.1093/brain/120.6.991

Mazzocchio, R., and Rossi, A. (2010). Role of Renshaw cells in amyotrophic lateral sclerosis. *Muscle Nerve.* 41, 441–443. doi: 10.1002/mus.21602

Murray, K. C., Nakae, A., Stephens, M. J., Rank, M., D'Amico, J., Harvey, P. J., et al. (2010). Recovery of motoneuron and locomotor function after spinal cord injury depends on constitutive activity in 5-HT. *Nat. Med.* 16, 694–700. doi: 10.1038/nm.2160

Murray, K. C., Stephens, M. J., Ballou, E. W., Heckman, C. J., and Bennett, D. J. (2011). Motoneuron excitability and muscle spasms are regulated by 5-HT2B and 5-HT2C receptor activity. *J. Neurophysiol.* 105, 731–748. doi: 10.1152/jn.00774.2010

Navarro, X., Vivó, M., and Valero-Cabré, A. (2007). Neural plasticity after peripheral nerve injury and regeneration. *Prog. Neurobiol.* 82, 163–201. doi: 10.1016/j.pneurobio.2007.06.005

Payne, J. A., Rivera, C., Voipio, J., and Kaila, K. (2003). Cation–chloride co-transporters in neuronal communication, development and trauma. *Trends Neurosci.* 26, 199–206. doi: 10.1016/S0166-2236(03)00068-7

Pieraut, S., Laurent-Matha, V., Sar, C., Hubert, T., Méchaly, I., Hilaire, C., et al. (2007). NKCC1 phosphorylation stimulates neurite growth of injured adult sensory neurons. *J. Neurosci.* 27, 6751–6759. doi: 10.1523/JNEUROSCI.1337-07.2007

Pieraut, S., Lucas, O., Sangari, S., Sar, C., Boudes, M., Bouffi, C., et al. (2011). An autocrine neuronal Interleukin-6 loop mediates chloride accumulation and NKCC1 phosphorylation in axotomized sensory neurons. *J. Neurosci.* 31, 13516–13526. doi: 10.1523/JNEUROSCI.3382-11.2011

Ripps, M. E., Huntley, G. W., Hof, P. R., Morrison, J. H., and Gordon, J. W. (1995). Transgenic mice expressing an altered murine superoxide dismutase gene provide an animal model of amyotrophic lateral sclerosis. *Proc. Natl. Acad. Sci. U.S.A.* 92, 689–693. doi: 10.1073/pnas.92.3.689

Rivera, C., Li, H., Thomas-Crusells, J., Lahtinen, H., Viitanen, T., Nanobashvili, A., et al. (2002). BDNF-induced TrkB activation down-regulates the K+-Cl- cotransporter KCC2 and impairs neuronal Cl- extrusion. *J. Cell Biol.* 159, 747–752. doi: 10.1083/jcb.200209011

Rivera, C., Voipio, J., Payne, J. A., Ruusuvuori, E., Lahtinen, H., Lamsa, K., et al. (1999). The K+/Cl- co-transporter KCC2 renders GABA hyperpolarizing during neuronal maturation. *Nature* 397, 251–255. doi: 10.1038/16697

Rosen, D. R. (1993). Mutations in Cu/Zn superoxide dismutase gene are associated with familial amyotrophic lateral sclerosis. *Nature* 364, 362. doi: 10.1038/362059a0

Saxena, S., Cabuy, E., and Caroni, P. (2009). A role for motoneuron subtype-selective ER stress in disease manifestations of FALS mice. *Nat. Neurosci.* 12, 627–636. doi: 10.1038/nn.2297

Schütz, B. (2005). Imbalanced excitatory to inhibitory synaptic input precedes motor neuron degeneration in an animal model of amyotrophic lateral sclerosis. *Neurobiol. Dis.* 20, 131–140. doi: 10.1016/j.nbd.2005.02.006

Stein, V., Hermans Borgmeyer, I., Jentsch, T. J., and Hübner, C. A. (2004). Expression of the KCl cotransporter KCC2 parallels neuronal maturation and the emergence of low intracellular chloride. *J. Comp. Neurol.* 468, 57–64. doi: 10.1002/cne.10983

Stil, A., Jean-Xavier, C., Liabeuf, S., Brocard, C., Delpire, E., Vinay, L., et al. (2011). Contribution of the potassium-chloride co-transporter KCC2 to the modulation of lumbar spinal networks in mice. *Eur. J. Neurosci.* 33, 1212–1222. doi: 10.1111/j.1460-9568.2010.07592.x

Tsujino, H., Kondo, E., Fukuoka, T., Dai, Y., Tokunaga, A., Miki, K., et al. (2000). Activating transcription factor 3 (ATF3) induction by axotomy in sensory and motoneurons: a novel neuronal marker of nerve injury. *Mol. Cell. Neurosci.* 15, 170–182. doi: 10.1006/mcne.1999.0814

Ulmann, L., Hatcher, J. P., Hughes, J. P., Chaumont, S., Green, P. J., Conquet, F., et al. (2008). Up-regulation of P2X4 receptors in spinal microglia after peripheral nerve injury mediates BDNF release and neuropathic pain. *J. Neurosci.* 28, 11263–11268. doi: 10.1523/JNEUROSCI.2308-08.2008

Valero-Cabré, A., and Navarro, X. (2001). H reflex restitution and facilitation after different types of peripheral nerve injury and repair. *Brain Res.* 919, 302–312. doi: 10.1016/S0006-8993(01)03052-9

Vlug, A. S., Teuling, E., Haasdijk, E. D., French, P., Hoogenraad, C. C., and Jaarsma, D. (2005). ATF3 expression precedes death of spinal motoneurons in amyotrophic lateral sclerosis-SOD1 transgenic mice and correlates with c-Jun phosphorylation, CHOP expression, somato-dendritic ubiquitination and Golgi fragmentation. *Eur. J. Neurosci.* 22, 1881–1894. doi: 10.1111/j.1460-9568.2005.04389.x

Wang, C., Shimizu-Okabe, C., Watanabe, K., Okabe, A., Matsuzaki, H., Ogawa, T., et al. (2002). Developmental changes in KCC1, KCC2, and NKCC1 mRNA expressions in the rat brain. *Dev. Brain Res.* 139, 59–66. doi: 10.1016/S0165-3806(02)00536-9

Wijesekera, L. C., and Leigh, P. N. (2009). Amyotrophic lateral sclerosis. *Orphan. J. Rare Dis.* 4, 3. doi: 10.1186/1750-1172-4-3

19

Phenotypic transition of microglia into astrocyte-like cells associated with disease onset in a model of inherited ALS

Emiliano Trias[1], Pablo Díaz-Amarilla[1], Silvia Olivera-Bravo[1], Eugenia Isasi[1], Derek A. Drechsel[2,3], Nathan Lopez[2,3], C. Samuel Bradford[2,3], Kyle E. Ireton[2,3,5], Joseph S. Beckman[2,3,4] and Luis Barbeito[5]*

[1] *Instituto de Investigaciones Biológicas Clemente Estable, Montevideo, Uruguay*
[2] *Department of Biochemistry and Biophysics, Oregon State University, Corvallis, OR, USA*
[3] *Environmental Health Sciences Center, Oregon State University, Corvallis, OR, USA*
[4] *Linus Pauling Institute, Oregon State University, Corvallis, OR, USA*
[5] *Institut Pasteur de Montevideo, Montevideo, Uruguay*

Edited by:
Ricardo Tapia, Universidad Nacional Autónoma de México, Mexico

Reviewed by:
Ricardo Tapia, Universidad Nacional Autónoma de México, Mexico
Jie Zhang, University of Texas Health Science Center at San Antonio, USA

****Correspondence:***
Luis Barbeito, Institut Pasteur de Montevideo, Mataojo 2020, Montevideo 11400, Uruguay
e-mail: barbeito@pasteur.edu.uy

Microglia and reactive astrocytes accumulate in the spinal cord of rats expressing the Amyotrophic lateral sclerosis (ALS)-linked SOD1^{G93A} mutation. We previously reported that the rapid progression of paralysis in ALS rats is associated with the appearance of proliferative astrocyte-like cells that surround motor neurons. These cells, designated as Aberrant Astrocytes (AbA cells) because of their atypical astrocytic phenotype, exhibit high toxicity to motor neurons. However, the cellular origin of AbA cells remains unknown. Because AbA cells are labeled with the proliferation marker Ki67, we analyzed the phenotypic makers of proliferating glial cells that surround motor neurons by immunohistochemistry. The number of Ki67^{+}AbA cells sharply increased in symptomatic rats, displaying large cell bodies with processes embracing motor neurons. Most were co-labeled with astrocytic marker GFAP concurrently with the microglial markers Iba1 and CD163. Cultures of spinal cord prepared from symptomatic SOD1^{G93A} rats yielded large numbers of microglia expressing Iba1, CD11b, and CD68. Cells sorted for CD11b expression by flow cytometry transformed into AbA cells within two weeks. During these two weeks, the expression of microglial markers largely disappeared, while GFAP and S100β expression increased. The phenotypic transition to AbA cells was stimulated by forskolin. These findings provide evidence for a subpopulation of proliferating microglial cells in SOD1^{G93A} rats that undergo a phenotypic transition into AbA cells after onset of paralysis that may promote the fulminant disease progression. These cells could be a therapeutic target for slowing paralysis progression in ALS.

Keywords: microglia, astrocytes, AbA cells, ALS, phenotypic transformation, neurodegeneration

INTRODUCTION

Amyotrophic lateral sclerosis (ALS) may be considered as a paradigm of neurodegeneration involving the progressive death of upper and lower motor neurons (Cleveland and Rothstein, 2001; Boillee et al., 2006a). A consistent neuropathological feature of ALS is the extensive inflammation around motor neurons and axonal degeneration, evidenced by the accumulation of reactive astrocytes, activated microglia and lymphocytes (Engelhardt et al., 1993; Barbeito et al., 2004; Ilieva et al., 2009; Graber et al., 2010). Neuroinflammation is evident in rodent models of inherited ALS overexpressing mutant Cu/Zn superoxide dismutase (SOD1) and in ALS human patients (Gurney et al., 1994; Bruijn et al., 1997; Howland et al., 2002; McGeer and McGeer, 2002; Appel, 2009). Several studies suggest that glial cells, including astrocytes and microglia, play a pathogenic role in ALS through promoting motor neuron death and spreading paralysis after disease onset (Hall et al., 1998; Barbeito et al., 2004; Sargsyan et al., 2005; Boillee et al., 2006b; Papadeas et al., 2011). These observations suggest that therapeutics targeting the inflammatory response of glial cells could slow ALS progression.

We have recently reported the isolation of astrocytes-like glial cells with an aberrant phenotype (AbA cells) from primary spinal cord cultures of symptomatic transgenic rats expressing the SOD1^{G93A} mutation (Diaz-Amarilla et al., 2011). Isolation was based on AbA cell's marked proliferative capacity and lack of replicative senescence. These cells secrete soluble factors that induce motor neuron death with a higher potency than neonatal transgenic astrocytes. Aberrant astrocytes only appear after disease onset in SOD1^{G93A} rats and are localized adjacent to motor neurons, suggesting a link between generation of AbA cells and the progression of paralysis. However, the origin of AbA cells remains unknown. Because AbA cells actively proliferate in the degenerating spinal cord, we hypothesized they could originate from glial progenitors with a high proliferative potential. Previous studies have identified phagocytic microglia as well as NG2^{+} glial progenitors that proliferate during the active phase of motor neuron degeneration in ALS mice and rats (Magnus et al., 2008; Kang et al., 2010; Sanagi et al., 2010). Because we have previously shown that AbA cells do not express NG2 (Diaz-Amarilla et al., 2011), we examined whether AbA cells might be derived from microglia proliferating adjacent to motoneurons. In this study, we have characterized both *in vivo* and *ex vivo* the phenotype of proliferating glial cells in symptomatic ALS rats and found evidence that neurotoxic AbA cells result from a phenotypic transition from activated microglial cells.

MATERIALS AND METHODS

ANIMALS

All procedures using laboratory animals were performed in accordance with the international guidelines for the use of live animals and were approved by the Institutional Animal Committee. Male hemizygous NTac:SD-TgN(SOD1^{G93A})L26H rats (Taconic), originally developed by Howland et al. (2002), were bred locally by crossing with wild-type Sprague–Dawley female rats. Male SOD1^{G93A} progenies were used for further breeding to maintain the line. Rats were housed in a centralized animal facility with a 12-h light-dark cycle with ad libitum access to food and water. Symptomatic disease onset was determined by periodic clinical examination for abnormal gait, typically expressed as subtle limping or dragging of one hind limb. Rats were killed when they reached the end stage of the disease. Both the onset of symptomatic disease (160–170 d) and lifespan (180–195 d) in our colony were delayed considerably compared with earlier reports (Howland et al., 2002). This study was carried out in strict accordance with the IIBCE Bioethics Committee's requirements and under the current ethical regulations of the Uruguayan Law N° 18.611 for animal experimentation that follows the Guide for the Care and Use of Laboratory Animals of the National Institutes of Health (USA). All surgery was performed under 90% ketamine – 10% xylazine anesthesia, and all efforts were made to minimize suffering, discomfort or stress.

CELL CULTURE FROM END-STAGE SYMPTOMATIC SOD1^{G93A} RATS

Microglia cells were obtained from adult spinal cord of symptomatic SOD1^{G93A} rats (175 d) according to the procedures described by Diaz-Amarilla et al. (2011) with minor modifications. Adult age-matched non-Tg rats were used as controls. Briefly, animals were killed by deeply anesthesia, and spinal cord was dissected on ice. After the meninges were removed carefully, spinal cord was chopped finely and dissociated with 0.25% trypsin in calcium-free buffer for 5 min at 37°C. Trypsin treatment was stopped by adding DMEM/10% (vol/vol) FBS in the presence of 50 μg/mL DNaseI and mechanical disaggregation by repeated pipetting. The resulting extract was passed through an 80-μm mesh to eliminate tissue debris and then was spun. The pellet was resuspended in culture medium [DMEM/10% (vol/vol) FBS, Hepes (3.6 g/L), penicillin (100 IU/mL), and streptomycin (100 μg/mL)] and then was plated in a 25-cm^2 tissue culture flask. Because large amounts of fat hindered cell counting, the cells isolated from individual spinal cords were plated in individual culture flasks. Culture medium was removed after 24 h and then was replaced every 48 h.

LEUCINE-METHYL ESTER TREATMENT

Leucine-Methyl Ester (Leu-OMe, Sigma) was prepared in DMEM, pH adjusted to 7.4. Cultures from transgenic symptomatic rats were treated 3 days after plated with 25 mM of Leu-OMe during 1 h. Then, the cells were washed three times with PBS and fixed with cold methanol during 5 min (n = 3).

IMMUNOCYTOCHEMICAL STAINING OF CULTURED CELLS

Cultured cells were fixed with absolute methanol at -20°C for 5 min on ice and then were washed three times with 10 mM PBS (pH 7.4). Non-specific binding was blocked by incubating fixed cells with 5% BSA in PBS for 1 h at room temperature. Corresponding primary antibodies were diluted in blocking solution and incubated overnight at 4°C in a wet closed chamber. The primary antibodies for microglia recognition were rabbit anti-Iba1 (1:200, Abcam), rabbit anti-CD11b (1:200, Abcam), and mouse anti-CD68 (1:300, Abcam). The antibodies used for astrocyte recognition were mouse anti-GFAP (1:500, Sigma), rabbit anti-GFAP (1:500, Sigma), mouse anti-S100β(1:400, Sigma). After washing, sections were incubated in a 1,000-fold dilution of secondary antibodies conjugated to Alexa Fluor 488 and/or Alexa Fluor 546 (1:1000, Invitrogen). Antibodies were detected by confocal microscopy using a confocal Olympus FV300 microscope.

ANALYSIS OF MICROGLIAL MARKERS EXPRESSION

After isolation of the symptomatic spinal cord, cells were plated in 35-mm dishes at 1.2×10^4 cells/cm^2. 7 days after plating, cells were fixed and stained with microglia specific markers as described above. The analysis was performed manually in using the cell counter tool of the Image J software. Values were expressed as a percentage (± SD) of the total number of DAPI$^+$ nuclei. Only healthy nuclei with clearly defined limiting membranes were counted. Cell counts were performed in duplicate.

FORSKOLIN TREATMENT

After 20 days *in vitro*, 35 mm dishes were treated with 10 μM of forskolin (FSK; Sigma) during 3 h. Then, the cells were fixed using cold methanol and stained as described above.

FLOW CYTOMETRIC ISOLATION

After 7 days *in vitro* the cells were incubated at 37°C with 0.25% trypsin without calcium. After 5 min, the cells were harvested in DMEM/10% (vol/vol) FBS and spun at $250 \times g$ for 10 min. The resultant pellet was washed three times in PBS at 37°C. After that, the cells were re-suspended in blocking solution (PBS; 5% FBS, and 1% BSA). The cells were labeled at 4°C for 15 min with mouse anti-CD11b-FITC (1:100, Abcam) and sorted using the MoFlo^{TM} XDP–Beckman Coulter. After sorting, the cells were re-plated in a 25 cm^2 bottle with DMEM/10% FBS.

IMMUNOHISTOCHEMICAL STAINING OF RAT SPINAL CORDS

Animals were deeply anesthetized and transcardial perfusion was performed with 0.9% saline and 4% paraformaldehyde in 0.1 M PBS (pH 7.2–7.4) at a constant flow of 1 mL/min. Fixed spinal cord was removed, post-fixed by immersion for 24 h, and then transverse sectioned serially (30–50 μm) on a vibrating microtome. Serial sections were collected in 100 mM PBS for immunohistochemistry. After citrate antigen retrieval, free-floating sections were permeabilized for 15 min at room temperature with 0.1% Triton X-100 in PBS, passed through washing buffered solutions, blocked with 5% BSA:PBS for 1 h at room temperature, and incubated overnight at 4°C in a solution of 0.1% Triton X-100 and PBS containing the primary antibodies, mouse anti-Iba1 (1:200, Abcam), mouse anti CD163 (1:100, Serotec) for microglia recognition, and rabbit anti-GFAP (1:500, Sigma) for astrocyte recognition. A rabbit anti-Ki67 (1:400, Abcam) was used as a proliferation marker. The expression of nitrotyrosine was recognized with a mouse anti-NO_2-Tyr (1:300, Millipore) antibody. The immunoreactivity was completely blocked by pre-incubation of the primary antibody with free nitrotyrosine (10 mM). No antigen retrieval was needed to detect nitrotyrosine. After washing, sections were incubated in 1:1,000-diluted secondary antibodies conjugated to Alexa Fluor 488 and/or Alexa Fluor 546 (Invitrogen). Antibodies were detected by confocal microscopy using a confocal Olympus FV300 microscope.

QUANTITATIVE ANALYSIS OF ABA CELLS IN THE DEGENERATING SPINAL CORD

The number of proliferating cells labeled with Ki67 and also stained for the astrocytic marker GFAP or microglial marker Iba1 was assessed by counting the respective double-positive cells in the gray matter of the lumbar cord of symptomatic or asymptomatic $SOD1^{G93A}$ rats. Quantification was performed only in the ventral horn, comparing the cell numbers in Rexed laminae VII and IX, which display low and high density of large motor neurons, respectively. Double-positive cells were counted in a perimeter of 100 μm, surrounding motor neurons. The analysis was performed manually in 10 histological sections per animal (two different rats for each condition) using the cell counter tool of the Image J software. Values were expressed as a ratio of double-positive cells per motor neuron. The number of double-positive cells labeled with Iba1 or CD163 and GFAP assessed by counting the respective double-positive cells in the gray matter of the lumbar cord of asymptomatic and symptomatic $SOD1^{G93A}$ rats. Quantification was performed only in the ventral horn, comparing the cell numbers in Rexed laminae VII and IX, which display low and high density of large motor neurons, respectively. Values were expressed as the number of double-positive cells per mm^2.

RESULTS

GLIAL PROLIFERATION ADJACENT TO DEGENERATING MOTOR NEURONS

The number of proliferating glia as identified by $Ki67^+$ nuclei sharply increased in the ventral horn of $SOD1^{G93A}$ symptomatic rats and accumulated near surviving motor neurons as well as at sites of apparent motor neuron loss (**Figure 1**). This population of $Ki67^+$ cells had large cell bodies (30–50 μm) with processes embracing motor neurons and expressed GFAP and Iba1 (**Figure 1A**, upper panels). Both Ki67/GFAP and Ki67/Iba1-positive cells displayed morphological features of AbA cells in culture (Diaz-Amarilla et al., 2011) and could be easily differentiated from astrocytes and microglia from non-transgenic or Tg asymptomatic rat's spinal cord. These large GFAP/Ki67 or Iba1/Ki67 cells were rarely observed in asymptomatic or non-transgenic rats (**Figure 1A**, lower panels). Due to the antigen retrieval procedure, motor neuron cell bodies were non-specifically labeled with Ki67 in all experimental conditions. The ratio of GFAP/Ki67 cells and Iba1/Ki67 cells to motor neurons in symptomatic rats was 2.7 and 2.9 respectively, whereas the ratio was < 0.3 in asymptomatic animals for both markers (**Figure 1B**).

CO-EXPRESSION OF MICROGLIAL AND ASTROCYTIC MARKERS IN ABA CELLS

While astrocytes and microglial cells constituted two separate cell populations in asymptomatic rats, being typically detected by GFAP and Iba1 respectively, most AbA cells surrounding the motor neurons in symptomatic rats were surprisingly co-labeled with both markers as well as CD163 (**Figure 2A**). 70% of the GFAP-positive AbA cells in the ventral horn exhibited microglial markers, as compared as <1% in asymptomatic rats. The number of cells labeled with Iba1/GFAP or CD163/GFAP was similar ($\sim$100 cells per mm^2) in symptomatic rats, suggesting the same cells expressed both microglial markers (**Figure 2B**). Detection of the microglial markers required the use of strong antigen retrieval methods, which made motor neuron to artifactually stained with CD163.

Both peri-neuronal AbA cells as well as motor neurons were strongly stained for nitrotyrosine in symptomatic rats, consistent with the production of peroxynitrite (**Figure 2C**). This immunoreactivity was completely blocked by preincubation of the primary antibody with free nitrotyrosine (data not shown).

CHARACTERIZATION OF FIRST STAGES OF ABA CELLS *IN VITRO*

Because AbA cells can be cultured from symptomatic rats (Diaz-Amarilla et al., 2011), we determined the time course of microglial and astrocytic marker expression. Soon after primary cultures of spinal cord were established (DIV2–DIV7), most of the cells displayed the morphology of phagocytic microglia and were fluorescently labeled with the microglia markers CD11b, CD68, and Iba1 (**Figure 3A**). The detailed morphology of cultured cells closely corresponded to the typical features of microglial cells previously reported (Kreutzberg, 1996; **Figure 3B**). No immunoreactivity for GFAP or S100β was detected in cultures since the establishment of cultures and until 10–12 DIV (data not shown). Microglial cells were also analyzed by flow cytometry (FACS) using FITC-labeled CD11b antibodies. FACS analysis showed that > 99% of cells of the primary spinal cord culture of symptomatic rats belonged to the microglia lineage. The purity of this culture was also determined by counting $CD68^+$ and $Iba1^+$ cells and found to be > 98% (**Figure 3C**).

PHENOTYPIC TRANSFORMATION OF MICROGLIA INTO ABA CELLS *IN VITRO*

To confirm that AbA cells were derived from microglia cell progenitors, $CD11b^+$ expressing cells were FACS-sorted and re-established in culture until DIV15. Sorted cells displayed the typical microglia morphology and phenotypic marker until DIV10. This population of cells progressively transitioned into astrocyte-like cells forming monolayers between DIV10 and DIV15, while losing the morphology and phenotypic markers of microglia (**Figure 4A**). At this time, transition zones in the border separating the microglial and the astrocyte-like cells expressed both microglial (Iba1 and CD11b) and astrocytic (GFAP) markers (**Figure 4B**). These transition zones were transient because most cells expressed S100β without microglial markers by DIV15. The treatment of

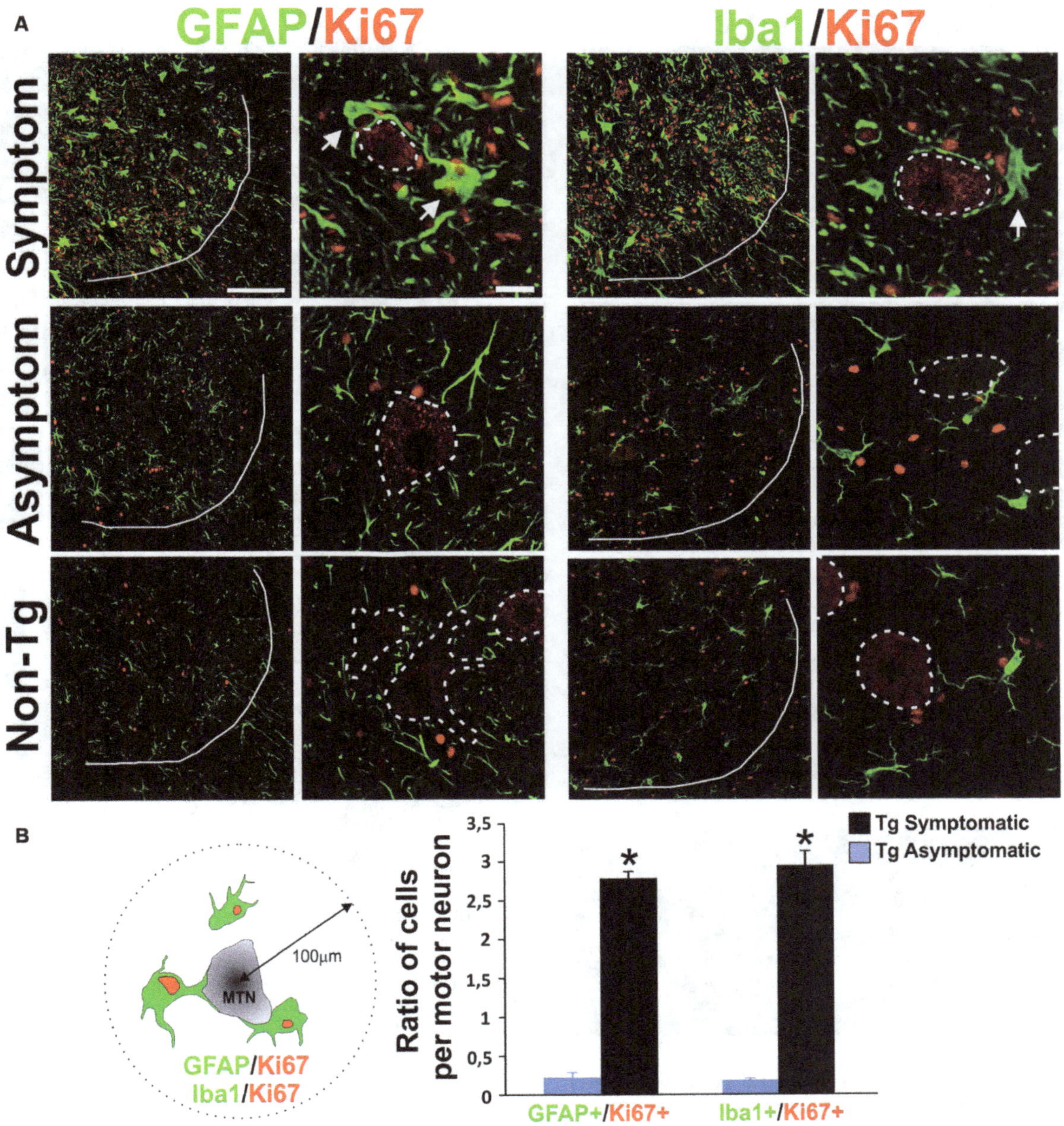

FIGURE 1 | Characterization of proliferative astrocytes and microglia in the degenerating lumbar spinal cord. (A) Photomicrographs showing GFAP/Ki67 and Iba1/Ki67 stained lumbar spinal cord sections measured in symptomatic (upper panels), asymptomatic (middle panels) SOD1^{G93A} rats, and non-transgenic rats (lower panels). Low magnification panels show the notorious increase in the number of Ki67$^+$ red nuclei and the appearance of large GFAP$^+$ and Iba1$^+$ cells (green) in the symptomatic rats, as compared to low cell proliferation in asymptomatic or non-Tg rats. A white line indicates the border between white and grey matter. The high magnification images show that GFAP/Ki67 and Iba1/Ki67 cells are typically located around the motor neurons (indicated as dotted lines) and their processes closely embrace the neuronal cell body. The arrows indicate double-labeled cells. Note the unspecific binding of Ki67 antibody to motor neuron cell bodies. **(B)** Ratio of GFAP/Ki67 and Iba1/Ki67-positive cells per motor neuron in symptomatic and asymptomatic rats. The scheme at the left shows the methods used to count the cells in a perimeter of 100 µm around motor neurons. The counting was performed in 10 histological sections per animal. Two different rats were used for each condition. Data are shown as mean ± SD; $^*P < 0.05$. Scale bars: 100 µm for low magnification panels; 20 µm for high magnification panels.

the cultures with 10 µM FSK, which is known to induce astrocytic processes growth and differentiation (Abe and Saito, 1997), accelerated the transition from microglia to AbA cells, while down-regulating the expression of Iba1 and promoting the growth of processes stained with GFAP (**Figure 4C**). To further confirm the microglia to astrocyte phenotypic switch, we treated the cultures with Leu-OMe, a compound used to selectively deplete microglia from primary cell cultures (Uliasz et al., 2012). **Figure 4D** shows that microglia from ALS rats were completely killed by 25 mM of Leu-OMe at DIV3, whereas there was no toxicity at DIV20 after the cells had undergone the phenotypic transition to an AbA morphology.

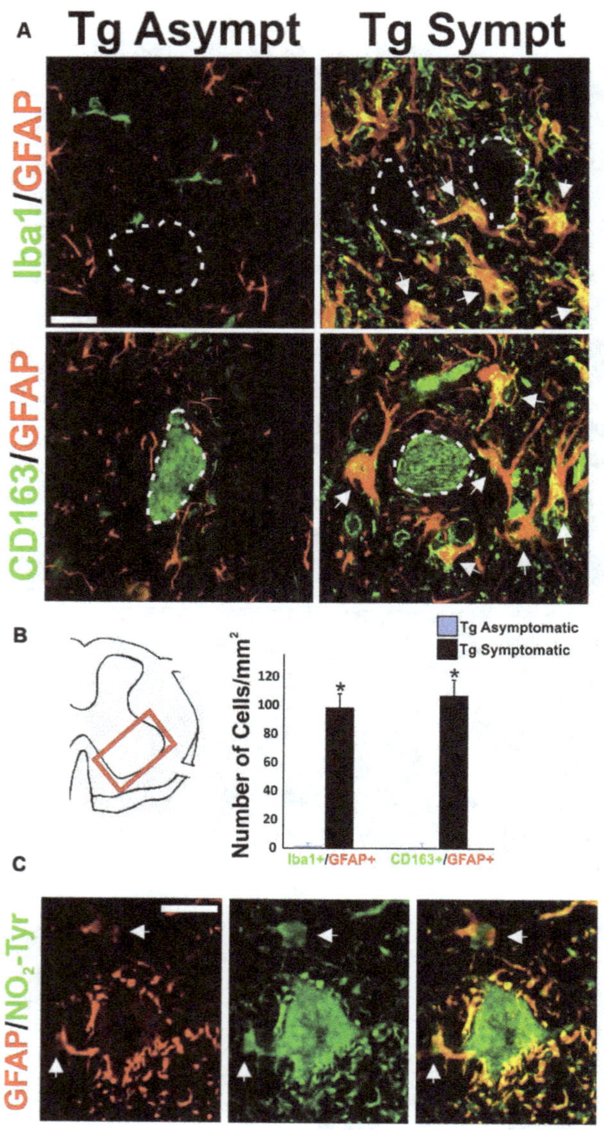

FIGURE 2 | Concurrent expression of microglia and astrocytic markers in AbA cells.(A) Representative image of GFAP (red), Iba1 (green), and CD163 (green) in lumbar spinal cord sections from transgenic asymptomatic (Tg-asymp) and symptomatic (Tg-sympt) SOD1^{G93A} rats. Dotted lines indicate motor neuron cells bodies, which artifactually stained for CD163. Note that microglia and astrocytes in asymptomatic rat expressed GFAP and Iba1 in well-segregated cell populations. In comparison, most of the Iba1$^+$ and CD163$^+$ cells also expressed GFAP in symptomatic animals (arrows). **(B)** Quantification of cells expressing Iba1/GFAP and CD163/GFAP in the lumbar spinal cord. The counting was performed in 10 histological sections per animal. Two different rats were used for each condition. Data are shown as mean ± SD; $*P < 0.05$. **(C)** Representative confocal immunostaining against GFAP (red) and nitrotyrosine (NO_2–Tyr, green) in the ventral horn of a symptomatic rat showing the intense nitration of Perineuronal AbA cells (arrows). Scale bars: 20 μm.

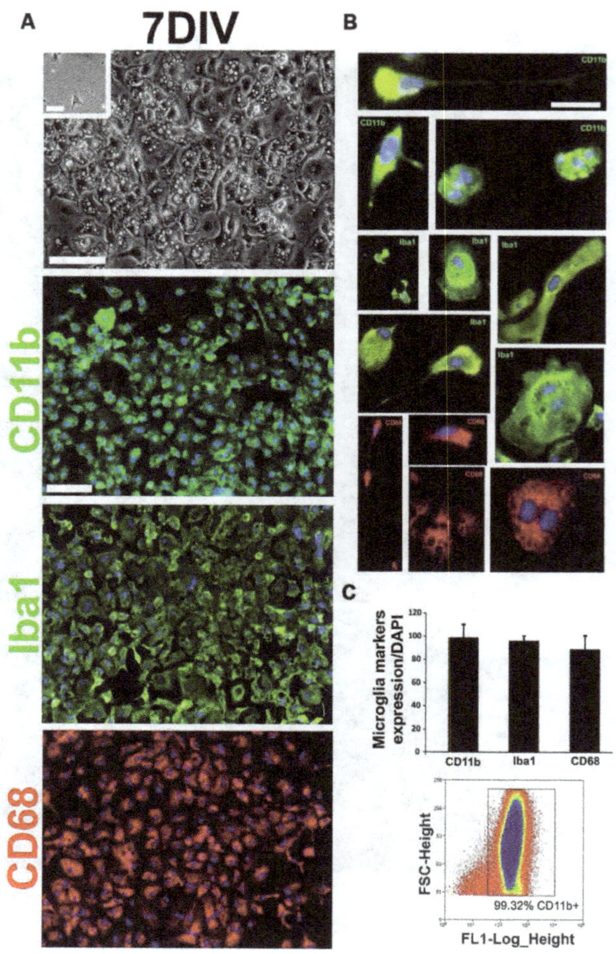

FIGURE 3 | Characterization of first stages of AbA cells *in vitro*. Primary cultures of the spinal cord of symptomatic rats were established as in (Diaz-Amarilla et al., 2011) and the cell phenotypes were analyzed on DIV7. **(A)** The upper panel shows a representative phase-contrast image of the culture at DIV7. The inset shows the same culture obtained from non-Tg littermates where no cells could be grown. The lower panels show confocal images of cells immunostained for typical microglia markers such as CD11b, CD68, and Iba1 at 7 DIV. Scale bars: 50 μm. **(B)** Characterization of different typical microglia phenotypes present at 7 DIV, cultured from Tg symptomatic rats. Scale bar: 25 μm. **(C)** Quantification of the microglia markers expression (CD11b, CD68, and Iba1) in culture at 7 DIV, counting cell positive for microglia marker respect to the total number of nuclei labeled with DAPI (upper panel). Typical data from flow cytometry showing that 99% of cells were CD11b$^+$. The data are representative of three independent experiments.

DISCUSSION

Glial cells expressing mutant SOD1 are now well established to be toxic to motor neurons in rodent models as well as in ALS patients (Barbeito et al., 2004; Nagai et al., 2007; Yamanaka et al., 2008; Haidet-Phillips et al., 2011). AbA cells are the most toxic cells yet identified to motor neurons (Diaz-Amarilla et al., 2011). These distinctive glial cells are directly associated with motor neuron disease, because they actively proliferate after the onset of progressive paralysis and make intimate contact with degenerating motor neurons. By analyzing the population of proliferating Ki67$^+$ glial cells in the ventral horn of symptomatic SOD1 rats, we found that AbA cells most likely originate from microglia. Notably, purified microglia isolated from the spinal cord of symptomatic rats spontaneously transformed into AbA cells.

The extremely rapid progression of paralysis in SOD1^{G93A} rats is characterized by prominent neuroinflammation associated with

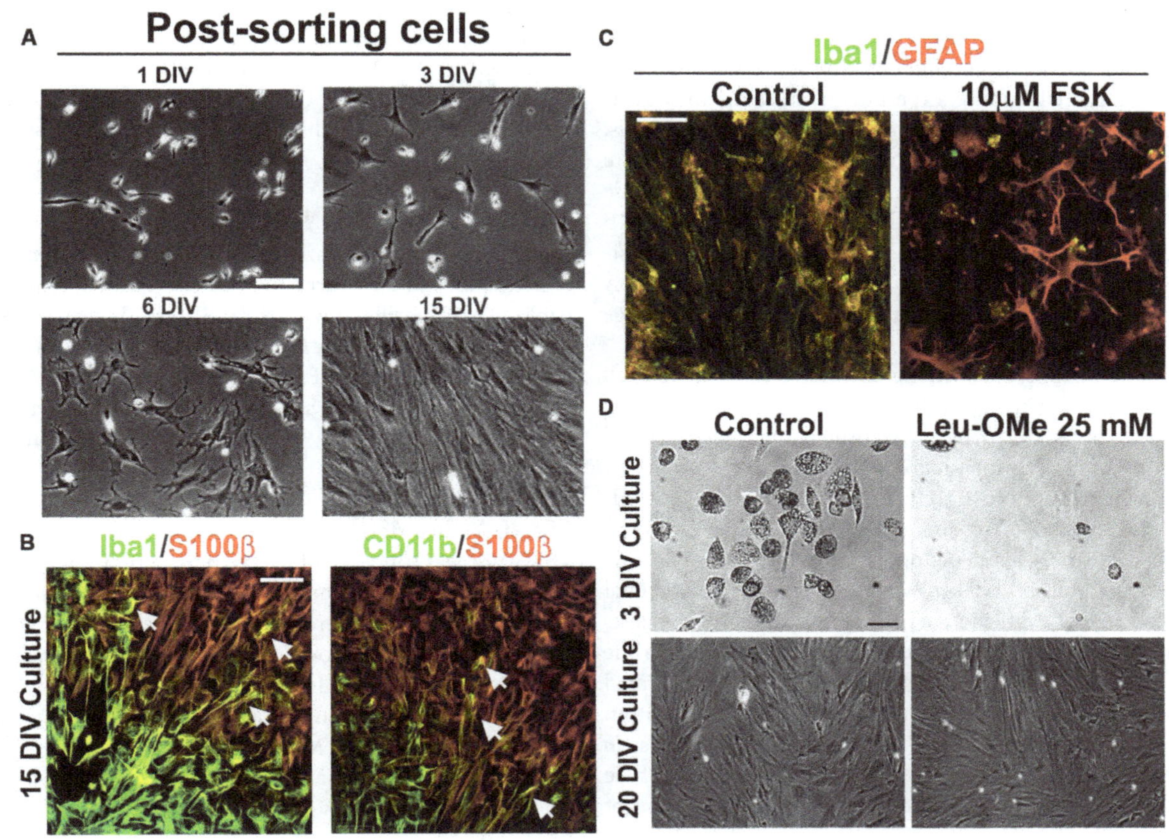

FIGURE 4 | Phenotypic transition of microglia into AbA cells in culture. **(A)** Microglia cell cultures (7 DIV) from symptomatic spinal cord were dissociated and stained with FITC-labeled CD11b. After FACS sorting, cells were re-plated and analyzed for phenotypic transition at DIV15. Scale bar: 50 μm. **(B)** Confocal image showing transition zones observed at 15 DIV. Note the segregation of astrocytic S100β staining with the microglia Iba1 or CD11b markers, which coincides with the morphological change of cells. The co-localization of astrocytic and microglia markers was found in a few cells in the border between these zones. Scale bar: 50 μm. **(C)** Treatment of cultures at DIV15 with foskolin (10 μM, 3 h) down regulated Iba1 expression and stimulated GFAP expression and growth of processes. Scale bars: 50 μm. **(D)** Differential effect of 25 μM of Leucine-Methyl Ester (Leu-OMe) before and after the phenotypic transition. Treatment with Leu-OMe was applied to cultures at DIV3 and DIV20 to assess the toxicity. Toxicity of Leu-OMe was restricted to the microglia phenotype. This experiment was repeated with three independent isolations of AbA cells. Scale bars: 20 μm

microglia activation (Sanagi et al., 2010; Philips and Robberecht, 2011). This inflammatory response is consistent with the sharp increase in cell proliferation others and we have observed with Ki67-staining in symptomatic animals (Schaefer et al., 2005; Pun et al., 2006). Previously, BrdU incorporation was used to demonstrate increased cell proliferation in ALS rats of NG2-positive glial progenitor cells (Magnus et al., 2008), which can potentially differentiate into astrocytes. Our results indicate that microglia more likely gave rise to AbA cells expressing astrocytic markers in regions adjacent to motor neurons.

The finding that spinal AbA cells co-express astrocytic GFAP with two different microglia markers Iba1 or CD163 was surprising because such a mixed phenotype is rarely observed. Co-expression of both markers has been observed in neoplastic glioblastoma multiforme cells (Huysentruyt et al., 2011; Persson and Englund, 2012). These human astroglial tumor cells seem to acquire phagocytic properties as a consequence of the dramatic inflammatory conditions occurring in tumors (Persson and Englund, 2012). Similarly, spinal AbA cells may originate from a phenotypic transition of inflammatory microglia into astrocytes-like cells in the degenerating cellular environment of the ventral horn. Other reports have shown aberrant features of microglial cells in symptomatic $SOD1^{G93A}$ rats, including formation of microglia clusters (Howland et al., 2002) and multi-nucleated giant cells (Fendrick et al., 2007). Based on the morphology, localization, high proliferation rate, and other phenotypic features, spinal AbA cells are distinct from previously described M1 or M2 microglia (Kigerl et al., 2009; Durafourt et al., 2012; Liao et al., 2012). It is uncertain whether the phenotypic transition is specific for mutant SOD1 microglia or might also be observed in other CNS insults where phagocytic microglia accumulate around dying neurons (Beyer et al., 2000; Sanagi et al., 2010; Neher et al., 2012). For example, ameboid microglia-like cells expressing markers of oligodendrocyte and monocyte lineages have been described in hippocampus following acute neuronal damage (Fiedorowicz et al., 2008). AbA cells represent a novel pathological phenotype of microglia/macrophages derived from their prominent plasticity following activation (Schwartz et al., 2006; Luo and Chen, 2012). This phenotypic transformation of microglia may explain why the ablation of dividing astrocytes did not alter astrogliosis in SOD1 mice (Lepore et al., 2008).

Further evidence that AbA cells derive from activated microglia was provided in cell culture experiments showing that purified endogenous microglia can transition to astrocyte-like cells. Microglia expressing CD11b, Iba1, and CD68 represented more than 98% of cells isolated from the spinal cord of symptomatic SOD1^{G93A} rats. Moreover, FACS sorting of these cells using CD11b antibodies resulted in typical microglia cultures that also transitioned to AbA cells after 2 weeks, showing not only that AbA cells are originated from microglia but also the phenotypic change occurs *in vitro*.

Because the phenotypic switch is associated to sustained cell proliferation and a critical cell density, we suggest that inflammatory mediators secreted by the activated microglia induced the transformation. Previous reports have shown the ability of microglia to be progenitors for different neural cell types, including astrocytes *in vitro* (Yokoyama et al., 2004). This property in turn may be related to their hematopoietic origin (Yokoyama et al., 2006). Compared to AbA cells growing in the degenerating spinal cord, the concurrent expression of astrocytic and microglia markers by cultured AbA cells is only transiently in restricted to the borders of the transition zones. Therefore, it appears that activated microglial cells in degenerating spinal cord are prone to transition to astrocyte-like phenotype both in culture conditions as well as *in vivo*, in the cellular niche surrounding the motor neurons. These cells may play a role in the killing and subsequent phagocytosis of motor neurons.

Spinal AbA cells also show a number of aberrant features including high levels of S100β and Cx43 expression (Diaz-Amarilla et al., 2011) that may be relevant for neuronal toxicity through secreted S100 proteins as well as extracellular ATP released through connexin hemichannels. Activation of the extracellular ATP receptor/channel P2X7 has recently been shown to induce motor neuron death and to induce the neurotoxic phenotypes of astrocytes in culture (Gandelman et al., 2010, 2013). Furthermore, endogenous nitration of tyrosine near the ATP binding pocket of HSP90 activates P2X7, which induces motor neuron apoptosis (Franco et al., 2013).

We also showed that spinal AbA cells are strongly stained for nitrotyrosine especially in the distal perineuronal processes, consistent with the production of peroxynitrite. Microglia bearing mutant SOD1 has been shown to damage motor neurons through the production of peroxynitrite (Thonhoff et al., 2012).Because their microglia origin, spinal AbA cells may have primed to generate superoxide and hence peroxynitrite on the exterior face of the plasma membrane in close proximity to motor neurons (Beckman et al., 2001).

CONCLUSION

Taken together, the present work supports the concept that aberrant astrocyte-like cells in the degenerating spinal cord are derived from activated microglia that proliferate around damaged motor neurons. The present study provides evidence that microglia isolated from the spinal cord of ALS–SOD rats developing paralysis have the potential to transition into an astrocyte-like phenotype. The proliferating spinal AbA cells concurrently express markers of both microglia and astrocytes lineages. Because the appearance of AbA cells is closely associated to the progression of paralysis in SOD1^{G93A} rats, a better understanding of the mediators inducing the phenotypic transition may provide another avenue of intervention to slow the progressive spread of disease in ALS patients.

AUTHOR CONTRIBUTIONS

Emiliano Trias, Pablo Díaz-Amarilla, Silvia Olivera-Bravo, Joseph S. Beckman, and Luis Barbeito designed research; Emiliano Trias, Pablo Díaz-Amarilla, Silvia Olivera-Bravo, Eugenia Isasi, Derek A. Drechsel, Nathan Lopez, C. Samuel Bradford, and Kyle E. Ireton performed research; Emiliano Trias, Pablo Díaz-Amarilla, C. Samuel Bradford, Joseph S. Beckman, and Luis Barbeito analyzed data; and Emiliano Trias, Joseph S. Beckman, and Luis Barbeito wrote the paper.

ACKNOWLEDGMENTS

This work was funded by the program for development of basic sciences (PEDECIBA), Innovation and Research National Agency (ANII), and FOCEM-Mercosur funding. Partial funding also came from National Institute on Environmental Health Sciences Grant P30ES000210, National Institute of Neurological Disorders and Stroke Grant R01NS058628A, and National Center for Complementary and Alternative Medicine Grant NCCAM P01AT002034; and from the ALS Association (to Joseph S. Beckman).

REFERENCES

Abe, K., and Saito, H. (1997). Developmental changes in cyclic AMP-stimulated stellation of cultured rat cortical astrocytes. *Jpn. J. Pharmacol.* 75, 433–438. doi: 10.1254/jjp.75.433

Appel, S. H. (2009). CD4+ T cells mediate cytotoxicity in neurodegenerative diseases. *J. Clin. Invest.* 119, 13–15. doi: 10.1172/JCI38096

Barbeito, L. H., Pehar, M., Cassina, P., Vargas, M. R., Peluffo, H., Viera, L., et al. (2004). A role for astrocytes in motor neuron loss in amyotrophic lateral sclerosis. *Brain Res. Brain Res. Rev.* 47, 263–274. doi: 10.1016/j.brainresrev.2004.05.003

Beckman, J. S., Estevez, A. G., Crow, J. P., and Barbeito, L. (2001). Superoxide dismutase and the death of motoneurons in ALS. *Trends Neurosci.* 24, S15–S20. doi: 10.1016/S0166-2236(01)00004-2

Beyer, M., Gimsa, U., Eyupoglu, I. Y., Hailer, N. P., and Nitsch, R. (2000). Phagocytosis of neuronal or glial debris by microglial cells: upregulation of MHC class II expression and multinuclear giant cell formation in vitro. *Glia* 31, 262–266. doi: 10.1002/1098-1136(200009)31:3<262::AID-GLIA70>3.0.CO;2-2

Boillee, S., Vande Velde, C., and Cleveland, D. W. (2006a). ALS: a disease of motor neurons and their non-neuronal neighbors. *Neuron* 52, 39–59. doi: 10.1016/j.neuron.2006.09.018

Boillee, S., Yamanaka, K., Lobsiger, C. S., Copeland, N. G., Jenkins, N. A., Kassiotis, G., et al. (2006b). Onset and progression in inherited ALS determined by motor neurons and microglia. *Science* 312, 1389–1392. doi: 10.1126/science.1123511

Bruijn, L. I., Becher, M. W., Lee, M. K., Anderson, K. L., Jenkins, N. A., Copeland, N. G., et al. (1997). ALS-linked SOD1 mutant G85R mediates damage to astrocytes and promotes rapidly progressive disease with SOD1-containing inclusions. *Neuron* 18, 327–338. doi: 10.1016/S0896-6273(00)80272-X

Cleveland, D. W., and Rothstein, J. D. (2001). From Charcot to Lou Gehrig: deciphering selective motor neuron death in ALS. *Nat. Rev. Neurosci.* 2, 806–819. doi: 10.1038/35097565

Diaz-Amarilla, P., Olivera-Bravo, S., Trias, E., Cragnolini, A., Martinez-Palma, L., Cassina, P., et al. (2011). Phenotypically aberrant astrocytes that promote motoneuron damage in a model of inherited amyotrophic lateral sclerosis. *Proc. Natl. Acad. Sci. U.S.A.* 108, 18126–18131. doi: 10.1073/pnas.1110689108

Durafourt, B. A., Moore, C. S., Zammit, D. A., Johnson, T. A., Zaguia, F., Guiot, M. C., et al. (2012). Comparison of polarization properties of human adult microglia and blood-derived macrophages. *Glia* 60, 717–727. doi: 10.1002/glia.22298

Engelhardt, J. I., Tajti, J., and Appel, S. H. (1993). Lymphocytic infiltrates in the spinal cord in amyotrophic lateral sclerosis. *Arch. Neurol.* 50, 30–36. doi: 10.1001/archneur.1993.00540010026013

Fendrick, S. E., Xue, Q. S., and Streit, W. J. (2007). Formation of multinucleated giant cells and microglial degeneration in rats expressing a mutant Cu/Zn superoxide dismutase gene. *J. Neuroinflammation* 4, 9. doi: 10.1186/1742-2094-4-9

Fiedorowicz, A., Figiel, I., Zaremba, M., Dzwonek, K., and Oderfeld-Nowak, B. (2008). The ameboid phenotype of NG2 (+) cells in the region of apoptotic dentate granule neurons in trimethyltin intoxicated mice shares antigen properties with microglia/macrophages. *Glia* 56, 209–222. doi: 10.1002/glia.20605

Franco, M. C., Ye, Y., Refakis, C. A., Feldman, J. L., Stokes, A. L., Basso, M., et al. (2013). Nitration of Hsp90 induces cell death. *Proc. Natl. Acad. Sci. U.S.A.* 110, E1102–E1111. doi: 10.1073/pnas.1215177110

Gandelman, M., Levy, M., Cassina, P., Barbeito, L., and Beckman, J. S. (2013). P2X7 receptor-induced death of motor neurons by a peroxynitrite/FAS-dependent pathway. *J. Neurochem.* 126, 382–388. doi: 10.1111/jnc.12286

Gandelman, M., Peluffo, H., Beckman, J. S., Cassina, P., and Barbeito, L. (2010). Extracellular ATP and the P2X7 receptor in astrocyte-mediated motor neuron death: implications for amyotrophic lateral sclerosis. *J. Neuroinflammation* 7, 33. doi: 10.1186/1742-2094-7-33

Graber, D. J., Hickey, W. F., and Harris, B. T. (2010). Progressive changes in microglia and macrophages in spinal cord and peripheral nerve in the transgenic rat model of amyotrophic lateral sclerosis. *J. Neuroinflammation* 7, 8. doi: 10.1186/1742-2094-7-8

Gurney, M. E., Pu, H., Chiu, A. Y., Dal Canto, M. C., Polchow, C. Y., Alexander, D. D., et al. (1994). Motor neuron degeneration in mice that express a human Cu,Zn superoxide dismutase mutation. *Science* 264, 1772–1775. doi: 10.1126/science.8209258

Haidet-Phillips, A. M., Hester, M. E., Miranda, C. J., Meyer, K., Braun, L., Frakes, A., et al. (2011). Astrocytes from familial and sporadic ALS patients are toxic to motor neurons. *Nat. Biotechnol.* 29, 824–828. doi: 10.1038/nbt.1957

Hall, E. D., Oostveen, J. A., and Gurney, M. E. (1998). Relationship of microglial and astrocytic activation to disease onset and progression in a transgenic model of familial ALS. *Glia* 23, 249–256. doi: 10.1002/(SICI)1098-1136(199807)23:3<249::AID-GLIA7>3.0.CO;2-#

Howland, D. S., Liu, J., She, Y., Goad, B., Maragakis, N. J., Kim, B., et al. (2002). Focal loss of the glutamate transporter EAAT2 in a transgenic rat model of SOD1 mutant-mediated amyotrophic lateral sclerosis (ALS). *Proc. Natl. Acad. Sci. U.S.A.* 99, 1604–1609. doi: 10.1073/pnas.032539299

Huysentruyt, L. C., Akgoc, Z., and Seyfried, T. N. (2011). Hypothesis: are neoplastic macrophages/microglia present in glioblastoma multiforme? *ASN Neuro.* 3, e00064. doi: 10.1042/AN20110011

Ilieva, H., Polymenidou, M., and Cleveland, D. W. (2009). Non-cell autonomous toxicity in neurodegenerative disorders: ALS and beyond. *J. Cell Biol.* 187, 761–772. doi: 10.1083/jcb.200908164

Kang, S. H., Fukaya, M., Yang, J. K., Rothstein, J. D., and Bergles, D. E. (2010). NG2+ CNS glial progenitors remain committed to the oligodendrocyte lineage in postnatal life and following neurodegeneration. *Neuron* 68, 668–681. doi: 10.1016/j.neuron.2010.09.009

Kigerl, K. A., Gensel, J. C., Ankeny, D. P., Alexander, J. K., Donnelly, D. J., and Popovich, P. G. (2009). Identification of two distinct macrophage subsets with divergent effects causing either neurotoxicity or regeneration in the injured mouse spinal cord. *J. Neurosci.* 29, 13435–13444. doi: 10.1523/JNEUROSCI.3257-09.2009

Kreutzberg, G. W. (1996). Microglia: a sensor for pathological events in the CNS. *Trends Neurosci.* 19, 312–318. doi: 10.1016/0166-2236(96)10049-7

Lepore, A. C., Dejea, C., Carmen, J., Rauck, B., Kerr, D. A., Sofroniew, M. V., et al. (2008). Selective ablation of proliferating astrocytes does not affect disease outcome in either acute or chronic models of motor neuron degeneration. *Exp. Neurol.* 211, 423–432. doi: 10.1016/j.expneurol.2008.02.020

Liao, B., Zhao, W., Beers, D. R., Henkel, J. S., and Appel, S. H. (2012). Transformation from a neuroprotective to a neurotoxic microglial phenotype in a mouse model of ALS. *Exp. Neurol.* 237, 147–152. doi: 10.1016/j.expneurol.2012.06.011

Luo, X. G., and Chen, S. D. (2012). The changing phenotype of microglia from homeostasis to disease. *Transl. Neurodegener.* 1:9. doi: 10.1186/2047-9158-1-9

Magnus, T., Carmen, J., Deleon, J., Xue, H., Pardo, A. C., Lepore, A. C., et al. (2008). Adult glial precursor proliferation in mutant SOD1G93A mice. *Glia* 56, 200–208. doi: 10.1002/glia.20604

McGeer, P. L., and McGeer, E. G. (2002). Inflammatory processes in amyotrophic lateral sclerosis. *Muscle Nerve* 26, 459–470. doi: 10.1002/mus.10191

Nagai, M., Re, D. B., Nagata, T., Chalazonitis, A., Jessell, T. M., Wichterle, H., et al. (2007). Astrocytes expressing ALS-linked mutated SOD1 release factors selectively toxic to motor neurons. *Nat. Neurosci.* 10, 615–622. doi: 10.1038/nn1876

Neher, J. J., Neniskyte, U., and Brown, G. C. (2012). Primary phagocytosis of neurons by inflamed microglia: potential roles in neurodegeneration. *Front. Pharmacol.* 3:27. doi: 10.3389/fphar.2012.00027

Papadeas, S. T., Kraig, S. E., O'Banion, C., Lepore, A. C., and Maragakis, N. J. (2011). Astrocytes carrying the superoxide dismutase 1 (SOD1G93A) mutation induce wild-type motor neuron degeneration in vivo. *Proc. Natl. Acad. Sci. U.S.A.* 108, 17803–17808. doi: 10.1073/pnas.1103141108

Persson, A., and Englund, E. (2012). Phagocytic properties in tumor astrocytes. *Neuropathology* 32, 252–260. doi: 10.1111/j.1440-1789.2011.01266.x

Philips, T., and Robberecht, W. (2011). Neuroinflammation in amyotrophic lateral sclerosis: role of glial activation in motor neuron disease. *Lancet Neurol.* 10, 253–263. doi: 10.1016/S1474-4422(11)70015-70011

Pun, S., Santos, A. F., Saxena, S., Xu, L., and Caroni, P. (2006). Selective vulnerability and pruning of phasic motoneuron axons in motoneuron disease alleviated by CNTF. *Nat. Neurosci.* 9, 408–419. doi: 10.1038/nn1653

Sanagi, T., Yuasa, S., Nakamura, Y., Suzuki, E., Aoki, M., Warita, H., et al. (2010). Appearance of phagocytic microglia adjacent to motoneurons in spinal cord tissue from a presymptomatic transgenic rat model of amyotrophic lateral sclerosis. *J. Neurosci. Res.* 88, 2736–2746. doi: 10.1002/jnr.22424

Sargsyan, S. A., Monk, P. N., and Shaw, P. J. (2005). Microglia as potential contributors to motor neuron injury in amyotrophic lateral sclerosis. *Glia* 51, 241–253. doi: 10.1002/glia.20210

Schaefer, A. M., Sanes, J. R., and Lichtman, J. W. (2005). A compensatory subpopulation of motor neurons in a mouse model of amyotrophic lateral sclerosis. *J. Comp. Neurol.* 490, 209–219. doi: 10.1002/cne.20620

Schwartz, M., Butovsky, O., Bruck, W., and Hanisch, U. K. (2006). Microglial phenotype: is the commitment reversible? *Trends Neurosci.* 29, 68–74. doi: 10.1016/j.tins.2005.12.005

Thonhoff, J. R., Gao, J., Dunn, T. J., Ojeda, L., and Wu, P. (2012). Mutant SOD1 microglia-generated nitroxidative stress promotes toxicity to human fetal neural stem cell-derived motor neurons through direct damage and noxious interactions with astrocytes. *Am. J. Stem Cells* 1, 2–21.

Uliasz, T. F., Hamby, M. E., Jackman, N. A., Hewett, J. A., and Hewett, S. J. (2012). Generation of primary astrocyte cultures devoid of contaminating microglia. *Methods Mol. Biol.* 814, 61–79. doi: 10.1007/978-1-61779-452-0_5

Yamanaka, K., Chun, S. J., Boillee, S., Fujimori-Tonou, N., Yamashita, H., Gutmann, D. H., et al. (2008). Astrocytes as determinants of disease progression in inherited amyotrophic lateral sclerosis. *Nat. Neurosci.* 11, 251–253. doi: 10.1038/nn2047

Yokoyama, A., Sakamoto, A., Kameda, K., Imai, Y., and Tanaka, J. (2006). NG2 proteoglycan-expressing microglia as multipotent neural progenitors in normal and pathologic brains. *Glia* 53, 754–768. doi: 10.1002/glia.20332

Yokoyama, A., Yang, L., Itoh, S., Mori, K., and Tanaka, J. (2004). Microglia, a potential source of neurons, astrocytes, and oligodendrocytes. *Glia* 45, 96–104. doi: 10.1002/glia.10306

20

A plural role for lipids in motor neuron diseases: energy, signaling and structure

Florent Schmitt[1,2], Ghulam Hussain[1,2], Luc Dupuis[1,2], Jean-Philippe Loeffler[1,2] and Alexandre Henriques[1,2]*

[1] Mécanismes Centraux et Périphériques de la Neurodégénerescence, INSERM U1118, Strasbourg, France
[2] UMRS1118, Fédération de Médecine Translationnelle de Strasbourg, Université de Strasbourg, France

Edited by:
Ricardo Tapia, Universidad Nacional Autónoma de México, Mexico

Reviewed by:
Ricardo Tapia, Universidad Nacional Autónoma de México, Mexico
Luis B. Tovar-y-Romo, Universidad Nacional Autónoma de México, Mexico

***Correspondence:**
Alexandre Henriques, Faculté de médecine, INSERM U1118, 11 rue Humann, 67085 Strasbourg, France
e-mail: henriques@unistra.fr

Motor neuron diseases (MNDs) are characterized by selective death of motor neurons and include mainly adult-onset amyotrophic lateral sclerosis (ALS) and spinal muscular atrophy (SMA). Neurodegeneration is not the single pathogenic event occurring during disease progression. There are multiple lines of evidence for the existence of defects in lipid metabolism at peripheral level. For instance, hypermetabolism is well characterized in ALS, and dyslipidemia correlates with better prognosis in patients. Lipid metabolism plays also a role in other MNDs. In SMA, misuse of lipids as energetic nutrients is described in patients and in related animal models. The composition of structural lipids in the central nervous system is modified, with repercussion on membrane fluidity and on cell signaling mediated by bioactive lipids. Here, we review the main epidemiologic and mechanistic findings that link alterations of lipid metabolism and motor neuron degeneration, and we discuss the rationale of targeting these modifications for therapeutic management of MNDs.

Keywords: ALS, motor neuron, lipid, metabolism, SMA, SBMA

INTRODUCTION

Motor neuron diseases (MNDs) are a group of incurable neurological disorders caused by the selective degeneration of motor neurons. Amyotrophic lateral sclerosis (ALS) is the most representative MNDs among adults with a incidence rate of 2–3 per 100,000 (Brooks et al., 2000). It is characterized by progressive muscle weakness and atrophy, loss of upper and lower motor neurons and death ensuing 3–5 years after diagnosis. Majority of ALS patients are of sporadic origin with unclear ethiopathology. Several mutations are associated with ALS, in particular in genes encoding superoxide dismutase 1 (*SOD-1*), TAR DNA binding protein of 43-kDa (*TDP-43*), fused in sarcoma (*FUS*) and chromosome 9 open reading frame 72 (*C9ORF72*) (Rosen et al., 1993; Mackenzie et al., 2007; Deng et al., 2010; Laaksovirta et al., 2010; Shatunov et al., 2010). Thus, several transgenic mouse models overexpressing various mutant genes have been developed, and the SOD1 model, overexpressing a mutated form of SOD1 gene, is the most studied in ALS (Ripps et al., 1995). Spinal muscular atrophy (SMA) is a genetic autosomal and recessive neuromuscular disease, caused by loss of functional survival motor neuron (SMN) gene 1. Patients suffer from degeneration of spinal motor neurons, muscle weakness leading to atrophy. Disease severity ranges from severe, with death of patients before the age of 10, to mild with moderate symptoms with no alteration of life expectancy. Spinal bulbar muscular atrophy (SBMA), also known as Kennedy's disease, is an X-linked recessive disease caused by a CAG-repeat expansion in the gene coding for the androgen receptor, leading to a poly-Q repeat expansion in the protein (Brooks and Fischbeck, 1995; Fischbeck et al., 1999). The disease affects mainly males, even though it has been described also in female patients. SBMA is characterized by progressive muscle atrophy and degeneration of lower motor neurons in the brain stem and spinal cord. Similarly to ALS, mouse models have been developed to study SMA and SBMA (Katsuno et al., 2003; Bebee et al., 2012).

Along with neuronal degeneration, several alterations of lipid metabolism are found in these diseases. Here, we review the role of lipids in MNDs, with a special attention on energy homeostasis, cell signaling and structure. We further discuss the rationale of targeting lipid metabolism for therapeutic management of MNDs.

ENERGETIC ALTERATIONS IN AMYOTROPHIC LATERAL SCLEROSIS

Multiple previously unrecognized phenotypes occur in ALS patients, in particular, the unbalance between food intake and energy (Braun et al., 2012; Muscaritoli et al., 2012). ALS patients often present with dyslipidemia, reduced body mass and increased resting energy expenditure (**Table 1**, Desport et al., 2001; Funalot et al., 2009; Dupuis et al., 2011). Energetic alterations are similarly found in transgenic animal models of ALS, the SOD1 mice. These mice are leaner than controls, hypermetabolic, hypolipidemic and present increased fatty acid uptake in muscles (**Table 2**, Dupuis et al., 2004; Fergani et al., 2007; Kim et al., 2011). Several lines of evidence point to lipid metabolism alterations being crucial for ALS progression. A first incidental event shed some light on the subject. During 2 years, a group of scientists remain in an isolated environment, and were submitted to long term caloric restriction (Walford et al., 2002). From eight members of the group, one died from ALS and another one developed progressive gait impairment and motor

Table 1 | Altered energetic metabolism in ALS patients.

Items	Cohort size (ALS patients)	Outcomes	References
BASAL METABOLISM IN ALS			
	$N = 62$	ALS patients are hypermetabolic.	Desport et al., 2001
	$N = 44$	ALS patients are hypermetabolic.	Funalot et al., 2009
EPIDEMIOLOGIC AND RISKS TO ALS			
	$N = 153$	High carbohydrates and low fat intakes increase ALS risk.	Okamoto et al., 2007
	$N = 222$	High prediagnostic body fat is associated with a decreased risk of ALS mortality.	Gallo et al., 2013
LIPIDS AND PROGNOSIS IN ALS			
	$N = 369$	High LDL/HDL ratio correlates to longer survival.	Dupuis et al., 2008
	$N = 658$	Hyperlipidemia does not correlate to longer survival.	Chio et al., 2009
	$N = 658$	Low level LDL/HDL ratio correlates to respiratory dysfunction.	Chio et al., 2009
	$N = 285$	Low BMI correlates to faster decline.	Jawaid et al., 2010
	$N = 92$	Poor nutritional status is associated with higher mortality.	Marin et al., 2011
	$N = 488$	High triglycerides or cholesterol correlates to longer survival.	Dorst et al., 2011
	$N = 427$	High BMI correlates to longer survival.	Paganoni et al., 2011
	$N = 77$	Fast reduction of BMI predicts faster decline.	Shimizu et al., 2012
	$N = 150$	High BMI correlate to slower ALSFRS score decline.	Reich-Slotky et al., 2013
	$N = 62$	High subcutaneous fat positively correlate to survival.	Lindauer et al., 2013

Table 2 | Altered energetic metabolism in mouse models of MNDs.

Model	Cohort size	Conclusion	References
ALS			
SOD1 G93A mice	$N = 8$	Altered composition of lipids in spinal cord.	Cutler et al., 2002
SOD1 G86Rand G93A mice	$N = 7–8$	Dramatic defect in energy homeostasis, hypermetabolism mainly of muscular origin.	Dupuis et al., 2004
	$N = 13$	High fat diet delays disease onset and extent survival.	Dupuis et al., 2004
SOD G93A mice	$N = 27$	The ketogenic diet protects against motor neuron death.	Zhao et al., 2006
SOD1 G86Rand G93A mice	$N = 10–15$	Hypolipidemia is found in SOD1 mice.	Fergani et al., 2007
SOD1 G93A mice	$N = 49$ females $N = 31$ males	Caloric restriction shortens lifespan through an increase in lipid peroxidation, inflammation and apoptosis.	Patel et al., 2010
SOD1 G93A mice	$N = 30$ males	Hypolipidemia is present at the presymptomatic stage of disease.	Kim et al., 2011
SOD1 G93A mice	$N =$ males	Medium chain triglycerides protect motoneurons survival but does not extent survival.	Zhao et al., 2012
SMA			
SMN1 deficient mice	$N = 30$ males	Hypolipidemia is present at the pre-symptomatic stage of disease.	Butchbach et al., 2010

neuron degeneration. Epidemiological studies went beyond this case study and documented an association between nutrition and the risk of developing ALS. First, a case control survey made in Japan in 2007 was conducted with the aim to study pre-illness nutritional habits of ALS patients. The authors identified that high carbohydrate and low fat intakes are associated with higher ALS risk (**Table 1**, Okamoto et al., 2007). More recently, another epidemiologic study focused on anthropometric characteristics of the general population with a follow up over 10 years. The investigators reached the conclusion that high fat content reduces the risk of developing ALS (Gallo et al., 2013). These clinical data are consistent with the reduced overall survival of SOD1 mice under caloric restriction (**Table 2**) (Hamadeh et al., 2005).

Conversely, increased energy intake is beneficial for SOD1 mice. The first evidence emerged in 2004 from our laboratory, when we fed SOD1 mice with a diet enriched in lipids. The treatment restored normal body mass and adiposity, delayed disease onset and motor neuron degeneration, and life expectancy was extended by 20% (Dupuis et al., 2004). The beneficial effects of high fat diet, or ketogenic diet, for SOD1 mice were confirmed by other groups (**Table 2**, Mattson et al., 2007; Zhao et al., 2006, 2012). In 2008, we aimed to study the link between lipids and disease progression, by quantifying circulating lipids in ALS patients. We found that dyslipidemia, defined by high LDL/HDL ratio, was a characteristic of the ALS group (Dupuis et al., 2008), and this dyslipidemia positively correlated with longer survival, increased by 13 months in the group of ALS patients with higher LDL/HDL ratio. Since then, others reported that either hyperlipidemia or high body mass index is a strong prognostic factor for survival (Dorst et al., 2011; Paganoni et al., 2011; Shimizu et al., 2012; Reich-Slotky et al., 2013). For instance, the median life expectancy was higher than 14 months in patients with high serum triglyceride levels (Dorst et al., 2011). Last, it was recently observed that subcutaneous fat positively correlated with survival of ALS patients (Lindauer et al., 2013). Conversely, lower LDL/HDL ratio has been linked to respiratory impairments (Chio et al., 2009), fast loss of BMI was associated with faster decline (Jawaid et al., 2010) and poor nutritional status is a negative prognosis factor (Marin et al., 2011).

These reports claim for a positive correlation between high circulating lipid levels of lipids or high fat mass and prognosis of ALS patients. The mechanisms in place deserve further investigation, to understand how peripheral lipids interfere with disease progression and how lipids can preserve motor axis integrity.

ENERGETIC SUBSTRATES AND MOTOR UNITS

The motor unit is an anatomical structure responsible for the control of muscle contraction and its destruction represents the first detectable event in ALS (Dupuis and Loeffler, 2009). The motor units are composed of different sorts of spinal motor neurons and muscles fibers, depending on their activity and energetic capacities. Fast fatigable motor units are composed of large alpha-motor neurons and glycolytic muscle fibers that burn preferentially glucose to exert heavy force on a short period. Conversely, slow motor units correspond to small alpha-motor neurons and oxidative muscle fibers, which store and use preferentially fatty acids to produce less intense but constant strength. Large alpha motor neurons are the first to degenerate in ALS models (Pun et al., 2006; Hegedus et al., 2007), and fast-twitch motor units are preferentially affected in both ALS patients and mouse models (Schmied et al., 1999; Atkin et al., 2005; Gordon et al., 2010). Stimulation of motor units via regular training was proposed to maintain and strengthen motor function in ALS (**Table 3**). Clinical investigations reported benefit for ALS patients whom followed moderate and mainly aerobic exercise program, which use lipids as energy source (de Almeida et al., 2012). In particular, specific training of the diaphragma preserved respiratory functions in ALS patients (Mahajan et al., 2012). It should be noted that these studies were not randomized and suffer from the small size of the cohorts. Moreover, higher release of reactive oxygen species during exercise was reported (Siciliano et al., 2002) and suggest that design for muscular training in ALS patients should be considered with caution (**Table 3**).

In an animal model of ALS, effects of high frequency and high amplitude training were compared to moderate and endurance training. SOD1 mice were subjected either to swimming-based training, targeting glycolytic motor units, or to running-based training, targeting oxidative motor units (Deforges et al., 2009). After training, the group of "swimmer" mice presented with benefits in terms of counts of motor neurons and survival, when compared to proper control. On the contrary, the "running"-trained mice presented a similar disease course compared to sedentary mice. Effect of training on SOD1 mice is not fully clarified. Others reported claimed that moderate exercise alone can improve outcomes in SOD1 mice (Carreras et al., 2010), and most importantly, Gerber and colleagues recently demonstrated that benefits of training in mice might come from the enrichment of the environment rather than mobilization of muscle fibers (Gerber et al., 2012). Therefore, the benefit after different types of training for SOD1 mice targeting different pool of motor units remains to be clarified. Currently, the effects of aerobic versus anaerobic exercises on vital capacity and muscular strength are under clinical investigations (**Table 4**, NCT01650818, NCT01521728). Additional work on this topic is required to understand the impact of different exercises, using different energetic sources, on motor units in ALS patients, and why glycolytic motor units are preferentially affected.

ENERGY, METABOLISM, AND MITOCHONDRIA

Taken separately, the two extremities of the motor units, the muscles and the motor neurons, show abnormal lipid metabolism. Indeed, early in the disease course, glycolytic muscles of SOD1 mice switch toward an oxidative phenotype, presumably due to the loss of their connection to large motor neurons and subsequent reinnervation by "slow" motor neurons (Sharp et al., 2005). The selective vulnerability of large motor neurons is potentially due to higher energetic needs that could either be not fulfilled or a source of oxidative stress. In case of higher needs, neurons can use ketone bodies as energetic substrate when glucose level becomes low (Guzman and Blazquez, 2004; LaManna et al., 2009). In this situation, astrocytes will use lipid to provide ketone bodies to neurons, and potentially motorneurons in ALS (Yi et al., 2011). Interestingly, medium chain triglycerides, precursors of ketone bodies, preserve motor functions and promote motorneuron survival in SOD1 mice through the enhancement of oxidative metabolism (**Table 2**, Zhao et al., 2012).

Moreover two recent studies have shown abnormally enhanced levels of ketone bodies, released by the breakdown of fatty acids, in the cerebrospinal fluid of ALS patients (Blasco et al., 2010; Kumar

Table 3 | Effect of exercise in ALS.

Cohort	Outcomes	References
SOD1 MICE G93A		
	High frequency and amplitude training support in motor neuron survival.	Deforges et al., 2009
	Moderate frequency and amplitude training support motor neurons survival.	Carreras et al., 2010
	Benefits of training might come from the enrichment of the environment.	Gerber et al., 2012
ALS PATIENTS		
	Regular moderate physical exercise should be recommended.	Drory et al., 2001
	Higher release of ROS during exercise suggests that design of training should be considered with caution.	Siciliano et al., 2002
	Benefits of moderate aerobic exercise.	Bello-Haas et al., 2007

Table 4 | Ongoing clinical trials in ALS.

Items	Clinical trial ID	Status	Study type	Intervention	Estimated enrollment	Study
EXERCISE						
	NCT01650818	Recruiting	Interventional	Endurance training	40	Aerobic exercise training in ALS
	NCT01521728	Recruiting	Interventional	Resistance exercise	60	Trial of resistance and endurance exercise in ALS
DIETARY SUPPLEMENT						
	NCT00983983	Completed	Interventional	Oxepa	30	High fat/high calorie trial in ALS
	NCT01016522	Terminated	Interventional	KetoCal	NA	Safety and tolerability of the ketogenic diet in ALS
BASAL METABOLISM						
	NCT00714220	Recruiting	Observational	/	150	Quantitative measurement of nutritional substrate utilization in patients with ALS
	NCT01592084	Completed	Observational	/	267	Hyperlipidemia and statin therapy in ALS
PHARMACOLOGY						
	NCT00690118	Terminated	Interventional	Pioglitazone (45 mg/day)	219	Study of pioglitazone in patients with Amyotrophic Lateral Sclerosis
	NCT00876772	Unknown	Interventional	Olanzapine (10 mg/day)	40	Olanzapine for the treatment of appetite loss in Amyotrophic Lateral Sclerosis (ALS)

Clinical trial IDs refer to the current nomenclature used at clinicaltrial.gov.

et al., 2010) that could account for an altered lipid beta oxidation in the CNS of ALS patients.

Higher energetic needs have been documented in muscle of SOD1 mice (Dupuis et al., 2004). In the animal model, the metabolic shift in muscle fibers (glycolytic to oxidative) could explain the pronounced appetence for fatty acids in SOD1 muscles, as well as the changes in the expression profile of genes involved in lipid metabolism (Fergani et al., 2007; Gonzalez de Aguilar et al., 2008; Thau et al., 2012). Interestingly, the predominance of oxidative metabolism goes along with deficiency in oxidative mitochondrial chain function, in particular in the muscles of ALS patients (Echaniz-Laguna et al., 2002; Dupuis et al., 2003; Crugnola et al., 2010). Mitochondria bioenergetic functions are impaired, as shown by Zhou and colleagues, whom described the presence of defective mitochondria in mass near the neuromuscular junctions that may contribute to the progression of muscle atrophy in ALS (Zhou et al., 2010). The origin of mitochondrial defect is under investigation. Several potential pathways are proposed to explain the shift in metabolism and the alterations of mitochondrial functions, and they concern the tuning of metabolic pathways.

Mitochondrial biogenesis and functions are orchestrated in part by peroxisome proliferator-activated receptor gamma coactivator (PGC)-1 alpha (Lin et al., 2002, 2005; Handschin, 2010). In ALS, the implication of PGC-1 alpha has been recently highlighted, as its expression is diminished in the muscles of patients and SOD1 mice (Thau et al., 2012). The downregulation of PGC-1 alpha triggers modification of lipid metabolism, and impacts the use of fatty acids (Barroso et al., 2011). Interestingly, we have very recently shown that deficiency in PGC1-alpha leads to hasten disease progression in the males of a mouse model of ALS (Eschbach et al., 2013), strengthening the relation between lipid metabolism alterations and disease progression, at least in SOD1 mice. When Da Cruz and collaborators overexpressed PGC1-alpha selectively in the muscles of SOD1 mice, they observed improved locomotor activity and reduced muscle atrophy, but no effects on the overall survival of this mouse line (Da Cruz et al., 2012). Their results suggest that improving muscle activity and reducing atrophy through increased PGC1-alpha could be used as a palliative treatment in ALS. In addition, the overexpression of PGC1-alpha selectively in the central nervous system (CNS) of SOD1 mice restored the activity of mitochondrial complexes in the spinal cord, supported motor functions and enhances survival by 8% (Zhao et al., 2011). Moreover sirtuin 3, a downstream target of PGC-1 alpha, protects neurons *in vitro* against SOD1 G85R toxicity (Song et al., 2013). General mitochondrial activity, including mitochondrial proliferation, is impaired in ALS and represents a promising therapeutic target for ALS as recently discussed (Cozzolino et al., 2013; Dupuis, 2013; Pasinetti et al., 2013).

Stearoyl-Coa desaturase 1 (SCD-1) is a key enzyme for the regulation of fatty acid metabolism, and it can impact fatty acid oxidation taking place in mitochondria. SCD-1 introduce a double bond in the carbon chain of saturated, to generated mono-unsaturated fatty acids that are more prone to be stored in fat tissues. We have recently reported a downregulation of SCD-1 in the muscle of SOD1 mice (Hussain et al., 2013), and in a subpopulation of ALS patients (Pradat et al., 2011). The function of SCD-1 is associated to regulation of energetic metabolism, and most particularly the management of lipid reserves. Downregulation of SCD-1 is known to trigger increased expression of genes involved in the beta-oxidation of fatty acids, increased energy expenditure and reduced fat storage, a metabolic phenotype exhibited by SOD1 mice (Ntambi et al., 2002; Dupuis et al., 2004). We aimed to study the impact of a low SCD-1 activity for the motor function. We recently described that knock-out mice for SCD-1, and non-transgenic mice treated with a SCD-1 inhibitor, present improved nerve regeneration after peripheral nerve injury (Hussain et al., 2013). Moreover, the products of SCD-1, the mono-unsaturated fatty acids, favor cytotoxic SOD-1 aggregation (Kim et al., 2005), and the accumulation of toxic lipid species such as ceramide

(Dobrzyn et al., 2005), suggesting that loss of SCD-1 activity could lower cytotoxicity in ALS. Further work is needed to understand the link between loss of SCD-1 activity and benefits for the motor units, especially in ALS. Aside from its role in energetic metabolism, SCD-1 is additionally required in the synthesis of more complex lipids, including phospholipids. Alterations in lipid metabolism will have repercussion not only on the energy homeostasis, but also on a wide range of cellular functions, including membrane fluidity and signaling.

A ROLE FOR LIPIDS BESIDE ENERGETIC METABOLISM

Lipids play a critical role in the structure of the central and peripheral nervous systems in particular at the cell membrane level. They control membrane fluidity, improve transmission of electrical signals and stabilize synapses.

MEMBRANE FLUIDITY

Basic cellular functions depend on the composition in lipids of plasmatic membranes. Enrichment of sphingolipids and cholesterol, as well as content in polyunsaturated fatty acids (PUFA), directly determines membrane fluidity and movement of membrane proteins in lipid rafts (Xu et al., 2001; Lang, 2007; Lingwood and Simons, 2010). Although the level of these lipids is altered in ALS patients and SOD1 mice, membrane fluidity *per se* has not been extensively investigated. One recent study described loss of membrane fluidity in the SOD1 mice at disease onset (Miana-Mena et al., 2011) presumably due to oxidative stress and lipid peroxidation. Membrane phospholipids in the CNS are rich in PUFA and in particular of docosahexaenoic acid (DHA). Interestingly, the profile of fatty acids in the brain cortex and spinal cord of ALS patients revealed an increase of DHA level with potential consequences on membrane fluidity (Ilieva et al., 2007). Changes in the membrane fluidity could affect wide range of cellular functions such as ligand-receptor signal transduction and membrane trafficking (Simons and Vaz, 2004), with consequences on cell functions and survival.

A DIRECT ROLE FOR LIPIDS IN MOTORNEURON SURVIVAL?

Back in 2002, the group of Pr. Mattson studied the lipid metabolites present in the spinal cord of both ALS patients and pre-symptomatic SOD1 mice, and reported higher amounts of sphingolipids and cholesterol associated with increased lipid peroxidation (Cutler et al., 2002). These findings are important as these lipid metabolites modulate vital cellular functions in the CNS that may be involved in ALS pathophysiology. Aberrant accumulation of ceramides is commonly seen as being toxic. It mediates neuron death by oxidative stress and apoptosis in animal models and patients of neurodegenerative diseases (Brugg et al., 1996; France-Lanord et al., 1997; Bras et al., 2008; Car et al., 2012; Filippov et al., 2012). Ceramides are precursor molecules at the crossroads of the sphingolipid metabolism and they can be converted into sphingomyelin, ceramide-1-phosphate and gangliosides. Abnormal repartition of gangliosides was described in the CNS of ALS patients and presence of antibodies anti-gangliosides has been described in their serum (Mizutani et al., 2003). Gangliosides are important for axonal function and regeneration, and neuronal survival (Akasako et al., 2011). In the 80's, clinicians initiated half-dozen trials in ALS with injection of gangliosides with the aim to protect the motor units, but lead to no benefit (Bradley, 1984; Hallett et al., 1984). These studies were however underpowered. Sphingomyelin is particularly abundant in the nervous systems and represents another lipid impacting motor neuron survival. Cutlers and colleagues proposed that the increase of sphingomyelin in the spinal cord of ALS patients mediates motor neuron death via oxidative stress (Cutler et al., 2002), and in 2007, another group reported that p75-mediated motor neuron death is stimulated upon sphingomyelin-associated ROS production in an animal model of ALS (Pehar et al., 2007).

SIGNALING MOLECULES

In addition to their role in the membrane structure, PUFA also have intrinsic functions on cell signaling, in particular on neuroinflammation and regulation of energetic metabolism. First, PUFA are known to bind to transcription factors, such as liver-X receptor and retinoic-X receptor (Yoshikawa et al., 2002), to stimulate the expression of genes involved in energy homeostasis and dysregulation of their levels could account for the altered metabolism in ALS.

PUFA can be also converted to active molecules. Depending on the location of the unsaturations, PUFA present either anti-inflammatory and neuroprotective effects, for the omega 3 fatty acids, or pro-inflammatory for omega 6 fatty acids (Schmitz and Ecker, 2008). For instance, eicosapentaenoic and arachidonic acids can be oxidized to give rise to prostanglandins or leukotrienes, and the oxidation of DHA produces the neuroprotectin D1, a signaling molecule that promotes beneficial effects on cell survival under stress (Bazan et al., 2011). Prostaglandin E2 (PGE2) is synthetized by cyclooxygenase-2 from the arachidonic acid, an omega 6 fatty acid, to promote inflammation after binding to its receptor. In ALS patients, level of PGE2 is increased in the serum and the cerebrospinal fluid (Ilzecka, 2003). Evidence from animal models also suggests a role for PGE2 in ALS physiopathology. Indeed, the pharmacological inhibition of PGE2 receptor or the silencing of the gene coding for cyclooxygenase-2 can lower neuroinflammation in SOD1 mice, preserve motor functions and extend survival (Pompl et al., 2003; Klivenyi et al., 2004; Liang et al., 2008).

The omega 3 fatty acids can be converted into anti-inflammatory and neuroprotective molecules. Many reports have shown that treatments based on omega 3 fatty acids exert beneficial effects in various animal models of neurodegenerative disease, such as Parkinson's or Alzheimer's diseases (Arsenault et al., 2011; Ozsoy et al., 2011). In a recent study, Michael-Titus and colleagues investigated the neuroprotective effect of eicosapentaenoic acid, an omega 3 fatty acid precursor for DHA, in SOD1 mice. Unexpectedly, the treatment resulted in enhancement of neuroinflammation, faster disease progression and hastened death for SOD1 mice (Yip et al., 2013). One explanation proposed by the authors is the greater susceptibility for PUFA to be peroxidized and therefore toxic (Kanner et al., 1987). Therefore, the increase in DHA of spinal cord from ALS patients could favor lipid peroxidability, and be potentially a toxic factor in ALS (Ilieva et al., 2007).

Taken together, all these results clearly argue for a strong relationship between lipid metabolism and motor neuron degeneration. Most of the findings originate from ALS, as it is the most studied MNDs. However, alterations of lipid metabolism are also present in other MNDs.

LIPID ALTERATIONS IN OTHER MOTOR NEURON DISEASES

Motor neuron degeneration is present in several diseases that complete the spectrum of MNDs with ALS. The role of lipids in those diseases is poorly understood, although some lines of evidence exist.

Progressive muscular atrophy (PMA) is rare subtype of ALS characterized by loss of lower motor neurons. To our knowledge, only one report described alterations of circulating lipids in two patients with a PMA syndrome (Yao et al., 1983). However, these patients suffer from other neurological disorders making difficult to reach a conclusion.

SBMA is characterized by progressive muscle atrophy and degeneration of lower motor neurons in the brain stem and spinal cord. Role and regulation of lipids have not been accessed in SBMA patients, although androgen receptors are known to modulate lipid metabolism (Singh et al., 2006). Indeed, the analysis of the muscle transcriptome of SBMA mice revealed that several differentially regulated genes relate to lipid metabolism, from an energetic and a structural point of view (Mo et al., 2010). For instance, the phospholipase A2, group VII (PLA_2g7) is downregulated in the muscles of SBMA mice. PLA_2g7 degrades phospholipids to release poly-unsaturated fatty acid and, in muscle, it is involved in the differentiation of myoblasts (Xiao et al., 2012) and reduction of adiposity (Rao et al., 2006). Ddit4l is another example of genes deregulated in SBMA mice. Ddit4l, also known as REDD2, is involved in muscle growth via stimulation of the IGF1/mTOR pathway and muscle fiber switch from oxidative to glycolytic metabolism (Pisani et al., 2005; Miyazaki and Esser, 2009; Mo et al., 2010).

SMA is a progressive, recessively inherited, neuromuscular disease. SMA is characterized by weakness and muscle atrophy due to loss of spinal cord motor neurons. Similarly to ALS, metabolic abnormality is part of pathophysiology of SMA. In SMA, an initial study reported normal body mass index in a mixed population of SMA patients with severe to moderate symptoms. However, in this cohort, the authors described a reduction in fat-free mass but an increase in total fat mass (Sproule et al., 2009). A second study, focusing only on the most severe form of the disease, described a lower calorie intake than the recommended dietary allowance in SMA patients, associated to higher fat mass (Poruk et al., 2012). These alterations potentially participate to failure to thrive described in SMA patients. The reason why SMA patients have high fat mass despite low caloric intake is unclear but strengthen the role of metabolism of lipids in the disease. Indeed, a misuse of lipids has been documented in SMA patients with various symptom severities, with an impaired mitochondrial fatty acid beta-oxidation and a loss of free circulating carnitine, arguing for impairment of fatty acid entry into mitochondria (Tein et al., 1995). Later, the same group of clinicians described fatty acid abnormalities in SMA, such as high dicarboxylic acid to ketone ratio in the plasma when fasting, or low C12:C14 fatty acid ratio, that further decreased within disease duration. These two parameters are strong markers for fatty acid beta oxidation defects (Crawford et al., 1999). The authors concluded that fatty acid abnormality in severe SMA is primary and general defect, directly caused by the loss of the SMN function.

Additionally, in a transgenic animal model of SMA, deficient for the SMN gene, pups survive longer when mothers were fed with a diet enriched in lipid content (**Table 2**). The treatment also corrected motor dysfunction despite lack of effect on motor neuron survival (Butchbach et al., 2010). Recently, a clinical trial investigated the effect of a combined treatment of valproic acid and L-carnitine in SMA patients, however, no to limited positive effects have been reported in ambulatory and non-ambulatory SMA patients (Swoboda et al., 2010; Kissel et al., 2011). However, further work is required to assess the role of lipids in SMA and their therapeutic potential.

PATHS TO EXPLORE

Clinical studies and basic research undoubtedly demonstrate a particular connection between lipid metabolism and ALS (**Table 4**). Contrary to that observed in other neurological diseases, such as Alzheimer's and Parkinson's diseases, or even ageing (Maswood et al., 2004; Patel et al., 2005), high level of lipids positively correlates to better prognosis in ALS. Preclinical data and clinical studies clearly show that dietary lipid supplementation is a promising strategy to treat ALS, although there is no extensive clinical research at this level.

We are aware of only three clinical trials based on nutritional intervention. In a recently published article, Dorst and colleagues aimed to stop weight loss in ALS patients with high caloric diets, either based on fats or carbohydrates. Both interventions were able to stabilize weight loss although the effect was larger in the high-fat diet group (Dorst et al., 2013). Another trial aims to correct malnutrition with high fat dietary supplement in ALS patients (NCT00983983). The second ongoing trial is a phase III that use high ketogenic supplementation (high fat and low carbohydrate) in ALS patients fed through a gastrostomy tube (NCT01016522). These studies are dedicated to the prevention of malnutrition in ALS patients, and are not designed to identify benefit on prognosis after high fat diet. In parallel, how patients on and off respiratory support use diverse nutritional substrates (e.g., lipids) is under investigation (NCT00714220), as well as the influence of lipid lowering therapy in ALS (NCT01592084). There are two additional trials based on pharmacological modulation of energetic metabolism, using pioglitazone or olanzapine. Pioglitazone is an anti-diabetic drug known to manage energetic metabolism and to lower level of circulating lipids in patients suffering from metabolic disorders. This phase II clinical trial has been stopped after interim analysis that revealed no benefit after treatment on primary and secondary outcomes (Dupuis et al., 2012, NCT00690118). A phase II/III using olanzapine is currently ongoing. Olanzapine is a neuroleptic drug with metabolic side effects, and investigators treated ALS patients with olanzapine, based on the weight-increasing effect of the drug (NCT00876772). Study results have not been released yet. The results of these trials will certainly help to determine whether modulation of lipids, though supplementation or pharmacology, is a feasible and rational treatment for ALS, and potentially for other MNDs.

As discussed in this review, the role of lipids in ALS and MND pathophysiology goes beyond energetic metabolism, to structure and signaling. These alterations, in particular those in the CNS, could represent an important source of therapeutic options in ALS. Indeed, there is a large spectrum of drugs targeting sphingolipids that are well characterized in terms of safety and bioavailability. They could be suitable for ALS patients, once clear targets are identified. A clinical trial has been very recently registered with the aim to test in ALS patients, the safety and tolerability of fingolimod, an agonist for sphingosine-1-phosphate receptors (NCT01786174), already used in multiple sclerosis to lower neuroinflammation in the CNS. In addition to pharmacological agents, dietary supplementation with neuroprotective and anti-inflammatory fatty acids, or derivatives, is worthy of further characterization. Altogether, alterations of lipid metabolism in MND deserve further work that will undoubtedly lead to new and interesting therapeutic options for patients.

ACKNOWLEDGMENTS

This work was supported by funds from European Community's Health Seventh Framework Programme under grant agreement no. 259867 (FP7/2007-2013) to Jean-Philippe Loeffler; Thierry Latran Foundation to Jean-Philippe Loeffler, and to Luc Dupuis (SpastALS); ALS Association (#2235) to Luc Dupuis; Agence Nationale de la Recherche (DyneMit) to Luc Dupuis; the Helmholtz Virtual Institute (RNA dysmetabolism in Amyotrophic Lateral Sclerosis and Frontotemporal Dementia) to Luc Dupuis; "Association Française contre les Myopathies" (AFM) to Florent Schmitt; Higher Education Commission of the Pakistani government to Ghulam Hussain; "Association pour la Recherche et le Développement de Moyens de Lutte contre les Maladies Neurodégénératives" (AREMANE); and "Association pour la Recherche sur la Sclérose latérale amyotrophique et autres maladies du motoneurone" (ARSLA). Alexandre Henriques is a research fellow receiving funds from FP7/2007-2013. We thank Dr. J.-L. Gonzalez de Aguilar for his critical reading of the manuscript and insightful comments.

REFERENCES

Akasako, Y., Nara, K., Nagai, Y., and Hashimoto, Y. (2011). Inhibition of ganglioside synthesis reduces the neuronal survival activity of astrocytes. *Neurosci. Lett.* 488, 199–203. doi: 10.1016/j.neulet.2010.11.029

Arsenault, D., Julien, C., Tremblay, C., and Calon, F. (2011). DHA improves cognition and prevents dysfunction of entorhinal cortex neurons in 3xTg-AD mice. *PLoS ONE* 6:e17397. doi: 10.1371/journal.pone.0017397

Atkin, J. D., Scott, R. L., West, J. M., Lopes, E., Quah, A. K., and Cheema, S. S. (2005). Properties of slow- and fast-twitch muscle fibres in a mouse model of amyotrophic lateral sclerosis. *Neuromuscul. Disord.* 15, 377–388. doi: 10.1016/j.nmd.2005.02.005

Barroso, E., Rodriguez-Calvo, R., Serrano-Marco, L., Astudillo, A. M., Balsinde, J., Palomer, X., et al. (2011). The PPARbeta/delta activator GW501516 prevents the down-regulation of AMPK caused by a high-fat diet in liver and amplifies the PGC-1alpha-Lipin 1-PPARalpha pathway leading to increased fatty acid oxidation. *Endocrinology* 152, 1848–1859. doi: 10.1210/en.2010-1468

Bazan, N. G., Musto, A. E., and Knott, E. J. (2011). Endogenous signaling by omega-3 docosahexaenoic acid-derived mediators sustains homeostatic synaptic and circuitry integrity. *Mol. Neurobiol.* 44, 216–222. doi: 10.1007/s12035-011-8200-6

Bebee, T. W., Dominguez, C. E., and Chandler, D. S. (2012). Mouse models of SMA: tools for disease characterization and therapeutic development. *Hum. Genet.* 131, 1277–1293. doi: 10.1007/s00439-012-1171-5

Bello-Haas, V. D., Florence, J. M., Kloos, A. D., Scheirbecker, J., Lopate, G., Hayes, S. M., et al. (2007). A randomized controlled trial of resistance exercise in individuals with alS. *Neurology* 68, 2003–2007. doi: 10.1212/01.wnl.0000264418.92308.a4

Blasco, H., Corcia, P., Moreau, C., Veau, S., Fournier, C., Vourc'h P., et al. (2010). 1H-NMR-based metabolomic profiling of CSF in early amyotrophic lateral sclerosis. *PLoS ONE* 5:e13223. doi: 10.1371/journal.pone.0013223

Bradley, W. G. (1984). Double-blind controlled trial of purified brain gangliosides in amyotrophic lateral sclerosis and experience with peripheral neuropathies. *Adv. Exp. Med. Biol.* 174, 565–573. doi: 10.1007/978-1-4684-1200-0_47

Bras, J., Singleton, A., Cookson, M. R., and Hardy, J. (2008). Emerging pathways in genetic Parkinson's disease: potential role of ceramide metabolism in Lewy body disease. *FEBS J.* 275, 5767–5773. doi: 10.1111/j.1742-4658.2008.06709.x

Braun, M. M., Osecheck, M., and Joyce, N. C. (2012). Nutrition assessment and management in amyotrophic lateral sclerosis. *Phys. Med. Rehabil. Clin. N. Am.* 23, 751–771. doi: 10.1016/j.pmr.2012.08.006

Brooks, B. P., and Fischbeck, K. H. (1995). Spinal and bulbar muscular atrophy: a trinucleotide-repeat expansion neurodegenerative disease. *Trends Neurosci.* 18, 459–461. doi: 10.1016/0166-2236(95)94497-S

Brooks, B. R., Juhasz-Poscine, K., Waclawik, A., Sanjak, M., Belden, D., Roelke, K., et al. (2000). Mosaic chemotherapy strategies for developing alS/MND therapeutic approaches: beta-2 adrenergic agonists. *Amyotroph. Lateral Scler. Other Motor Neuron Disord.* 1(Suppl. 4), 45–53. discussion: 53–54. doi: 10.1080/14660820050515700-1

Brugg, B., Michel, P. P., Agid, Y., and Ruberg, M. (1996). Ceramide induces apoptosis in cultured mesencephalic neurons. *J. Neurochem.* 66, 733–739. doi: 10.1046/j.1471-4159.1996.66020733.x

Butchbach, M. E., Rose, F. F. Jr., Rhoades, S., Marston, J., McCrone, J. T., Sinnott, R., et al. (2010). Effect of diet on the survival and phenotype of a mouse model for spinal muscular atrophy. *Biochem. Biophys. Res. Commun.* 391, 835–840. doi: 10.1016/j.bbrc.2009.11.148

Car, H., Zendzian-Piotrowska, M., Fiedorowicz, A., Prokopiuk, S., Sadowska, A., and Kurek, K. (2012). [The role of ceramides in selected brain pathologies: ischemia/hypoxia, Alzheimer disease]. *Postepy Hig. Med. Dosw. (Online)* 66, 295–303. doi: 10.5604/17322693.999024

Carreras, I., Yuruker, S., Aytan, N., Hossain, L., Choi, J. K., Jenkins, B. G., et al. (2010). Moderate exercise delays the motor performance decline in a transgenic model of alS. *Brain Res.* 1313, 192–201. doi: 10.1016/j.brainres.2009.11.051

Chio, A., Calvo, A., Ilardi, A., Cavallo, E., Moglia, C., Mutani, R., et al. (2009). Lower serum lipid levels are related to respiratory impairment in patients with alS. *Neurology* 73, 1681–1685. doi: 10.1212/WNL.0b013e3181c1df1e

Cozzolino, M., Ferri, A., Valle, C., and Carri, M. T. (2013). Mitochondria and alS: implications from novel genes and pathways. *Mol. Cell. Neurosci.* 55, 44–49. doi: 10.1016/j.mcn.2012.06.001

Crawford, T. O., Sladky, J. T., Hurko, O., Besner-Johnston, A., and Kelley, R. I. (1999). Abnormal fatty acid metabolism in childhood spinal muscular atrophy. *Ann. Neurol.* 45, 337–343. doi: 10.1002/1531-8249(199903)45:3<337::AID-ANA9>3.0.CO;2-U

Crugnola, V., Lamperti, C., Lucchini, V., Ronchi, D., Peverelli, L., Prelle, A., et al. (2010). Mitochondrial respiratory chain dysfunction in muscle from patients with amyotrophic lateral sclerosis. *Arch. Neurol.* 67, 849–854. doi: 10.1001/archneurol.2010.128

Cutler, R. G., Pedersen, W. A., Camandola, S., Rothstein, J. D., and Mattson, M. P. (2002). Evidence that accumulation of ceramides and cholesterol esters mediates oxidative stress-induced death of motor neurons in amyotrophic lateral sclerosis. *Ann. Neurol.* 52, 448–457. doi: 10.1002/ana.10312

Da Cruz, S., Parone, P. A., Lopes, V. S., Lillo, C., McAlonis-Downes, M., Lee, S. K., et al. (2012). Elevated PGC-1alpha activity sustains mitochondrial biogenesis and muscle function without extending survival in a mouse model of inherited alS. *Cell Metab.* 15, 778–786. doi: 10.1016/j.cmet.2012.03.019

de Almeida, J. P., Silvestre, R., Pinto, A. C., and de Carvalho, M. (2012). Exercise and amyotrophic lateral sclerosis. *Neurol. Sci.* 33, 9–15. doi: 10.1007/s10072-011-0921-9

Deforges, S., Branchu, J., Biondi, O., Grondard, C., Pariset, C., Lecolle, S., et al. (2009). Motoneuron survival is promoted by specific exercise in a mouse model of amyotrophic lateral sclerosis. *J. Physiol.* 587, 3561–3572. doi: 10.1113/jphysiol.2009.169748

Deng, H. X., Zhai, H., Bigio, E. H., Yan, J., Fecto, F., Ajroud, K., et al. (2010). FUS-immunoreactive inclusions are a common feature in sporadic and non-SOD1 familial amyotrophic lateral sclerosis. *Ann. Neurol.* 67, 739–748. doi: 10.1002/ana.22051

Desport, J. C., Preux, P. M., Magy, L., Boirie, Y., Vallat, J. M., Beaufrere, B., et al. (2001). Factors correlated with hypermetabolism in patients with amyotrophic lateral sclerosis. *Am. J. Clin. Nutr.* 74, 328–334.

Dobrzyn, A., Dobrzyn, P., Lee, S. H., Miyazaki, M., Cohen, P., Asilmaz, E., et al. (2005). Stearoyl-CoA desaturase-1 deficiency reduces ceramide synthesis by downregulating serine palmitoyltransferase and increasing beta-oxidation in skeletal muscle. *Am. J. Physiol. Endocrinol. Metab.* 288, E599–E607. doi: 10.1152/ajpendo.00439.2004

Dorst, J., Cypionka, J., and Ludolph, A. C. (2013). High-caloric food supplements in the treatment of amyotrophic lateral sclerosis: a prospective interventional study. *Amyotroph. Lateral Scler. Frontotemporal Degener.* 14, 533–536. doi: 10.3109/21678421.2013.823999

Dorst, J., Kuhnlein, P., Hendrich, C., Kassubek, J., Sperfeld, A. D., and Ludolph, A. C. (2011). Patients with elevated triglyceride and cholesterol serum levels have a prolonged survival in amyotrophic lateral sclerosis. *J. Neurol.* 258, 613–617. doi: 10.1007/s00415-010-5805-z

Drory, V. E., Goltsman, E., Reznik, J. G., Mosek, A., and Korczyn, A. D. (2001). The value of muscle exercise in patients with amyotrophic lateral sclerosis. *J. Neurol. Sci.* 191, 133–137. doi: 10.1016/S0022-510X(01)00610-4

Dupuis, L. (2013). Mitochondrial quality control in neurodegenerative diseases. *Biochimie.* doi: 10.1016/j.biochi.2013.07.033. [Epub ahead of print].

Dupuis, L., Corcia, P., Fergani, A., Gonzalez De Aguilar, J. L., Bonnefont-Rousselot, D., Bittar, R., et al. (2008). Dyslipidemia is a protective factor in amyotrophic lateral sclerosis. *Neurology* 70, 1004–1009. doi: 10.1212/01.wnl.0000285080.70324.27

Dupuis, L., Dengler, R., Heneka, M. T., Meyer, T., Zierz, S., Kassubek, J., et al. (2012). A randomized, double blind, placebo-controlled trial of pioglitazone in combination with riluzole in amyotrophic lateral sclerosis. *PLoS ONE* 7:e37885. doi: 10.1371/journal.pone.0037885

Dupuis, L., and Loeffler, J. P. (2009). Neuromuscular junction destruction during amyotrophic lateral sclerosis: insights from transgenic models. *Curr. Opin. Pharmacol.* 9, 341–346. doi: 10.1016/j.coph.2009.03.007

Dupuis, L., Oudart, H., Rene, F., Gonzalez de Aguilar, J. L., and Loeffler, J. P. (2004). Evidence for defective energy homeostasis in amyotrophic lateral sclerosis: benefit of a high-energy diet in a transgenic mouse model. *Proc. Natl. Acad. Sci. U.S.A.* 101, 11159–11164. doi: 10.1073/pnas.0402026101

Dupuis, L., Pradat, P. F., Ludolph, A. C., and Loeffler, J. P. (2011). Energy metabolism in amyotrophic lateral sclerosis. *Lancet Neurol.* 10, 75–82. doi: 10.1016/S1474-4422(10)70224-6

Dupuis, L., di Scala, F., Rene, F., de Tapia, M., Oudart, H., Pradat, P. F., et al. (2003). Up-regulation of mitochondrial uncoupling protein 3 reveals an early muscular metabolic defect in amyotrophic lateral sclerosis. *FASEB J.* 17, 2091–2093. doi: 10.1096/fj.02-1182fje

Echaniz-Laguna, A., Zoll, J., Ribera, F., Tranchant, C., Warter, J. M., Lonsdorfer, J., et al. (2002). Mitochondrial respiratory chain function in skeletal muscle of alS patients. *Ann. Neurol.* 52, 623–627. doi: 10.1002/ana.10357

Eschbach, J., Schwalenstocker, B., Soyal, S., Bayer, H., Wiesner, D., Akimoto, C., et al. (2013). PGC-1alpha is a male-specific disease modifier of human and experimental amyotrophic lateral sclerosis. *Hum. Mol. Genet.* 22, 3477–3484. doi: 10.1093/hmg/ddt202

Fergani, A., Oudart, H., Gonzalez De Aguilar, J. L., Fricker, B., Rene, F., Hocquette, J. F., et al. (2007). Increased peripheral lipid clearance in an animal model of amyotrophic lateral sclerosis. *J. Lipid Res.* 48, 1571–1580. doi: 10.1194/jlr.M700017-JLR200

Filippov, V., Song, M. A., Zhang, K., Vinters, H. V., Tung, S., Kirsch, W. M., et al. (2012). Increased ceramide in brains with Alzheimer's and other neurodegenerative diseases. *J. Alzheimers. Dis.* 29, 537–547. doi: 10.3233/JAD-2011-111202

Fischbeck, K. H., Lieberman, A., Bailey, C. K., Abel, A., and Merry, D. E. (1999). Androgen receptor mutation in Kennedy's disease. *Philos. Trans. R. Soc. Lond. B Biol. Sci.* 354, 1075–1078. doi: 10.1098/rstb.1999.0461

France-Lanord, V., Brugg, B., Michel, P. P., Agid, Y., and Ruberg, M. (1997). Mitochondrial free radical signal in ceramide-dependent apoptosis: a putative mechanism for neuronal death in Parkinson's disease. *J. Neurochem.* 69, 1612–1621. doi: 10.1046/j.1471-4159.1997.69041612.x

Funalot, B., Desport, J. C., Sturtz, F., Camu, W., and Couratier, P. (2009). High metabolic level in patients with familial amyotrophic lateral sclerosis. *Amyotroph. Lateral Scler.* 10, 113–117. doi: 10.1080/17482960802295192

Gallo, V., Wark, P. A., Jenab, M., Pearce, N., Brayne, C., Vermeulen, R., et al. (2013). Prediagnostic body fat and risk of death from amyotrophic lateral sclerosis: the EPIC cohort. *Neurology* 80, 829–838. doi: 10.1212/WNL.0b013e3182840689

Gerber, Y. N., Sabourin, J. C., Hugnot, J. P., and Perrin, F. E. (2012). Unlike physical exercise, modified environment increases the lifespan of SOD1G93A mice however both conditions induce cellular changes. *PLoS ONE* 7:e45503. doi: 10.1371/journal.pone.0045503

Gonzalez de Aguilar, J. L., Niederhauser-Wiederkehr, C., Halter, B., De Tapia, M., Di Scala, F., Demougin, P., et al. (2008). Gene profiling of skeletal muscle in an amyotrophic lateral sclerosis mouse model. *Physiol. Genomics* 32, 207–218. doi: 10.1152/physiolgenomics.00017.2007

Gordon, T., Tyreman, N., Li, S., Putman, C. T., and Hegedus, J. (2010). Functional over-load saves motor units in the SOD1-G93A transgenic mouse model of amyotrophic lateral sclerosis. *Neurobiol. Dis.* 37, 412–422. doi: 10.1016/j.nbd.2009.10.021

Guzman, M., and Blazquez, C. (2004). Ketone body synthesis in the brain: possible neuroprotective effects. *Prostaglandins Leukot. Essent. Fatty Acids* 70, 287–292. doi: 10.1016/j.plefa.2003.05.001

Hallett, M., Harrington, H., Tyler, H. R., Flood, T., and Slater, N. (1984). Trials of ganglioside therapy for amyotrophic lateral sclerosis and diabetic neuropathy. *Adv. Exp. Med. Biol.* 174, 575–579. doi: 10.1007/978-1-4684-1200-0_48

Hamadeh, M. J., Rodriguez, M. C., Kaczor, J. J., and Tarnopolsky, M. A. (2005). Caloric restriction transiently improves motor performance but hastens clinical onset of disease in the Cu/Zn-superoxide dismutase mutant G93A mouse. *Muscle Nerve* 31, 214–220. doi: 10.1002/mus.20255

Handschin, C. (2010). Regulation of skeletal muscle cell plasticity by the peroxisome proliferator-activated receptor gamma coactivator 1alpha. *J. Recept. Signal Transduct. Res.* 30, 376–384. doi: 10.3109/10799891003641074

Hegedus, J., Putman, C. T., and Gordon, T. (2007). Time course of preferential motor unit loss in the SOD1 G93A mouse model of amyotrophic lateral sclerosis. *Neurobiol. Dis.* 28, 154–164. doi: 10.1016/j.nbd.2007.07.003

Hussain, G., Schmitt, F., Henriques, A., Lequeu, T., Rene, F., Bindler, F., et al. (2013). Systemic down-regulation of delta-9 desaturase promotes muscle oxidative metabolism and accelerates muscle function recovery following nerve injury. *PLoS ONE* 8:e64525. doi: 10.1371/journal.pone.0064525

Ilieva, E. V., Ayala, V., Jove, M., Dalfo, E., Cacabelos, D., Povedano, M., et al. (2007). Oxidative and endoplasmic reticulum stress interplay in sporadic amyotrophic lateral sclerosis. *Brain* 130, 3111–3123. doi: 10.1093/brain/awm190

Ilzecka, J. (2003). Prostaglandin E2 is increased in amyotrophic lateral sclerosis patients. *Acta Neurol. Scand.* 108, 125–129. doi: 10.1034/j.1600-0404.2003.00102.x

Jawaid, A., Murthy, S. B., Wilson, A. M., Qureshi, S. U., Amro, M. J., Wheaton, M., et al. (2010). A decrease in body mass index is associated with faster progression of motor symptoms and shorter survival in alS. *Amyotroph. Lateral Scler.* 11, 542–548. doi: 10.3109/17482968.2010.482592

Kanner, J., German, J. B., and Kinsella, J. E. (1987). Initiation of lipid peroxidation in biological systems. *Crit. Rev. Food Sci. Nutr.* 25, 317–364. doi: 10.1080/10408398709527457

Katsuno, M., Adachi, H., Inukai, A., and Sobue, G. (2003). Transgenic mouse models of spinal and bulbar muscular atrophy (SBMA). *Cytogenet. Genome Res.* 100, 243–251. doi: 10.1159/000072860

Kim, S. M., Kim, H., Kim, J. E., Park, K. S., Sung, J. J., Kim, S. H., et al. (2011). Amyotrophic lateral sclerosis is associated with hypolipidemia at the presymptomatic stage in mice. *PLoS ONE* 6:e17985. doi: 10.1371/journal.pone.0017985

Kim, Y. J., Nakatomi, R., Akagi, T., Hashikawa, T., and Takahashi, R. (2005). Unsaturated fatty acids induce cytotoxic aggregate formation of amyotrophic lateral sclerosis-linked superoxide dismutase 1 mutants. *J. Biol. Chem.* 280, 21515–21521. doi: 10.1074/jbc.M502230200

Kissel, J. T., Scott, C. B., Reyna, S. P., Crawford, T. O., Simard, L. R., Krosschell, K. J., et al. (2011). SMA CARNIVal TRIal PART II: a prospective, single-armed trial of L-carnitine and valproic acid in ambulatory children with spinal muscular atrophy. *PLoS ONE* 6:e21296. doi: 10.1371/journal.pone.0021296

Klivenyi, P., Kiaei, M., Gardian, G., Calingasan, N. Y., and Beal, M. F. (2004). Additive neuroprotective effects of creatine and cyclooxygenase 2 inhibitors in a transgenic mouse model of amyotrophic lateral sclerosis. *J. Neurochem.* 88, 576–582. doi: 10.1046/j.1471-4159.2003.02160.x

Kumar, A., Bala, L., Kalita, J., Misra, U. K., Singh, R. L., Khetrapal, C. L., et al. (2010). Metabolomic analysis of serum by (1) H NMR spectroscopy in amyotrophic lateral sclerosis. *Clin. Chim. Acta* 411, 563–567. doi: 10.1016/j.cca.2010.01.016

Laaksovirta, H., Peuralinna, T., Schymick, J. C., Scholz, S. W., Lai, S. L., Myllykangas, L., et al. (2010). Chromosome 9p21 in amyotrophic lateral sclerosis in Finland: a genome-wide association study. *Lancet Neurol.* 9, 978–985. doi: 10.1016/S1474-4422(10)70184-8

LaManna, J. C., Salem, N., Puchowicz, M., Erokwu, B., Koppaka, S., Flask, C., et al. (2009). Ketones suppress brain glucose consumption. *Adv. Exp. Med. Biol.* 645, 301–306. doi: 10.1007/978-0-387-85998-9_45

Lang, T. (2007). SNARE proteins and "membrane rafts." *J. Physiol.* 585, 693–698. doi: 10.1113/jphysiol.2007.134346

Liang, X., Wang, Q., Shi, J., Lokteva, L., Breyer, R. M., Montine, T. J., et al. (2008). The prostaglandin E2 EP2 receptor accelerates disease progression and inflammation in a model of amyotrophic lateral sclerosis. *Ann. Neurol.* 64, 304–314. doi: 10.1002/ana.21437

Lin, J., Handschin, C., and Spiegelman, B. M. (2005). Metabolic control through the PGC-1 family of transcription coactivators. *Cell Metab.* 1, 361–370. doi: 10.1016/j.cmet.2005.05.004

Lin, J., Wu, H., Tarr, P. T., Zhang, C. Y., Wu, Z., Boss, O., et al. (2002). Transcriptional co-activator PGC-1 alpha drives the formation of slow-twitch muscle fibres. *Nature* 418, 797–801. doi: 10.1038/nature00904

Lindauer, E., Dupuis, L., Muller, H. P., Neumann, H., Ludolph, A. C., and Kassubek, J. (2013). Adipose tissue distribution predicts survival in amyotrophic lateral sclerosis. *PLoS ONE* 8:e67783. doi: 10.1371/journal.pone.0067783

Lingwood, D., and Simons, K. (2010). Lipid rafts as a membrane-organizing principle. *Science* 327, 46–50. doi: 10.1126/science.1174621

Mackenzie, I. R., Bigio, E. H., Ince, P. G., Geser, F., Neumann, M., Cairns, N. J., et al. (2007). Pathological TDP-43 distinguishes sporadic amyotrophic lateral sclerosis from amyotrophic lateral sclerosis with SOD1 mutations. *Ann. Neurol.* 61, 427–434. doi: 10.1002/ana.21147

Mahajan, K. R., Bach, J. R., Saporito, L., and Perez, N. (2012). Diaphragm pacing and noninvasive respiratory management of amyotrophic lateral sclerosis/motor neuron disease. *Muscle Nerve* 46, 851–855. doi: 10.1002/mus.23663

Marin, B., Desport, J. C., Kajeu, P., Jesus, P., Nicolaud, B., Nicol, M., et al. (2011). Alteration of nutritional status at diagnosis is a prognostic factor for survival of amyotrophic lateral sclerosis patients. *J. Neurol. Neurosurg. Psychiatry* 82, 628–634. doi: 10.1136/jnnp.2010.211474

Maswood, N., Young, J., Tilmont, E., Zhang, Z., Gash, D. M., Gerhardt, G. A., et al. (2004). Caloric restriction increases neurotrophic factor levels and attenuates neurochemical and behavioral deficits in a primate model of Parkinson's disease. *Proc. Natl. Acad. Sci. U.S.A.* 101, 18171–18176. doi: 10.1073/pnas.0405831102

Mattson, M. P., Cutler, R. G., and Camandola, S. (2007). Energy intake and amyotrophic lateral sclerosis. *Neuromolecular Med.* 9, 17–20. doi: 10.1385/NMM:9:1:17

Miana-Mena, F. J., Piedrafita, E., Gonzalez-Mingot, C., Larrode, P., Munoz, M. J., Martinez-Ballarin, E., et al. (2011). Levels of membrane fluidity in the spinal cord and the brain in an animal model of amyotrophic lateral sclerosis. *J. Bioenerg. Biomembr.* 43, 181–186. doi: 10.1007/s10863-011-9348-5

Miyazaki, M., and Esser, K. A. (2009). REDD2 is enriched in skeletal muscle and inhibits mTOR signaling in response to leucine and stretch. *Am. J. Physiol. Cell Physiol.* 296, C583–C592. doi: 10.1152/ajpcell.00464.2008

Mizutani, K., Oka, N., Kusunoki, S., Kaji, R., Kanda, M., Akiguchi, I., et al. (2003). Amyotrophic lateral sclerosis with IgM antibody against gangliosides GM2 and GD2. *Intern. Med.* 42, 277–280. doi: 10.2169/internalmedicine.42.277

Mo, K., Razak, Z., Rao, P., Yu, Z., Adachi, H., Katsuno, M., et al. (2010). Microarray analysis of gene expression by skeletal muscle of three mouse models of Kennedy disease/spinal bulbar muscular atrophy. *PLoS ONE* 5:e12922. doi: 10.1371/journal.pone.0012922

Muscaritoli, M., Kushta, I., Molfino, A., Inghilleri, M., Sabatelli, M., and Rossi Fanelli, F. (2012). Nutritional and metabolic support in patients with amyotrophic lateral sclerosis. *Nutrition* 28, 959–966. doi: 10.1016/j.nut.2012.01.011

Ntambi, J. M., Miyazaki, M., Stoehr, J. P., Lan, H., Kendziorski, C. M., Yandell, B. S., et al. (2002). Loss of stearoyl-CoA desaturase-1 function protects mice against adiposity. *Proc. Natl. Acad. Sci. U.S.A.* 99, 11482–11486. doi: 10.1073/pnas.132384699

Okamoto, K., Kihira, T., Kondo, T., Kobashi, G., Washio, M., Sasaki, S., et al. (2007). Nutritional status and risk of amyotrophic lateral sclerosis in Japan. *Amyotroph. Lateral Scler.* 8, 300–304. doi: 10.1080/17482960701472249

Ozsoy, O., Seval-Celik, Y., Hacioglu, G., Yargicoglu, P., Demir, R., Agar, A., et al. (2011). The influence and the mechanism of docosahexaenoic acid on a mouse model of Parkinson's disease. *Neurochem. Int.* 59, 664–670. doi: 10.1016/j.neuint.2011.06.012

Paganoni, S., Deng, J., Jaffa, M., Cudkowicz, M. E., and Wills, A. M. (2011). Body mass index, not dyslipidemia, is an independent predictor of survival in amyotrophic lateral sclerosis. *Muscle Nerve* 44, 20–24. doi: 10.1002/mus.22114

Pasinetti, G. M., Bilski, A. E., and Zhao, W. (2013). Sirtuins as therapeutic targets of alS. *Cell Res.* 23, 1073–1074. doi: 10.1038/cr.2013.94

Patel, B. P., Safdar, A., Raha, S., Tarnopolsky, M. A., and Hamadeh, M. J. (2010). Caloric restriction shortens lifespan through an increase in lipid peroxidation, inflammation and apoptosis in the G93A mouse, an animal model of alS. *PLoS ONE* 5:e9386. doi: 10.1371/journal.pone.0009386

Patel, N. V., Gordon, M. N., Connor, K. E., Good, R. A., Engelman, R. W., Mason, J., et al. (2005). Caloric restriction attenuates Abeta-deposition in Alzheimer transgenic models. *Neurobiol. Aging* 26, 995–1000. doi: 10.1016/j.neurobiolaging.2004.09.014

Pehar, M., Vargas, M. R., Robinson, K. M., Cassina, P., Diaz-Amarilla, P. J., Hagen, T. M., et al. (2007). Mitochondrial superoxide production and nuclear factor erythroid 2-related factor 2 activation in p75 neurotrophin receptor-induced motor neuron apoptosis. *J. Neurosci.* 27, 7777–7785. doi: 10.1523/JNEUROSCI.0823-07.2007

Pisani, D. F., Leclerc, L., Jarretou, G., Marini, J. F., and Dechesne, C. A. (2005). SMHS1 is involved in oxidative/glycolytic-energy metabolism balance of muscle fibers. *Biochem. Biophys. Res. Commun.* 326, 788–793. doi: 10.1016/j.bbrc.2004.11.111

Pompl, P. N., Ho, L., Bianchi, M., McManus, T., Qin, W., and Pasinetti, G. M. (2003). A therapeutic role for cyclooxygenase-2 inhibitors in a transgenic mouse model of amyotrophic lateral sclerosis. *FASEB J.* 17, 725–727. doi: 10.1096/fj.02-0876fje

Poruk, K. E., Davis, R. H., Smart, A. L., Chisum, B. S., Lasalle, B. A., Chan, G. M., et al. (2012). Observational study of caloric and nutrient intake, bone density, and body composition in infants and children with spinal muscular atrophy type, I. *Neuromuscul. Disord.* 22, 966–973. doi: 10.1016/j.nmd.2012.04.008

Pradat, P. F., Dubourg, O., de Tapia, M., di Scala, F., Dupuis, L., Lenglet, T., et al. (2011). Muscle gene expression is a marker of amyotrophic lateral sclerosis severity. *Neurodegener. Dis.* 9, 38–52. doi: 10.1159/000329723

Pun, S., Santos, A. F., Saxena, S., Xu, L., and Caroni, P. (2006). Selective vulnerability and pruning of phasic motoneuron axons in motoneuron disease alleviated by CNTF. *Nat. Neurosci.* 9, 408–419. doi: 10.1038/nn1653

Rao, A., Asadi-Lari, M., Walsh, J., Wilcox, R., and Gray, D. (2006). Quality of life in patients with signs and symptoms of heart failure–does systolic function matter? *J. Card. Fail.* 12, 677–683. doi: 10.1016/j.cardfail.2006.08.004

Reich-Slotky, R., Andrews, J., Cheng, B., Buchsbaum, R., Levy, D., Kaufmann, P., et al. (2013). Body mass index (BMI) as predictor of alSFRS-R score decline in alS patients. *Amyotroph. Lateral Scler. Frontotemporal Degener.* 14, 212–216. doi: 10.3109/21678421.2013.770028

Ripps, M. E., Huntley, G. W., Hof, P. R., Morrison, J. H., and Gordon, J. W. (1995). Transgenic mice expressing an altered murine superoxide dismutase gene provide an animal model of amyotrophic lateral sclerosis. *Proc. Natl. Acad. Sci. U.S.A.* 92, 689–693. doi: 10.1073/pnas.92.3.689

Rosen, D. R., Siddique, T., Patterson, D., Figlewicz, D. A., Sapp, P., Hentati, A., et al. (1993). Mutations in Cu/Zn superoxide dismutase gene are associated with familial amyotrophic lateral sclerosis. *Nature* 362, 59–62. doi: 10.1038/362059a0

Schmied, A., Pouget, J., and Vedel, J. P. (1999). Electromechanical coupling and synchronous firing of single wrist extensor motor units in sporadic amyotrophic lateral sclerosis. *Clin. Neurophysiol.* 110, 960–974. doi: 10.1016/S1388-2457(99)00032-2

Schmitz, G., and Ecker, J. (2008). The opposing effects of n-3 and n-6 fatty acids. *Prog. Lipid Res.* 47, 147–155. doi: 10.1016/j.plipres.2007.12.004

Sharp, P. S., Dick, J. R., and Greensmith, L. (2005). The effect of peripheral nerve injury on disease progression in the SOD1(G93A) mouse model of amyotrophic lateral sclerosis. *Neuroscience* 130, 897–910. doi: 10.1016/j.neuroscience.2004.09.069

Shatunov, A., Mok, K., Newhouse, S., Weale, M. E., Smith, B., Vance, C., et al. (2010). Chromosome 9p21 in sporadic amyotrophic lateral sclerosis in the UK and seven other countries: a genome-wide association study. *Lancet Neurol.* 9, 986–994. doi: 10.1016/S1474-4422(10)70197-6

Shimizu, T., Nagaoka, U., Nakayama, Y., Kawata, A., Kugimoto, C., Kuroiwa, Y., et al. (2012). Reduction rate of body mass index predicts prognosis for survival in amyotrophic lateral sclerosis: a multicenter study in Japan. *Amyotroph. Lateral Scler.* 13, 363–366. doi: 10.3109/17482968.2012.678366

Siciliano, G., D'Avino, C., Del Corona, A., Barsacchi, R., Kusmic, C., Rocchi, A., et al. (2002). Impaired oxidative metabolism and lipid peroxidation in exercising muscle from alS patients. *Amyotroph. Lateral Scler. Other Motor Neuron Disord.* 3, 57–62. doi: 10.1080/146608202760196011

Simons, K., and Vaz, W. L. (2004). Model systems, lipid rafts, and cell membranes. *Annu. Rev. Biophys. Biomol. Struct.* 33, 269–295. doi: 10.1146/annurev.biophys.32.110601.141803

Singh, R., Artaza, J. N., Taylor, W. E., Braga, M., Yuan, X., Gonzalez-Cadavid, N. F., et al. (2006). Testosterone inhibits adipogenic differentiation in 3T3-L1 cells: nuclear translocation of androgen receptor complex with beta-catenin and T-cell factor 4 may bypass canonical Wnt signaling to down-regulate adipogenic transcription factors. *Endocrinology* 147, 141–154. doi: 10.1210/en.2004-1649

Song, Y., Nagy, M., Ni, W., Tyagi, N. K., Fenton, W. A., Lopez-Giraldez, F., et al. (2013). Molecular chaperone Hsp110 rescues a vesicle transport defect produced by an alS-associated mutant SOD1 protein in squid axoplasm. *Proc. Natl. Acad. Sci. U.S.A.* 110, 5428–5433. doi: 10.1073/pnas.1303279110

Sproule, D. M., Montes, J., Montgomery, M., Battista, V., Koenigsberger, D., Shen, W., et al. (2009). Increased fat mass and high incidence of overweight despite low body mass index in patients with spinal muscular atrophy. *Neuromuscul. Disord.* 19, 391–396. doi: 10.1016/j.nmd.2009.03.009

Swoboda, K. J., Scott, C. B., Crawford, T. O., Simard, L. R., Reyna, S. P., Krosschell, K. J., et al. (2010). SMA CARNI-Val trial part I: double-blind, randomized, placebo-controlled trial of L-carnitine and valproic acid in spinal muscular atrophy. *PLoS ONE* 5:e12140. doi: 10.1371/journal.pone.0012140

Tein, I., Sloane, A. E., Donner, E. J., Lehotay, D. C., Millington, D. S., and Kelley, R. I. (1995). Fatty acid oxidation abnormalities in childhood-onset spinal muscular atrophy: primary or secondary defect(s)? *Pediatr. Neurol.* 12, 21–30. doi: 10.1016/0887-8994(94)00100-G

Thau, N., Knippenberg, S., Korner, S., Rath, K. J., Dengler, R., and Petri, S. (2012). Decreased mRNA expression of PGC-1alpha and PGC-1alpha-regulated factors in the SOD1G93A alS mouse model and in human sporadic alS. *J. Neuropathol. Exp. Neurol.* 71, 1064–1074. doi: 10.1097/NEN.0b013e318275df4b

Walford, R. L., Mock, D., Verdery, R., and MacCallum, T. (2002). Calorie restriction in biosphere 2: alterations in physiologic, hematologic, hormonal, and biochemical parameters in humans restricted for a 2-year period. *J. Gerontol. A Biol. Sci. Med. Sci.* 57, B211–B224. doi: 10.1093/gerona/57.6.B211

Xiao, Q., Pepe, A. E., Wang, G., Luo, Z., Zhang, L., Zeng, L., et al. (2012). Nrf3-Pla2g7 interaction plays an essential role in smooth muscle differentiation from stem cells. *Arterioscler. Thromb. Vasc. Biol.* 32, 730–744. doi: 10.1161/ATVBAHA.111.243188

Xu, X., Bittman, R., Duportail, G., Heissler, D., Vilcheze, C., and London, E. (2001). Effect of the structure of natural sterols and sphingolipids on the formation of ordered sphingolipid/sterol domains (rafts). Comparison of cholesterol to plant, fungal, and disease-associated sterols and comparison of sphingomyelin, cerebrosides, and ceramide. *J. Biol. Chem.* 276, 33540–33546. doi: 10.1074/jbc.M104776200

Yao, J. K., Cannon, K. P., Holman, R. T., and Dyck, P. J. (1983). Effects of polyunsaturated fatty acid diets on plasma lipids of patients with adrenomultineuronal degeneration, hepatosplenomegaly and fatty acid derangement. *J. Neurol. Sci.* 62, 67–75. doi: 10.1016/0022-510X(83)90190-9

Yi, C. X., Habegger, K. M., Chowen, J. A., Stern, J., and Tschop, M. H. (2011). A role for astrocytes in the central control of metabolism. *Neuroendocrinology* 93, 143–149. doi: 10.1159/000324888

Yip, P. K., Pizzasegola, C., Gladman, S., Biggio, M. L., Marino, M., Jayasinghe, M., et al. (2013). The omega-3 Fatty Acid eicosapentaenoic Acid accelerates disease progression in a model of amyotrophic lateral sclerosis. *PLoS ONE* 8:e61626. doi: 10.1371/journal.pone.0061626

Yoshikawa, T., Shimano, H., Yahagi, N., Ide, T., Amemiya-Kudo, M., Matsuzaka, T., et al. (2002). Polyunsaturated fatty acids suppress sterol regulatory element-binding protein 1c promoter activity by inhibition of liver X receptor (LXR) binding to LXR response elements. *J. Biol. Chem.* 277, 1705–1711. doi: 10.1074/jbc.M105711200

Zhao, W., Varghese, M., Vempati, P., Dzhun, A., Cheng, A., Wang, J., et al. (2012). Caprylic triglyceride as a novel therapeutic approach to effectively improve the performance and attenuate the symptoms due to the motor neuron loss in alS disease. *PLoS ONE* 7:e49191. doi: 10.1371/journal.pone.0049191

Zhao, W., Varghese, M., Yemul, S., Pan, Y., Cheng, A., Marano, P., et al. (2011). Peroxisome proliferator activator receptor gamma coactivator-1alpha (PGC-1alpha) improves motor performance and survival in a mouse model of amyotrophic lateral sclerosis. *Mol. Neurodegener.* 6, 51. doi: 10.1186/1750-1326-6-51

Zhao, Z., Lange, D. J., Voustianiouk, A., MacGrogan, D., Ho, L., Suh, J., et al. (2006). A ketogenic diet as a potential novel therapeutic intervention in amyotrophic lateral sclerosis. *BMC Neurosci.* 7:29. doi: 10.1186/1471-2202-7-29

Zhou, J., Yi, J., Fu, R., Liu, E., Siddique, T., Rios, E., et al. (2010). Hyperactive intracellular calcium signaling associated with localized mitochondrial defects in skeletal muscle of an animal model of amyotrophic lateral sclerosis. *J. Biol. Chem.* 285, 705–712. doi: 10.1074/jbc.M109.041319

21

Attitudes toward assisted suicide and life-prolonging measures in Swiss ALS patients and their caregivers

Ralf Stutzki[1]*, Ursula Schneider[2], Stella Reiter-Theil[1] and Markus Weber[2]

[1] *Clinical Ethics Support and Accompanying Research, University Hospital Basel/Psychiatric University Hospitals Basel, Institut für Bio- und Medizin Ethik, University of Basel, Basel, Switzerland*

[2] *Muskelzentrum/ALS Clinic, Kantonsspital St. Gallen, St. Gallen, Switzerland*

Edited by:
Francesco Pagnini, Catholic University of Milan, Italy

Reviewed by:
Gian Mauro Manzoni, Istituto Auxologico Italiano IRCCS, Italy
Francesco Pagnini, Catholic University of Milan, Italy

Correspondence:
Ralf Stutzki, Clinical Ethics Support and Accompanying Research, Universitäre Psychiatrische Kliniken, Schanzenstrasse 13, 4056 Basel, Switzerland.
e-mail: ralf.stutzki@unibas.ch

Objectives: In Switzerland, assisted suicide (AS) is legal, provided that the person seeking assistance has decisional capacity and the person assisting is not motivated by reasons of self-interest. However, in this particular setting nothing is known about patients' and their caregivers' attitudes toward AS and life-prolonging measures. **Methods:** Data was retrieved through validated questionnaires and personal interviews in 33 patients and their caregivers covering the following domains: physical function according to the revised Amyotrophic Lateral Sclerosis Functional Rating Scale (ALSFRS-R), demographic data, quality of life, anxiety, depression, social situation, spirituality, burden of disease, life-prolonging, and life-shortening acts. **Results:** In patients the median time after diagnosis was 9 months (2–90) and the median Amyotrophic Lateral Sclerosis (ALS) FRS-R score was 37 (22–48). The majority of patients (94%; $n = 31$) had no desire to hasten death. Patients' and caregivers' attitudes toward Percutaneous Endoscopic Gastrostomy (PEG) and Non-Invasive Ventilation (NIV) differed. Significantly more patients than caregivers (21.2 versus 3.1%) stated that they were against NIV ($p = 0.049$) and against PEG (27.3 versus 3.1%; $p = 0.031$). Answers regarding tracheotomy were not significantly different ($p = 0.139$). Caregivers scored significantly higher levels of "suffering" ($p = 0.007$), "loneliness" ($p = 0.006$), and "emotional distress" answering the questionnaires ($p < 0.001$). Suffering ($p < 0.026$) and loneliness ($p < 0.016$) were related to the score of the Hospital Anxiety and Depression Scale (HADS) in patients. **Conclusion:** A liberal legal setting does not necessarily promote the wish for AS. However, the desire to discuss AS is prevalent in ALS patients. There is a higher level of suffering and loneliness on the caregivers' side. A longitudinal study is warranted.

Keywords: ALS, motor neuron disease, quality of life, depression, end of life

INTRODUCTION

During the course of the disease, Amyotrophic Lateral Sclerosis (ALS) patients may suffer from depression, hopelessness, the feeling of loneliness, and loss of control (Rabkin et al., 2000, 2005; Albert et al., 2005; Olney and Lomen-Hoerth, 2005). In the terminal phase respiratory distress, anxiety, and other distressing symptoms may occur (Mandler et al., 2001). Given the suffering associated with the disease, some patients choose to decline life-prolonging measures such as Percutaneous Endoscopic Gastrostomy (PEG) and Non-Invasive Ventilation (NIV) and/or wish to hasten death (Ganzini et al., 1998; Veldink et al., 2002; Fang et al., 2008; Maessen et al., 2009). In an early study from Oregon, about 56% of all ALS patients considered physician-assisted suicide (PAS; legalized after 1997) during the terminal phase and 73% of caregivers and patients had similar attitudes toward PAS (Ganzini et al., 1998). In the Netherlands, during the 2000–2005 period 16.8% of ALS patients decided for euthanasia or PAS (Maessen et al., 2009), while in Sweden (where PAS is not legalized), ALS patients have a sixfold increased risk of committing suicide (Fang et al., 2008). Factors such as depression, hopelessness, loss of meaning, and purpose in life have been discussed to be associated with the wish to hasten death, whereas the contrary applies to religious faith and spiritual beliefs (Rabkin et al., 2000, 2005; Albert et al., 2005; Olney and Lomen-Hoerth, 2005). These findings are not consistent between different countries (Maessen et al., 2009). Moreover, there is a lack of longitudinal studies analyzing changes of these factors over time. It is also unclear whether the legal background in different countries influences patients' attitudes toward assisted suicide (AS) as comparative studies are lacking.

In Switzerland, however, assistance in committing suicide by a physician or a lay person is not explicitly regulated by law, but article 115 of the Swiss Penal Code allows assistance in suicide provided that the person seeking assistance has decisional capacity and the person assisting – physician or lay person – is not motivated by reasons of self-interest. Based on this article, Swiss "right to die" organizations offer assistance to commit suicide (Fischer et al., 2008). A recent study from the City of Zurich revealed that between 2001 and 2004 "Dignitas or Exit Deutsche Schweiz" had facilitated a total of 421 cases of AS (Fischer et al., 2008). Amongst the patients, 60% had been non-residents in Switzerland emphasizing the problem of "suicide tourism." Twenty-four percent of ASs were patients with "neurological disorders" including

ALS. However, no information is available about the total number of ALS patients, their motivation and associated factors that had made them choose this exit strategy.

The objective of this study is to analyze patients' and caregivers' attitudes toward AS, life-prolonging measures as well as associated factors (e.g., depression, quality of life (QoL), loneliness, suffering, education, profession, family status, living situation, Amyotrophic Lateral Sclerosis Functional Rating Scale (ALSFRS, and time after diagnosis) in a country with a comparatively easy access to AS.

METHODS AND PARTICIPANTS

PARTICIPANTS

Swiss patients and their primary caregivers were recruited from a tertiary referral center (Muskelzentrum/ALS clinic) at the Kantonsspital St. Gallen. Patients and caregivers attended the ALS outpatient clinic on a regular basis (usually every 3 months). Patients and caregivers had to be at least 18 years old. Further inclusion criteria for patients were a diagnosis of definitive, probable, or probable laboratory supported ALS according to the revised El Escorial Criteria (Brooks et al., 2000). Patients were only eligible if they had been informed about their ALS diagnosis, disease progression, prognosis, and therapeutic options including PEG insertion and different forms of ventilation (e.g., NIV, tracheotomy). The discussion about PEG and ventilation was usually triggered by clinical decline that resulted in use of PEG or NIV. Both issues are part of ALS – specific advanced directives which are routinely applied during this discussion (Benditt et al., 2001). Patients who inquired about these interventions shortly after diagnosis were also eligible. The study was approved by the local ethics committee and all patients and caregivers gave written informed consent.

For this study inclusion criteria, exclusion criteria, variables, and statistical analysis were pre-specified. Data were retrieved through questionnaires and personal interviews during home visits. The data collection took place as soon as patients had been informed about life-prolonging measures. Interviews were carried out by a researcher trained in interview technique, experienced in pastoral care, and medical ethics, not involved in clinical care of the patients and their primary caregivers. Patients and caregivers filled in the questionnaires simultaneously. In case the patient was unable to complete the questionnaire by his/her own hand due to weakness, the interviewer completed the questionnaire according to the patient's statements. The mean duration of the interview was approximately 60 min. After the interview, the primary caregiver/relative had the opportunity to clarify any issues that may have arisen during completion of the questionnaire. Specifically the following data and questionnaires were retrieved/applied:

Demographic data

The collection of data included age, sex, living situation, education, profession, and religious confession.

Numerical rating scale

(Eleven-point format; 0–10) asking the following questions: (1) What is your current QoL?; (2) How much are you suffering from your disease/from the disease of your partner?; (3) How lonely do you feel?; (4) How strong is your current desire to ask others for help to end your life prematurely?; (5) How distressing or how helpful was it for you to speak about such issues?

Hospital anxiety and depression scale (HADS)

A self-assessment scale to quantify patients' anxiety and depression by choosing one response from four given. The range is from 0 to 42 with the maximum score indicating a high level of depression and anxiety (Bjelland et al., 2002).

Questions regarding life-prolonging measures and hastening death

Patients' and caregivers' opinions were assessed with regards to tracheotomy, NIV, and PEG within a four-point response format. The following questions were asked: What is your attitude toward the following life-prolonging measures: (a) Tracheotomy; (b) NIV; (c) PEG? Possible answers to each item were: (a) I am not sure; (b) I am absolutely in favor of it; (c) I am in favor of it under certain circumstances; (d) I am against it.

Questions in yes/no format included: (1) Have you ever thought about committing suicide after receiving your diagnosis?; (2) Can you imagine a future scenario in which a physician prescribes a fatal drug which you administer yourself?; (3) Can you imagine a future scenario in which a physician prescribes and administers to you a fatal drug?; (4) Have you ever discussed suicide with others?; (5) Would you like to discuss suicide with a physician?

Idler index of religiosity (IRR)

The IRR assesses both public and private religiosity: (1) summing up attendance at religious meetings and services and the number of church members known to the patient; (2) self-assessment of personal religiosity as well as the amount of strength and comfort provided by personal faith (Robbins et al., 2001).

STATISTICAL ANALYSIS

For continuous variables (e.g., age) the mean of the differences between "patient" and "caregiver" was calculated by the t-test. Variables applying scores were compared by the Wilcoxon signed rank tests providing the median difference and its 95% confidence limits. Differences of ordered categorical variables (four-point response format) were tested by the Fishers exact test and the McNemar's Chi-squared test. For analyzing possible associations between the paired samples ("patient," "caregiver") the Spearman's rho correlation coefficient was applied. The level of significance was $p < 0.05$.

In order to predict score ratios between patients and caregiver, generalized linear mixed-effects models with group ("patient" and "caregiver") and given variables as fixed factors (sex, age, education, profession, family status, living situation, children, ALSFRS, time after diagnosis, and QoL) and subject ("patient") as random factor were performed either as multivariate or univariate model (for each parameter as a separate model). In order to predict dichotomous variables (yes versus no) concerning suicidal ideation for patients, logistic regression models were performed providing odds ratios (OR) and 95% confidence intervals (CI) with corresponding p-values.

All analyses were performed using R version 2.12.2 (R Development Core Team, 2011).

RESULTS

DEMOGRAPHIC DATA

During the recruitment period from 2008 to 2010 a total of 59 patients and caregivers were asked whether they would participate in this study. Twenty-six patients declined, 33 patients and their caregivers agreed to participate. The most frequent reason for declining participation was "no interest" and reluctance toward the themes of religiosity and spirituality. **Table 1** summarizes the epidemiological data, social status, and religious denominations of patients and their caregivers. Mean age of patients was 59.6 and mean age of caregivers was 56.9 (paired t-test; $p = 0{,}065$). The median time after diagnosis at which the first interview took place was 9 months (2–90) and the median ALSFRS-R was 37 (22–48).

ASSISTED SUICIDE/HASTENING DEATH

Thirteen patients (39%) answered that during the course of the disease they had thought about the possibility of committing suicide (**Table 2**). However, at the time of the interview, 31 of the patients (94%) expressed no wish to hasten death by AS. Thirty-three percent of the patients would like to discuss the issue "suicide" with a physician. Fifty-four percent of the patients could imagine asking a physician in the future to prescribe a fatal drug that they could take themselves; 57% could imagine a physician administer such a drug to them in the future. Logistic regression revealed that for patients QoL was the major predictor toward suicidal ideation (OR: 0.58, CI: 0.35–0.99) and the wish to discuss suicide with a physician (OR: 0.32, CI: 0.13–0.81, **Table 2**). The number of children (OR: 0.54, CI: 0.28–1.04) and HADS score (OR: 1.2, CI: 0.99–1.45) was also predictive of the wish to discuss suicide with a physician. Other analyzed factors (education, profession, family status, living situation, ALSFRS, and time after diagnosis) were not associated.

LIFE-PROLONGING MEASURES

The majority of patients (57.6%) and caregivers (50.0%) were against tracheotomy (**Table 3**). As verified by the McNemar test no significant difference was detected between the coincident answers of the two study groups ($p = 0.37$). No patient and no caregiver were generally in favor of its application, only "under certain circumstances" (27.3 patients versus 25.0% caregivers). The remaining interviewees were "unsure" about tracheotomy. Within the four-point response format attitudes between patients and caregivers regarding NIV and PEG differed (Fishers exact test). Significantly more patients than caregivers (21.2 versus 3.1%) stated that they were against NIV ($p = 0.049$) and against PEG (27.3 versus 3.1%; $p = 0.031$).

Table 1 | Demographic data.

	Patients % (n)	Caregivers % (n)
Age (mean, range)	59.6 (38–79)	56.9 (31–79)
Sex		
Female	36.4 (12)	62.5 (20)
Male	63.6 (21)	37.5 (12)
Living situation		
Alone	9.1 (3)	3.1 (1)
With spouse	57.6 (19)	59.4 (19)
With spouse and child(ren)	33.3 (11)	37.5 (12)
Religious confession		
Roman-catholic	51.5 (17)	46.9 (15)
Protestant	33.3 (11)	25.0 (8)
No confession	15.2 (5)	28.1 (9)

QUALITY OF LIFE AND BURDEN OF DISEASE

The median of QoL rated on a 11-point scale was six for patients and caregivers ($p = 0.68$). "Suffering," "loneliness," and "emotional distress answering the questionnaire" were significantly higher on the caregivers' than on the patients' side (**Table 4**). The mean HADS score of patients was 10.6 ± 5.1. Univariate analysis by a general linear mixed-effects model revealed a significant influence of the HADS on "suffering" (OR: 1.04 (95% CI: 1.01–1.07, $p = 0.027$) and "loneliness" (OR: 1.17 (95% CI: 1.04–1.33, $p = 0.017$) for coincident answers of patients and caregivers. Other analyzed factors (sex, age, education, profession, family status, living situation, children, ALSFRS-R, time after diagnosis, and QoL) did not show a significant effect, both in univariate and multivariate analysis (data not shown).

RELIGIOSITY

With regard to publicly practiced or private religiosity patients considered themselves to be more religious than their caregivers ($p < 0.001$) and derived more strength and comfort from their faith ($p < 0.01$).

DISCUSSION

The most important finding of the study is that at the time of the interview 94% of the patients had no intention to hasten death. This seems notable as the Swiss legal situation is liberal regarding assistance to commit suicide and the society is tolerating the practice of lay organizations offering the assistance through the collaboration of physicians and lay persons (van der Heide et al., 2003; Reiter-Theil, 2006). In contrast, a comparable study from Germany on ALS patients revealed that 37% of patients wished to hasten death (Jox et al., 2007). Germany is characterized by a liberal regulation of AS in penal law, but at the same time by a restrictive regulation and prohibition of PAS in the medical law (Reiter-Theil, 2006). The only difference between the Swiss and the German study methodology was that our patients were interviewed at home, whereas in the German study the interviews took place in the outpatient clinical. This difference, however, is unlikely to account for the imbalance and suggests that not the legal background as such (e.g., a more liberal legal situation promotes AS), but other factors must be responsible for the wish to hasten death. Previous studies from Oregon and the Netherlands where PAS is also legal, revealed a high prevalence of AS and euthanasia among ALS patients (Ganzini et al., 1998, 2002; Veldink et al., 2002; Albert et al., 2005; Maessen et al., 2009). This contrasts with our findings where only a minority of patients expressed a wish to hasten death. However, a comparison of our results with the Oregonian and Dutch studies is difficult as they were either retrospective (Veldink et al., 2002; Maessen et al., 2009) or interviews took place at a late to terminal stage (Ganzini et al., 2002; Albert et al., 2005). Longitudinal studies analyzing attitudes toward AS

Table 2 | Patient suicidality; n.s., no significant effect.

	Yes % (*n*)	No % (*n*)	No answer % (*n*)	Associated factors (adjusted for gender and age)
Thought about suicide after receiving diagnosis	39.4 (13)	60.6 (20)	0	n.s.
Can imagine future scenario: committing suicide by means of a prescribed drug	54.5 (18)	45.5 (15)	0	Quality of life ($p=0.026$)
Can imagine future scenario: suicide with the help of physician administering fatal drug	57.6 (19)	42.4 (14)	0	n.s.
Have already discussed suicide with others	33.3 (11)	66.7 (22)	0	n.s.
Would like to discuss suicide with a physician	33.3 (11)	60.6 (20)	6.1 (2)	Number of children ($p=0.048$), quality of life ($p<0.001$), HADS ($p=0.037$)

Table 3 | Live-prolonging measures: "what is your attitude toward the following life-prolonging measures?" *p*-values derived from McNemar test.

	Not sure% (*n*)	Absolutely yes % (*n*)	Yes under certain circumstances % (*n*)	Against % (*n*)	*p*
Tracheotomy					0.37
Patients	15.2 (5)	0	27.3 (9)	57.6 (19)	
Caregivers	25.0 (8)	0	25 (8)	50.0 (16)	
NIV					0.17
Patients	3.0 (1)	42.4 (14)	33.3 (11)	21.2 (7)	
Caregivers	18.8 (6)	43.8 (14)	34.4 (11)	3.1 (1)	
PEG					0.75
Patients	12.1 (4)	24.2 (8)	36.4 (12)	27.3 (9)	
Caregivers	25.0 (8)	18.8 (6)	53.1 (17)	3.1 (1)	

Table 4 | Quality of life and burden of disease variables rated on self-rating scales (0–10).

Parameters	Patients (median, IQR)	Caregivers (median, IQR)	Difference of medians	Lower 95% CI	Upper % 95 CI	*p*-value
Quality of life	6 (5–8)	6 (5–7)	0.25	−1.0	1.5	0.68
Loneliness	0 (0–1)	2 (0–6)	−3.25	−5.5	−1.5	0.003
Emotional distress	0 (0–1)	3 (0.8–5)	−4.25	−5.5	−3.0	<0.001
Suffering	5 (3–6)	6.5 (5–8)	−2.25	−3.5	−0.5	0.006

Differences determined by Wilcoxon signed rank test. IQR, inter quartile range.

have not been published yet, but are important to understand whether these attitudes depend on the degree of disability.

With respect to preferences for life-prolonging and ameliorative technologies it seems that ALS patients make choices consistent with preferences expressed shortly after diagnosis (Albert et al., 1999). It is unclear whether this also applies to attitudes toward AS. Nevertheless, more than one-third (39%) of our patients had thought about the possibility of committing suicide after being diagnosed with ALS and 33% of the patients expressed the wish to discuss suicide with their physician. Even 58% said they could imagine a future scenario in which a physician would not only prescribe, but also administer a fatal drug (i.e., euthanasia which is prohibited in Switzerland) to them. This mirrors other studies which have shown that the themes of assisted dying and suicide are prevalent in ALS patients (Ganzini et al., 1998, 2002; Albert et al., 2005; Palmieri et al., 2010). The wish of patients to discuss suicide with a physician was associated with poorer QoL and a higher HADS score. It can be concluded that medical caregivers need to develop an openness and willingness to discuss with and inform patients about suicide and to deal with the fact that a considerable number of patients facing end of life may ask for their physician's active involvement in hastening death (Bascom and Tolle, 2002; Jox et al., 2007; Moore et al., 2007; Oliver et al., 2007). The prevalence for a physician's active involvement in hastening death in the future corresponds with a retrospective study (Lofmark et al., 2008) which reports that 37% of the Swiss physicians ($n=1397$) had received a patient request to hasten death.

Patients' and caregivers' attitudes regarding life-prolonging measures were largely concordant. Fifty-eight percent of patients and 50% of caregivers were against tracheotomy. However, caregivers (mean: 22.2%) in general were considerably more unsure about NIV, PEG, and tracheotomy than patients (mean: 9.8%). Furthermore significantly more patients than caregivers were strictly against PEG and NIV. This confirms a fundamental need for more information and discussion about life-prolonging measures as has also been shown by other studies (Albert et al., 1999; Trail et al., 2003).

Another important finding of this study is that caregivers scored significantly higher in the domains of suffering, loneliness, and distress filling out the questionnaires compared to patients, despite overall QoL being not different between patients and their caregivers. The only associated factor was patients' depression and anxiety as measured by HADS. Sex, age, education, profession, family status, living situation, children, ALSFRS, time after diagnosis, and QoL were not related. Previous studies also revealed that depression in patients is associated with caregiver burden (Chio et al., 2005) and that patients' and caregivers' well-being are interrelated (Pagnini et al., 2011). Other examined factors such as time since diagnosis and degree of disability were not related in our as in previous studies (Rabkin et al., 2000; Chio et al., 2005). This is in contrast with studies that have shown that caregiver burden and distress are associated with the degree of disability (Hecht et al., 2003; Chio et al., 2005; Lo Coco et al., 2005). However, it needs to be taken into account that the patients in our study had only mild to moderate handicap as compared to other studies. A prospective longitudinal study may help to resolve this discrepancy and would also reveal dynamic changes as disease and disability progress.

This study has several limitations. Patients were recruited from a single center and may therefore not be representative for all Swiss ALS patients. At our ALS Clinic patient care is strictly adhering to international guidelines (Miller et al., 2009; Andersen et al., 2012) which may not be the case in all Swiss centers. Each follow-up consultation lasts 2 h allowing ample time to discuss end of life decisions and related issues that may have influenced the results. Second, since spirituality and religiosity were part of the study, this may have introduced a self-selection bias toward couples that tend to be more religious which is known to be inversely related to the wish to hasten death (Albert et al., 2005). The themes of religiosity/spirituality may also contribute for the relatively high non-participate rate of 44%. However, these problems are inherent in almost all of the published interview studies.

CONCLUSION

In summary the "liberal" Swiss legal setting does not promote the wish for AS, but the wish to discuss AS is prevalent amongst ALS patients even in moderately advanced stages of the disease. This wish is associated with poorer QoL and degree of depression.

ACKNOWLEDGMENTS

We are thankful to patients and caregivers for participating in this study and to Urs Simmen, biostatistician, for designing and conducting the statistical analysis. Funding: This work was supported by a grant from the Swiss Academy of Medical Sciences, Käthe Zingg Schwichtenberg Fonds in Basel.

AUTHOR NOTE

This study was approved by the ethics committee of St. Gallen.

REFERENCES

Albert, S. M., Murphy, P. L., Del Bene, M. L., and Rowland, L. P. (1999). A prospective study of preferences and actual treat- ment choices in ALS. *Neurology* 53, 278–283.

Albert, S. M., Rabkin, J. G., Del Bene, M. L., Tider, T., O'sullivan, I., Row- land, L. P., et al. (2005). Wish to die in end-stage ALS. *Neurology* 65, 68–74.

Andersen, P. M., Abrahams, S., Bora- sio, G. D., De Carvalho, M., Chio, A., Van Damme, P., et al. (2012). EFNS guidelines on the clinical manage- ment of amyotrophic lateral sclero-sis (MALS) – revised report of an EFNS task force. *Eur. J. Neurol.* 19, 360–375.

Bascom, P. B., and Tolle, S. W. (2002). Responding to requests for physician-assisted suicide: "these are uncharted waters for both of us...." *JAMA* 288, 91–98.

Benditt, J. O., Smith, T. S., and Tonelli, M. R. (2001). Empowering the individual with ALS at the end-of-life: disease-specific advance care plan- ning. *Muscle Nerve* 24, 1706–1709.

Bjelland, I., Dahl, A. A., Haug, T. T., and Neckelmann, D. (2002). The validity of the hospital anxiety and depression scale. An updated liter- ature review. *J. Psychosom. Res.* 52, 69–77.

Brooks, B. R., Miller, R. G., Swash, M., and Munsat, T. L. (2000). El escorial revisited: revised criteria for the diagnosis of amyotrophic lateral sclerosis. *Amyotroph. Lateral Scler. Other Motor Neuron Disord.* 1, 293–299.

Chio, A., Gauthier, A., Calvo, A., Ghiglione, P., and Mutani, R. (2005). Caregiver burden and patients' perception of being a burden in ALS. *Neurology* 64, 1780–1782.

Fang, F., Valdimarsdottir, U., Furst, C. J., Hultman, C., Fall, K., Sparen, P., et al. (2008). Suicide among patients with amyotrophic lateral sclerosis. *Brain* 131, 2729–2733.

Fischer, S., Huber, C. A., Imhof, L., Mahrer Imhof, R., Furter, M., Ziegler, S. J., et al. (2008). Sui- cide assisted by two Swiss right-to- die organisations. *J. Med. Ethics* 34, 810–814.

Ganzini, L., Johnston, W. S., Mcfar- land, B. H., Tolle, S. W., and Lee, M. A. (1998). Attitudes of patients with amyotrophic lateral sclero- sis and their care givers toward assisted suicide. *N. Engl. J. Med.* 339, 967–973.

Ganzini, L., Silveira, M. J., and John- ston, W. S. (2002). Predictors and correlates of interest in assisted sui- cide in the final month of life among ALS patients in Oregon and Wash- ington. *J. Pain Symptom. Manage.* 24, 312–317.

Hecht, M. J., Graesel, E., Tigges, S., Hillemacher, T., Winterholler, M., Hilz, M. J., et al. (2003). Burden of care in amyotrophic lateral sclerosis. *Palliat. Med.* 17, 327–333.

Jox, R., Haarmann-Doetkotte, S., Was-ner, M., and Borasio, G. D. (2007). The wish to hasten death among ALS patients in a palliative care program. *Amyotroph. Lateral. Scler.* 8(Suppl. 1), 87–88.

Lo Coco, G., Lo Coco, D., Cicero, V., Oliveri, A., Lo Verso, G., Pic- coli, F., et al. (2005). Individual and health-related quality of life assess- ment in amyotrophic lateral sclero- sis patients and their caregivers. *J. Neurol. Sci.* 238, 11–17.

Lofmark, R., Nilstun, T., Cartwright, C., Fischer, S., Van Der Heide, A., Mortier, F., et al. (2008). Physi- cians' experiences with end-of- life decision-making: survey in 6 European countries and Australia. *BMC Med.* 6, 4. doi:10.1186/1741-7015-6-4

Maessen, M., Veldink, J. H., Onwuteaka- Philipsen, B. D., De Vries, J. M., Wokke, J. H., Van Der Wal, G., et al. (2009). Trends and determinants of end-of-life practices in ALS in the Netherlands. *Neurology* 73, 954–961.

Mandler, R. N., Anderson, F. A. Jr., Miller, R. G., Clawson, L., Cudkow- icz, M., and Del Bene, M. (2001). The ALS patient care database: insights into end-of-life care in ALS. *Amy- otroph. Lateral Scler. Other Motor Neuron Disord.* 2, 203–208.

Miller, R. G., Jackson, C. E., Kasarskis, E. J., England, J. D., Forshew, D., Johnston, W., et al. (2009). Prac- tice parameter update: the care of the patient with *amyotrophic* lat- eral sclerosis: multidisciplinary care, symptom management, and cog- nitive/behavioral impairment (an evidence-based review): report of the quality standards subcommittee of the American academy of neurol- ogy. *Neurology* 73, 1227–1233.

Moore, M., Sadeghi, R., Gawel, M., Web-ster, P., Baryshnik, D., and Zinman, L. (2007). Advance care directives in ALS: when is the right time to talk? *Amyotroph. Lateral. Scler.* 8(Suppl. 1), 13.

Oliver, D., Campbell, C., Sloan, R., Sykes, N., Tallon, C., Webb, S., et al. (2007). End-of-life care and deci- sion making in ALS/MND: a cross- cultural study. *Amyotroph. Lateral. Scler.* 8(Suppl. 1), 13.

Olney, R. K., and Lomen-Hoerth, C. (2005). Exit strategies in ALS: an influence of depression or despair? *Neurology* 65, 9–10.

Pagnini, F., Lunetta, C., Rossi, G., Banfi, P., Gorni, K., Cellotto, N., et al. (2011). Existential well-being and spirituality of individuals with amy- otrophic lateral sclerosis is related to psychological well-being of their caregivers. *Amyotroph. Lateral Scler.* 12, 105–108.

Palmieri, A., Soraru, G., Albertini, E., Semenza, C., Vottero-Ris, F., D'ascenzo, C., et al. (2010). Psy- chopathological features and suici- dal ideation in amyotrophic lateral sclerosis patients. *Neurol. Sci.* 31, 735–740.

R Development Core Team. (2011). *R: A Language and Environment for Sta- tistical Computing*. Vienna: R Foun- dation for Statistical Computing.

Rabkin, J. G., Albert, S. M., Del Bene, M. L., O'sullivan, I., Tider, T., Rowland, L. P., et al. (2005). Prevalence of depressive disorders and change over time in late-stage ALS. *Neurology* 65, 62–67.

Rabkin, J. G., Wagner, G. J., and Del Bene, M. (2000). Resilience and distress among amyotrophic lateral sclerosis patients and caregivers. *Psy- chosom. Med.* 62, 271–279.

Reiter-Theil, S. (2006). Aerztliche Bei- hilfe zum Suizid oder "Laienhilfe?" Ein Vergleich zwischen der Schweiz, Oregon und den Niederlanden. *Vorgänge Heft* 3, 117–135.

Robbins, R. A., Simmons, Z., Bremer, B. A., Walsh, S. M., and Fischer, S. (2001). Quality of life in ALS is maintained as physical function declines. *Neurology* 56, 442–444.

Trail, M., Nelson, N. D., Van, J. N., Appel, S. H., and Lai, E. C. (2003). A study comparing patients with amy- otrophic lateral sclerosis and their caregivers on measures of quality of life, depression, and their attitudes toward treatment options. *J. Neurol. Sci.* 209, 79–85.

van der Heide, A., Deliens, L., Faisst, K., Nilstun, T., Norup, M., Paci, E., et al. (2003). End-of-life decision- making in six European coun- tries: descriptive study. *Lancet* 362, 345–350.

Veldink, J. H., Wokke, J. H., Van Der Wal, G., Vianney De Jong, J. M., and Van Den Berg, L. H. (2002). Euthanasia and physician- assisted suicide among patients with amyotrophic lateral sclerosis in the Netherlands. *N. Engl. J. Med.* 346, 1638–1644.

22

An emerging role for misfolded wild-type SOD1 in sporadic ALS pathogenesis

Melissa S. Rotunno and Daryl A. Bosco*

Department of Neurology, University of Massachusetts Medical Center, Worcester, MA, USA

Edited by:
Ricardo Tapia, Universidad Nacional Autónoma de México, Mexico

Reviewed by:
Yoshiaki Furukawa, Keio University, Japan
Anne Bertolotti, MRC Laboratory of Molecular Biology, UK

****Correspondence:***
Daryl A. Bosco, Department of Neurology, University of Massachusetts Medical Center, 55 Lake Ave. North, Worcester, MA 01655, USA
e-mail: daryl.bosco@umassmed.edu

Amyotrophic lateral sclerosis (ALS) is a fatal neurodegenerative disorder that targets motor neurons, leading to paralysis and death within a few years of disease onset. While several genes have been linked to the inheritable, or familial, form of ALS, much less is known about the cause(s) of sporadic ALS, which accounts for ~90% of ALS cases. Due to the clinical similarities between familial and sporadic ALS, it is plausible that both forms of the disease converge on a common pathway and, therefore, involve common factors. Recent evidence suggests the Cu,Zn-superoxide dismutase (SOD1) protein to be one such factor that is common to both sporadic and familial ALS. In 1993, mutations were uncovered in SOD1 that represent the first known genetic cause of familial ALS. While the exact mechanism of mutant-SOD1 toxicity is still not known today, most evidence points to a gain of toxic function that stems, at least in part, from the propensity of this protein to misfold. In the wild-type SOD1 protein, non-genetic perturbations such as metal depletion, disruption of the quaternary structure, and oxidation, can also induce SOD1 to misfold. In fact, these aforementioned post-translational modifications cause wild-type SOD1 to adopt a "toxic conformation" that is similar to familial ALS-linked SOD1 variants. These observations, together with the detection of misfolded wild-type SOD1 within human post-mortem sporadic ALS samples, have been used to support the controversial hypothesis that misfolded forms of wild-type SOD1 contribute to sporadic ALS pathogenesis. In this review, we present data from the literature that both support and contradict this hypothesis. We also discuss SOD1 as a potential therapeutic target for both familial and sporadic ALS.

Keywords: amyotrophic lateral sclerosis (ALS), sporadic amyotrophic lateral sclerosis, SOD1, protein misfolding, immunotherapy

INTRODUCTION

Amyotrophic lateral sclerosis (ALS) is the most common motor neuron disease and is clinically characterized by the degeneration of motor neurons in the brain and spinal cord, culminating in paralysis and death within 2–5 years. The only available treatment is riluzole, which in the best cases extends survival by only a few months (Glicksman, 2011). In 1993, mutations in the *SOD1* gene encoding Cu,Zn superoxide dismutase-1 were reported as the first genetic link to familial, or inherited, forms of ALS (FALS) (Rosen et al., 1993). Because of the high incidence of *SOD1* mutations, which account for 20–25% of FALS cases, *SOD1* has been one of the most intensely studied genes in the ALS field and continues to be a primary therapeutic target (Bosco and Landers, 2010).

Much of what we understand about the pathomechanisms of ALS is based on *in vivo* studies with transgenic rodent models expressing FALS-linked SOD1 variants. These FALS-SOD1 animal models recapitulate many key features of the human disease, including motor neuron degeneration, paralysis and shortened life-span (Turner and Talbot, 2008). Moreover, FALS-SOD1 animal models reveal the complex nature of this disease, which involves oxidative stress, a loss of proteostasis (i.e., protein aggregation with defective protein clearance), mitochondrial dysfunction, impaired axonal transport, and glutamate excitotoxicity (Rothstein, 2009). While motor neurons are the primary target in ALS, ALS may actually represent a non-cell autonomous disorder for which glia play an active role (Ilieva et al., 2009). Despite decades of research on FALS-SOD1 *in vitro* and *in vivo*, the exact mechanism of SOD1 in ALS pathogenesis remains unknown (Pasinelli and Brown, 2006; Ling et al., 2013). However, as will be discussed throughout this review, a substantial body of literature points to a gain of toxic function for FALS-SOD1 that stems, at least in part, from SOD1 misfolding.

In contrast to FALS, much less is known about the etiology of sporadic ALS (SALS), which accounts for 90% of ALS cases. Pathological aggregates composed of the TAR DNA-binding protein 43 (TDP-43) are detected in CNS tissues for a majority of SALS cases (Neumann et al., 2006), providing strong evidence for an association of misfolded TDP-43 with ALS pathogenesis (Xu, 2012). Mutations in TDP-43 have also been linked to SALS and FALS (Sreedharan et al., 2008), further establishing a role for this protein in disease. Another RNA-binding protein called fused in sarcoma/translocated in liposarcoma (FUS/TLS) has also been linked to FALS and SALS (Kwiatkowski et al., 2009; Vance et al., 2009). Although the association of FUS/TLS with pathological aggregates in SALS has been reported (Deng et al., 2010), this association is not as common as for TDP-43.

The inheritable nature of FALS facilitates the identification of causal genes, because many FALS-linked genes, such as *SOD1*, *TDP-43* and *FUS/TLS*, are autosomal dominant and segregate according to Mendelian genetics within an ALS family. In an effort to identify genetic susceptibility factors associated with SALS, several genome-wide association studies (GWAS) have been performed. However, by and large these studies have failed to generate confirmed SALS-susceptibility genes (Bosco and Landers, 2010). More recently, repeat expansions within the genome that are associated with different forms of ALS have been identified. Hexanucleotide repeat expansions in the *C9ORF72* gene were linked to familial frontotemporal lobar degeneration (FTLD)/ALS, FALS as well as to SALS (Dejesus-Hernandez et al., 2011; Renton et al., 2011), making this gene the most common factor in all of ALS. Moreover, repeat expansions in ataxin-2 (*ATXN2*) represent a susceptibility factor in SALS (Elden et al., 2010). Despite these advances in the genetics of SALS, the etiology remains unknown for a majority of SALS cases, likely a reflection of the complex nature of SALS. In fact, SALS may arise from genetic as well as environmental and behavioral factors. Smoking, diet, excessive exercise, injury and exposure to environmental toxins have all been implicated in SALS (D'Amico et al., 2013), although none have been shown to unequivocally cause disease. Although FALS is inheritable and SALS is not, the fact that FALS and SALS are clinically indistinguishable raises the possibility that they do in fact emerge from a common source and/or involve similar toxicity factors.

Recent evidence supports SOD1 as a toxic factor that is common to a subset of both FALS and SALS. This evidence is largely based on the observation that aberrant conformations of WT SOD1, induced by oxidation, demetallation and other altered post-translational modifications, cause WT SOD1 to acquire the same toxic functions that are observed for FALS-associated SOD1 variants (Ezzi et al., 2007; Bosco et al., 2010; Guareschi et al., 2012). Moreover, by employing conformation specific antibodies that are selective for SOD1 only when it is mutated or has altered post-translational modifications, misfolded "mutant-like" WT SOD1 has been detected in human post-mortem tissues from SALS individuals (Bosco et al., 2010; Forsberg et al., 2010, 2011; Pokrishevsky et al., 2012), suggesting that such species are in fact pathogenic. The concept that critical proteins can become pathogenic via both germline mutations and non-Mendelian post-translational modifications is not novel, but rather has strong precedence in neurodegeneration with examples including the α-synuclein (Beyer and Ariza, 2013), tau (Mandelkow et al., 1996) and TDP-43 proteins (Arai et al., 2010). The concept that WT SOD1 could play a role in SALS is controversial, since not all conformation specific antibodies employed to date have detected aberrant WT SOD1 species in SALS (Furukawa, 2012; Ling et al., 2013). However, such a role should be strongly considered and fully explored as it has important therapeutic implications for treating both familial and sporadic forms of ALS.

NORMAL PROPERTIES AND CELLULAR FUNCTIONS OF SOD1

Long before SOD1 was identified as a causative factor in FALS (Rosen et al., 1993), the anti-oxidizing and catalytic properties of native SOD1 were being investigated (McCord and Fridovich, 1969). While the role of SOD1 as an anti-oxidizing enzyme is well known and accepted, the role of SOD1 as a signaling molecule has been relatively underappreciated. Herein we discuss what is known regarding the normal functions of SOD1 in the context of both anti-oxidation and signaling. The normal physiological properties of SOD1 are discussed in order to establish a foundation for the following sections that describe how both FALS-linked mutations and post-translational modifications alter the structure and function of the protein.

SOD1: LOCATION, ACTIVITY, AND STRUCTURE

Copper,zinc- superoxide dismutase-1 (SOD1) is a member of the human SOD family of proteins, which also includes SOD2 and SOD3. While all three proteins function as anti-oxidizing enzymes that catalyze the dismutation of superoxide radicals ($O_2\bullet^-$) to hydrogen peroxide (H_2O_2), they are distinct proteins with unique characteristics (Zelko et al., 2002). SOD1 is highly abundant, comprising ~1% of total protein in the cell (Pardo et al., 1995), and resides mainly in the cytosol with some degree of localization in the mitochondrial inner membrane space (Fukai and Ushio-Fukai, 2011). The mitochondrion is also home to SOD2, which is localized to the mitochondrial matrix. In contrast to both SOD1 and SOD2, SOD3 is predominately located outside the cell in the extracellular matrix. Other key differences amongst the SOD proteins include their quaternary structures and mechanism of superoxide dismutation: SOD1 is a homodimer while SOD2 and SOD3 are homotetrameric proteins; SOD1 and SOD3 catalyze the dismutation of $O_2\bullet^-$ through the alternate reduction and reoxidation of Cu^{2+}, whereas SOD2 utilizes manganese (Mn) as a redox active transition metal for this purpose. The role of SOD in FALS, which will be discussed in detail below, is specific to the SOD1 isoform as there is no compelling evidence supporting the involvement of either SOD2 or SOD3 in FALS pathogenesis (Tomkins et al., 2001).

While coordination of copper to SOD1 is required for dismutation of $O_2\bullet^-$, other post-translational modifications, such as Zn^{2+} coordination (Kayatekin et al., 2008) and disulfide oxidation, help create a mature and structurally stable protein. The 32 kDa homodimeric SOD1 protein adopts an eight-stranded Greek key beta-barrel structural motif (**Figure 1A**). Two functional loops are present in SOD1: the electrostatic loop that guides superoxide into the redox active site where Cu^{2+} is located and the zinc-binding loop. All tolled, each SOD1 molecule coordinates two copper and two zinc atoms, one of each per subunit. A unique functional feature of SOD1 is the presence of an intra-subunit disulfide bond between Cys57 and Cys146 (C57–C146), which is unusual for proteins that reside in the highly reducing environment of the cytosol. Both copper coordination and formation of C57-C146 is facilitated by the cytosolic copper carrier protein CCS (copper chaperone for SOD1) (Furukawa et al., 2004; Seetharaman et al., 2009). A recent study utilizing both electrospray ionization mass spectrometry (ESI-MS) and nuclear magnetic resonance (NMR) spectroscopy support a step-wise model for SOD1 maturation: (i) SOD1 is loaded with Zn, (ii) heterodimerization between SOD1 and CCS, (iii) Cu is transferred from CCS to SOD1, (iv) C57–C146 is formed, and (v) SOD1 homodimerization (Banci et al., 2012). Together these

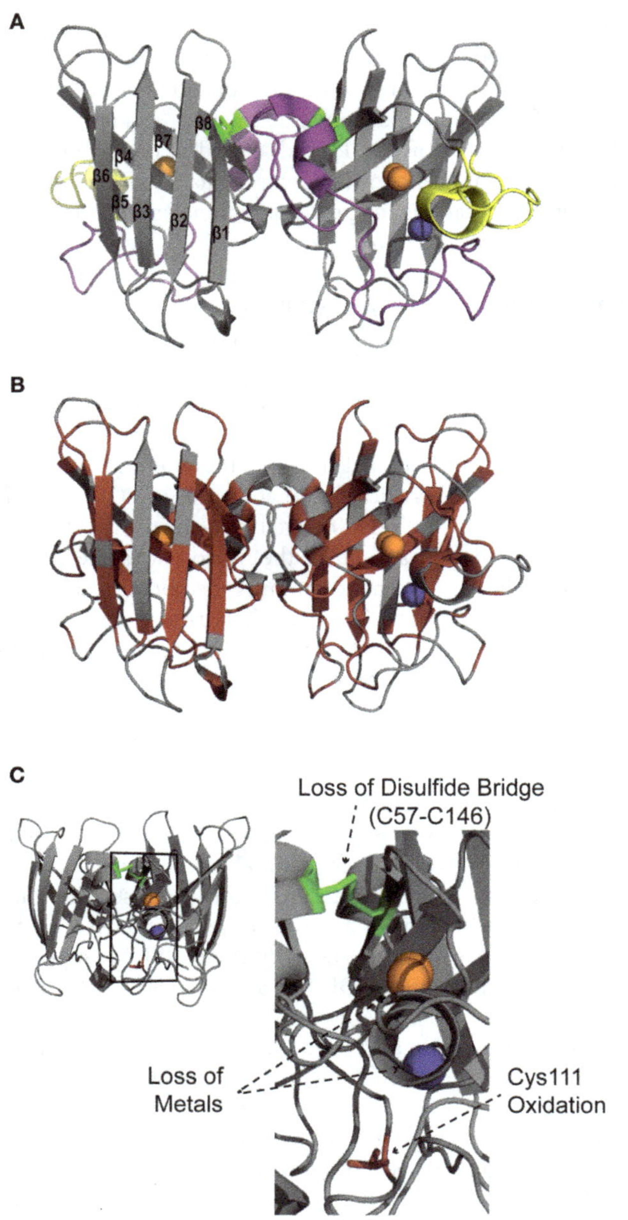

FIGURE 1 | Structural features of SOD1. SOD1 is a homodimer with one copper (orange) and one zinc (blue) per subunit (PDB:2C9V). **(A)** SOD1 consists of eight beta sheets that form the beta barrel core. The major functional loops are the zinc binding loop (purple; residues 49–81) and electrostatic loop (yellow; residues 124–139). An intramolecular disulfide bond (C57–C146; green) stabilizes the protein structure. **(B)** Mapping the ALS-linked mutations (red) onto the structure of SOD1 illustrates that these mutations are present throughout the entire protein. **(C)** Alterations to normal post-translational modifications, such as loss of the disulfide bridge (C57–C146; green), demetallation and monomerization (not shown), as well as aberrant modifications such as oxidation of amino acid side chains (shown for Cys 111; red), cause WT SOD1 to misfold.

post-translational modifications produce a highly stable protein, as evidenced by a high melting temperature (T_m) of ~92°C and resistance to denaturation in both 6 M GdmCl and 4% SDS (Forman and Fridovich, 1973; Bartnikas and Gitlin, 2003). Demetalation of SOD1 and/or reduction of C57–C146 destabilizes the protein and drastically decreases the melting temperature (Forman and Fridovich, 1973; Furukawa and O'Halloran, 2005). As will be discussed below, these post-translational modifications are compromised by both FALS-linked mutations and oxidation, which in turn destabilize SOD1 in the context of disease.

SOD1 IN SIGNAL TRANSDUCTION

The physiological relevance of SOD1 catalysis extends beyond oxidative stress protection. In fact, SOD1 catalysis plays a key role in signal transduction, a function that is largely underappreciated compared to its role as an anti-oxidizing enzyme (**Figure 2**). For instance, H_2O_2 generated by SOD1 can reversibly and specifically react with proteins, generally by oxidizing Cys residues. Cys oxidation in turn alters the biochemical and functional properties of those proteins in a redox dependent manner (Georgiou, 2002). A variety of signal transduction pathways are modulated by H_2O_2, including but not limited to gene expression, cell proliferation, differentiation and death (Rhee, 2006; Brown and Griendling, 2009). NADPH oxygenases (Nox) function as upstream regulators of these signal transduction pathways through the production of $O_2\bullet^-$, which is either converted to H_2O_2 spontaneously or catalytically by SOD1. SOD1 comes into close proximity with Nox2-derived $O_2\bullet^-$ at the surface of endosomes in response to proinflammatory cytokines (Harraz et al., 2008). A report by Harraz et al. (2008) demonstrated that SOD1 not only acts downstream of Nox2 but can also modulate Nox function through an interaction with Rac1. SOD1 directly binds and stabilizes the active form of Rac1 in its GTP-bound state, leading to Nox2 activation and $O_2\bullet^-$ production. Interestingly, H_2O_2 generated by SOD1 serves as a negative feedback of Nox2 activity: H_2O_2 induces the dissociation of the SOD1/Rac1 complex, thereby inactivating Rac1 and Nox2 (Harraz et al., 2008). The mechanism for how H_2O_2 disrupts the interaction between SOD1 and Rac1 has not been elucidated. One possibility is that the H_2O_2 generated by SOD1, which is in close proximity to Rac1, oxidatively modifies Cys residues within Rac1 in such a way that disrupts the SOD1/Rac1 binding interaction.

Another example of SOD1 redox-sensing and signaling activity is in the context of respiratory repression, which occurs during aerobic fermentation in proliferating cells, including in the context of some cancers. In *Saccharomyces cerevisiae*, a loss of SOD1 activity impairs respiratory repression (Sehati et al., 2011). SOD1 was shown to modulate respiratory repression through binding and stabilizing Yck1p and Yck2p, two casein kinase 1-gamma homologs in yeast that inhibit respiration (Reddi and Culotta, 2013). The authors speculate that SOD1 stabilizes Yck1p/Yck2p through the action of the reaction product H_2O_2, where oxidative modification of lysine residues within Yck1p/Yck2p by H_2O_2 prevents their ubiquitination and degradation by the ubiquitin-proteasome system. Therefore, both the Rac1/Nox2 and Yck1p/Yck2p interactions with SOD1 demonstrate that the catalytic action of SOD1 can direct the modification and activity of specific protein substrates. In this manner, SOD1 catalyzes a "molecular redox switch" that ultimately controls protein function and signaling, much like phosphorylation.

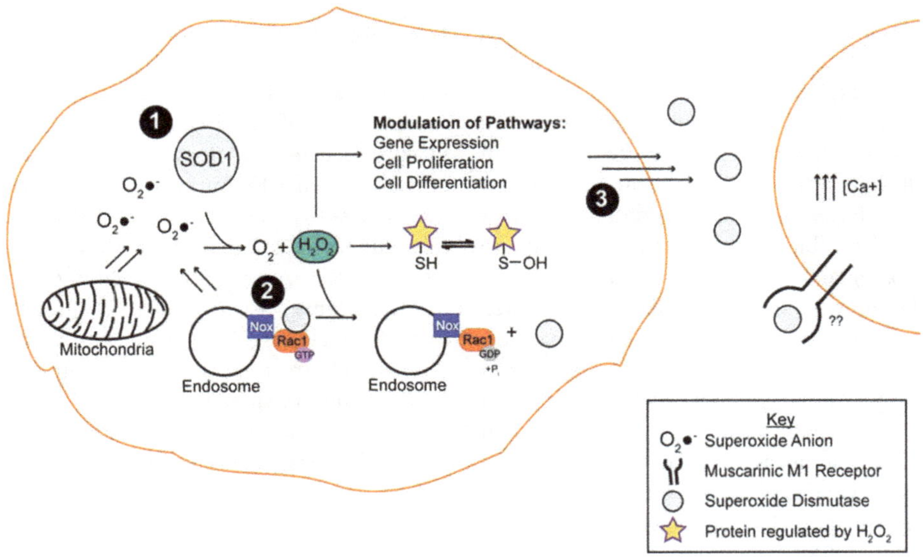

FIGURE 2 | The putative normal function of the native WT SOD1 protein. (**1**) SOD1 is responsible for converting the toxic superoxide anion ($O_2\bullet^-$) into oxygen (O_2) and hydrogen peroxide (H_2O_2), the latter of which is involved in the modulation of multiple pathways through oxidation of exposed thiols. (**2**) SOD1 binds and stabilizes Rac1 in its active, GTP bound state, resulting in Nox2 (Nox) activation and superoxide production. The hydrogen peroxide by-product of the dismutase reaction of SOD1 and superoxide anion promotes the disassociation of SOD1 from the Rac1 complex, resulting in Nox inactivation. **(3)** Secreted SOD1 plays a role in extracellular signaling processes. The presence of extracellular SOD1 leads to an increase in intracellular calcium via a mechanism involving the phospholipase C/protein kinase C pathway.

While the catalytic activity of SOD1 is required for these interactions, it is not simply to remove $O_2\bullet^-$ from circulation, but rather to modulate signaling pathways in a redox sensitive manner. One can imagine that redox signaling needs to be regulated, as an excess of either $O_2\bullet^-$ or H_2O_2 would have deleterious effects on the cell. The levels of H_2O_2 in the cell are further controlled by the antioxidant enzymes catalase, peroxiredoxins and glutathione peroxidases (Fukai and Ushio-Fukai, 2011), which convert H_2O_2 into water and oxygen.

Extracellular SOD1 has also been shown to play a role in signaling. Although SOD1 is predominately localized to the cytoplasm, multiple reports have demonstrated that SOD1 is secreted (Mondola et al., 1996, 1998, 2003; Cimini et al., 2002; Turner et al., 2005). The presence of extracellular SOD1 can in turn increase intracellular calcium levels (Mondola et al., 2004), a phenomena shown to have neuroprotective effects on cerebellar granular neurons exposed to a dopaminergic toxin (Polazzi et al., 2012). This increase in intracellular calcium results from SOD1 activating the phospholipase C/protein kinase C pathway, a pathway implicated in calcium homeostasis (Mondola et al., 2004) through a mechanism involving signal transduction of the muscarinic acetylcholine M1 receptor (M1) (Damiano et al., 2013). Moreover, M1 activation in response to extracellular SOD1 jumpstarts downstream pathways such as the extracellular regulated protein kinase (ERK 1/2) and the Akt signaling cascades (Damiano et al., 2013). Unlike the previous SOD1 signaling pathways discussed above, the activation of the M1 receptor does not appear to be dependent upon the production of $O_2\bullet^-$, as the ROS scavenger N-acetylcysteine did not alter the signaling effect of SOD1 in this context.

SOD1 MISFOLDING: LESSONS FROM FAMILIAL ALS

For the past 20 years, mutant-SOD1 has been the most intensely studied molecule in the ALS field. Studies in animal and cell culture models, as well as extensive biochemical and biophysical analyses of recombinant mutant-SOD1 proteins have collectively revealed a gain-of-toxic mechanism for mutant-SOD1 in ALS that is linked to its propensity to misfold. Aberrantly modified WT SOD1 adapts a conformation and toxic nature much like FALS-linked SOD1 mutants, and is therefore proposed as a pathogenic factor in SALS. Below we introduce what is known about the structure and aberrant properties of FALS-SOD1.

FALS-LINKED SOD1 MUTATIONS: EFFECT ON STRUCTURE AND CONFORMATION

Currently, 171 mutations have been identified within SOD1 that are linked to ALS (http://alsod.iop.kcl.ac.uk/) (Abel et al., 2012). Approximately 20–25% of FALS cases and 6% of all ALS cases are caused by mutations in *SOD1* (Pasinelli and Brown, 2006). The majority of these mutations (>80%) result in amino acid substitutions while the remaining lesions are a combination of insertions, polymorphisms, and deletions. FALS-linked mutations are not localized to one portion of SOD1, but rather span the entire protein (**Figure 1B**). Moreover, relatively conservative amino acid substitutions within SOD1 can cause ALS, suggesting that even minor alterations severely affect SOD1 structure and/or function. Much effort has been focused on determining the common "toxic" feature within SOD1 that is induced by all of these ALS-linked mutations. Except for the mutations that directly interfere with metal coordination, as copper coordination is required for catalytic activity, many ALS-linked mutations have no effect on SOD1 dismutase activity (Borchelt et al., 1994; Bowling et al., 1995; Hayward et al., 2002; Potter and Valentine, 2003). The effect of ALS-linked mutations on SOD1 signaling activity remains largely unexplored. However, in the context of Nox2 signaling, FALS-linked SOD1 mutations were shown to alter the SOD1/Rac1 interaction, resulting in persistent activation of Nox2 and abnormally high levels of ROS (Harraz et al., 2008).

A general feature of FALS-linked SOD1 mutants is that they are destabilized and exhibit reductions in T_m relative to WT SOD1 (Stathopulos et al., 2006; Vassall et al., 2006). In fact, FALS-linked SOD1 mutants are further destabilized when normal post-translational modifications such as Cu/Zn coordination and C57–C146 oxidation are impaired (Furukawa and O'Halloran, 2005; Rodriguez et al., 2005; Kayatekin et al., 2010; Svensson et al., 2010), demonstrating interconnection between normal post-translational modifications and the stability of SOD1. Additionally, mutant SOD1 exhibits an altered tertiary structure, evidenced by enhanced hydrophobicity compared to WT SOD1 (Tiwari et al., 2005; Munch and Bertolotti, 2010). While X-ray crystallography has failed to reveal significant structural differences between WT- and mutant-SOD1 proteins, (Hart et al., 1998; Elam et al., 2003; Hough et al., 2004; Cao et al., 2008; Galaleldeen et al., 2009), solution-based structural studies indicate that FALS-linked mutations induce some degree of SOD1 unfolding, or "misfolding" (**Figure 3**), within the electrostatic and/or zinc loops (**Figure 1**). For example, NMR relaxation experiments reveal an overall increase in protein dynamics for SOD1 G93A compared to WT SOD1 (Shipp et al., 2003). The region proximal to the G93A mutation, termed the "β-barrel plug," as well as residues within the zinc-binding loop exhibited the greatest increase in mobility, whereas the dynamics within the electrostatic loop were comparable between SOD1 G93A and WT (Shipp et al., 2003). Similarly, β-strands 3 and 4, which contain the β-barrel plug, displayed high deuterium exchange rates as assessed by mass spectrometry for several demetallated mutant forms of SOD1 (Durazo et al., 2009). In a separate study using similar methodology but with metallated forms of SOD1, only 1 out of the 13 mutants exhibited relatively high deuterium exchange rates in the β-barrel plug (Molnar et al., 2009). However, this study detected a 10–31% increase in deuterium exchange within the electrostatic loop for 7 out of 8 "WT-like" ALS-linked SOD1 mutants (i.e., mutant-SOD1 proteins that coordinate Cu and Zn), including A4V. Deuterium exchange increased within both the electrostatic and zinc binding loops for those SOD1 mutants with impaired metal binding (Molnar et al., 2009).

The generation of conformation specific antibodies has also provided important insights into the misfolded nature of FALS-linked mutant-SOD1 proteins. Most conformation specific antibodies reported to date are selectively reactive for mutant SOD1 over WT SOD1, consistent with the notion that mutations induce some degree of misfolding that exposes linear sequences or conformational epitopes that are otherwise buried in the intact, native protein (Rakhit et al., 2007; Urushitani et al., 2007; Liu et al., 2009; Bosco et al., 2010; Forsberg et al., 2010; Gros-Louis et al., 2010; Grad et al., 2011; Brotherton et al., 2012; Fujisawa et al., 2012; Broering et al., 2013) (**Figure 4**, **Table 1**). For example, the conformation specific antibodies B8H10, D3H5, and A5C3 that were generated against apo-SOD1 G93A do not immunoprecipitate WT SOD1, but rather exhibit differential reactivity for various mutant-SOD1 proteins (G93A, G37R, G85R, G127X, and D90A) from spinal cord lysates derived from the respective ALS mouse models. That B8H10, D3H5, and A5C3

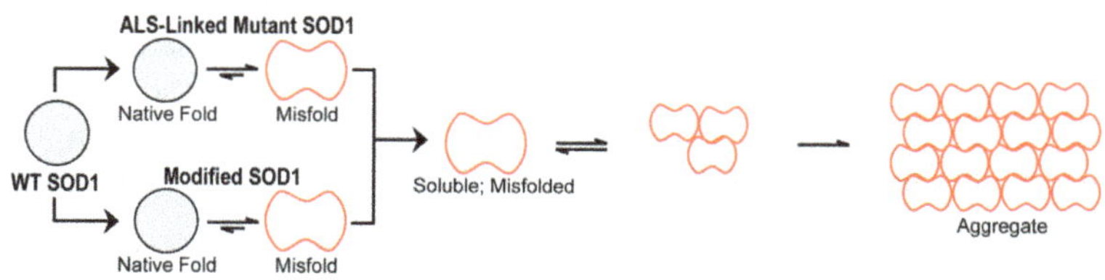

FIGURE 3 | Misfolded vs. aggregated SOD1. Misfolded SOD1 results from both ALS-linked mutations and aberrant post-translational modifications. Throughout the review, the term "misfolding" refers to the structural loosening of SOD1 due to a mutation and/or altered post-translational modification within a soluble form of the protein. Misfolded, soluble SOD1 can engage in aberrant protein-interactions and acquire new toxic functions (illustrated in **Figure 5**). Misfolded SOD1 can also assemble into aggregates. In this review, "aggregates" refer to those insoluble species characteristic of end-stage pathological inclusions present in human post-mortem CNS tissues.

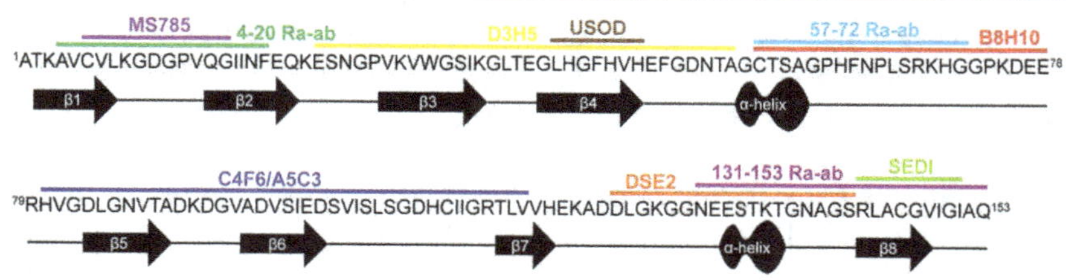

FIGURE 4 | Conformation specific antibodies highlight regions exposed in SOD1 upon misfolding. The primary sequence for WT SOD1 is shown with the secondary structure displayed below. The binding regions of 11 antibodies specific for misfolded SOD1 are depicted above the sequence (see **Table 1** for antibody details).

Table 1 | Conformation specific antibodies recognize regions of SOD1 exposed upon misfolding.

Antibody	SOD1 epitope (aa)	Reactive for FALS SOD1	Reactive for SALS SOD1		Therapeutic benefits	Reference
			Patient tissue	*Modified SOD1*		
B8H10[e]	57–78[a]	+	nd[b]	nd	nd	Gros-Louis et al., 2010; Pickles et al., 2013
C4F6[e]	80–118	+	+	+ (ox)	nd	Urushitani et al., 2006; Bosco et al., 2010; Prudencio and Borchelt, 2011; Brotherton et al., 2012; Pickles et al., 2013
MS785	6–16	+	nd	+[c]	nd	Fujisawa et al., 2012
D3H5	24–55[a]	+	nd	+ (apo)	+	Gros-Louis et al., 2010
A5C3[e]	80–118[a]	+	nd	nd	–	Gros-Louis et al., 2010
SEDI	143–151	+	–	+ (ox)	+[d]	Rakhit et al., 2007; Liu et al., 2009, 2012; Kerman et al., 2010; Prudencio and Borchelt, 2011; Mulligan et al., 2012
USOD	42–48	+	–	– (ox)	nd	Kerman et al., 2010; Mulligan et al., 2012
DSE2 (3H1)	125–142	+	+	nd	nd	Vande Velde et al., 2008; Grad et al., 2011; Pokrishevsky et al., 2012
4–20Ra-ab	4–20	+	+	nd	nd	Jonsson et al., 2004; Forsberg et al., 2010
57–72Ra-ab	57–72	+	+	nd	nd	Stewart et al., 2006; Forsberg et al., 2010, 2011
131–153Ra-ab	131–153	+	+	nd	nd	Jonsson et al., 2004; Forsberg et al., 2010, 2011

Misfolded SOD1-specific antibodies highlight regions in SOD1 that become exposed as a result of misfolding.

[a] *Determined using similar methodology as in C4F6 epitope mapping (Bosco et al., 2010) (unpublished data, Bosco DA).*

[b] *nd, Not determined.*

[c] *Serum starvation in cultured cells results in SOD1 reactivity with antibody.*

[d] *Benefits observed from active immunization with SOD1 peptide recognized by SEDI.*

[e] *Commercially Available.*

become reactive for denatured WT SOD1 is consistent with a linear epitope within natively folded WT SOD1 that is exposed only upon SOD1 unfolding (Gros-Louis et al., 2010). The C4F6 antibody is also selective for FALS-linked SOD1 mutants G37R, G85R, G93A (Urushitani et al., 2007) A4V (Brotherton et al., 2012) over WT SOD1 when these proteins are in their native state but exhibits weak reactivity for denatured SOD1 proteins, suggesting that this antibody recognizes a conformational epitope (Bosco et al., 2010). Interestingly, both D3H5 (Gros-Louis et al., 2010) and C4F6 (Brotherton et al., 2012) immunoreactivity for SOD1 G93A directly correlates with disease progression in the transgenic SOD1 G93A ALS mouse model, indicating that these antibodies report on the presence of "toxic," misfolded forms of SOD1 G93A.

In contrast to the aforementioned antibodies, for which the epitope within SOD1 remains unknown, several conformation specific antibodies have been generated against sequences that are predicted to become exposed only upon SOD1 misfolding (Rakhit et al., 2007; Grad et al., 2011; Fujisawa et al., 2012). One such antibody, MS785, targets amino acids 6-16 at the N-terminus of SOD1. This portion of mutant SOD1 is implicated in binding Derlin-1, a protein involved with ER associated degradation, and is thus referred to as the Derlin-1 binding region (DBR). Fujisawa et al., demonstrated through immunoprecipitation experiments that mutant-SOD1 associates with Derlin-1 when coexpressed in HEK cells. Their comprehensive immunoprecipitation strategy assessed the interaction between Derlin-1 and 132 ALS-linked SOD1 mutants, of which 124 were found to associate with Derlin-1. Further, MS785 selectively immunoprecipitated SOD1 from B-lymphocytes derived from all 14 SOD1 positive ALS cases examined but not from 11 healthy controls (Fujisawa et al., 2012). An alternative antibody called SEDI was created against an epitope at the opposite end of the SOD1 molecule. SEDI stands for SOD1 Exposed Dimer Interface and was raised against the amino acids 143–151 located at the dimer interface in SOD1 (Rakhit et al., 2007). SEDI reactivity is specific for mutant SOD1 over native WT SOD1 in the context of transgenic mouse tissue [G37R, G93A, and G85R (Rakhit et al., 2007)] and human post-mortem tissues harboring SOD1 mutations [A4V (Rakhit et al., 2007), A4T, V14M, ΔG27/P28, and I113T (Liu et al., 2009)]. Therefore, MS785 and SEDI antibodies report on misfolding events within the N- and C-termini, respectively, that are induced by ALS-linked mutations.

A direct consequence of mutation-induced misfolding of SOD1 is aggregation, which refers to the irreversible assembly of misfolded SOD1 species into an insoluble structure (**Figure 3**). SOD1 aggregation has been extensively investigated *in vivo*, both in ALS human post-mortem tissues and in mutant-SOD1 transgenic mice. The enhanced aggregation propensities of FALS-linked SOD1 mutants have also been comprehensively examined in cell culture and in other *in vitro* assays. We refer the reader to many excellent reviews and original works that detail current models of mutant-SOD1 aggregation (Durham et al., 1997; Bruijn et al., 1998; Johnston et al., 2000; Stathopulos et al., 2003;

Furukawa et al., 2006; Wang et al., 2008; Prudencio et al., 2009) Review: (Chattopadhyay and Valentine, 2009; Turner and Talbot, 2008).

Although it remains unclear whether SOD1 aggregation is a causative or protective factor in disease progression, several recent reports demonstrate that misfolded SOD1 species can spread from cell to cell in a prion-like fashion (Grad et al., 2011; Munch et al., 2011; Sundaramoorthy et al., 2013). Munch et al demonstrated that the uptake of aggregated ALS-linked SOD1 mutants in cultured neuronal cells seeded aggregation of endogenous mutant-SOD1. These endogenous SOD1 aggregates persisted well after (>30 days) the original aggregates dissipated from cell division, consistent with a prion-like propagation of aggregated SOD1 (Munch et al., 2011). More recently, uptake of both misfolded mutant-SOD1 as well as aggregated mutant-SOD1 was shown to induce aggregation of the native WT SOD1 protein (Sundaramoorthy et al., 2013). This latter report demonstrates how misfolded SOD1 can alter the conformation of otherwise normally folded SOD1, however, it remains to be determined whether this spreading of misfolded and aggregated SOD1 directly impacts ALS pathogenesis *in vivo* (Guest et al., 2011).

MISFOLDED FALS-LINKED SOD1 EXERTS A GAIN OF TOXIC FUNCTION IN ALS

Studies using transgenic rodent models have generated the majority of data pointing to a gain of toxic mechanism for mutant-SOD1 in FALS (Turner and Talbot, 2008). Several transgenic mouse models have been engineered to overexpress ALS-linked SOD1 mutants. Mutant-SOD1 transgenic mice develop an ALS-like phenotype that includes motor neuron degeneration, neuroinflammation, severe paralysis and premature death (Gurney et al., 1994; Dal Canto and Gurney, 1995; Wong et al., 1995; Bruijn et al., 1997; Dal Canto and Gurney, 1997). In addition, cytosolic SOD1-containing ubiquitinated aggregates are detected within CNS tissues from these mice, recapitulating the pathological features of the human disease (Gurney et al., 1994; Dal Canto and Gurney, 1995; Bruijn et al., 1997; Dal Canto and Gurney, 1997; Watanabe et al., 2001). These mice express endogenous murine SOD1, and yet develop motor neuron disease upon expression of exogenous human mutant-SOD1, providing evidence that SOD1 mutations lead to a gain of toxic function. Further, SOD1-deficient mice develop normally with no overt signs of neurodegeneration (Reaume et al., 1996). However, it is noted that SOD1 null mice are more susceptible to axonal (Reaume et al., 1996) and ischemic brain (Kondo et al., 1997) injuries, and therefore a complete loss of SOD1 may be disadvantageous, especially in the context of disease (van Blitterswijk et al., 2011).

Because the aforementioned SOD1 pathological aggregates are a downstream consequence of SOD1 misfolding, the presence of such aggregates in human post-mortem tissues and ALS-mice argues for a role of misfolded SOD1 in disease. This notion is supported by immunization strategies that both target misfolded SOD1 species and have therapeutic outcome in ALS mice. A passive immunization strategy with the D3H5 antibody that specifically reacts with misfolded SOD1 extended survival in SOD1 G93A transgenic mice (Gros-Louis et al., 2010)(**Figure 4**, **Table 1**). A greater therapeutic impact was shown in active immunization trials with the SOD1 G37R transgenic mouse model, using both recombinant apo-SOD1 G93A (Urushitani et al., 2007) and the SEDI (SOD1 exposed dimer interface) peptide (Liu et al., 2012) as immunogens. Use of SEDI increased survival and delayed disease onset to a greater extent than the full-length SOD1 immunogen, likely due to specific targeting of a misfolded toxic epitope within mutant-SOD1 (Liu et al., 2009, 2012). While these studies provide a direct correlation between misfolded SOD1 species and disease in mice, a survival benefit was not realized using humanized SOD1 antibodies in SOD1 transgenic mice (Broering et al., 2013). Going forward, immunotherapeutic strategies in humans may require the specific targeting of regions within SOD1 that are only exposed upon misfolding. Moreover, these regions should mediate some toxic effect *in vivo*, so that antibodies have the potential to neutralize or otherwise block that "toxic epitope." The latter criterion is important in light of the fact that not all mutant-specific antibodies have produced a therapeutic outcome in SOD1 transgenic mice (Gros-Louis et al., 2010).

The immunization studies described above demonstrate that misfolded SOD1 can impact the disease course in ALS mice. What evidence supports a toxic role of misfolded and/or aggregated SOD1 in the human disease? Wang et al., found an inverse correlation between SOD1 aggregation propensity and disease duration in human ALS cases (i.e., mutants that are more aggregation prone are associated with cases that exhibit relatively short survival) using the Chiti-Dobson equation (Wang et al., 2008). A complementary study determined the relative aggregation propensities of 30 SOD1 mutants in a cell culture assay and also reported an indirect correlation between SOD1 aggregation propensity and disease duration (Prudencio et al., 2009). However, this correlation was not statistically significant, possibly due to the limited number of SOD1 mutants that could be included in this type of analysis that utilizes patient data (Prudencio et al., 2009). Nonetheless, these studies implicate misfolded SOD1 as a factor in human ALS pathogenesis.

TOXIC, SOLUBLE MISFOLDED FALS-SOD1 SPECIES IN DISEASE

While end-stage pathological aggregates composed of insoluble mutant-SOD1 are detected in ALS-mouse models and in the human disease, emerging evidence suggests that the toxic SOD1 species is in fact a misfolded, soluble form of the protein (**Figure 3**). One can imagine that an aggregated, insoluble form of SOD1, much like what is found at end stage of disease, is isolated and unable to diffuse within the cell. Conversely, a non-aggregated misfolded form of SOD1 is soluble, accessible, and able to engage in aberrant interactions, thereby enabling a gain of toxic function. To enumerate all of the aberrant functions and interactions that have been observed for mutant-SOD1 is beyond the scope of this review and therefore we refer the reader to excellent reviews that cover this topic (Cleveland and Rothstein, 2001; Bruijn et al., 2004; Pasinelli and Brown, 2006; Joyce et al., 2011). Herein, we will focus on those gain-of-toxic functions for FALS-linked mutants that are thought to involve misfolded, soluble SOD1 and that may also have relevance to sporadic ALS (**Figure 5**).

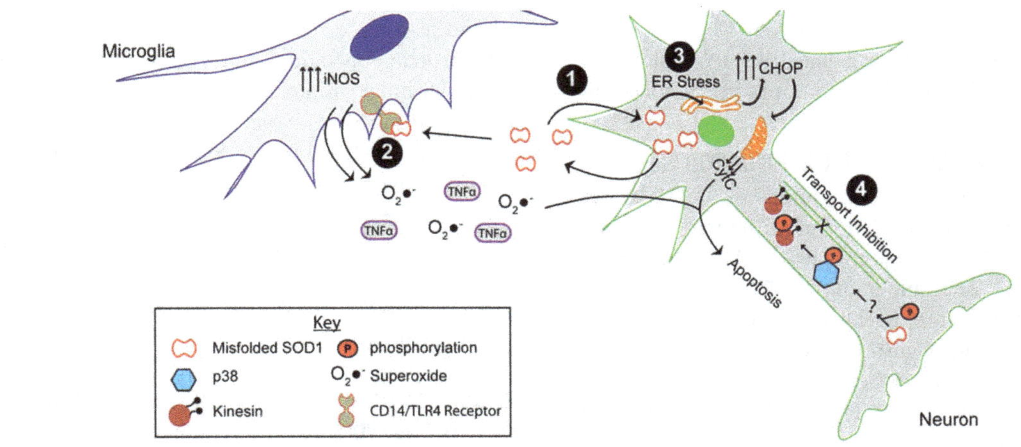

FIGURE 5 | The toxic properties shared by ALS-linked mutant SOD1 and modified WT SOD1. As shown, misfolded SOD1, resulting from mutations or aberrant post-translational modifications, causes the protein to engage in aberrant interactions. **(1)** Misfolded SOD1 is both secreted, possibly through chromogranins, and taken up from the extracellular environment. **(2)** Extracellular misfolded SOD1 activates microglia by binding to the CD14/TLR4 receptor, thereby elevating nitric oxide synthase (iNOS) activity as well as secretion of superoxide anion ($O_2\bullet^-$) and proinflammatory cytokines (e.g., TNFα). **(3)** Expression and uptake of misfolded SOD1 leads to ER stress, which elevates the pro-apoptotic CHOP protein and induces mitochondrial damage. **(4)** The presence of misfolded SOD1 in the axon results in axonal transport inhibition through a mechanism involving the phosphorylation of p38 MAPK and the kinesin motor. All of these aberrant functions compromise the integrity of the motor neuron, and potentially contribute to both FALS and SALS pathogenesis.

Support for a soluble misfolded form of SOD1 comes from studies in both SOD1 animal models and cell culture. Zetterstrom et al., identified an accumulation of soluble misfolded SOD1 that was enriched in the spinal cord of SOD1 G93A transgenic mice. The fraction of soluble misfolded SOD1 was quantified with hydrophobic interaction chromatography (HIC) (Zetterstrom et al., 2007). Interestingly, not only is the solubility of FALS-linked SOD1 variants enhanced upon heterodimerization with WT SOD1, but the toxicity of these variants is also enhanced, consistent with the toxic SOD1 species being soluble-misfolded rather than insoluble-aggregated (Witan et al., 2008, 2009). In CHO cells, the fraction of soluble SOD1 was found to correlate with cellular toxicity (Brotherton et al., 2013). This cellular toxicity was attenuated upon expression of exogenous hsp70 (Brotherton et al., 2013), a chaperone that refolds misfolded proteins, although it is not clear whether this is due solely to a reduced load of misfolded SOD1 or whether the anti-apoptotic function of hsp70 also contributed to this effect (Beckmann et al., 1990; Beere et al., 2000; Luders et al., 2000).

Misfolded mutant SOD1 can have downstream effects both outside and inside the cell. Although WT SOD1 is known to be secreted normally (Mondola et al., 1996, 1998, 2003; Cimini et al., 2002; Turner et al., 2005; Urushitani et al., 2006; Santillo et al., 2007), Urushitani et al. demonstrated that mutant-SOD1 can be secreted by an alternate pathway that involves the secretory chromogranin proteins (Urushitani et al., 2006). In contrast, Turner et al., demonstrated an impaired secretion of mutant SOD1 compared to WT SOD1 (Turner et al., 2005). The discrepancy between these studies may de due to the different cell types employed. Nonetheless, both studies are consistent with a dysregulation of mutant-SOD1 secretion compared to native WT SOD1. Once secreted into the extracellular space, mutant-SOD1 activates microglia though a mechanism that involves binding to the CD14/TLR receptor (Zhao et al., 2010), resulting in a typical proinflammatory response (i.e., increased levels of TNFα and IL-1β). This mode of microglia activation leads to motor neuron death (Urushitani et al., 2006; Zhao et al., 2010).

Inside the cell, mutant SOD1 can induce stress in the context of various pathways. For example, primary neurons derived from SOD1 G93A transgenic mice, as well as cell culture models of mutant-SOD1, exhibit signs of ER stress including spliced XBP1 and induction of CHOP (Nishitoh et al., 2008; Prell et al., 2012). ER stress has been shown to be a major player in ALS pathogenesis [reviewed in Kanekura et al. (2009), Matus et al. (2011)]. It should be noted that endogenous expression of mutant-SOD1 is not required for activation of the ER stress response pathway. Uptake of extracellular SOD1 G93A is sufficient to induce ER stress and neuronal toxicity (Sundaramoorthy et al., 2013). Thus, the combination of mutant-SOD1 uptake and intracellular expression in neurons could exacerbate ER stress, and tilt the scale from the UPR coping mechanism toward apoptosis *in vivo*. Mitochondria represent an additional intracellular compartment that is affected by mutant-SOD1 (Pickles et al., 2013). Recent evidence indicates that mutant-SOD1 directly interacts with Bcl-2, leading to exposure of the toxic BH3 domain, which in turn causes mitochondrial damage (Pasinelli et al., 2004; Pedrini et al., 2010). Interestingly, enhanced exposure of the BH3 domain has been detected in FALS SOD1 A4V patient spinal cord homogenates, and increases as a function of disease in spinal cords of SOD1 G93A transgenic mice (Pedrini et al., 2010). Finally, much evidence suggests that mutant-SOD1 impairs the process of axonal transport in different model systems (Morfini et al., 2009). In studies of fast axonal transport (FAT) performed in squid axoplasm, there is compelling evidence that it is a soluble misfolded form of mutant-SOD1 that inhibits transport in the anterograde direction (Morfini et al., 2009, 2013; Song et al., 2013). Moreover, these studies were extended to explore the role of WT SOD1 in SALS, which is the topic of the following section.

MISFOLDED WILD-TYPE SOD1: IMPLICATIONS FOR SALS

Since the discovery of FALS-linked mutations in SOD1 (Rosen et al., 1993), there has been speculation that the wild-type version of the protein could play a role in sporadic ALS (Selverstone Valentine et al., 2005; Kabashi et al., 2007). It has become increasingly clear that alterations of the normal post-translational modifications of SOD1 and/or introduction of aberrant modifications in WT SOD1 cause this otherwise stable protein to misfold and adapt properties similar to FALS-linked SOD1 mutants (**Figure 1C**). Until recently, however, there was a lack of direct evidence for aberrant forms of WT SOD1 in SALS. This is probably because the field lacked the appropriate tools and methodologies to detect such species. Below we describe modifications of WT SOD1 that cause this protein to become misfolded and "toxic." We also present evidence, largely from the use of conformation specific antibodies that recognize misfolded SOD1 species, that support or contradict the hypothesis that WT SOD1 plays a role in sporadic ALS.

LOSS OF NATIVE SOD1 POST-TRANSLATIONAL MODIFICATIONS LEADS TO WT SOD1 MISFOLDING

As discussed above, coordination of Zn, oxidation of the C57–C146 intrasubunit disulfide bond and homodimerization of SOD1 contribute to the structural stability of the molecule. A loss in integrity of any one of these normal post-translational modifications compromises the stability of WT SOD1 and contributes to its misfolding and aggregation (**Figures 1C, 3**). For example, a reduction of WT SOD1 stability upon demetallation is a widely documented observation (Stathopulos et al., 2003; Lynch et al., 2004; Furukawa and O'Halloran, 2005; Ding and Dokholyan, 2008). Interestingly, demetallation of WT SOD1 induces similar conformational perturbations within the zinc binding and the electrostatic loops (loops IV and VII, respectively, **Figure 1**) as do FALS-linked SOD1 mutations (Strange et al., 2003, 2007; Ding and Dokholyan, 2008; Durazo et al., 2009; Molnar et al., 2009). A direct comparison of NMR backbone chemical shifts for apo dimeric WT SOD1 vs. holo dimeric WT SOD1 revealed the largest structural variations within the electrostatic loop (Banci et al., 2009). These structural alterations were accompanied by pronounced changes in backbone dynamics that further support demetallation-induced misfolding (Banci et al., 2009). Molecular dynamics (Ding and Dokholyan, 2008) and H/D exchange by mass spectrometry (Durazo et al., 2009) also report enhanced flexibility within the aforementioned loops of apo WT SOD1 compared to holo SOD1, but in addition these studies also detect misfolding within the beta barrel of SOD1 upon demetallation (Ding and Dokholyan, 2008; Durazo et al., 2009). Furthermore, the misfolding of WT SOD1 induced by demetallation leads to aggregation of the protein (Banci et al., 2007), which may be driven by the exposure of hydrophobic regions within misfolded SOD1 that are otherwise buried in the native protein (Tiwari et al., 2009).

In addition to demetallation, reduction of the C57–C146 disulfide bond also has a destabilizing effect on WT SOD1 that can lead to protein misfolding and aggregation in a manner similar to FALS-linked mutant SOD1 (**Figure 3**) (Furukawa et al., 2008; Chan et al., 2013). Several studies have demonstrated that a reduction of C57–C146 in apo-SOD1 shifts the monomer-dimer equilibrium toward the monomeric state. Addition of zinc or oxidation of C57–C146 shifts the equilibrium back to the dimeric state, demonstrating interdependence between Zn coordination, C57–C146 bond integrity, and dimerization on the structural stability of SOD1 (Arnesano et al., 2004; Lindberg et al., 2004; Hornberg et al., 2007).

INTRODUCTION OF ABERRANT POST-TRANSLATIONAL MODIFICATIONS INDUCE WT SOD1 MISFOLDING

In addition to alterations of the normal post-translational modifications of SOD1, WT SOD1 misfolding and aggregation can be induced by the formation of aberrant modifications. Oxidation of SOD1 side chains represents one such modification that has been postulated to play a significant causal role in both FALS and SALS (Kabashi et al., 2007). In the context of WT SOD1, which has relevance to SALS, metal catalyzed oxidation with $CuCl_2$ and ascorbic acid leads to oxidative modification of SOD1 histidine residues and subsequent SOD1 aggregation (Rakhit et al., 2002, 2004). This mode of oxidation-induced SOD1 aggregation proceeds by way of SOD1 dimer dissociation/monomer formation, demonstrating interdependence between aberrant and normal SOD1 post-translational modifications (Rakhit et al., 2004). Cys111 within SOD1 is particularly susceptible to H_2O_2 induced oxidation (**Figure 1C**). Prolonged exposure of SOD1 to H_2O_2 results in the irreversible conversion of the Cys111 sulfhydryl group to sulfonic acid (Fujiwara et al., 2007; Bosco et al., 2010; Auclair et al., 2013), which may be detrimental since WT SOD1 oxidized by H_2O_2 (hereafter referred to as SOD1ox) exhibits an enhanced propensity to misfold and aggregate (Ezzi et al., 2007; Fujiwara et al., 2007; Bosco et al., 2010; Chen et al., 2012). Interestingly, modifications such as β-mercaptoethanol (Fujiwara et al., 2007), persulfide (de Beus et al., 2004) and cysteinylation (Auclair et al., 2013) on Cys111 protect SOD1 against oxidation and possibly against subsequent misfolding.

ABERRANTLY MODIFIED WT SOD1 PROTEINS ARE TOXIC AND MIMIC FALS-LINKED SOD1 MUTANTS

The observation that zinc depleted WT SOD1 exerts a toxic effect onto motor neurons by a mechanism involving nitric oxide provided one of the first clues that modified WT SOD1 species are toxic and may contribute to SALS pathogenesis (Estevez et al., 1999; Beckman et al., 2001). More recently, zinc-deficient SOD1 was shown to exhibit a toxic effect related to mitochondrial dysfunction in *Drosophila* (Bahadorani et al., 2013). That metal deficient WT SOD1 can be induced to misfold and exhibit a toxic nature analogous to FALS-linked SOD1 is supported by the immunization trial in ALS mice reported by Takeuchi et al. Low copy SOD1 G93A transgenic mice vaccinated with the apo WT SOD1 immunogen exhibited delayed disease onset and prolonged survival compared to control mice injected with saline/adjuvant, and importantly, to a similar degree as mice vaccinated with apo

SOD1 G93A (Takeuchi et al., 2010). This study also implicates WT SOD1 as a viable therapeutic target for SALS.

In recent years, several reports have demonstrated a toxic effect of SOD1ox in the context of ALS relevant pathways and processes (**Figure 5**). For example, SOD1ox acquires aberrant protein-interactions that are also observed for FALS-linked SOD1 mutants. SOD1ox interacts with the heat shock protein Hsc70 that plays a role in refolding misfolded proteins (Ezzi et al., 2007), the secretory protein chromagranin B that actively secretes misfolded forms of SOD1 (Urushitani et al., 2006; Ezzi et al., 2007), and the anti-apoptotic protein Bcl-2 in a manner that induces mitochondrial damage (Pasinelli et al., 2004; Guareschi et al., 2012). SOD1ox was also shown to mimic FALS-linked SOD1 mutants in the inhibition of anterograde FAT in squid axoplasm. These studies demonstrated that the inhibitory effect of SOD1ox and mutant SOD1 was mediated by activated p38 MAPK, indicating that misfolded SOD1 can trigger kinase-dependent signaling cascades (Morfini et al., 2009; Bosco et al., 2010; Morfini et al., 2013; Song et al., 2013). Extracellular derived WT SOD1 can also induce a toxic effect onto cells. SOD1ox applied to cell culture media activates immortalized microglia (Ezzi et al., 2007), which in turn may cause motor neuron death (Ezzi et al., 2007; Zhao et al., 2010). Furthermore, uptake of aggregated WT SOD1 species by macropinocytosis in neuronal cells caused ER stress and seeded the aggregation of intracellular, endogenous SOD1 (Sundaramoorthy et al., 2013).

Studies in various SOD1 transgenic ALS mouse models have provided direct evidence for WT SOD1 mediated toxicity *in vivo*. Intriguingly, an ALS-like phenotype was only observed in transgenic mice expressing the human SOD1 A4V variant, a mutation that corresponds to an aggressive ALS phenotype in humans, when these mice expressed the human WT version of SOD1 (Deng et al., 2006). This paradoxical result may be explained by heterodimerization of WT and A4V subunits, affording a "stabilized" and thus more toxic version of SOD1 A4V that would otherwise be degraded (Witan et al., 2008, 2009). A similar phenomenon was observed in double-transgenic mice expressing human SOD1 WT and G85R, where disease onset was hastened relative to single-transgenic SOD1 G85R mice (Wang et al., 2009). Recently, a transgenic mouse model was developed that over-expresses human WT SOD1 at similar levels to the established high-copy SOD1 G93A mouse model (Gurney et al., 1994; Graffmo et al., 2013). Compared to transgenic mice expressing fewer copies of the human WT SOD1 gene, the mice generated by Graffmo et al exhibit an ALS-like phenotype that includes significant weight loss, SOD1 aggregation, neurodegeneration, gliosis, and a shortened life-span of ~360 days (Graffmo et al., 2013). The authors posit that the ALS-like phenotype is not a general effect of SOD1 overexpression *per se*, but rather a direct consequence of a substoichiometric population of misfolded SOD1. Although the exact mechanism for WT SOD1 mediated toxicity is not well understood in these models, and the extent to which WT SOD1 is post-translationally modified has not been addressed, these studies clearly demonstrate a link between WT SOD1 and motor neuron degeneration characteristic of ALS.

EVIDENCE FOR MISFOLDED, TOXIC WT SOD1 SPECIES IN SALS

There is accumulating evidence that WT SOD1 can misfold *in vitro* and exert a toxic effect *in vivo*. That genetic mutations in SOD1 are sufficient to cause ALS raises the possibility that modified forms of WT SOD1 may cause SALS, especially because modified WT SOD1 closely mimics the toxic behavior of FALS-linked SOD1 mutants in the context of numerous assays described above. To date, there is no animal model for SALS. Therefore, investigations into the relevance of WT SOD1 in SALS are focused on biological samples from individuals with this disease.

Early immunohistochemistry (IHC) studies using pan-SOD1 antibodies detected SOD1 within Lewy body-like inclusions in spinal cord sections from individuals with SALS (Shibata et al., 1994, 1996), implicating WT SOD1 in SALS pathology. However, pan-SOD1 antibodies failed to detect SOD1 containing aggregates in every IHC study that included SALS cases (Watanabe et al., 2001). In recent years, conformation specific antibodies have been developed that discriminate between native WT SOD1 and mutant and/or misfolded SOD1. These antibodies are being employed using IHC to address whether misfolded WT SOD1 is in fact present in post-mortem SALS tissues [**Figure 4**, **Table 1**, reviewed in Bosco et al. (2011), Furukawa (2012)]. Forsberg et al generated multiple polyclonal antibodies against small peptide sequences spanning the entire SOD1 protein. Two antibodies targeted to amino acids 4–20 within β-strands 1 and 2, and amino acids 131–153 that includes both the electrostatic loop and the SOD1 dimer interface [i.e., the same sequence used to develop the SEDI antibody Rakhit et al. (2007)] were shown to detect SOD1-containing aggregates within the motor neurons of all 29 sporadic cases examined and punctate staining in only 2 out of 19 non-neurological controls (Forsberg et al., 2010). The C4F6 conformation specific antibody introduced earlier was shown to react with misfolded WT SOD1 in a subset (4 out of 9) of SALS spinal cord sections (Bosco et al., 2010), but produced a diffuse staining pattern as opposed to a punctate pattern that would be consistent with insoluble aggregates (Bosco et al., 2010; Brotherton et al., 2012). The DSE2 antibody, which recognizes a "Disease-Specific Epitope" located within the electrostatic loop that is only exposed when SOD1 is misfolded (Vande Velde et al., 2008), was shown to detect misfolded SOD1 within SALS cases that also exhibit TDP-43 pathology (Pokrishevsky et al., 2012). Although these conformation specific antibodies appear to recognize different types of WT SOD1 species (i.e., soluble misfolded vs. aggregated), these reports collectively implicate SOD1 in SALS.

However, not all SOD1 conformation specific antibodies have detected misfolded or aggregated SOD1 in SALS cases. The USOD antibody, which was generated against residues 42–48 within "Unfolded SOD1" failed to detect misfolded SOD1 in SALS cases as did the SEDI antibody, whereas both antibodies detected aggregated SOD1 in FALS (Liu et al., 2009; Kerman et al., 2010). Furthermore, some antibody studies have produced conflicting results. While Bosco et al did not detect C4F6 reactivity in 17 control spinal cord sections, Brotherton et al., reported C4F6 reactivity in SALS tissues as well as tissues from controls (Brotherton et al., 2012). The source of these discrepancies is not clear, and may stem from technical differences in the experimental procedures, inherent variations in the nature of these antibodies (i.e., different epitopes) or inconsistancies amongst the SALS cases utilized across studies.

Biochemistry-based methods offer an alternative approach to IHC for the investigation of misfolded WT SOD1 in SALS. One study reported that SOD1 present in FALS and SALS spinal cord extracts is more susceptible to forming a 32 kDa cross-linked species upon treatment with a biotinylation reagent, suggestive of a misfolded SOD1 molecule that is common to FALS and SALS (Gruzman et al., 2007). This 32 kDa species, however, was later identified as carbonic anhydrase and not misfolded SOD1 (Liu et al., 2010). Subsequently, SOD1 immunopurified from SALS spinal cord tissues was shown to inhibit FAT in squid axoplasm to the same extent as recombinant forms of both oxidized WT and FALS-linked mutant SOD1 (Bosco et al., 2010). Although misfolded SOD1 has been detected in SALS tissues with different antibodies by IHC, this study demonstrated that SOD1 derived from SALS tissues could in fact exert a "toxic" effect in an ALS-relevant assay (Bosco et al., 2010; Yates, 2010). Importantly, this effect was blocked by C4F6 (Bosco et al., 2010), indicating that C4F6 reports on the toxic region within SOD1 and therefore may be useful for designing immunotherapeutic strategies for humans with ALS.

Haidet-Phillips et al. further demonstrated the toxic nature of SOD1 in the context of SALS, as astrocytes derived from human SALS spinal cords exert a toxic effect onto motor neurons only when they expressed near-endogenous levels of SOD1 (Haidet-Phillips et al., 2011). This is consistent with the observation of misfolded SOD1 in glia (Forsberg et al., 2011). Moreover, an ELISA designed for the detection of auto-SOD1 antibodies in human sera demonstrated that these antibodies can influence the SALS disease course. Elevated auto-SOD1 antibodies reactive for the misfolded oxidized form of WT SOD1 conferred a survival benefit within the SALS cohort examined, whereas those cases with elevated auto-SOD1 antibodies against the native WT SOD1 exhibited shorter survival (van Blitterswijk et al., 2011). These data are consistent with a toxic effect of misfolded SOD1 in human SALS, but also indicate a disadvantage to lowering endogenous levels of normal WT SOD1 in SALS. Therefore, it may be necessary to avoid immunotherapeutic and anti-sense oligonucleotide strategies that reduce levels of the normal, native WT SOD1 protein.

The actual molecular nature of "toxic" WT SOD1 species within the aforementioned human SALS studies was not addressed, and therefore it is not clear whether WT SOD1 in SALS exhibits aberrant post-translational modifications. It is intriguing that the H_2O_2 product of the dismutation reaction that is catalyzed by SOD1 (**Figure 2**) can also induce the conversion of this otherwise normal protein into a misfolded, toxic species (Ezzi et al., 2007; Bosco et al., 2010). A report by Guareschi et al., may shed some light onto the nature of the SOD1 modifications *in vivo*, as elevated levels of carbonylated SOD1 species were detected in lymphoblast cell lines from a subset of SALS patients with bulbar onset (Guareschi et al., 2012). An over-oxidized form of WT SOD1 that could explain both SOD1 misfolding and toxicity in SALS is reasonable, considering that oxidative stress is a pathological hallmark of SALS (D'Amico et al., 2013).

While there is compelling data supporting that misfolded and/or aggregated WT SOD1 is *associated* with SALS, it is still unclear whether WT SOD1 can *cause* SALS. The existing data cannot exclude the possibility that misfolded SOD1 is simply a downstream effect of disease. In fact, oxidized SOD1 has been detected in the brains of individuals with Alzheimer's and Parkinson's disease (Choi et al., 2005). Moreover, the conformation specific antibodies that detect misfolded and aggregated SOD1 in SALS also detect misfolded SOD1 in SOD1-negative FALS cases as well as in the context of other neurodegenerative disorders (Forsberg et al., 2010, 2011; Brotherton et al., 2012; Pokrishevsky et al., 2012). Therefore, misfolded SOD1 may represent a general consequence of aging and disease. Nonetheless, one would still expect the presence of misfolded SOD1, whether it be the mutant or WT form, to exacerbate disease based on all of the data demonstrating the toxic effects associated with these proteins. Several therapies are under development, with some in clinical trials, that target SOD1 (Glicksman, 2011). It will be important to determine whether any SOD1-based therapies can confer a therapeutic benefit to those individuals with SALS as well as FALS. Such an outcome would provide unequivocal evidence that SOD1 is indeed a pro-active factor is SALS pathogenesis.

FUTURE OUTLOOK

There is an indisputable role for mutant-SOD1 in FALS; however, whether there is an analogous role for WT SOD1 in the context of SALS is unclear and controversial. The evidence that misfolded WT SOD1 is present in human post-mortem SALS samples, together with two decades worth of evidence that misfolded SOD1 can exert a toxic effect onto cells, supports the hypothesis that WT SOD1 is a causal factor in SALS. However, the presence of misfolded WT SOD1 may simply represent a downstream, non-specific consequence of aging and disease. Because SALS accounts for 90% of ALS cases, and the field is lacking an effective therapy for this devastating disease, a role for misfolded WT SOD1 in the pathogenesis of SALS should be considered. Such a role may include an upstream trigger of the disease, and/or a factor that promotes disease progression. As therapies become available to treat SOD1 in the context of FALS, it will be important to assess whether these therapies can also be applied to all or at least a subset of SALS.

ACKNOWLEDGMENTS

We are very grateful to Drs. Jill Zitzewitz (University of Massachusetts Medical School) and Joseph Salisbury (Northeastern University) for their critical review of the manuscript, and Dr. John Landers (University of Massachusetts Medical School) for helpful discussion.

REFERENCES

Abel, O., Powell, J. F., Andersen, P. M., and Al-Chalabi, A. (2012). ALSoD: a user-friendly online bioinformatics tool for amyotrophic lateral sclerosis genetics. *Hum. Mutat.* 33, 1345–1351. doi: 10.1002/humu.22157

Arai, T., Hasegawa, M., Nonoka, T., Kametani, F., Yamashita, M., Hosokawa, M., et al. (2010). Phosphorylated and cleaved TDP-43 in ALS, FTLD and other neurodegenerative disorders and in cellular models of TDP-43 proteinopathy. *Neuropathology* 30, 170–181. doi: 10.1111/j.1440-1789.2009.01089.x

Arnesano, F., Banci, L., Bertini, I., Martinelli, M., Furukawa, Y., and O'Halloran, T. V. (2004). The unusually stable quaternary structure of human Cu, Zn-superoxide dismutase 1 is controlled by both metal occupancy and disulfide status. *J. Biol. Chem.* 279, 47998–48003. doi: 10.1074/jbc.M406021200

Auclair, J. R., Johnson, J. L., Liu, Q., Salisbury, J. P., Rotunno, M., Petsko, G. A., et al. (2013). Post-translational modification by cysteine protects Cu/Zn-superoxide dismutase from oxidative damage. *Biochemistry* 52, 6137–6144. doi: 10.1021/bi4006122

Bahadorani, S., Mukai, S. T., Rabie, J., Beckman, J. S., Phillips, J. P., and Hilliker, A. J. (2013). Expression of zinc-deficient human superoxide dismutase in Drosophila neurons produces a locomotor defect linked to mitochondrial dysfunction. *Neurobiol. Aging* 34, 2322–2330. doi: 10.1016/j.neurobiolaging.2013.03.024

Banci, L., Bertini, I., Boca, M., Calderone, V., Cantini, F., Girotto, S., et al. (2009). Structural and dynamic aspects related to oligomerization of apo SOD1 and its mutants. *Proc. Natl. Acad. Sci. U.S.A.* 106, 6980–6985. doi: 10.1073/pnas.0809845106

Banci, L., Bertini, I., Cantini, F., Kozyreva, T., Massagni, C., Palumaa, P., et al. (2012). Human superoxide dismutase 1 (hSOD1) maturation through interaction with human copper chaperone for SOD1 (hCCS). *Proc. Natl. Acad. Sci. U.S.A.* 109, 13555–13560. doi: 10.1073/pnas.1207493109

Banci, L., Bertini, I., Durazo, A., Girotto, S., Gralla, E. B., Martinelli, M., et al. (2007). Metal-free superoxide dismutase forms soluble oligomers under physiological conditions: a possible general mechanism for familial ALS. *Proc. Natl. Acad. Sci. U.S.A.* 104, 11263–11267. doi: 10.1073/pnas.0704307104

Bartnikas, T. B., and Gitlin, J. D. (2003). Mechanisms of biosynthesis of mammalian copper/zinc superoxide dismutase. *J. Biol. Chem.* 278, 33602–33608. doi: 10.1074/jbc.M305435200

Beckman, J. S., Estevez, A. G., Crow, J. P., and Barbeito, L. (2001). Superoxide dismutase and the death of motoneurons in ALS. *Trends Neurosci.* 24, S15–S20. doi: 10.1016/S0166-2236(00)01981-0

Beckmann, R. P., Mizzen, L. E., and Welch, W. J. (1990). Interaction of Hsp 70 with newly synthesized proteins: implications for protein folding and assembly. *Science* 248, 850–854. doi: 10.1126/science.2188360

Beere, H. M., Wolf, B. B., Cain, K., Mosser, D. D., Mahboubi, A., Kuwana, T., et al. (2000). Heat-shock protein 70 inhibits apoptosis by preventing recruitment of procaspase-9 to the Apaf-1 apoptosome. *Nat. Cell Biol.* 2, 469–475. doi: 10.1038/35019501

Beyer, K., and Ariza, A. (2013). Alpha-synuclein posttranslational modification and alternative splicing as a trigger for neurodegeneration. *Mol. Neurobiol.* 47, 509–524. doi: 10.1007/s12035-012-8330-5

Borchelt, D. R., Lee, M. K., Slunt, H. S., Guarnieri, M., Xu, Z. S., Wong, P. C., et al. (1994). Superoxide dismutase 1 with mutations linked to familial amyotrophic lateral sclerosis possesses significant activity. *Proc. Natl. Acad. Sci. U.S.A.* 91, 8292–8296. doi: 10.1073/pnas.91.17.8292

Bosco, D. A., and Landers, J. E. (2010). Genetic determinants of amyotrophic lateral sclerosis as therapeutic targets. *CNS Neurol. Disord. Drug Targets* 9, 779–790. doi: 10.2174/187152710793237494

Bosco, D. A., LaVoie, M. J., Petsko, G. A., and Ringe, D. (2011). Proteostasis and movement disorders: Parkinson's disease and amyotrophic lateral sclerosis. *Cold Spring Harbor. Perspect. Biol.* 3:007500. doi: 10.1101/cshperspect.a007500

Bosco, D. A., Morfini, G., Karabacak, N. M., Song, Y., Gros-Louis, F., Pasinelli, P., et al. (2010). Wild-type and mutant SOD1 share an aberrant conformation and a common pathogenic pathway in ALS. *Nat. Neurosci.* 13, 1396–1403. doi: 10.1038/nn.2660

Bowling, A. C., Barkowski, E. E., McKenna-Yasek, D., Sapp, P., Horvitz, H. R., Beal, M. F., et al., Jr. (1995). Superoxide dismutase concentration and activity in familial amyotrophic lateral sclerosis. *J. Neurochem.* 64, 2366–2369. doi: 10.1046/j.1471-4159.1995.64052366.x

Broering, T. J., Wang, H., Boatright, N. K., Wang, Y., Baptista, K., Shayan, G., et al. (2013). Identification of human monoclonal antibodies specific for human SOD1 recognizing distinct epitopes and forms of SOD1. *PLoS ONE* 8:e61210. doi: 10.1371/journal.pone.0061210

Brotherton, T. E., Li, Y., and Glass, J. D. (2013). Cellular toxicity of mutant SOD1 protein is linked to an easily soluble, non-aggregated form *in vitro*. *Neurobiol. Dis.* 49C, 49–56. doi: 10.1016/j.nbd.2012.08.010

Brotherton, T. E., Li, Y., Cooper, D., Gearing, M., Julien, J. P., Rothstein, J. D., et al. (2012). Localization of a toxic form of superoxide dismutase 1 protein to pathologically affected tissues in familial ALS. *Proc. Natl. Acad. Sci. U.S.A.* 109, 5505–5510. doi: 10.1073/pnas.1115009109

Brown, D. I., and Griendling, K. K. (2009). Nox proteins in signal transduction. *Free Radic. Biol. Med.* 47, 1239–1253. doi: 10.1016/j.freeradbiomed.2009.07.023

Bruijn, L. I., Houseweart, M. K., Kato, S., Anderson, K. L., Anderson, S. D., Ohama, E., et al. (1998). Aggregation and motor neuron toxicity of an ALS-linked SOD1 mutant independent from wild-type SOD1. *Science* 281, 1851–1854. doi: 10.1126/science.281.5384.1851

Bruijn, L. I., Miller, T. M., and Cleveland, D. W. (2004). Unraveling the mechanisms involved in motor neuron degeneration in ALS. *Annu. Rev. Neurosci.* 27, 723–749. doi: 10.1146/annurev.neuro.27.070203.144244

Bruijn, L. I., Becher, M. W., Lee, M. K., Anderson, K. L., Jenkins, N. A., Copeland, N. G., et al. (1997). ALS-linked SOD1 mutant G85R mediates damage to astrocytes and promotes rapidly progressive disease with SOD1-containing inclusions. *Neuron* 18, 327–338. doi: 10.1016/S0896-6273(00)80272-X

Cao, X., Antonyuk, S. V., Seetharaman, S. V., Whitson, L. J., Taylor, A. B., Holloway, S. P., et al. (2008). Structures of the G85R variant of SOD1 in familial amyotrophic lateral sclerosis. *J. Biol. Chem.* 283, 16169–16177. doi: 10.1074/jbc.M801522200

Chan, P. K., Chattopadhyay, M., Sharma, S., Souda, P., Gralla, E. B., Borchelt, D. R., et al. (2013). Structural similarity of wild-type and ALS-mutant superoxide dismutase-1 fibrils using limited proteolysis and atomic force microscopy. *Proc. Natl. Acad. Sci. U.S.A.* 110, 10934–10939. doi: 10.1073/pnas.1309613110

Chattopadhyay, M., and Valentine, J. S. (2009). Aggregation of copper-zinc superoxide dismutase in familial and sporadic, ALS. *Antioxid. Redox Signal.* 11, 1603–1614. doi: 10.1089/ARS.2009.2536

Chen, X., Shang, H., Qiu, X., Fujiwara, N., Cui, L., Li, X. M., et al. (2012). Oxidative modification of cysteine 111 promotes disulfide bond-independent aggregation of SOD1. *Neurochem. Res.* 37, 835–845. doi: 10.1007/s11064-011-0679-8

Choi, J., Rees, H. D., Weintraub, S. T., Levey, A. I., Chin, L. S., and Li, L. (2005). Oxidative modifications and aggregation of Cu, Zn-superoxide dismutase associated with Alzheimer and Parkinson diseases. *J. Biol. Chem.* 280, 11648–11655. doi: 10.1074/jbc.M414327200

Cimini, V., Ruggiero, G., Buonomo, T., Seru, R., Sciorio, S., Zanzi, C., et al. (2002). CuZn-superoxide dismutase in human thymus: immunocytochemical localisation and secretion in thymus-derived epithelial and fibroblast cell lines. *Histochem. Cell Biol.* 118, 163–169. doi: 10.1007/s00418-002-0429-8

Cleveland, D. W., and Rothstein, J. D. (2001). From Charcot to Lou Gehrig: deciphering selective motor neuron death in ALS. *Nat. Rev. Neurosci.* 2, 806–819. doi: 10.1038/35097565

Dal Canto, M. C., and Gurney, M. E. (1995). Neuropathological changes in two lines of mice carrying a transgene for mutant human Cu, Zn, SOD, and in mice overexpressing wild type human SOD: a model of familial amyotrophic lateral sclerosis (FALS). *Brain Res.* 676, 25–40. doi: 10.1016/0006-8993(95)00063-V

Dal Canto, M. C., and Gurney, M. E. (1997). A low expressor line of transgenic mice carrying a mutant human Cu, Zn superoxide dismutase (SOD1) gene develops pathological changes that most closely resemble those in human amyotrophic lateral sclerosis. *Acta Neuropathol* 93, 537–550. doi: 10.1007/s004010050650

Damiano, S., Petrozziello, T., Ucci, V., Amente, S., Santillo, M., and Mondola, P. (2013). Cu-Zn superoxide dismutase activates muscarinic acetylcholine M1 receptor pathway in neuroblastoma cells. *Mol. Cell. Neurosci.* 52, 31–37. doi: 10.1016/j.mcn.2012.11.001

D'Amico, E., Factor-Litvak, P., Santella, R. M., and Mitsumoto, H. (2013). Clinical perspective on oxidative stress in sporadic amyotrophic lateral sclerosis. *Free Radic. Biol. Med.* 65C, 509–527. doi: 10.1016/j.freeradbiomed.2013.06.029

de Beus, M. D., Chung, J., and Colon, W. (2004). Modification of cysteine 111 in Cu/Zn superoxide dismutase results in altered spectroscopic and biophysical properties. *Protein Sci.* 13, 1347–1355. doi: 10.1110/ps.03576904

Dejesus-Hernandez, M., Mackenzie, I. R., Boeve, B. F., Boxer, A. L., Baker, M., Rutherford, N. J., et al. (2011). Expanded GGGGCC hexanucleotide repeat in noncoding region of C9ORF72 causes chromosome 9p-linked FTD and ALS. *Neuron* 72, 245–256. doi: 10.1016/j.neuron.2011.09.011

Deng, H. X., Zhai, H., Bigio, E. H., Yan, J., Fecto, F., Ajroud, K., et al. (2010). FUS-immunoreactive inclusions are a common feature in sporadic and non-SOD1 familial amyotrophic lateral sclerosis. *Ann. Neurol.* 67, 739–748. doi: 10.1002/ana.22051

Deng, H. X., Shi, Y., Furukawa, Y., Zhai, H., Fu, R., Liu, E., et al. (2006). Conversion to the amyotrophic lateral sclerosis phenotype is associated with intermolecular linked insoluble aggregates of SOD1 in mitochondria. *Proc. Natl. Acad. Sci. U.S.A.* 103, 7142–7147. doi: 10.1073/pnas.0602046103

Ding, F., and Dokholyan, N. V. (2008). Dynamical roles of metal ions and the disulfide bond in Cu, Zn superoxide dismutase folding and aggregation. *Proc. Natl. Acad. Sci. U.S.A.* 105, 19696–19701. doi: 10.1073/pnas.0803266105

Durazo, A., Shaw, B. F., Chattopadhyay, M., Faull, K. F., Nersissian, A. M., Valentine, J. S., et al. (2009). Metal-free superoxide dismutase-1 and three different ALS variants share a similar partially unfolded {beta}-barrel at physiological temperature. *J. Biol. Chem.* 284, 34382–34389. doi: 10.1074/jbc.M109.052076

Durham, H. D., Roy, J., Dong, L., and Figlewicz, D. A. (1997). Aggregation of mutant Cu/Zn superoxide dismutase proteins in a culture model of ALS. *J. Neuropathol. Exp. Neurol.* 56, 523–530. doi: 10.1097/00005072-199705000-00008

Elam, J. S., Taylor, A. B., Strange, R., Antonyuk, S., Doucette, P. A., Rodriguez, J. A., et al. (2003). Amyloid-like filaments and water-filled nanotubes formed by SOD1 mutant proteins linked to familial ALS. *Nat. Struct. Biol.* 10, 461–467. doi: 10.1038/nsb935

Elden, A. C., Kim, H. J., Hart, M. P., Chen-Plotkin, A. S., Johnson, B. S., Fang, X., et al. (2010). Ataxin-2 intermediate-length polyglutamine expansions are associated with increased risk for ALS. *Nature* 466, 1069–1075. doi: 10.1038/nature09320

Estevez, A. G., Crow, J. P., Sampson, J. B., Reiter, C., Zhuang, Y., Richardson, G. J., et al. (1999). Induction of nitric oxide-dependent apoptosis in motor neurons by zinc-deficient superoxide dismutase. *Science* 286, 2498–2500. doi: 10.1126/science.286.5449.2498

Ezzi, S. A., Urushitani, M., and Julien, J. P. (2007). Wild-type superoxide dismutase acquires binding and toxic properties of ALS-linked mutant forms through oxidation. *J. Neurochem.* 102, 170–178. doi: 10.1111/j.1471-4159.2007.04531.x

Forman, H. J., and Fridovich, I. (1973). On the stability of bovine superoxide dismutase. The effects of metals. *J. Biol. Chem.* 248, 2645–2649.

Forsberg, K., Andersen, P. M., Marklund, S. L., and Brannstrom, T. (2011). Glial nuclear aggregates of superoxide dismutase-1 are regularly present in patients with amyotrophic lateral sclerosis. *Acta Neuropathol.* 121, 623–634. doi: 10.1007/s00401-011-0805-3

Forsberg, K., Jonsson, P. A., Andersen, P. M., Bergemalm, D., Graffmo, K. S., Hultdin, M., et al. (2010). Novel antibodies reveal inclusions containing non-native SOD1 in sporadic ALS patients. *PLoS ONE* 5:e11552. doi: 10.1371/journal.pone.0011552

Fujisawa, T., Homma, K., Yamaguchi, N., Kadowaki, H., Tsuburaya, N., Naguro, I., et al. (2012). A novel monoclonal antibody reveals a conformational alteration shared by amyotrophic lateral sclerosis-linked SOD1 mutants. *Ann. Neurol.* 72, 739–749. doi: 10.1002/ana.23668

Fujiwara, N., Nakano, M., Kato, S., Yoshihara, D., Ookawara, T., Eguchi, H., et al. (2007). Oxidative modification to cysteine sulfonic acid of Cys111 in human copper-zinc superoxide dismutase. *J. Biol. Chem.* 282, 35933–35944. doi: 10.1074/jbc.M702941200

Fukai, T., and Ushio-Fukai, M. (2011). Superoxide dismutases: role in redox signaling, vascular function, and diseases. *Antioxid. Redox Signal.* 15, 1583–1606. doi: 10.1089/ars.2011.3999

Furukawa, Y. (2012). Pathological roles of wild-type cu, zn-superoxide dismutase in amyotrophic lateral sclerosis. *Neurol. Res. Int.* 2012:323261. doi: 10.1155/2012/323261

Furukawa, Y., Fu, R., Deng, H. X., Siddique, T., and O'Halloran, T. V. (2006). Disulfide cross-linked protein represents a significant fraction of ALS-associated Cu, Zn-superoxide dismutase aggregates in spinal cords of model mice. *Proc. Natl. Acad. Sci. U.S.A.* 103, 7148–7153. doi: 10.1073/pnas.0602048103

Furukawa, Y., Kaneko, K., Yamanaka, K., O'Halloran, T. V., and Nukina, N. (2008). Complete loss of post-translational modifications triggers fibrillar aggregation of SOD1 in the familial form of amyotrophic lateral sclerosis. *J. Biol. Chem.* 283, 24167–24176. doi: 10.1074/jbc.M802083200

Furukawa, Y., and O'Halloran, T. V. (2005). Amyotrophic lateral sclerosis mutations have the greatest destabilizing effect on the apo- and reduced form of SOD1, leading to unfolding and oxidative aggregation. *J. Biol. Chem.* 280, 17266–17274. doi: 10.1074/jbc.M500482200

Furukawa, Y., Torres, A. S., and O'Halloran, T. V. (2004). Oxygen-induced maturation of SOD1: a key role for disulfide formation by the copper chaperone CCS. *EMBO J.* 23, 2872–2881. doi: 10.1038/sj.emboj.7600276

Galaleldeen, A., Strange, R. W., Whitson, L. J., Antonyuk, S. V., Narayana, N., Taylor, A. B., et al. (2009). Structural and biophysical properties of metal-free pathogenic SOD1 mutants A4V and G93A. *Arch. Biochem. Biophys.* 492, 40–47. doi: 10.1016/j.abb.2009.09.020

Georgiou, G. (2002). How to flip the (redox) switch. *Cell* 111, 607–610. doi: 10.1016/S0092-8674(02)01165-0

Glicksman, M. A. (2011). The preclinical discovery of amyotrophic lateral sclerosis drugs. *Expert Opin. Drug Discov.* 6, 1127–1138. doi: 10.1517/17460441.2011.628654

Grad, L. I., Guest, W. C., Yanai, A., Pokrishevsky, E., O'Neill, M. A., and Gibbs, E. (2011). Intermolecular transmission of superoxide dismutase 1 misfolding in living cells. *Proc. Natl. Acad. Sci. U.S.A.* 108, 16398–16403. doi: 10.1073/pnas.1102645108

Graffmo, K. S., Forsberg, K., Bergh, J., Birve, A., Zetterstrom, P., Andersen, P. M., et al. (2013). Expression of wild-type human superoxide dismutase-1 in mice causes amyotrophic lateral sclerosis. *Hum. Mol. Genet.* 22, 51–60. doi: 10.1093/hmg/dds399

Gros-Louis, F., Soucy, G., Lariviere, R., and Julien, J. P. (2010). Intracerebroventricular infusion of monoclonal antibody or its derived Fab fragment against misfolded forms of SOD1 mutant delays mortality in a mouse model of ALS. *J. Neurochem.* 113, 1188–1199. doi: 10.1111/j.1471-4159.2010.06683.x

Gruzman, A., Wood, W. L., Alpert, E., Prasad, M. D., Miller, R. G., Rothstein, J. D., et al. (2007). Common molecular signature in SOD1 for both sporadic and familial amyotrophic lateral sclerosis. *Proc. Natl. Acad. Sci. U.S.A.* 104, 12524–12529. doi: 10.1073/pnas.0705044104

Guareschi, S., Cova, E., Cereda, C., Ceroni, M., Donetti, E., Bosco, D. A., et al. (2012). An over-oxidized form of superoxide dismutase found in sporadic amyotrophic lateral sclerosis with bulbar onset shares a toxic mechanism with mutant SOD1. *Proc. Natl. Acad. Sci. U.S.A.* 109, 5074–5079. doi: 10.1073/pnas.1115402109

Guest, W. C., Silverman, J. M., Pokrishevsky, E., O'Neill, M. A., Grad, L. I., and Cashman, N. R. (2011). Generalization of the prion hypothesis to other neurodegenerative diseases: an imperfect fit. *J. Toxicol. Environ. Health. A* 74, 1433–1459. doi: 10.1080/15287394.2011.618967

Gurney, M. E., Pu, H., Chiu, A. Y., Dal Canto, M. C., Polchow, C. Y., Alexander, D. D., et al. (1994). Motor neuron degeneration in mice that express a human Cu, Zn superoxide dismutase mutation. *Science* 264, 1772–1775. doi: 10.1126/science.8209258

Haidet-Phillips, A. M., Hester, M. E., Miranda, C. J., Meyer, K., Braun, L., Frakes, A., et al. (2011). Astrocytes from familial and sporadic ALS patients are toxic to motor neurons. *Nat. Biotechnol.* 29, 824–828. doi: 10.1038/nbt.1957

Harraz, M. M., Marden, J. J., Zhou, W., Zhang, Y., Williams, A., Sharov, V. S., et al. (2008). SOD1 mutations disrupt redox-sensitive Rac regulation of NADPH oxidase in a familial ALS model. *J. Clin. Invest.* 118, 659–670.

Hart, P. J., Liu, H., Pellegrini, M., Nersissian, A. M., Gralla, E. B., Valentine, J. S., et al. (1998). Subunit asymmetry in the three-dimensional structure of a human CuZnSOD mutant found in familial amyotrophic lateral sclerosis. *Protein Sci.* 7, 545–555. doi: 10.1002/pro.5560070302

Hayward, L. J., Rodriguez, J. A., Kim, J. W., Tiwari, A., Goto, J. J., Cabelli, D. E., et al. (2002). Decreased metallation and activity in subsets of mutant superoxide dismutases associated with familial amyotrophic lateral sclerosis. *J. Biol. Chem.* 277, 15923–15931. doi: 10.1074/jbc.M112087200

Hornberg, A., Logan, D. T., Marklund, S. L., and Oliveberg, M. (2007). The coupling between disulphide status, metallation and dimer interface strength in Cu/Zn superoxide dismutase. *J. Mol. Biol.* 365, 333–342. doi: 10.1016/j.jmb.2006.09.048

Hough, M. A., Grossmann, J. G., Antonyuk, S. V., Strange, R. W., Doucette, P. A., Rodriguez, J. A., et al. (2004). Dimer destabilization in superoxide dismutase may result in disease-causing properties: structures of motor neuron disease mutants. *Proc. Natl. Acad. Sci. U.S.A.* 101, 5976–5981. doi: 10.1073/pnas.0305143101

Ilieva, H., Polymenidou, M., and Cleveland, D. W. (2009). Non-cell autonomous toxicity in neurodegenerative disorders: ALS and beyond. *J. Cell Biol.* 187, 761–772. doi: 10.1083/jcb.200908164

Johnston, J. A., Dalton, M. J., Gurney, M. E., and Kopito, R. R. (2000). Formation of high molecular weight complexes of mutant Cu, Zn-superoxide dismutase in a mouse model for familial amyotrophic lateral sclerosis. *Proc. Natl. Acad. Sci. U.S.A.* 97, 12571–12576. doi: 10.1073/pnas.220417997

Jonsson, P. A., Ernhill, K., Andersen, P. M., Bergemalm, D., Brannstrom, T., Gredal, O., et al. (2004). Minute quantities of misfolded mutant superoxide dismutase-1 cause amyotrophic lateral sclerosis. *Brain* 127, 73–88. doi: 10.1093/brain/awh005

Joyce, P. I., Fratta, P., Fisher, E. M., and Acevedo-Arozena, A. (2011). SOD1 and TDP-43 animal models of amyotrophic lateral sclerosis: recent advances in understanding disease toward the development of clinical treatments. *Mamm. Genome* 22, 420–448. doi: 10.1007/s00335-011-9339-1

Kabashi, E., Valdmanis, P. N., Dion, P., and Rouleau, G. A. (2007). Oxidized/misfolded superoxide dismutase-1: the cause of all amyotrophic lateral sclerosis. *Ann. Neurol.* 62, 553–559. doi: 10.1002/ana.21319

Kanekura, K., Suzuki, H., Aiso, S., and Matsuoka, M. (2009). ER stress and unfolded protein response in amyotrophic lateral sclerosis. *Mol. Neurobiol.* 39, 81–89. doi: 10.1007/s12035-009-8054-3

Kayatekin, C., Zitzewitz, J. A., and Matthews, C. R. (2008). Zinc binding modulates the entire folding free energy surface of human Cu, Zn superoxide dismutase. *J. Mol. Biol.* 384, 540–555. doi: 10.1016/j.jmb.2008.09.045

Kayatekin, C., Zitzewitz, J. A., and Matthews, C. R. (2010). Disulfide-reduced ALS variants of Cu, Zn superoxide dismutase exhibit increased populations of unfolded species. *J. Mol. Biol.* 398, 320–331. doi: 10.1016/j.jmb.2010.02.034

Kerman, A., Liu, H. N., Croul, S., Bilbao, J., Rogaeva, E., Zinman, L., et al. (2010). Amyotrophic lateral sclerosis is a non-amyloid disease in which extensive misfolding of SOD1 is unique to the familial form. *Acta Neuropathol.* 119, 335–344. doi: 10.1007/s00401-010-0646-5

Kondo, T., Reaume, A. G., Huang, T. T., Carlson, E., Murakami, K., Chen, S. F., et al. (1997). Reduction of CuZn-superoxide dismutase activity exacerbates neuronal cell injury and edema formation after transient focal cerebral ischemia. *J. Neurosci.* 17, 4180–4189.

Kwiatkowski, T. J. Jr., et al. (2009). Mutations in the FUS/TLS gene on chromosome 16 cause familial amyotrophic lateral sclerosis. *Science* 323, 1205–1208. doi: 10.1126/science.1166066

Lindberg, M. J., Normark, J., Holmgren, A., and Oliveberg, M. (2004). Folding of human superoxide dismutase: disulfide reduction prevents dimerization and produces marginally stable monomers. *Proc. Natl. Acad. Sci. U.S.A.* 101, 15893–15898. doi: 10.1073/pnas.0403979101

Ling, S. C., Polymenidou, M., and Cleveland, D. W. (2013). Converging mechanisms in ALS and FTD: disrupted RNA and protein homeostasis. *Neuron* 79, 416–438. doi: 10.1016/j.neuron.2013.07.033

Liu, H. N., Sanelli, T., Horne, P., Pioro, E. P., Strong, M. J., Rogaeva, E., et al. (2009). Lack of evidence of monomer/misfolded superoxide dismutase-1 in sporadic amyotrophic lateral sclerosis. *Ann. Neurol.* 66, 75–80. doi: 10.1002/ana.21704

Liu, H. N., Tjostheim, S., Dasilva, K., Taylor, D., Zhao, B., Rakhit, R., et al. (2012). Targeting of monomer/misfolded SOD1 as a therapeutic strategy for amyotrophic lateral sclerosis. *J. Neurosci.* 32, 8791–8799. doi: 10.1523/JNEUROSCI.5053-11.2012

Liu, J., Akhavan, A., Lu, M., Gruzman, A., Lingappa, V. R., An, J., et al. (2010). Carbonic anhydrase I is recognized by an SOD1 antibody upon biotinylation of human spinal cord extracts. *Int. J. Mol. Sci.*11, 4051–4062. doi: 10.3390/ijms11104051

Luders, J., Demand, J., and Hohfeld, J. (2000). The ubiquitin-related BAG-1 provides a link between the molecular chaperones Hsc70/Hsp70 and the proteasome. *J. Biol. Chem.* 275, 4613–4617. doi: 10.1074/jbc.275.7.4613

Lynch, S. M., Boswell, S. A., and Colon, W. (2004). Kinetic stability of Cu/Zn superoxide dismutase is dependent on its metal ligands: implications for ALS. *Biochemistry* 43, 16525–16531. doi: 10.1021/bi048831v

Mandelkow, E. M., Schweers, O., Drewes, G., Biernat, J., Gustke, N., Trinczek, B., et al. (1996). Structure, microtubule interactions, and phosphorylation of tau protein. *Ann. N.Y. Acad. Sci.* 777, 96–106. doi: 10.1111/j.1749-6632.1996.tb34407.x

Matus, S., Glimcher, L. H., and Hetz, C. (2011). Protein folding stress in neurodegenerative diseases: a glimpse into the ER. *Curr. Opin. Cell Biol.* 23, 239–252. doi: 10.1016/j.ceb.2011.01.003

McCord, J. M., and Fridovich, I. (1969). Superoxide dismutase. An enzymic function for erythrocuprein (hemocuprein). *J. Biol. Chem.* 244, 6049–6055.

Molnar, K. S., Karabacak, N. M., Johnson, J. L., Wang, Q., Tiwari, A., Hayward, L. J., et al. (2009). A common property of amyotrophic lateral sclerosis-associated variants: destabilization of the Cu/Zn superoxide dismutase electrostatic loop. *J. Biol. Chem.* 284, 30965–30973. doi: 10.1074/jbc.M109.023945

Mondola, P., Annella, T., Santillo, M., and Santangelo, F. (1996). Evidence for secretion of cytosolic CuZn superoxide dismutase by Hep G2 cells and human fibroblasts. *Int. J. Biochem. Cell Biol.* 28, 677–681. doi: 10.1016/1357-2725(96)00004-0

Mondola, P., Annella, T., Seru, R., Santangelo, F., Iossa, S., Gioielli, A., et al. (1998). Secretion and increase of intracellular CuZn superoxide dismutase content in human neuroblastoma SK-N-BE cells subjected to oxidative stress. *Brain Res. Bull.* 45, 517–520. doi: 10.1016/S0361-9230(97)00438-3

Mondola, P., Ruggiero, G., Seru, R., Damiano, S., Grimaldi, S., Garbi, C., et al. (2003). The Cu, Zn superoxide dismutase in neuroblastoma SK-N-BE cells is exported by a microvesicles dependent pathway. *Brain Res. Mol. Brain Res.* 110, 45–51. doi: 10.1016/S0169-328X(02)00583-1

Mondola, P., Santillo, M., Seru, R., Damiano, S., Alvino, C., Ruggiero, G., et al. (2004). Cu, Zn superoxide dismutase increases intracellular calcium levels via a phospholipase C-protein kinase C pathway in SK-N-BE neuroblastoma cells. *Biochem. Biophys. Res. Commun.* 324, 887–892. doi: 10.1016/j.bbrc.2004.09.131

Morfini, G. A., Burns, M., Binder, L. I., Kanaan, N. M., LaPointe, N., Bosco, D. A., et al. (2009). Axonal transport defects in neurodegenerative diseases. *J. Neurosci.* 29, 12776–12786. doi: 10.1523/JNEUROSCI.3463-09.2009

Morfini, G. A., Bosco, D. A., Brown, H., Gatto, R., Kaminska, A., Song, Y., et al. (2013). Inhibition of fast axonal transport by pathogenic SOD1 involves activation of p38 MAP kinase. *PLoS ONE* 8:e65235. doi: 10.1371/journal.pone.0065235

Mulligan, V. K., Kerman, A., Laister, R. C., Sharda, P. R., Arslan, P. E., Chakrabartty, A. (2012). Early steps in oxidation-induced SOD1 misfolding: implications for non-amyloid protein aggregation in familial ALS. *J. Mol. Biol.* 421, 631–652. doi: 10.1016/j.jmb.2012.04.016

Munch, C., and Bertolotti, A. (2010). Exposure of hydrophobic surfaces initiates aggregation of diverse ALS-causing superoxide dismutase-1 mutants. *J. Mol. Biol.* 399, 512–525. doi: 10.1016/j.jmb.2010.04.019

Munch, C., O'Brien, J., and Bertolotti, A. (2011). Prion-like propagation of mutant superoxide dismutase-1 misfolding in neuronal cells. *Proc. Natl. Acad. Sci. U.S.A.* 108, 3548–3553. doi: 10.1073/pnas.1017275108

Neumann, M., Sampathu, D. M., Kwong, L. K., Truax, A. C., Micsenyi, M. C., Chou, T. T., et al. (2006). Ubiquitinated TDP-43 in frontotemporal lobar degeneration and amyotrophic lateral sclerosis. *Science* 314, 130–133. doi: 10.1126/science.1134108

Nishitoh, H., Kadowaki, H., Nagai, A., Maruyama, T., Yokota, T., Fukutomi, H., et al. (2008). ALS-linked mutant SOD1 induces ER stress- and ASK1-dependent motor neuron death by targeting Derlin-1. *Genes Dev.* 22, 1451–1464. doi: 10.1101/gad.1640108

Pardo, C. A., Xu, Z., Borchelt, D. R., Price, D. L., Sisodia, S. S., and Cleveland, D. W. (1995). Superoxide dismutase is an abundant component in cell bodies, dendrites, and axons of motor neurons and in a subset of other neurons. *Proc. Natl. Acad. Sci. U.S.A.* 92, 954–958. doi: 10.1073/pnas.92.4.954

Pasinelli, P., and Brown, R. H. (2006). Molecular biology of amyotrophic lateral sclerosis: insights from genetics. *Nat. Rev. Neurosci.* 7, 710–723. doi: 10.1038/nrn1971

Pasinelli, P., Belford, M. E., Lennon, N., Bacskai, B. J., Hyman, B. T., Trotti, D., et al. (2004). Amyotrophic lateral sclerosis-associated SOD1 mutant proteins bind and aggregate with Bcl-2 in spinal cord mitochondria. *Neuron* 43, 19–30. doi: 10.1016/j.neuron.2004.06.021

Pedrini, S., Sau, D., Guareschi, S., Bogush, M., Brown, R. H. Jr., Naniche, N., et al. (2010). ALS-linked mutant SOD1 damages mitochondria by promoting conformational changes in Bcl-2. *Hum. Mol. Genet.* 19, 2974–2986. doi: 10.1093/hmg/ddq202

Pickles, S., Destroismaisons, L., Peyrard, S. L., Cadot, S., Rouleau, G. A., Brown, R. H., et al. (2013). Mitochondrial damage revealed by immunoselection for ALS-linked misfolded SOD1. *Hum. Mol. Genet.* 22, 3947–3959. doi: 10.1093/hmg/ddt249

Pokrishevsky, E., Grad, L. I., Yousefi, M., Wang, J., Mackenzie, I. R., Cashman, N. R. (2012). Aberrant localization of FUS and TDP43 is associated with misfolding of SOD1 in amyotrophic lateral sclerosis. *PLoS ONE* 7:e35050. doi: 10.1371/journal.pone.0035050

Polazzi, E., Mengoni, I., Caprini, M., Pena-Altamira, E., Kurtys, E., and Monti, B. (2012). Copper-zinc superoxide dismutase (SOD1) is released by microglial cells and confers neuroprotection against 6-OHDA neurotoxicity. *Neurosignals* 21, 112–128. doi: 10.1159/000337115

Potter, S. Z., and Valentine, J. S. (2003). The perplexing role of copper-zinc superoxide dismutase in amyotrophic lateral sclerosis (Lou Gehrig's disease). *J. Biol. Inorg. Chem.* 8, 373–380. doi: 10.1007/s00775-003-0447-6

Prell, T., Lautenschlager, J., Witte, O. W., Carri, M. T., and Grosskreutz, J. (2012). The unfolded protein response in models of human mutant G93A amyotrophic lateral sclerosis. *Eur. J. Neurosci.* 35, 652–660. doi: 10.1111/j.1460-9568.2012.08008.x

Prudencio, M., and Borchelt, D. R. (2011). Superoxide dismutase 1 encoding mutations linked to ALS adopts a spectrum of misfolded states. *Mol. Neurodegener.* 6, 77. doi: 10.1186/1750-1326-6-77

Prudencio, M., Hart, P. J., Borchelt, D. R., and Andersen, P. M. (2009). Variation in aggregation propensities among ALS-associated variants of SOD1: correlation to human disease. *Hum. Mol. Genet.* 18, 3217–3226. doi: 10.1093/hmg/ddp260

Rakhit, R., Crow, J. P., Lepock, J. R., Kondejewski, L. H., Cashman, N. R., and Chakrabartty, A. (2004). Monomeric Cu, Zn-superoxide dismutase is a common misfolding intermediate in the oxidation models of sporadic and familial amyotrophic lateral sclerosis. *J. Biol. Chem.* 279, 15499–15504. doi: 10.1074/jbc.M313295200

Rakhit, R., Cunningham, P., Furtos-Matei, A., Dahan, S., Qi, X. F., Crow, J. P., et al. (2002). Oxidation-induced misfolding and aggregation of superoxide dismutase and its implications for amyotrophic lateral sclerosis. *J. Biol. Chem.* 277, 47551–47556. doi: 10.1074/jbc.M207356200

Rakhit, R., Robertson, J., Velde, C. V., Horne, P., Ruth, D. M., Griffin, J., et al. (2007). An immunological epitope selective for pathological monomer-misfolded SOD1 in ALS. *Nat. Med.* 13, 754–759. doi: 10.1038/nm1559

Reaume, A. G., Elliott, J. L., Hoffman, E. K., Kowall, N. W., Ferrante, R. J., Siwek, D. F., et al. (1996). Motor neurons in Cu/Zn superoxide dismutase-deficient mice develop normally but exhibit enhanced cell death after axonal injury. *Nat. Genet.* 13, 43–47. doi: 10.1038/ng0596-43

Reddi, A. R., and Culotta, V. C. (2013). SOD1 integrates signals from oxygen and glucose to repress respiration. *Cell* 152, 224–235. doi: 10.1016/j.cell.2012.11.046

Renton, A. E., Majounie, E., Waite, A., Simon-Sanchez, J., Rollinson, S., Gibbs, J. R., et al. (2011). A Hexanucleotide repeat expansion in C9ORF72 Is the cause of chromosome 9p21-linked ALS-FTD. *Neuron* 72, 257–268. doi: 10.1016/j.neuron.2011.09.010

Rhee, S. G. (2006). Cell signaling. H2O2, a necessary evil for cell signaling. *Science* 312, 1882–1883. doi: 10.1126/science.1130481

Rodriguez, J. A., Shaw, B. F., Durazo, A., Sohn, S. H., Doucette, P. A., Nersissian, A. M., et al. (2005). Destabilization of apoprotein is insufficient to explain Cu, Zn-superoxide dismutase-linked ALS pathogenesis. *Proc. Natl. Acad. Sci. U.S.A.* 102, 10516–10521. doi: 10.1073/pnas.0502515102

Rosen, D. R., Siddique, T., Patterson, D., Figlewicz, D. A., Sapp, P., Hentati, A., et al. (1993). Mutations in Cu/Zn superoxide dismutase gene are associated with familial amyotrophic lateral sclerosis. *Nature* 362, 59–62. doi: 10.1038/362059a0

Rothstein, J. D. (2009). Current hypotheses for the underlying biology of amyotrophic lateral sclerosis. *Ann. Neurol.* 65(Suppl. 1), S3–S9. doi: 10.1002/ana.21543

Santillo, M., Secondo, A., Seru, R., Damiano, S., Garbi, C., Taverna, E., et al. (2007). Evidence of calcium- and SNARE-dependent release of CuZn superoxide dismutase from rat pituitary GH3 cells and synaptosomes in response to depolarization. *J. Neurochem.* 102, 679–685. doi: 10.1111/j.1471-4159.2007.04538.x

Seetharaman, S. V., Prudencio, M., Karch, C., Holloway, S. P., Borchelt, D. R., Hart, P. J. (2009). Immature copper-zinc superoxide dismutase and familial amyotrophic lateral sclerosis. *Exp. Biol. Med.* 234, 1140–1154. doi: 10.3181/0903-MR-104

Sehati, S., Clement, M. H., Martins, J., Xu, L., Longo, V. D., Valentine, J. S., et al. (2011). Metabolic alterations in yeast lacking copper-zinc superoxide dismutase. *Free Radic. Biol. Med.* 50, 1591–1598. doi: 10.1016/j.freeradbiomed.2011.03.004

Selverstone Valentine, J., Doucette, P. A., and Zittin Potter, S. (2005). Copper-zinc superoxide dismutase and amyotrophic lateral sclerosis. *Annu. Rev. Biochem.* 74, 563–593. doi: 10.1146/annurev.biochem.72.121801.161647

Shibata, N., Asayama, K., Hirano, A., and Kobayashi, M. (1996). Immunohistochemical study on superoxide dismutases in spinal cords from autopsied patients with amyotrophic lateral sclerosis. *Dev. Neurosci.* 18, 492–498. doi: 10.1159/000111445

Shibata, N., Hirano, A., Kobayashi, M., Sasaki, S., Kato, T., Matsumoto, S., et al. (1994). Cu/Zn superoxide dismutase-like immunoreactivity in Lewy body-like inclusions of sporadic amyotrophic lateral sclerosis. *Neurosci. Lett.* 179, 149–152. doi: 10.1016/0304-3940(94)90956-3

Shipp, E. L., Cantini, F., Bertini, I., Valentine, J. S., and Banci, L. (2003). Dynamic properties of the G93A mutant of copper-zinc superoxide dismutase as detected by NMR spectroscopy: implications for the pathology of familial amyotrophic lateral sclerosis. *Biochemistry* 42, 1890–1899. doi: 10.1021/bi026704y

Song, Y., Nagy, M., Ni, W., Tyagi, N. K., Fenton, W. A., Lopez-Giraldez, F., et al. (2013). Molecular chaperone Hsp110 rescues a vesicle transport defect produced by an ALS-associated mutant SOD1 protein in squid axoplasm. *Proc. Natl. Acad. Sci. U.S.A.* 110, 5428–5433. doi: 10.1073/pnas.1303279110

Sreedharan, J., Blair, I. P., Tripathi, V. B., Hu, X., Vance, C., Rogelj, B., et al. (2008). TDP-43 mutations in familial and sporadic amyotrophic lateral sclerosis. *Science* 319, 1668–1672. doi: 10.1126/science.1154584

Stathopulos, P. B., Rumfeldt, J. A., Karbassi, F., Siddall, C. A., Lepock, J. R., and Meiering, E. M. (2006). Calorimetric analysis of thermodynamic stability and aggregation for apo and holo amyotrophic lateral sclerosis-associated Gly-93 mutants of superoxide dismutase. *J. Biol. Chem.* 281, 6184–6193. doi: 10.1074/jbc.M509496200

Stathopulos, P. B., Rumfeldt, J. A., Scholz, G. A., Irani, R. A., Frey, H. E., Hallewell, R. A., et al. (2003). Cu/Zn superoxide dismutase mutants associated with amyotrophic lateral sclerosis show enhanced formation of aggregates *in vitro*. *Proc. Natl. Acad. Sci. U.S.A.* 100, 7021–7026. doi: 10.1073/pnas.1237797100

Stewart, H. G., Mackenzie, I. R., Eisen, A., Brannstrom, T., Marklund, S. L., and Andersen, P. M. (2006). Clinicopathological phenotype of ALS with a novel G72C SOD1 gene mutation mimicking a myopathy. *Muscle Nerve* 5, 701–706. doi: 10.1002/mus.20495

Strange, R. W., Antonyuk, S., Hough, M. A., Doucette, P. A., Rodriguez, J. A., Hart, P. J., et al. (2003). The structure of holo and metal-deficient wild-type human Cu, Zn superoxide dismutase and its relevance to familial amyotrophic lateral sclerosis. *J. Mol. Biol.* 328, 877–891. doi: 10.1016/S0022-2836(03)00355-3

Strange, R. W., Yong, C. W., Smith, W., and Hasnain, S. S. (2007). Molecular dynamics using atomic-resolution structure reveal structural fluctuations that may lead to polymerization of human Cu-Zn superoxide dismutase. *Proc. Natl. Acad. Sci. U.S.A.* 104, 10040–10044. doi: 10.1073/pnas.0703857104

Sundaramoorthy, V., Walker, A. K., Yerbury, J., Soo, K. Y., Farg, M. A., Hoang, V., et al. (2013). Extracellular wildtype and mutant SOD1 induces ER-Golgi pathology characteristic of amyotrophic lateral sclerosis in neuronal cells. *Cell. Mol. Life Sci.* 70, 4181–4195. doi: 10.1007/s00018-013-1385-2

Svensson, A. K., Bilsel, O., Kayatekin, C., Adefusika, J. A., Zitzewitz, J. A., and Matthews, C. R. (2010). Metal-free ALS variants of dimeric human Cu, Zn-superoxide dismutase have enhanced populations of monomeric species. *PLoS ONE* 5:e10064. doi: 10.1371/journal.pone.0010064

Takeuchi, S., Fujiwara, N., Ido, A., Oono, M., Takeuchi, Y., Tateno, M., et al. (2010). Induction of protective immunity by vaccination with wild-type apo superoxide dismutase 1 in mutant SOD1 transgenic mice. *J. Neuropathol. Exp. Neurol.* 69, 1044–1056. doi: 10.1097/NEN.0b013e3181f4a90a

Tiwari, A., Liba, A., Sohn, S. H., Seetharaman, S. V., Bilsel, O., Matthews, C. R., et al. (2009). Metal deficiency increases aberrant hydrophobicity of mutant superoxide dismutases that cause amyotrophic lateral sclerosis. *J. Biol. Chem.* 284, 27746–27758. doi: 10.1074/jbc.M109.043729

Tiwari, A., Xu, Z., and Hayward, L. J. (2005). Aberrantly increased hydrophobicity shared by mutants of Cu, Zn-superoxide dismutase in familial amyotrophic lateral sclerosis. *J. Biol. Chem.* 280, 29771–29779. doi: 10.1074/jbc.M504039200

Tomkins, J., Banner, S. J., McDermott, C. J., and Shaw, P. J. (2001). Mutation screening of manganese superoxide dismutase in amyotrophic lateral sclerosis. *Neuroreport* 12, 2319–2322. doi: 10.1097/00001756-200108080-00008

Turner, B. J., Atkin, J. D., Farg, M. A., Zang, D. W., Rembach, A., Lopes, E. C., et al. (2005). Impaired extracellular secretion of mutant superoxide dismutase 1 associates with neurotoxicity in familial amyotrophic lateral sclerosis. *J. Neurosci.* 25, 108–117. doi: 10.1523/JNEUROSCI.4253-04.2005

Turner, B. J., and Talbot, K. (2008). Transgenics, toxicity and therapeutics in rodent models of mutant SOD1-mediated familial ALS. *Prog. Neurobiol.* 85, 94–134. doi: 10.1016/j.pneurobio.2008.01.001

Urushitani, M., Ezzi, S. A., and Julien, J. P. (2007). Therapeutic effects of immunization with mutant superoxide dismutase in mice models of amyotrophic lateral sclerosis. *Proc. Natl. Acad. Sci. U.S.A.* 104, 2495–2500. doi: 10.1073/pnas.0606201104

Urushitani, M., Sik, A., Sakurai, T., Nukina, N., Takahashi, R., and Julien, J. P. (2006). Chromogranin-mediated secretion of mutant superoxide dismutase proteins linked to amyotrophic lateral sclerosis. *Nat. Neurosci.* 9, 108–118. doi: 10.1038/nn1603

van Blitterswijk, M., Gulati, S., Smoot, E., Jaffa, M., Maher, N., Hyman, B. T., et al. (2011). Anti-superoxide dismutase antibodies are associated with survival in patients with sporadic amyotrophic lateral sclerosis. *Amyotroph. Lateral Scler.* 12, 430–438. doi: 10.3109/17482968.2011.585163

Vance, C., Rogelj, B., Hortobagyi, T., De Vos, K. J., Nishimura, A. L., Sreedharan, J., et al. (2009). Mutations in FUS, an RNA processing protein, cause familial amyotrophic lateral sclerosis type 6. *Science* 323, 1208–1211. doi: 10.1126/science.1165942

Vande Velde, C., Miller, T. M., Cashman, N. R., and Cleveland, D. W. (2008). Selective association of misfolded ALS-linked mutant SOD1 with the cytoplasmic face of mitochondria. *Proc. Natl. Acad. Sci. U.S.A.* 105, 4022–4027. doi: 10.1073/pnas.0712209105

Vassall, K. A., Stathopulos, P. B., Rumfeldt, J. A., Lepock, J. R., and Meiering, E. M. (2006). Equilibrium thermodynamic analysis of amyotrophic lateral sclerosis-associated mutant apo Cu, Zn superoxide dismutases. *Biochemistry* 45, 7366–7379. doi: 10.1021/bi0600953

Wang, L., Deng, H. X., Grisotti, G., Zhai, H., Siddique, T., and Roos, R. P. (2009). Wild-type SOD1 overexpression accelerates disease onset of a G85R SOD1 mouse. *Hum. Mol. Genet.* 18, 1642–1651. doi: 10.1093/hmg/ddp085

Wang, Q., Johnson, J. L., Agar, N. Y., and Agar, J. N. (2008). Protein aggregation and protein instability govern familial amyotrophic lateral sclerosis patient survival. *PLoS Biol.* 6:e170. doi: 10.1371/journal.pbio.0060170

Watanabe, M., Dykes-Hoberg, M., Culotta, V. C., Price, D. L., Wong, P. C., and Rothstein, J. D. (2001). Histological evidence of protein aggregation in mutant SOD1 transgenic mice and in amyotrophic lateral sclerosis neural tissues. *Neurobiol. Dis.* 8, 933–941. doi: 10.1006/nbdi.2001.0443

Witan, H., Gorlovoy, P., Kaya, A. M., Koziollek-Drechsler, I., Neumann, H., Behl, C., et al. (2009). Wild-type Cu/Zn superoxide dismutase (SOD1) does not facilitate, but impedes the formation of protein aggregates of amyotrophic lateral sclerosis causing mutant SOD1. *Neurobiol. Dis.* 36, 331–342. doi: 10.1016/j.nbd.2009.07.024

Witan, H., Kern, A., Koziollek-Drechsler, I., Wade, R., Behl, C., and Clement, A. M. (2008). Heterodimer formation of wild-type and amyotrophic lateral sclerosis-causing mutant Cu/Zn-superoxide dismutase induces toxicity independent of protein aggregation. *Hum. Mol. Genet.* 17, 1373–1385. doi: 10.1093/hmg/ddn025

Wong, P. C., Pardo, C. A., Borchelt, D. R., Lee, M. K., Copeland, N. G., Jenkins, N. A., et al. (1995). An adverse property of a familial ALS-linked SOD1 mutation causes motor neuron disease characterized by vacuolar degeneration of mitochondria. *Neuron* 14, 1105–1116. doi: 10.1016/0896-6273(95)90259-7

Xu, Z. S. (2012). Does a loss of TDP-43 function cause neurodegeneration. *Mol. Neurodegener.* 7:27. doi: 10.1186/1750-1326-7-27

Yates, D. (2010). Motor neuron disease: misfolded wild-type SOD1 may link sporadic and familial ALS. *Nat. Rev. Neurol.* 6, 645. doi: 10.1038/nrneurol.2010.169

Zelko, I. N., Mariani, T. J., and Folz, R. J. (2002). Superoxide dismutase multigene family: a comparison of the CuZn-SOD (SOD1), Mn-SOD (SOD2), and EC-SOD (SOD3) gene structures, evolution, and expression. *Free Radic. Biol. Med.* 33, 337–349. doi: 10.1016/S0891-5849(02)00905-X

Zetterstrom, P., Stewart, H. G., Bergemalm, D., Jonsson, P. A., Graffmo, K. S., Andersen, P. M., et al. (2007). Soluble misfolded subfractions of mutant superoxide dismutase-1s are enriched in spinal cords throughout life in murine ALS models. *Proc. Natl. Acad. Sci. U.S.A.* 104, 14157–14162. doi: 10.1073/pnas.0700477104

Zhao, W., Beers, D. R., Henkel, J. S., Zhang, W., Urushitani, M., Julien, J. P., et al. (2010). Extracellular mutant SOD1 induces microglial-mediated motoneuron injury. *Glia* 58, 231–243. doi: 10.1002/glia.20919

23

Early gene expression changes in spinal cord from SOD1^{G93A} amyotrophic lateral sclerosis animal model

Gabriela P. de Oliveira, Chrystian J. Alves and Gerson Chadi*

Department of Neurology, Neuroregeneration Center, University of São Paulo School of Medicine, São Paulo, Brazil

Edited by:
Ricardo Tapia, Universidad Nacional Autónoma de México, Mexico

Reviewed by:
Hermona Soreq, The Hebrew University of Jerusalem, Israel
Takumi Takizawa, Gunma University, Japan

***Correspondence:**
Gerson Chadi, Department of Neurology, University of São Paulo, Av. Dr. Arnaldo, 455, 2nd floor, room 2119, 01246-903-São Paulo, Brazil
e-mail: gerchadi@usp.br

Amyotrophic Lateral Sclerosis (ALS) is an adult-onset and fast progression neurodegenerative disease that leads to the loss of motor neurons. Mechanisms of selective motor neuron loss in ALS are unknown. The early events occurring in the spinal cord that may contribute to motor neuron death are not described, neither astrocytes participation in the pre-symptomatic phases of the disease. In order to identify ALS early events, we performed a microarray analysis employing a whole mouse genome platform to evaluate the gene expression pattern of lumbar spinal cords of transgenic SOD1^{G93A} mice and their littermate controls at pre-symptomatic ages of 40 and 80 days. Differentially expressed genes were identified by means of the Bioconductor packages Agi4×44Preprocess and limma. FunNet web based tool was used for analysis of over-represented pathways. Furthermore, immunolabeled astrocytes from 40 and 80 days old mice were submitted to laser microdissection and RNA was extracted for evaluation of a selected gene by qPCR. Statistical analysis has pointed to 492 differentially expressed genes (155 up and 337 down regulated) in 40 days and 1105 (433 up and 672 down) in 80 days old ALS mice. KEGG analysis demonstrated the over-represented pathways tight junction, antigen processing and presentation, oxidative phosphorylation, endocytosis, chemokine signaling pathway, ubiquitin mediated proteolysis and glutamatergic synapse at both pre-symptomatic ages. *Ube2i* gene expression was evaluated in astrocytes from both transgenic ages, being up regulated in 40 and 80 days astrocytes enriched samples. Our data points to important early molecular events occurring in pre-symptomatic phases of ALS in mouse model. Early SUMOylation process linked to astrocytes might account to non-autonomous cell toxicity in ALS. Further studies on the signaling pathways presented here may provide new insights to better understand the events triggering motor neuron death in this devastating disorder.

Keywords: ALS, SOD1^{G93A}, pre-symptomatic, spinal cord, microarray, laser microdissection, astrocytes

INTRODUCTION

Amyotrophic Lateral Sclerosis (ALS) is a fast disabling neurodegenerative disease characterized by upper and lower motor neuron loss of motor cortex, brainstem, and spinal cord leading to respiratory insufficiency and death (Turner et al., 2013). The incidence of ALS ranges from 1.7 to 2.3 cases per 100,000 population per year worldwide (Beghi et al., 2006). The mechanisms underlying neurodegeneration in ALS are multifactorial, and seem to involve neurons and non-neuronal cells (Boillee et al., 2006a,b; Yamanaka et al., 2008; Wang et al., 2011a) as well as several molecular pathways (Boillee et al., 2006a; Ferraiuolo et al., 2011b; Kiernan et al., 2011; Usuki et al., 2012). Approximately 5% of ALS cases are familial, and 20% of these have been linked to mutations in Cu/Zn superoxide dismutase 1 (SOD1) (Rosen et al., 1993; Andersen and Al-Chalabi, 2011). The first symptoms define the beginning of the clinical phase of the diagnosed cases of the more prevalent sporadic forms, consisting in muscle atrophy, weakness, fasciculations, and spasticity (Brooks et al., 2000). There is a lack of pathological studies on post mortem spinal cord from ALS patients that could add information about the triggering, initial time of motor neuron death and mechanisms of the disease. In fact, Fischer et al. (2004) reported the post-mortem evaluation in a patient with a short history of ALS, whose electromyography showed signs of acute and chronic denervation, coming out with an unexpected die without peripheral and central motor neuron death together with autolytic changes and a little axonal degeneration. Histological evaluations at the neuromuscular junctions and also electrophysiological analysis at the peripheral nerves in ALS patients have allowed authors to claim that motor neuron death correlates to the begging of clinical classical symptoms (Veugelers et al., 1996; Liu et al., 2013).

As the majority of familial ALS cases are linked to the mutations in SOD1 gene (Dion et al., 2009), transgenic mice expressing human mutant SOD1 (mSOD1) developing age-dependent clinical and pathological features of human ALS are current largely employed in the physiopathological studies of the disorder (Turner and Talbot, 2008). Using this mouse model, we previously described early behavior and electrophysiological alterations, prior the classical neurological symptoms and the beginning of motor neuron death (Alves et al., 2011). In fact, several early events demonstrated in animal models seemed to precede the neuronal death, remarkably the activation of glial cells (microglia and astrocytes) close to motor neurons (Graber et al., 2010; Wang et al., 2011b; Gerber et al., 2012), retraction of motor neuron fibers and neuromuscular junction displacement (Fischer et al., 2004; De Winter et al., 2006; Narai et al., 2009). It is still unknown whether the most claimed pathogenic processes for ALS, for instance oxidative stress, mitochondrial and neurofilament dysfunction, excitotoxicity, inflammation, non-autonomous cell toxicity, protein misfolding and abnormal RNA processing (Rothstein et al., 1992; Bergeron et al., 1994; Boillee et al., 2006a; Lemmens et al., 2010; Bendotti et al., 2012; Richardson et al., 2013) are taking place at the pre-symptomatic period of the disease.

The central question in understanding ALS facing therapeutic target development involves a further knowledge about the toxic mechanisms that trigger motor neuron death (Boillee et al., 2006a). Until scientific technology approaches do not overstep ethical limitations of clinical studies, the mutant SOD1-expressing mouse model may offer opportunity for a detailed analysis of intra and intercellular signaling-related to motor neuron toxicity.

The profiling of gene expression using different platforms have been largely employed in the ALS model in several stages of the disease course (Olsen et al., 2001; Dangond et al., 2004; Malaspina and De Belleroche, 2004; Jiang et al., 2005; Perrin et al., 2005; Ferraiuolo et al., 2007, 2011a; Yamamoto et al., 2007; Offen et al., 2009; Brockington et al., 2010; D'arrigo et al., 2010; Guipponi et al., 2010; Saris et al., 2013b; Yu et al., 2013), including the early symptomatic phase (Olsen et al., 2001; Yoshihara et al., 2002; Ferraiuolo et al., 2007; Yu et al., 2013), however, there is a lack of information on differential gene expression taking place before classical clinical symptoms (Olsen et al., 2001; Yoshihara et al., 2002; Ferraiuolo et al., 2007; Guipponi et al., 2010). Olsen et al. (2001) inaugurated that issue by looking at patterns of gene expression from SOD1^{G93A} spinal cord by means of a murine restricted platform of oligonucleotide microarray and by describing negligible changes in the transcript profile at the pre-symptomatic phases. Other authors that have examined gene profiling in pre-symptomatic phases of ALS disease employed restricted platforms of cDNA arrays, used animals with an uncommon symptom onset (Yoshihara et al., 2002; Guipponi et al., 2010) or evaluated gene profiling in specific spinal cord cells (Ferraiuolo et al., 2007, 2011a). Authors have encountered gene expressions related to inflammation, apoptosis, oxidative stress, ATP biosynthesis, myelination, axonal transport as candidates of biological processes taking place in the pre-symptomatic periods of ALS.

By means of a high-density oligonucleotide microarrays linked to specific tools capable to identify enriched pathways, the aim of this work was to identify early molecular changes in the pre-symptomatic stage in the spinal cord of the SOD1^{G93A} mouse model. The data showed important alterations at early 40 days pre-symptomatic period of disease and in 80 days old pre-symptomatic mice.

MATERIALS AND METHODS

SAMPLES

Specific pathogen-free male SOD1^{G93A} mice of preclinical 40 and 80 days old mice and their age-paired non-transgenic wild-type controls, 20–25 g body weight, from University of São Paulo Medical School (São Paulo, Brazil) were used in the experiments. A total of 5 animals were used in each group in microarray experiments, while in the verification experiments by quantitative polymerase chain reaction (qPCR) and laser microdissection, each group was comprised for 6 and 3 different animals, respectively. Animals were kept under standardized lighting conditions (lights on at 7:00 h and off at 19:00 h), at a constant temperature of 23°C and with free access to food pellets and tap water. The colony was derived from Jackson Laboratories (Bar Harbor, ME, USA) from G93A mutant mice with 25 ± 1.5 copies of the human SOD1 transgene (Gurney, 1994). Mouse identification (SOD^{G93A} or WT) in our colony was performed by genotyping (Scorisa et al., 2010). Animals were killed by decapitation and their lumbar spinal cords were collected for molecular analysis. The study was conducted according protocols approved by the Animal Care and Use of Ethic Committee at the University of São Paulo and in accordance with the Guide for Care and Use of Laboratory Animals adopted by the National Institutes of Health.

RNA EXTRACTION

Total RNA was isolated using the MiniSpin kit for RNA extraction (GE Healthcare, USA) according to the manufacturer's instructions. RNA quantity and integrity were assessed by spectrophotometry (Nanodrop, Thermo Scientific, USA) and microfluidics—based electrophoresis (Agilent 2100 Bioanalyzer, Agilent Technologies, USA), respectively. RNA samples with OD 260/280 of approximately 2.0 and RIN > 7.0 were used for microarray experiments and qPCR. A pool of RNAs from neonatal organs (heart, kidney, liver) was employed as reference sample. A representative eletropherogram from Bioanalyzer evaluation of RNA integrity is shown in supplementary material (Figure S1).

MICROARRAY EXPERIMENTS

For samples and reference, respectively, 250 and 500 ng of RNA were reverse transcribed by the Low-input RNA Linear Amplification Kit (Agilent Technologies) and then transcribed to Cy3-labeled (samples) or Cy5-labeled (reference) cRNA according to the manufacturer. The labeled cRNA was purified (Minispin kit, GE Life Sciences), and the dye content and concentration of cRNA were measured by a NanoDrop ND-1000 spectrophotometer (Thermo Scientific). A total of 850 ng of Cy3-labeled cRNA was hybridized together with the same amount of Cy5-labeled reference to Whole Mouse Genome Oligo 4×44 K microarrays overnight at 65°C, and then the slides were washed and treated with Stabilizing and Drying Solution (Agilent Technologies) and scanned by Agilent Microarray Scanner. All steps were performed according to the manufacturer (Agilent Technologies).

The raw data from hybridizations and experimental conditions are available on the Gene Expression Omnibus website under accession number GSE50642.

DATA ANALYSES

The Feature Extraction Software v9.1.3.1 (Agilent Technologies) was used to extract and analyze the assay signals and subsequently determine the signal-to-noise ratios from the microarray images. Microarrays without enough quality were taken out from further analysis. The analysis proceeded with 4 samples for each group. Microarray raw data (.txt files) were imported into R v. 3.0.1 (Team RDC, 2012) and analyzed with the Bioconductor (Gentleman et al., 2004) packages Agi4×44PreProcess and limma (Smyth, 2005). Briefly, after quality check, the microarray probes were filtered and their median foreground intensity was normalized within and between arrays according to Agi4×44Preprocess and limma user guides, respectively. Finally, the probes were tested for differential expression using a linear model followed by Bayes moderated t-test (Smyth, 2005) for the comparisons of interest. Genes with nominal $p < 0.05$ were accepted to be differentially expressed and further considered in the analysis.

FunNet ANALYSIS

In order to further identify over-represented pathways and biological process, the lists with differentially expressed genes for both 40 and 80 days old mice were split into lists of up and down regulated genes and submitted to FunNet web based tool (Functional Analysis of Transcriptional Networks), using Kyoto Encyclopedia of Genes and Genomes (KEGG) and Gene Ontology (GO) annotations (Prifti et al., 2008).

LASER MICRODISSECTION OF ASTROCYTES

The lumbar spinal cord of mice were rapidly removed and immediately frozen in ice cold isopentane at −45°C and stored at −80°C until use. The labeling procedure was performed as described previously (De Oliveira et al., 2009) and modified according to our experience. Frozen sections (5μm) were rapidly defrosted for 30 s and fixed with ice cold acetone, for 3 min. Sections were then incubated during 3 min in phosphate buffered saline (PBS) containing 3% Triton X-100 and then incubated with primary antibody, a polyclonal rabbit anti-glial fibrillary acidic protein (GFAP; Dako Cytomation; 1:100) diluted in 0.3% Triton X-100 containing 1% BSA for 5 min. Sections were then washed in PBS for 3 times of 15 s and then incubated with texas red-conjugated goat-anti-rabbit secondary antibody, in the same diluent than primary antibody, in a final concentration of 1:50 during 5 min in the dark and at room temperature. Sections were rinsed carefully three times with PBS for 15 s and immediately submitted to laser microdissection.

Around 200 astrocytes were isolated from each 40 and 80 days old mice lumbar spinal cords using P.A.L.M. Microlaser Technologies (Zeiss). RNA was extracted using PicoPure RNA isolation kit (Arcturus) and linear amplification of RNA was performed following Eberwine's procedure (Van Gelder et al., 1990) using the RiboampHSplus kit (Arcturus) according to the manufacturer's protocol. The quantity (NanoDrop 1000 Spectrophotometer) and quality (Agilent 2100 bioanalyser, RNA 6000 Pico LabChip) of amplified RNA was analyzed as described above. Also, the astrocytes enriched samples were submitted to PCRs in order to access contamination from other cell types. Protocol and results of astrocyte samples enrichment are presented in the supplementary material (Figure S2).

QUANTITATIVE PCR

A proportion of genes identified as differentially expressed were selected for verification by qPCR, on the basis of robust microarray data confirming differential gene expression. The genes were chosen for verification based on their possible involvement in ALS related mechanisms. Verification addresses the possibility of false positive microarray signals, due to cross-hybridization with related genes, concern about the accuracy of array probe sets, and uncertainty about the hybridization kinetics of multiple reactions occurring on the miniature scale of an array chip. The qPCR verification of microarray results were performed on independent sample, as described above. cDNA was synthesized from 1 μg of total RNA treated with DNAse by a reverse transcription reagent kit (Applied Biosystems Life Technologies) according to manufacturer. qPCR reactions were carried out in duplicate with 40 ng cDNA, the DyNAmo ColorFlash SYBR Green qPCR kit (Thermo Scientific, USA) and 400 nM of each primer in a final volume reaction of 20 μl, by using the PikoReal Real-Time PCR System (Thermo Scientific). The information for SYBR primers can be found in **Table 1**. For astrocytes enriched samples, 1 μg of amplified RNA was reverse transcribed to cDNA by a reverse transcription reagent kit (Applied Biosystems Life Technologies) modified from original protocol in order to improve efficiency. Briefly, Oligo(dT)$_{16}$ primer was added to samples and incubated at 70°C during 5 min, then the other required reagents, such as reaction buffer, $MgCl_2$, dNTPs, RNAse inhibitor, in the same concentrations than manufacturer protocol, and 156,25 U of Reverse transcriptase (Multiscribe), were added to reaction and incubated at 37°C for 60 min followed by 95°C for 5 min. qPCR reactions were carried out in duplicate using Taqman master mix and the

Table 1 | Information for primers used in SYBR qPCR experiments of 40 and 80 days old pre-symptomatic SOD1^{G93A} and wild-type mice.

Gene ID	Primer sequences (5′-3′)	Amplicon (bp)
Glg1	F: GAGTGAGATTGCAGCCAGAG R:CAGGATGTAGTTCTTTGAGGGAG	143
Aqp4	F: GCTCGATCTTTTGGACCCG R: AGACATACTCATAAAGGGCACC	112
Calca	F: TGCAGATGAAAGCCAGGG R: CTTCACCACACCTCCTGATC	149
Eef2	F: CATGTTTGTGGTCAAGGCATAC R:TTGTCAAAAGGATCCCCAGG	141
Nsg1	F: AAGTGTACAAGTATGACCGCG R: GACAGTGTAAAATTTCTCCCGG	128
Syt10	F: AGACCATTGGAACGAGATGC R: TGGAGGCTTTTATGGTGTGG	148
NORMALYZER		
Gapdh	F: GAGTAAGAAACCCTGGACCAC R: TCTGGGATGGAAATTGTGAGG	109

The Glg1, Aqp4, Calca genes and Eef2, Nsg1, Syt10 genes were verified in 40 and 80 days mice, respectively, according to microarray results.

following assays were used: *Ube2i* (Mm04243971_g1) and *Gapdh* (Mm99999915_g1).

For SYBR reactions the cycling was composed by an initial denaturation at 95°C for 10 min, templates were amplified by 40 cycles of 95°C for 15 s and 60°C for 30 s. A dissociation curve was then generated to ensure amplification of a single product, and absence of primer dimers. For each primer pair, a standard curve was generated to determine the efficiency of the PCR reaction over a range of template concentrations from 0.032 ng/μl to 20 ng/μl, using cDNA synthesized from mouse reference RNA. The efficiency for each set of primers was 100 ± 5%. For Taqman reactions, cycling was composed by an initial step of 50°C for 2 min, followed by denaturation at 95°C for 10 min, templates were amplified by 40 cycles of 95°C for 15 s and 60°C for 1 min. Gene expressions, normalized to *Gapdh*, could be determined using the ΔΔCt mathematical model (ABI PRISM 7700 Sequence Detection System protocol; Applied Biosystems). One-tailed unpaired *t*-test was used to determine the statistical significance of any differences in gene expression [GraphPad (San Diego, CA) Prism 5]. *Gapdh* was chosen as a housekeeping gene to normalize the qPCR values because the microarray analysis showed that its expression was stable across samples.

RESULTS

GENERAL FEATURES OF DIFFERENTIAL GENE EXPRESSION BETWEEN SOD1^{G93A} AND WILD-TYPE MICE

Statistical analysis has pointed to 492 differentially expressed genes at the lumbar region of 40 days SOD1^{G93A}, compared to the age matched wild-type mice, being 155 up and 337 down regulated genes, respectively, while 1105 genes were found differentially expressed by 80 days old ALS mice compared to age matched controls, being 433 up and 672 down regulated genes, respectively. The whole list with differentially expressed gene for both age mice can be found in Tables S1 and S2 in the Supplementary material. Of interest, among differentially expressed genes, 66 are common to both ages; they are presented in the **Table 2**.

VERIFICATION OF MICROARRAY RESULTS BY qPCR

The results of qPCR verification for the six representative genes are shown in Table S3 (Supplementary material). The up and down regulations of the verified genes in the 40 days and 80 days old SOD1^{G93A} mice by means of qPCR were coincident and supported the microarray findings of correspondent animal ages (Table S3).

FunNet ANALYSIS

KEGG terms which were significantly enriched (at level $p < 0.05$) amongst differentially expressed genes between SOD1^{G93A} and wild-type mice were identified for both 40 days and 80 days old pre-symptomatic ALS mice. Over-represented KEGG pathways and respective genes taking part of them are given in **Tables 3, 4.** Of importance, differentially expressed genes from 40 and 80 days old mice allowed to recognize 7 pathways common among both periods (**Figure 1**). Those were glutamatergic synapse, ubiquitin mediated proteolysis, chemokine signaling pathway, endocytosis, oxidative phosphorylation, antigen processing and presentation and tight junction. The number of transcripts in each pathway

Table 2 | Differentially expressed genes common to both gene lists of 40 and 80 days old pre-symptomatic SOD1^{G93A} and wild-type mice.

Gene symbol	Fold change 40 days	Fold change 80 days
Ocel1	−1.68	−1.92
Fam32a	−1.45	−1.61
Trim37	1.22	−1.34
Lsm6	−1.3	−1.29
Map1a	1.2	−1.15 and −1.28
Bmpr2	1.21	−1.26
Eif3j2	1.29	−1.26
Foxn3	1.28	−1.25
Plekha5	1.17	−1.25
Rfxank	−1.12	−1.22
Malat1	1.1	−1.21
Ddx6	1.3	−1.19
Huwe1	1.12	−1.19
Snx27	1.19	−1.19
Srrm3	1.18	−1.19
Dzip1	1.14	−1.17
Hook3	1.14	−1.17
Nemf	1.15	−1.16
Pdlim5	1.09	−1.16
Plvap	−1.14	−1.16
Thrap3	1.15	−1.16
Srsf11	−1.1	−1.15
Azin1	1.12	−1.14
Eif5b	1.19	−1.14
Hspa4	1.1	−1.14
Kras	1.19	−1.14
Sp4	1.12	−1.14
Tusc3	−1.1	−1.14
Vegfa	1.12	−1.14
Fam133b	1.09	−1.13
Fam81a	1.12	−1.13
Prkrir	−1.1	−1.13
Ptrf	−1.3	−1.13
6330411E07Rik	1.09	−1.12
Gria4	1.18	−1.12
Zfp866	1.07	−1.12
Marc-2	−1.07	−1.11
Hadh	1.12	−1.11
Mtf2	1.1	−1.11
Dhps	−1.09	−1.1
Nsd1	1.12	−1.1
Mier1	1.13	−1.09
U2surp	1.13	−1.09
2610507B11Rik	1.07	1.1
Ncam1	1.17	1.12
Rtn1	−1.17	1.12
Chd5	1.12	1.13
Dhcr7	−1.08	1.15
Strbp	1.15	1.15
Synm	−1.12	1.15
Map7d1	1.14	1.16
Specc1	1.1	1.17

(Continued)

Table 2 | Continued

Gene symbol	Fold change 40 days	Fold change 80 days
Maea	1.1	1.19
Ncl	1.1 and −1.1	1.19
Glg1	1.29	1.2
Dnajc27	1.17	1.21
Ncdn	1.14	1.21
Lpcat2	1.16	1.22
D17Wsu92e	1.11	1.24
Nisch	1.08	1.24
Tkt	−1.1	1.25
Tmem59l	1.29	1.26
Mast3	1.24	1.28
Plac9a	−1.45	1.35
Nsg1	−1.17	1.22 and 1.35
Trappc3	−1.2	1.32 and 1.41

Map1a, Ncl, Nsg1, and Trappc3 genes were represented by an additional probe.

is also shown in **Figure 1**. Moreover, other interesting pathways could also be identified to appear only in 40 days (**Table 3**) or 80 days old SOD1^{G93A} mice (**Table 4**). Furthermore, among pathways common to both ages, ubiquitin mediated proteolysis, chemokine signaling pathway and endocytosis were over-represented by up regulated genes and oxidative phosphorylation was pointed by down regulated genes (**Figure 1**). Furthermore, glutamatergic synapse and tight junction were pointed by the genes that were up regulated in 40 days and also up or down regulated in 80 days gene expression lists (**Figure 1**). Finally, antigen processing and presentation was pointed for down regulated genes in 40 days and up regulated genes in 80 days lists (**Figure 1**).

Some pathways pointed by FunNet were omitted from table because they were composed by genes already presented in other pathways and also genes apparently not related to ALS. They were melanoma, measles, hepatitis C, melanogenesis, pathways in cancer and prostate cancer at 40 days and viral myocarditis and melanogenesis in 80 days results.

The results for GO enriched terms can be found in Tables S4 and S5 in Supplementary material.

LASER MICRODISSECTION OF ASTROCYTES AND qPCR EXPERIMENT

The profile for GFAP immunofluorescence for specific identification of astrocytes can be found in **Figure 2**. Our protocol allowed easily identifying the astrocytic profiles (**Figure 2A**) to be microdissected (**Figure 2B**). The procedure allowed a complete microdissection of the desired cell type (**Figure 2C**), the astrocytes in our case. The results of qPCR for *Ube2i*, using the two cycle amplified RNA, from 40 and 80 days mouse laser microdissected astrocytes have shown increased gene expressions in transgenic mice of both pre-symptomatic ages (**Figure 3**). The *Ube2i* expression was increased by 5.53-fold in the astrocytes from 40 days old SOD1^{G92A} mice and by 1.77-fold change in astrocytes from 80 days old SOD1^{G92A} mice compared to respective age matched wild-type samples.

Table 3 | KEGG pathways enriched amongst differentially expressed up or down regulated genes at 40 days old mice.

Gene ID	Gene symbol	Gene name
PATHWAYS POINTED BY UP REGULATED GENES		
Fructose and manose metabolism		
170768	*Pfkfb3*	6-Phosphofructo-2-kinase/fructose-2,6-biphosphatase 3
18640	*Pfkfb2*	6-Phosphofructo-2-kinase/fructose-2,6-biphosphatase 2
18642	*Pfkm*	Phosphofructokinase, muscle
230163	*Aldob*	Aldolase B, fructose-bisphosphate
54384	*Mtmr7*	Myotubularin related protein 7
Tight junction		
14677	*Gnai1*	Guanine nucleotide binding protein (G protein), alpha inhibiting 1
16653	*Kras*	v-Ki-ras2 Kirsten rat sarcoma viral oncogene homolog
18176	*Nras*	Neuroblastoma ras oncogene
18417	*Cldn11*	Claudin 11
192195	*Ash1l*	Ash1 (absent, small, or homeotic)-like (Drosophila)
Glutamatergic synapse		
140919	*Slc17a6*	Solute carrier family 17 (sodium-dependent inorganic phosphate cotransporter), member 6
14677	*Gnai1*	Guanine nucleotide binding protein (G protein), alpha inhibiting 1
14802	*Gria4*	Glutamate receptor, ionotropic, AMPA4 (alpha 4)
14810	*Grin1*	Glutamate receptor, ionotropic, NMDA1 (zeta 1)
20511	*Slc1a2*	Solute carrier family 1 (glial high affinity glutamate transporter), member 2
Axon guidance		
12767	*Cxcr4*	Chemokine (C-X-C motif) receptor 4
14677	*Gnai1*	Guanine nucleotide binding protein (G protein), alpha inhibiting 1
16653	*Kras*	v-Ki-ras2 Kirsten rat sarcoma viral oncogene homolog
18176	*Nras*	Neuroblastoma ras oncogene
22253	*Unc5c*	Unc-5 homolog C (*C. elegans*)
56637	*Gsk3b*	Glycogen synthase kinase 3 beta
Ubiquitin mediated proteolysis		
107568	*Wwp1*	WW domain containing E3 ubiquitin protein ligase 1
17999	*Nedd4*	Neural precursor cell expressed, developmentally down-regulated 4
22210	*Ube2b*	Ubiquitin-conjugating enzyme E2B
59026	*Huwe1*	HECT, UBA and WWE domain containing 1
68729	*Trim37*	Tripartite motif-containing 37
70790	*Ubr5*	Ubiquitin protein ligase E3 component n-recognin 5
Chemokine signaling pathway		
12767	*Cxcr4*	Chemokine (C-X-C motif) receptor 4
14677	*Gnai1*	Guanine nucleotide binding protein (G protein), alpha inhibiting 1

(Continued)

Table 3 | Continued

Gene ID	Gene symbol	Gene name
16653	*Kras*	v-Ki-ras2 Kirsten rat sarcoma viral oncogene homolog
18176	*Nras*	Neuroblastoma ras oncogene
18708	*Pik3r1*	Phosphatidylinositol 3-kinase, regulatory subunit, polypeptide 1 (p85 alpha)
56637	*Gsk3b*	Glycogen synthase kinase 3 beta
73178	*Wasl*	Wiskott-Aldrich syndrome-like (human)
Endocytosis		
107568	*Wwp1*	WW domain containing E3 ubiquitin protein ligase 1
12767	*Cxcr4*	Chemokine (C-X-C motif) receptor 4
13854	*Epn1*	Epsin 1
17999	*Nedd4*	Neural precursor cell expressed, developmentally down-regulated 4
193740	*Hspa1a*	Heat shock protein 1A
26431	*Git2*	G protein-coupled receptor kinase-interactor 2
78618	*Acap2*	ArfGAP with coiled-coil, ankyrin repeat and PH domains 2
PATHWAYS POINTED BY DOWN REGULATED GENES		
Nucleotide excision repair		
19718	*Rfc2*	Replication factor C (activator 1) 2
66979	*Pole4*	Polymerase (DNA-directed), epsilon 4 (p12 subunit)
DNA replication		
19718	*Rfc2*	Replication factor C (activator 1) 2
66979	*Pole4*	Polymerase (DNA-directed), epsilon 4 (p12 subunit)
Fatty acid metabolism		
11363	*Acadl*	Acyl-Coenzyme A dehydrogenase, long-chain
74205	*Acsl3*	Acyl-CoA synthetase long-chain family member 3
TGF-beta signaling pathway		
12167	*Bmpr1b*	Bmpr1b bone morphogenetic protein receptor, type 1B
15902	*Id2*	Inhibitor of DNA binding 2
19651	*Rbl2*	Retinoblastoma-like 2
Antigen processing and presentation		
12010	*B2m*	Beta-2 microglobulin
12317	*Calr*	Calreticulin
19727	*Rfxank*	Regulatory factor X-associated ankyrin-containing protein
ECM-receptor interaction		
11603	*Agrn*	Agrin
12814	*Col11a1*	Collagen, type XI, alpha 1
16773	*Lama2*	Laminin, alpha 2
GnRH signaling pathway		
12314	*Calm2*	Calmodulin 2
16440	*Itpr3*	Inositol 1,4,5-triphosphate receptor 3
16476	*Jun*	Jun oncogene
17390	*Mmp2*	Matrix metallopeptidase 2

(Continued)

Table 3 | Continued

Gene ID	Gene symbol	Gene name
Parkinson's disease		
104130	*Ndufb11*	NADH dehydrogenase (ubiquinone) 1 beta subcomplex, 11
12857	*Cox4i1*	Cytochrome c oxidase subunit IV isoform 1
66576	*Uqcrh*	Ubiquinol-cytochrome c reductase hinge protein
67264	*Ndufb8*	NADH dehydrogenase (ubiquinone) 1 beta subcomplex 8
Oxidative phosphorylation		
104130	*Ndufb11*	NADH dehydrogenase (ubiquinone) 1 beta subcomplex, 11
12857	*Cox4i1*	Cytochrome c oxidase subunit IV isoform 1
66576	*Uqcrh*	Ubiquinol-cytochrome c reductase hinge protein
67264	*Ndufb8*	NADH dehydrogenase (ubiquinone) 1 beta subcomplex 8
Alzheimer's disease		
104130	*Ndufb11*	NADH dehydrogenase (ubiquinone) 1 beta subcomplex, 11
12314	*Calm2*	Calmodulin 2
12857	*Cox4i1*	Cytochrome c oxidase subunit IV isoform 1
16440	*Itpr3*	Inositol 1,4,5-triphosphate receptor 3
66576	*Uqcrh*	Ubiquinol-cytochrome c reductase hinge protein
67264	*Ndufb8*	NADH dehydrogenase (ubiquinone) 1 beta subcomplex 8

DISCUSSION

Gene-expression profiling studies have been conducted in the search of molecular pathways related to motor neuron death in ALS by employing animal models in different phases of the disease and human post mortem material at the very end stage of motor neuron degeneration (Olsen et al., 2001; Dangond et al., 2004; Malaspina and De Belleroche, 2004; Jiang et al., 2005; Perrin et al., 2005; Ferraiuolo et al., 2007, 2011a; Yamamoto et al., 2007; Offen et al., 2009; Brockington et al., 2010; D'arrigo et al., 2010; Guipponi et al., 2010; Saris et al., 2013b).

The analysis of the mechanisms that trigger motor neuron death in the ALS may include evaluation of the altered molecular pathways that are taking place in compromised regions before the occurrence of cell death. Previous works have attempted to describe gene profiling in the pre-symptomatic phases of ALS animal model by employing distinct methodologies (Ferraiuolo et al., 2007; D'arrigo et al., 2010; Guipponi et al., 2010). This is the first work to analyze gene expression profile in the whole lumbar spinal cord of early 40 and 80 days old pre-symptomatic SOD1^{G93A} mouse in a whole genome array platform, which allowed depicting enriched pathways related to possible mechanisms of neuronal toxicity in ALS. Our analysis has pointed to up to 1105 differentially expressed genes in pre-symptomatic periods of SOD1^{G93A} mouse model, a larger number of than described elsewhere (Perrin et al., 2005, 2006). It should be pointed that the average of fold change described in previous publications is about 3, which is higher than that found in our microarray analysis. However, it must be emphasized that

Table 4 | KEGG pathways enriched amongst differentially expressed up or down regulated genes at 80 days old mice.

Gene ID	Gene symbol	Gene name
PATHWAYS POINTED BY UP REGULATED GENES		
Vascular smooth muscle contraction		
104111	*Adcy3*	Adenylate cyclase 3
12315	*Calm3*	Calmodulin 3
14673	*Gna12*	Guanine nucleotide binding protein, alpha 12
14674	*Gna13*	Guanine nucleotide binding protein, alpha 13
18751	*Prkcb*	Protein kinase C, beta
213498	*Arhgef11*	Rho guanine nucleotide exchange factor (GEF) 11
224129	*Adcy5*	Adenylate cyclase 5
26413	*Mapk1*	Mitogen-activated protein kinase 1
Antigen processing and presentation		
14963	*H2-Bl*	Histocompatibility 2, blastocyst
14972	*H2-K1*	Histocompatibility 2, K1, K region
15006	*H2-Q1*	Histocompatibility 2, Q region locus 1
15007	*H2-Q10*	Histocompatibility 2, Q region locus 10
15013	*H2-Q2*	Histocompatibility 2, Q region locus 2
15018	*H2-Q7*	Histocompatibility 2, Q region locus 7
15039	*H2-T22*	Histocompatibility 2, T region locus 22
15040	*H2-T23*	Histocompatibility 2, T region locus 23
15481	*Hspa8*	Heat shock protein 8
21355	*Tap2*	Transporter 2, ATP-binding cassette, sub-family B (MDR/TAP)
Tight junction		
11465	*Actg1*	Actin, gamma, cytoplasmic 1
13043	*Cttn*	Cortactin
13821	*Epb4.1l1*	Erythrocyte protein band 4.1-like 1
13822	*Epb4.1l2*	Erythrocyte protein band 4.1-like 2
14924	*Magi1*	Membrane associated guanylate kinase, WW and PDZ domain containing 1
16897	*Llgl1*	Lethal giant larvae homolog 1
17475	*Mpdz*	Multiple PDZ domain protein
18751	*Prkcb*	Protein kinase C, beta
67374	*Jam2*	Junction adhesion molecule 2
71960	*Myh14*	Myosin, heavy polypeptide 14
Chemokine signaling pathway		
104111	*Adcy3*	Adenylate cyclase 3
14083	*Ptk2*	PTK2 protein tyrosine kinase 2
14688	*Gnb1*	Guanine nucleotide binding protein (G protein), beta 1
14693	*Gnb2*	Guanine nucleotide binding protein (G protein), beta 2
14697	*Gnb5*	Guanine nucleotide binding protein (G protein), beta 5
14701	*Gng12*	Guanine nucleotide binding protein (G protein), gamma 12
14708	*Gng7*	Guanine nucleotide binding protein (G protein), gamma 7
18751	*Prkcb*	Protein kinase C, beta

(Continued)

Table 4 | Continued

Gene ID	Gene symbol	Gene name
224129	*Adcy5*	Adenylate cyclase 5
26413	*Mapk1*	Mitogen-activated protein kinase 1
277360	*Prex1*	Phosphatidylinositol-3,4,5-trisphosphate-dependent Rac exchange factor 1
Ubiquitin mediated proteolysis		
103583	*Fbxw11*	F-box and WD-40 domain protein 11
15204	*Herc2*	Hect (homologous to the E6-AP (UBE3A) carboxyl terminus) domain and RCC1 (CHC1)-like domain (RLD) 2
17237	*Mgrn1*	Mahogunin, ring finger 1
19823	*Rnf7*	Ring finger protein 7
217342	*Ube2o*	Ubiquitin-conjugating enzyme E2O
22192	*Ube2m*	Ubiquitin-conjugating enzyme E2M
22196	*Ube2i*	Ubiquitin-conjugating enzyme E2I
22213	*Ube2g2*	Ubiquitin-conjugating enzyme E2G 2
229615	*Pias3*	Protein inhibitor of activated STAT 3
50754	*Fbxw7*	F-box and WD-40 domain protein 7
63958	*Ube4b*	Ubiquitination factor E4B, UFD2 homolog (S. cerevisiae)
Regulation of actin cytoskeleton		
11465	*Actg1*	Actin, gamma, cytoplasmic 1
14083	*Ptk2*	PTK2 protein tyrosine kinase 2
14673	*Gna12*	Guanine nucleotide binding protein, alpha 12
14674	*Gna13*	Guanine nucleotide binding protein, alpha 13
14701	*Gng12*	Guanine nucleotide binding protein (G protein), gamma 12
18717	*Pip5k1c*	Phosphatidylinositol-4-phosphate 5-kinase, type 1 gamma
192897	*Itgb4*	Integrin beta 4
226970	*Arhgef4*	Rho guanine nucleotide exchange factor (GEF) 4
227753	*Gsn*	Gelsolin
26413	*Mapk1*	Mitogen-activated protein kinase 1
67771	*Arpc5*	Actin related protein 2/3 complex, subunit 5
71960	*Myh14*	Myosin, heavy polypeptide 14
Glutamatergic synapse		
104111	*Adcy3*	Adenylate cyclase 3
110637	*Grik4*	Glutamate receptor, ionotropic, kainate 4
14645	*Glul*	Glutamate-ammonia ligase (glutamine synthetase)
14688	*Gnb1*	Guanine nucleotide binding protein (G protein), beta 1
14693	*Gnb2*	Guanine nucleotide binding protein (G protein), beta 2
14697	*Gnb5*	Guanine nucleotide binding protein (G protein), beta 5
14701	*Gng12*	Guanine nucleotide binding protein (G protein), gamma 12
14708	*Gng7*	Guanine nucleotide binding protein (G protein), gamma 7
18751	*Prkcb*	Protein kinase C, beta
216456	*Gls2*	Glutaminase 2 (liver, mitochondrial)
224129	*Adcy5*	Adenylate cyclase 5
26413	*Mapk1*	Mitogen-activated protein kinase 1

(Continued)

Table 4 | Continued

Gene ID	Gene symbol	Gene name
Phagosome		
11465	*Actg1*	Actin, gamma, cytoplasmic 1
14963	*H2-Bl*	Histocompatibility 2, blastocyst
14972	*H2-K1*	Histocompatibility 2, K1, K region
15006	*H2-Q1*	Histocompatibility 2, Q region locus 1
15007	*H2-Q10*	Histocompatibility 2, Q region locus 10
15013	*H2-Q2*	Histocompatibility 2, Q region locus 2
15018	*H2-Q7*	Histocompatibility 2, Q region locus 7
15039	*H2-T22*	Histocompatibility 2, T region locus 22
15040	*H2-T23*	Histocompatibility 2, T region locus 23
15239	*Hgs*	HGF-regulated tyrosine kinase substrate
17113	*M6pr*	Mannose-6-phosphate receptor, cation dependent
21355	*Tap2*	Transporter 2, ATP-binding cassette, sub-family B (MDR/TAP)
22142	*Tuba1a*	Tubulin, alpha 1A
22151	*Tubb2a*	Tubulin, beta 2A class IIA
Protein processing in endoplasmic reticulum		
100037258	*Dnajc3*	DnaJ (Hsp40) homolog, subfamily C, member 3
108687	*Edem2*	ER degradation enhancer, mannosidase alpha-like 2
12955	*Cryab*	Crystallin, alpha B
15481	*Hspa8*	Heat shock protein 8
20014	*Rpn2*	Ribophorin II
20338	*Sel1l*	Sel-1 suppressor of lin-12-like (C. elegans)
216440	*Os9*	Amplified in osteosarcoma
22213	*Ube2g2*	Ubiquitin-conjugating enzyme E2G 2
269523	*Vcp*	Valosin containing protein
50907	*Preb*	Prolactin regulatory element binding
54197	*Rnf5*	Ring finger protein 5
56453	*Mbtps1*	Membrane-bound transcription factor peptidase, site 1
56812	*Dnajb2*	DnaJ (Hsp40) homolog, subfamily B, member 2
63958	*Ube4b*	Ubiquitination factor E4B, UFD2 homolog (S. cerevisiae)
Cell adhesion molecules (CAMS)		
14963	*H2-Bl*	Histocompatibility 2, blastocyst
14972	*H2-K1*	Histocompatibility 2, K1, K region
15006	*H2-Q1*	Histocompatibility 2, Q region locus 1
15007	*H2-Q10*	Histocompatibility 2, Q region locus 10
15013	*H2-Q2*	Histocompatibility 2, Q region locus 2
15018	*H2-Q7*	Histocompatibility 2, Q region locus 7
15039	*H2-T22*	Histocompatibility 2, T region locus 22
15040	*H2-T23*	Histocompatibility 2, T region locus 23
17967	*Ncam1*	Neural cell adhesion molecule 1
18007	*Neo1*	Neogenin
19274	*Ptprm*	Protein tyrosine phosphatase, receptor type, M
20340	*Glg1*	Golgi apparatus protein 1
20970	*Sdc3*	Syndecan 3
58235	*Pvrl1*	Poliovirus receptor-related 1
67374	*Jam2*	Junction adhesion molecule 2

(Continued)

Table 4 | Continued

Gene ID	Gene symbol	Gene name
Endocytosis		
11771	*Ap2a1*	Adaptor-related protein complex 2, alpha 1 subunit
12757	*Clta*	Clathrin, light polypeptide (Lca)
13196	*Asap1*	ArfGAP with SH3 domain, ankyrin repeat and PH domain1
13429	*Dnm1*	Dynamin 1
14963	*H2-Bl*	Histocompatibility 2, blastocyst
14972	*H2-K1*	Histocompatibility 2, K1, K region
15006	*H2-Q1*	Histocompatibility 2, Q region locus 1
15007	*H2-Q10*	Histocompatibility 2, Q region locus 10
15013	*H2-Q2*	Histocompatibility 2, Q region locus 2
15018	*H2-Q7*	Histocompatibility 2, Q region locus 7
15039	*H2-T22*	Histocompatibility 2, T region locus 22
15040	*H2-T23*	Histocompatibility 2, T region locus 23
15239	*Hgs*	HGF-regulated tyrosine kinase substrate
15481	*Hspa8*	Heat shock protein 8
16835	*Ldlr*	Low density lipoprotein receptor
18717	*Pip5k1c*	Phosphatidylinositol-4-phosphate 5-kinase, type 1 gamma
234852	*Chmp1a*	Charged multivesicular body protein 1A
243621	*Iqsec3*	IQ motif and Sec7 domain 3
67588	*Rnf41*	Ring finger protein 41
98366	*Smap1*	Stromal membrane-associated protein 1
PATHWAYS POINTED BY DOWN REGULATED GENES		
VEGF signaling pathway		
11651	*Akt1*	Thymoma viral proto-oncogene 1
16653	*Kras*	v-Ki-ras2 Kirsten rat sarcoma viral oncogene homolog
19056	*Ppp3cb*	Protein phosphatase 3, catalytic subunit, beta isoform
22339	*Vegfa*	Vascular endothelial growth factor A
Long-term depression		
14678	*Gnai2*	Guanine nucleotide binding protein (G protein), alpha inhibiting 2
14683	*Gnas*	GNAS (guanine nucleotide binding protein, alpha stimulating) complex locus
16653	*Kras*	v-Ki-ras2 Kirsten rat sarcoma viral oncogene homolog
18795	*Plcb1*	Phospholipase C, beta 1
60596	*Gucy1a3*	Guanylate cyclase 1, soluble, alpha 3
Gap junction		
14678	*Gnai2*	Guanine nucleotide binding protein (G protein), alpha inhibiting 2
14683	*Gnas*	GNAS (guanine nucleotide binding protein, alpha stimulating) complex locus
16653	*Kras*	v-Ki-ras2 Kirsten rat sarcoma viral oncogene homolog
18795	*Plcb1*	Phospholipase C, beta 1
60596	*Gucy1a3*	Guanylate cyclase 1, soluble, alpha 3

(Continued)

Table 4 | Continued

Gene ID	Gene symbol	Gene name
RNA degradation		
104625	*Cnot6*	CCR4-NOT transcription complex, subunit 6
13209	*Ddx6*	DEAD (Asp-Glu-Ala-Asp) box polypeptide 6
66373	*Lsm5*	LSM5 homolog, U6 small nuclear RNA associated (S. cerevisiae)
72662	*Dis3*	DIS3 mitotic control homolog (S. cerevisiae)
78651	*Lsm6*	LSM6 homolog, U6 small nuclear RNA associated (S. cerevisiae)
Parkinson's disease		
12866	*Cox7a2*	Cytochrome c oxidase subunit VIIa 2
333182	*Cox6b2*	Cytochrome c oxidase subunit VIb polypeptide 2
66142	*Cox7b*	Cytochrome c oxidase subunit VIIb
66495	*Ndufb3*	NADH dehydrogenase (ubiquinone) 1 beta subcomplex 3
66916	*Ndufb7*	NADH dehydrogenase (ubiquinone) 1 beta subcomplex, 7
68202	*Ndufa5*	NADH dehydrogenase (ubiquinone) 1 alpha subcomplex, 5
Oxidative phosphorylation		
12866	*Cox7a2*	Cytochrome c oxidase subunit VIIa 2
333182	*Cox6b2*	Cytochrome c oxidase subunit VIb polypeptide 2
66142	*Cox7b*	Cytochrome c oxidase subunit VIIb
66495	*Ndufb3*	NADH dehydrogenase (ubiquinone) 1 beta subcomplex 3
66916	*Ndufb7*	NADH dehydrogenase (ubiquinone) 1 beta subcomplex, 7
68202	*Ndufa5*	NADH dehydrogenase (ubiquinone) 1 alpha subcomplex, 5
Tight junction		
11651	*Akt1*	Thymoma viral proto-oncogene 1
14678	*Gnai2*	Guanine nucleotide binding protein (G protein), alpha inhibiting 2
16653	*Kras*	v-Ki-ras2 Kirsten rat sarcoma viral oncogene homolog
17888	*Myh6*	Myosin, heavy polypeptide 6, cardiac muscle, alpha
30960	*Vapa*	Vesicle-associated membrane protein, associated protein A
58187	*Cldn10*	Claudin 10
Glutamatergic synapse		
14678	*Gnai2*	Guanine nucleotide binding protein (G protein), alpha inhibiting 2
14683	*Gnas*	GNAS (guanine nucleotide binding protein, alpha stimulating) complex locus
14702	*Gng2*	Guanine nucleotide binding protein (G protein), gamma 2
14802	*Gria4*	Glutamate receptor, ionotropic, AMPA4 (alpha 4)
14805	*Grik1*	Glutamate receptor, ionotropic, kainate 1
18795	*Plcb1*	Phospholipase C, beta 1
19056	*Ppp3cb*	Protein phosphatase 3, catalytic subunit, beta isoform
216227	*Slc17a8*	Solute carrier family 17 (sodium-dependent inorganic phosphate cotransporter), member 8

(Continued)

Table 4 | Continued

Gene ID	Gene symbol	Gene name
Huntington's disease		
12866	*Cox7a2*	Cytochrome c oxidase subunit VIIa 2
18795	*Plcb1*	Phospholipase C, beta 1
333182	*Cox6b2*	Cytochrome c oxidase subunit VIb polypeptide 2
66142	*Cox7b*	Cytochrome c oxidase subunit VIIb
66495	*Ndufb3*	NADH dehydrogenase (ubiquinone) 1 beta subcomplex 3
66916	*Ndufb7*	NADH dehydrogenase (ubiquinone) 1 beta subcomplex, 7
68202	*Ndufa5*	NADH dehydrogenase (ubiquinone) 1 alpha subcomplex, 5
69920	*Polr2i*	Polymerase (RNA) II (DNA directed) polypeptide I
Alzheimer's disease		
11820	*App*	Amyloid beta (A4) precursor protein
12866	*Cox7a2*	Cytochrome c oxidase subunit VIIa 2
18795	*Plcb1*	Phospholipase C, beta 1
19056	*Ppp3cb*	Protein phosphatase 3, catalytic subunit, beta isoform
333182	*Cox6b2*	Cytochrome c oxidase subunit VIb polypeptide 2
66142	*Cox7b*	Cytochrome c oxidase subunit VIIb
66495	*Ndufb3*	NADH dehydrogenase (ubiquinone) 1 beta subcomplex 3
66916	*Ndufb7*	NADH dehydrogenase (ubiquinone) 1 beta subcomplex, 7
68202	*Ndufa5*	NADH dehydrogenase (ubiquinone) 1 alpha subcomplex, 5
Ribosome		
19951	*Rpl32*	Ribosomal protein L32
19981	*Rpl37a*	Ribosomal protein L37a
19982	*Rpl36a*	Ribosomal protein L36A
20068	*Rps17*	Ribosomal protein S17
20085	*Rps19*	Ribosomal protein S19
22186	*Uba52*	Ubiquitin A-52 residue ribosomal protein fusion product 1
57294	*Rps27*	Ribosomal protein S27
66489	*Rpl35*	Ribosomal protein L35
67945	*Rpl41*	Ribosomal protein L41
68028	*Rpl22l1*	Ribosomal protein L22 like 1
75617	*Rps25*	Ribosomal protein S25

subtle changes in gene expression are exactly those that occur in initial stages of disease before the onset of clinical symptoms (Druyan et al., 2008). Moreover, some authors have argued that even small differences can be biologically relevant (Pedotti et al., 2008). Indeed, our qPCR verification analysis revealed higher fold changes than in the microarray, reaching values higher than 2 in the 80 days pre-symptomatic phase, which is closer to the symptom onset. The use of qPCR analysis to qualitatively verify the microarray results is largely accepted in the literature. However, it is well recognized that both methods have quantitative differences (Chuaqui et al., 2002), which are

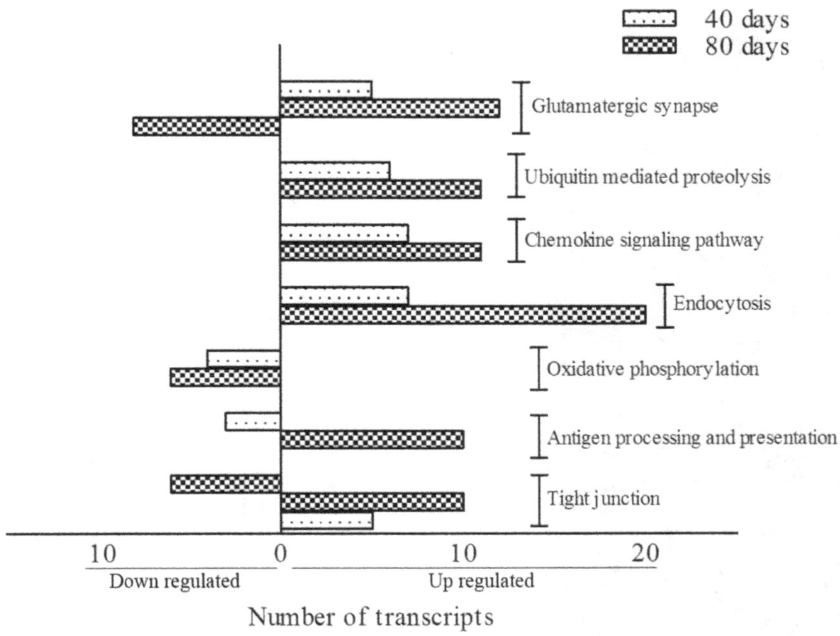

FIGURE 1 | KEGG pathways classification showing the number of transcripts up regulated and down regulated per category in 40 and 80 days pre-symptomatic SOD1^{G93A} mice in relation to age matched wild-types. Bars on the left indicate the number of down regulated genes, and bars on the right indicate the number of up regulated genes, for each category.

thought to be related to the variation in the hybridization kinetics of the technologies, low fold changes or lack of concordance between transcripts accessed in each method. The number of genes employed in qPCR validation is comparable to that found by other studies (Dallas et al., 2005; Brockington et al., 2010).

The differentially expressed genes with a p-value lower than 0.05 were submitted to enrichment analyses based on GO and KEGG databases, which correlated genes to already described related pathways and processes. Modulated genes based on GO evidenced more general biological processes that might be implicated in the ALS mechanisms. Of interest, regulation of astrocyte differentiation, protein retention in endoplasmatic reticulum lumen, Golgi vesicle transport and fructose metabolism, among others, were pointed at the pre-symptomatic 40 days old transgenic mice. At later pre-symptomatic phase of 80 days, the pattern of gene expression identified the GO terms post-Golgi vesicle-mediated transport, tricarboxylic acid cycle (TCA) and mRNA processing, among others. GO database analyses have been largely employed in the ALS research in several phases of the disease (Ferraiuolo et al., 2007, 2011a; Brockington et al., 2010).

Authors have also used the KEGG database to identify over-represented pathways based on differentially expressed genes obtained by the microarray technique (Mougeot et al., 2011; Kalathur et al., 2012). The KEGG database analysis in the present work pointed to pathways that might be related to ALS mechanism at the pre-symptomatic ages of SOD1^{G93A} mice. Some pathways were found to be common to both pre-symptomatic periods, emphasizing the putative toxic triggering that may last before the onset of classical ALS symptoms with possible significance to mechanisms of initiation of motor neuron degeneration.

Those pathways are going to be discussed below. It should be mentioned that alternative splicing have been recently implicated in ALS mechanisms (Lenzken et al., 2011; Singh and Cooper, 2012), however we could not access this biological event because the present analysis employed a platform designed to gene expression studies on 3′UTR that does not allow evaluation of alternative splicing variants.

GLUTAMATERGIC SYNAPSE

The microarray profiling study by means of KEEG enriched analysis pointed to the category of glutamatergic synapse pathway in the lumbar spinal cord of ALS SOD1^{G93A}. The large number of up regulated genes at 40 and 80 days underlines the excitotoxicity estate mediated by glutamatergic synapse of motor neurons in the pre-symptomatic condition of ALS disease (Bendotti et al., 2001; Gibb et al., 2007; Zhao et al., 2008; Jiang et al., 2009; Sunico et al., 2011). The modulation of GluR4, by means of *Gria4* findings in our microarray analysis, might reflect the dynamic state of the AMPA receptor subunit in the course of pre-symptomatic stages of ALS. At the early phases of the pre-symptomatic period, highly expressed *Gria4* gene might contribute to the AMPA receptor-mediated motor neuron toxicity, being a very early mechanism of the disease. The down regulation of the *Gria4* at the late pre-symptomatic stage could reflect a transient reactive mechanism to excitotoxic condition preceding motor neuron death. Reductions of GluR4 have been described at cellular level in the late disease stage of SOD1 mice, without alterations at the pre-symptomatic periods (Petri et al., 2005) thus, reflecting a disappearance of GluR4 containing neurons. In fact, imbalance of excitatory to inhibitory synaptic function precedes motor neuron degeneration

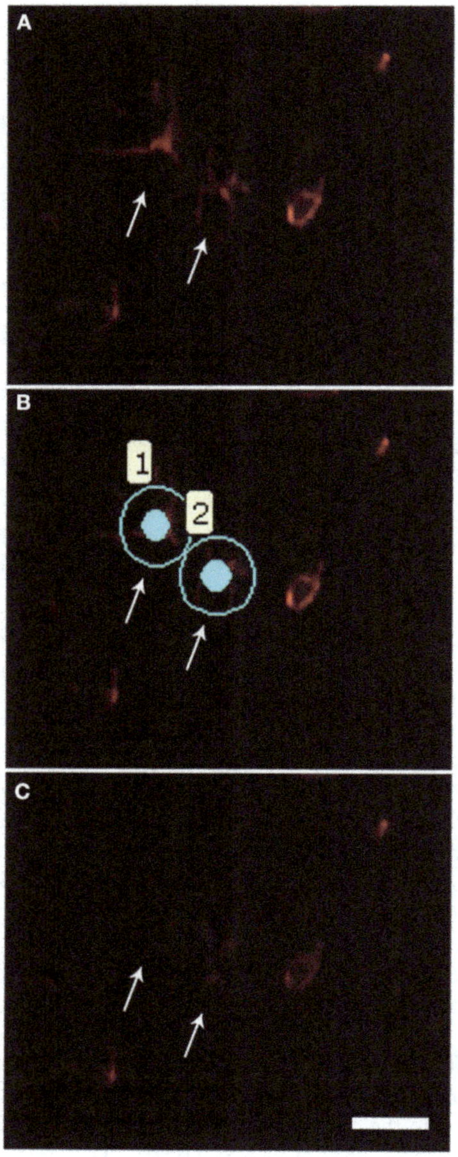

FIGURE 2 | Photomicrographs illustrating astrocyte laser microdissection process. (A) The quick GFAP immunofluorescence allows recognizing the astrocytic profiles (arrows). **(B)** Astrocytes (1 and 2) were then selected for microdissection. **(C)** After laser firing and microdissection, selected cells (arrows) can no longer be visualized in the tissue. Scale bars of 20 μm.

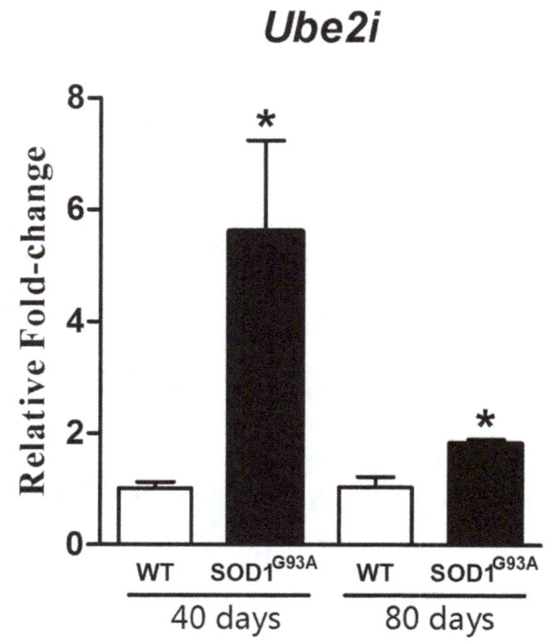

FIGURE 3 | Graph shows relative fold change values for *Ube2i* in microdissected astrocytes from 40 and 80 days old SOD1^{G93A} mice compared to the age matched wild-type controls (WT). Significant increases are seen in both transgenic astrocytes enriched samples. Results are presented as means ± s.e.m. from 3 samples used for each group. **p*-value < 0.05, according to unpaired *t*-test.

as described in the spinal cord motor neurons in the late stage of pre-symptomatic phase of SOD1 ALS model by means of cellular analyses (Schutz, 2005). It should be mentioned that Ca^{2+} permeability of the AMPA receptor seems to occur mainly by the presence of the GluR2 subunit in the receptor complex. In fact, GluR2 deficiency clearly accelerated the motor neuron degeneration and shortened the life span of mutant SOD1^{G93A} double transgenic mice (Tateno et al., 2004). Synaptic GluR1 increases/mRNA up regulation, and decreases of synaptic and total GluR2 were found at early ages prior to disease onset thus prompting motor neurons to a higher Ca^{2+}-permeable AMPA receptors -induced excitotoxicity (Zhao et al., 2008). The variant C-terminus of GluR4 (GluR4c), an alternative splicing isoform, stabilizes and locates AMPA receptors in the cell membrane, and also seems to potentate actions of GluR2 (Kawahara et al., 2004), thus highlighting the pivotal role of GluR4 subunit in regulating channel properties and trafficking of AMPA receptors. It must be then further clarified the role of GluR4 in the ALS mechanisms and possible dynamic interaction with that subunit with other AMPA receptor subtypes, especially GluR2.

The regulation of *Slc1a2* glial glutamate transporter (named EAAT2 or glial glutamate transporter GLT1) has not been evaluated in details. Excitotoxicity caused by a down-regulation of EAAT2 is thought to be a contributing factor to motor neuron death in ALS. Several mechanisms may account for impairment of EAAT2 function, for instance altered transcription/splicing, post-translational modifications, accelerated degradation, intracellular trafficking and inactivation by caspase-3 cleavage (Heath and Shaw, 2002; Boston-Howes et al., 2006) but not directly to gene regulation processes. It is possible that the impaired EAAT2 function could take place at the very early period of the pre-symptomatic stage, a matter that remains to be elucidated (Bendotti et al., 2001; Sasaki et al., 2001), thus, explaining the *Slc1a2* expression possibly related to motor neuron protection at those ages. The absence of this genomic process in the late pre-symptomatic period might potentiate loss of function of GLT1 thus culminating with the motor neuron death in ALS. Furthermore, the vesicular glutamate transporter 2 (VGLUT2), codified by *Slc17a6* gene, was found to be regulated and related to neuronal death in the pre-symptomatic stage of ALS model (Schutz, 2005; Sunico et al., 2011). The genetic reduction of VGLUT2 protein level in the ALS mouse model accounted for motor neuron rescue without modifying functional impairment (Wootz et al., 2010). It is possible that the up regulation of the *Slc17a6* gene at the early pre-symptomatic stage of the 40 days old SOD1^{G93A} mice potentiates the toxic state of motor neurons.

UBIQUITIN MEDIATED PROTEOLYSIS AND OXIDATIVE PHOSPHORYLATION

A recent meta-analysis study of the reported gene lists has described the evidences for a shared dysfunction in protein turnover in the ubiquitin-proteasome system in ALS mouse models and ALS patients (Saris et al., 2013a). Moreover, constitutive proteasome was decreased in motor neurons at the pre-symptomatic stage of SOD1^{G93A} (Cheroni et al., 2005), an alternative processes to decrease aggregate formation, thus an attempt to neuroprotect motor neurons of preclinical SOD1^{G93A} mice before the onset of clinical symptoms (Bendotti et al., 2012). That should be the case of *Nedd4* and *Fbxw7* expressions described here, whose encoded molecules have been already correlated to neuroprotection in ALS (Nateri et al., 2004; Matsumoto et al., 2011; Kwak et al., 2012). Moreover, it should be taken into attention the elevation of *Ubc12* in the spinal cord of SOD1^{G93A} mice at the pre-symptomatic phase (Massignan et al., 2007). *Ubc12* is an ubiquitin E2 ligase that adds NEDD-8 to substrates. *Ubc12* elevation in pre-symptomatic ALS was correlated to a tentative response to protein aggregation (Massignan et al., 2007). Interestingly, *Nedd8* gene was down regulated in our microarray analysis only in 80 days old mice, possibly representing a failure of the above described process close to the period of clinical onset.

The down regulation of genes over-representing the oxidative phosphorylation category at both pre-symptomatic ages of ALS mice seen in this work may be related to the progressive deteriorations of mitochondrial function and oxidative phosphorylation system described at pre-symptomatic ALS phases (Lin et al., 2009; Chen et al., 2010; Martin, 2010, 2011; Koopman et al., 2013), thus triggering reactive oxygen species (ROS) production (Manfredi and Xu, 2005) and motor neuron vulnerability before the onset of clinical symptoms. It is also interesting to notice that the TCA was seen as an over-represented GO term (Table S5, Supplementary material) in the up-regulated 80 days gene expression list. The TCA cycle is responsible to provide substrate to oxidative phosphorylation (Koopman et al., 2013) and its up regulation was previously seen in laser microdissected motor neurons from a VEGF model of ALS already in the pre-symptomatic period (Brockington et al., 2010). All in all, a possible mechanism of oxidative phosphorylation in the astrocyte-neuronal unit taking place in pre-symptomatic ALS might amplify motor neuron vulnerability to ROS damage.

CHEMOKINE SIGNALING PATHWAY AND TIGHT JUNCTION

The up regulation of all genes in the category chemokine signaling pathway in the pathogenesis of ALS is in agreement to previous publications (Henkel et al., 2006; Zhang et al., 2006; Rentzos et al., 2007; Kuhle et al., 2009; Sargsyan et al., 2009; Tateishi et al., 2010; Gupta et al., 2012). The up regulation of *Cxcr4* and *Pik3r1* described in this work is an important finding because the genes might be involved in non-autonomous toxicity in the early phase of ALS (Shideman et al., 2006; Luo et al., 2007; Manzano et al., 2011). Furthermore, disruption of blood-brain barrier and blood-spinal cord barrier are described as early events in ALS, thus impairing neurovascular unit prior motor neuron degeneration (Garbuzova-Davis et al., 2011, 2012; Grammas et al., 2011; Miyazaki et al., 2011). Indeed, reduced levels of adhesion molecules and the tight junction proteins zona occludens-1, occludin and claudin-5 are shown in post mortem tissue from patients and in ALS animal models (Zhong et al., 2008; Arhart, 2010; Garbuzova-Davis et al., 2012).

Our KEGG enriched analysis also demonstrated the modulation of tight junction related genes. Of substantial interest, we might point out the up regulation of *Cldn11* at 40 days and the down regulation of *Cldn10* at 80 days pre-symptomatic ALS mice, in agreement to previous description on differential regulation of tight junction genes related to specific characteristics of ALS clinical evolution (Henkel et al., 2009).

It is also important to highlight the particular modulation of the *Kras* gene, which has been up regulated at the age of 40 days and down regulated at the age of 80 days. The *Kras* gene is an oncogene that was located in the tight junction category by the KEGG analysis probably due its relation to topography of invading/proliferating cells in the scenario of neurodegenerative processes. Moreover, Kras proteins regulate cell activities such as proliferation, differentiation, apoptosis, and cell migration, those taking place in neurodegenerative processes-induced astroglial/microglial activation as well as expression of inflammatory and neurotrophic/neurotoxic mediators (Rotshenker, 2009). There is a marked proliferation/activation of both microglia and astrocytes at specific disease stages in ALS mouse models (Hall et al., 1998; Weydt et al., 2002) leading to the production of neuroprotective or pro-inflammatory molecules, which can decrease or increase the rate of primary motor neuron degeneration, respectively. Taken all together, up regulation of *Kras* gene at the early pre-symptomatic phase is in line with the early glial proliferative and reactivity events that will initiate the toxic triggering of non-autonomous cells and also the glial neuroprotective mechanisms to maintain temporarily the motor neurons. Later in that period, still before neuronal degeneration taking place, *Kras* gene down regulation might allow glial cells to drive toxic insult.

ENDOCYTOSIS AND ANTIGEN PROCESSING AND PRESENTATION

Endocytosis was an additional over-represented pathway in the pre-symptomatic stage of ALS. Genes found before clinical onset pointing to endocytosis have been related to clathrin-dependent/independent endocytosis, autophagy and also neurotransmission (Massey et al., 2006; Luo et al., 2007; Kon and Cuervo, 2010; McMahon and Boucrot, 2011; Elmer and McAllister, 2012), thus, related to extracellular turnover, repair of molecular processes and neuroprotection (Le Roy and Wrana, 2005; Doherty and McMahon, 2009; McMahon and Boucrot, 2011; Polymenidou and Cleveland, 2011). Disruption of these processes has been implicated as a general feature in the pathogenesis of ALS (Otomo et al., 2012), whereas there is a lack of information on that issue in pre-symptomatic periods

(Morimoto et al., 2007; Tian et al., 2011). Clathrin-mediated endocytosis has a range of different physiological functions, remarkably the regulation of surface proteins, nutrition, activation of signaling pathways, protein trafficking and degradation of membrane components, in fact, mechanisms that might occur at the pre-symptomatic phases of ALS.

It is likely that the regulation of the genes for the heat shock proteins *Hspa1a* and *Hspa8* (also known as Hsp70-3 and Hsc70, respectively), described in our work is related to neuroprotective events before neurodegeneration, once treatment with recombinant human Hsp70 was able to both increase lifespan (Gifondorwa et al., 2007) and decrease neuromuscular junction denervation (Gifondorwa et al., 2012) in the SOD1^{G93A} mouse model. This protective role of Hsp70 has been also supported by other authors (Bruening et al., 1999; Takeuchi et al., 2002; Kieran et al., 2004). Actually, the increase of Hsc70 in the spinal cord of transgenic mice at pre-symptomatic ages of disease (Basso et al., 2009) and the demonstration of ubiquitinated Hsc70-induced degradation of mutant SOD1 (Urushitani et al., 2004) emphasized the possible neuroprotective role of heat shock protein regulation described in our work.

Furthermore, antigen processing and presentation pathway was also pointed as enriched among down regulated genes in 40 days old and up regulated genes in 80 days old pre-symptomatic SOD1^{G93A} mice. Genes presented in 40 and 80 days lists are mostly related to major histocompatibility complex (MHC) class I (*H2-Bl, H2-K1, H2-Q1, H2-Q10, H2-Q2, H2-Q7, H2-T22, H2-T23*—80 days ALS mice), molecules necessary for peptide loading (*Tap2*—80 days ALS mice) and to surface expression (*B2m*—40 days ALS mice) (Kimura and Griffin, 2000). *B2m* gene, possibly via cell surface MHC class I molecules, has been implicated in the synaptic plasticity at dendrites and axonal regeneration after peripheral nerve axotomy (Oliveira et al., 2004). It is possible that the down regulation of *B2m* in spinal cord from SOD1^{G93A}at pre-symptomatic ages is related to axonal and dendritic retractions and displacement of neuromuscular junction described as one of the earliest events faced by motor neurons in ALS models (Fischer et al., 2004). Our findings are in line with a description of down regulation of B2m protein reported in cerebrospinal fluid of ALS patients (Brettschneider et al., 2008), thus emphasizing the importance of its regulation in ALS. Additionally, *Rfxank* was down regulated at 40 days in our analysis, which is in agreement to a loss of MHC-II neuronal expression concurrent with abundant MHCII-positive microglia surrounding motor neurons in the pre-symptomatic SOD1^{G93A} mice (Casas et al., 2013), thus, interfering with the neuroimmunemodulation mediated by microglia (Graber et al., 2010; Sanagi et al., 2010). All in all, dysregulation of genes related to antigen processing and presentation might account for a number of intercellular mechanisms able to amplify the harmful non-autonomous cell toxicity at the pre-symptomatic stages of ALS.

LASER MICRODISSECTION OF ASTROCYTES

We performed laser microdissection of GFAP positive astrocytes from lumbar spinal cord ventral horn of SOD1^{G93A} transgenic and wild-type mice in the same pre-symptomatic ages of microarray analysis. The use of laser microdissection has been gained importance in recent years, once it allows specific cell enrichment from complex tissues, revealing to be a powerful tool in the study of neurodegenerative disorders in which individual cell types are known to be differentially involved in disease stages. The advantage of the methodology is the possibility to address molecular biology in the context of *in vivo* cellular analysis. The method is of substantial importance to evaluate changes in the astrocytes, the glial cell involved remarkably in toxic mechanisms of ALS. A previous study has employed laser microdissection of astrocytes to perform microarray experiments in ALS mouse model (Ferraiuolo et al., 2011a). The pattern of gene expression was first evaluated in the lumbar regions of the spinal cord in the present analysis, thus, taking into account all cell types from tissue. The depicted pathways represented the state of intercellular interaction in the pre-symptomatic studied periods of the ALS mouse model. The selected genes to be evaluated in type-specific cell, which is the case of *Ube2i* in the laser microdissected astrocytes described herein, would allow a closer analysis of astrocyte participation in the context of the neighbor cell toxicity. The *Ube2i* gene was then chosen for further evaluation in astrocytes by qPCR because astrocytes exert a non-autonomous cell toxicity to motor neurons and because SUMOylation pathway has gained importance in ALS mechanisms recently (for review, see Dangoumau et al., 2013). Increases of gene expression for *Ube2i* were found in enriched astrocytes samples from 40 and 80 days old pre-symptomatic mice, a regulation still not presented in the literature in that stage of disease, thus, entering in the context of ALS pathogenesis. In fact, conjugation of small ubiquitin-like modifier (SUMO) molecules involves a series of steps, being the ubiquitin conjugating enzyme E2, codified by *Ube2i* gene, responsible for the recognition of the target protein. SUMOylation is involved in the cellular response to oxidative stress, hypoxia, glutamate excitotoxicity and proteasome impairment, events that have been linked to motor neuron toxicity in ALS (Xu et al., 2011). Moreover, studies are required to determine the precise implication of the SUMO pathway in regulating the balance between cellular adaptive and neuroprotective response to stress (Fei et al., 2006; Dangoumau et al., 2013) with a special importance to motor neuron in the pre-symptomatic stage of ALS. Nevertheless, as discussed previously in this report, glutamate astroglial excitotoxicity faced by motor neurons in ALS is also hamfull by the cleavage of EAAT2 in the ventral horn of the spinal cord (Martin et al., 2007; Foran et al., 2011). The proteolytic fragments may be SUMOylated and accumulated in the nucleus of astrocytes (Boston-Howes et al., 2006; Foran et al., 2011) as described in SOD1^{G93A} mice, worsening the gliotoxic effects of astrocytes to motor neurons (Foran et al., 2011). Taking together, SUMOylation process and expression of *Ube2i* might participate in complex events related to the astrocyte-neuron unit in ALS, and future works are required to address specific cellular events.

In conclusion, the present work gives further evidence about molecular events taking place in the spinal cord from ALS mouse model before the onset of classical symptoms. The gene expression changes reflect responses for both neuroprotection and toxicity at the spinal cord in the evaluated periods. Indeed, the study of Ube2i expression in astrocytes adds novel insights for the participation of this cell type on the early mechanisms in ALS.

AUTHOR CONTRIBUTIONS

Gabriela Pintar de Oliveira and Chrystian J. Alves performed the experiments. All authors designed the study, analyzed the results and wrote the manuscript. All authors read and approved the final manuscript.

ACKNOWLEDGMENTS

Grant #2010/20457-7, São Paulo Research Foundation (FAPESP). I would like to thanks Dr. Jessica Ruivo Maximino for establishing the SOD1^{G93A} mouse colony in the Animal Facility of FMUSP and advices on animal handling and tissue processing. We also thanks Drs. Dirce Maria Carraro and Alex Fiorini de Carvalho from Laboratory of Genomics and Molecular Biology, A.C. Camargo Hospital, São Paulo, Brazil, for expertise on microarray experiments and Dr. Chin Jia Lin, responsible for Laser Microdissection Microscope Facility at FMUSP, for his expertise on laser microdissection experiments. Indeed, we thank Dr. Pamela J Shaw, from Sheffield University, and her research team for the support in the microarray analysis.

REFERENCES

Alves, C. J., De Santana, L. P., Dos Santos, A. J., De Oliveira, G. P., Duobles, T., Scorisa, J. M., et al. (2011). Early motor and electrophysiological changes in transgenic mouse model of amyotrophic lateral sclerosis and gender differences on clinical outcome. *Brain Res.* 1394, 90–104. doi: 10.1016/j.brainres.2011.02.060

Andersen, P. M., and Al-Chalabi, A. (2011). Clinical genetics of amyotrophic lateral sclerosis: what do we really know? *Nat. Rev. Neurol.* 7, 603–615. doi: 10.1038/nrneurol.2011.150

Arhart, R. W. (2010). A possible haemodynamic mechanism for amyotrophic lateral sclerosis. *Med. Hypotheses* 75, 341–346. doi: 10.1016/j.mehy.2010.03.017

Basso, M., Samengo, G., Nardo, G., Massignan, T., D'alessandro, G., Tartari, S., et al. (2009). Characterization of detergent-insoluble proteins in ALS indicates a causal link between nitrative stress and aggregation in pathogenesis. *PLoS ONE* 4:e8130. doi: 10.1371/journal.pone.0008130

Beghi, E., Logroscino, G., Chio, A., Hardiman, O., Mitchell, D., Swingler, R., et al. (2006). The epidemiology of ALS and the role of population-based registries. *Biochim. Biophys. Acta* 1762, 1150–1157. doi: 10.1016/j.bbadis.2006.09.008

Bendotti, C., Marino, M., Cheroni, C., Fontana, E., Crippa, V., Poletti, A., et al. (2012). Dysfunction of constitutive and inducible ubiquitin-proteasome system in amyotrophic lateral sclerosis: implication for protein aggregation and immune response. *Prog. Neurobiol.* 97, 101–126. doi: 10.1016/j.pneurobio.2011.10.001

Bendotti, C., Tortarolo, M., Suchak, S. K., Calvaresi, N., Carvelli, L., Bastone, A., et al. (2001). Transgenic SOD1 G93A mice develop reduced GLT-1 in spinal cord without alterations in cerebrospinal fluid glutamate levels. *J. Neurochem.* 79, 737–746. doi: 10.1046/j.1471-4159.2001.00572.x

Bergeron, C., Beric-Maskarel, K., Muntasser, S., Weyer, L., Somerville, M. J., and Percy, M. E. (1994). Neurofilament light and polyadenylated mRNA levels are decreased in amyotrophic lateral sclerosis motor neurons. *J. Neuropathol. Exp. Neurol.* 53, 221–230. doi: 10.1097/00005072-199405000-00002

Boillee, S., Vande Velde, C., and Cleveland, D. W. (2006a). ALS: a disease of motor neurons and their nonneuronal neighbors. *Neuron* 52, 39–59. doi: 10.1016/j.neuron.2006.09.018

Boillee, S., Yamanaka, K., Lobsiger, C. S., Copeland, N. G., Jenkins, N. A., Kassiotis, G., et al. (2006b). Onset and progression in inherited ALS determined by motor neurons and microglia. *Science* 312, 1389–1392. doi: 10.1126/science.1123511

Boston-Howes, W., Gibb, S. L., Williams, E. O., Pasinelli, P., Brown, R. H. Jr., and Trotti, D. (2006). Caspase-3 cleaves and inactivates the glutamate transporter EAAT2. *J. Biol. Chem.* 281, 14076–14084. doi: 10.1074/jbc.M600653200

Brettschneider, J., Mogel, H., Lehmensiek, V., Ahlert, T., Sussmuth, S., Ludolph, A. C., et al. (2008). Proteome analysis of cerebrospinal fluid in amyotrophic lateral sclerosis (ALS). *Neurochem. Res.* 33, 2358–2363. doi: 10.1007/s11064-008-9742-5

Brockington, A., Heath, P. R., Holden, H., Kasher, P., Bender, F. L., Claes, F., et al. (2010). Downregulation of genes with a function in axon outgrowth and synapse formation in motor neurones of the VEGFdelta/delta mouse model of amyotrophic lateral sclerosis. *BMC Genomics* 11:203. doi: 10.1186/1471-2164-11-203

Brooks, B. R., Miller, R. G., Swash, M., and Munsat, T. L. (2000). El Escorial revisited: revised criteria for the diagnosis of amyotrophic lateral sclerosis. *Amyotroph. Lateral Scler. Other Motor Neuron Disord.* 1, 293–299. doi: 10.1080/146608200300079536

Bruening, W., Roy, J., Giasson, B., Figlewicz, D. A., Mushynski, W. E., and Durham, H. D. (1999). Up-regulation of protein chaperones preserves viability of cells expressing toxic Cu/Zn-superoxide dismutase mutants associated with amyotrophic lateral sclerosis. *J. Neurochem.* 72, 693–699. doi: 10.1046/j.1471-4159.1999.0720693.x

Casas, C., Herrando-Grabulosa, M., Manzano, R., Mancuso, R., Osta, R., and Navarro, X. (2013). Early presymptomatic cholinergic dysfunction in a murine model of amyotrophic lateral sclerosis. *Brain Behav* 3, 145–158. doi: 10.1002/brb3.104

Chen, K., Northington, F. J., and Martin, L. J. (2010). Inducible nitric oxide synthase is present in motor neuron mitochondria and Schwann cells and contributes to disease mechanisms in ALS mice. *Brain Struct. Funct.* 214, 219–234. doi: 10.1007/s00429-009-0226-4

Cheroni, C., Peviani, M., Cascio, P., Debiasi, S., Monti, C., and Bendotti, C. (2005). Accumulation of human SOD1 and ubiquitinated deposits in the spinal cord of SOD1G93A mice during motor neuron disease progression correlates with a decrease of proteasome. *Neurobiol. Dis.* 18, 509–522. doi: 10.1016/j.nbd.2004.12.007

Chuaqui, R. F., Bonner, R. F., Best, C. J., Gillespie, J. W., Flaig, M. J., Hewitt, S. M., et al. (2002). Post-analysis follow-up and validation of microarray experiments. *Nat. Genet.* 32(Suppl.), 509–514. doi:10.1038/ng1034

Dallas, P. B., Gottardo, N. G., Firth, M. J., Beesley, A. H., Hoffmann, K., Terry, P. A., et al. (2005). Gene expression levels assessed by oligonucleotide microarray analysis and quantitative real-time RT-PCR—how well do they correlate? *BMC Genomics* 6:59. doi:10.1186/1471-2164-6-59

Dangond, F., Hwang, D., Camelo, S., Pasinelli, P., Frosch, M. P., Stephanopoulos, G., et al. (2004). Molecular signature of late-stage human ALS revealed by expression profiling of postmortem spinal cord gray matter. *Physiol. Genomics* 16, 229–239. doi: 10.1152/physiolgenomics.00087.2001

Dangoumau, A., Veyrat-Durebex, C., Blasco, H., Praline, J., Corcia, P., Andres, C. R., et al. (2013). Protein SUMOylation, an emerging pathway in amyotrophic lateral sclerosis. *Int. J. Neurosci.* 123, 366–374. doi: 10.3109/00207454.2012.761984

D'arrigo, A., Colavito, D., Pena-Altamira, E., Fabris, M., Dam, M., Contestabile, A., et al. (2010). Transcriptional profiling in the lumbar spinal cord of a mouse model of amyotrophic lateral sclerosis: a role for wild-type superoxide dismutase 1 in sporadic disease? *J. Mol. Neurosci.* 41, 404–415. doi: 10.1007/s12031-010-9332-2

De Oliveira, G. P., Maximino, J. R., Lin, C. J., and Chadi, G. (2009). A method to immunolabel rodent spinal cord neurons and glia for molecular study in specific laser microdissected cells involved in neurodegenerative disorders. *J. Mol. Histol.* 40, 217–225. doi: 10.1007/s10735-009-9233-2

De Winter, F., Vo, T., Stam, F. J., Wisman, L. A., Bar, P. R., Niclou, S. P., et al. (2006). The expression of the chemorepellent Semaphorin 3A is selectively induced in terminal Schwann cells of a subset of neuromuscular synapses that display limited anatomical plasticity and enhanced vulnerability in motor neuron disease. *Mol. Cell. Neurosci.* 32, 102–117. doi: 10.1016/j.mcn.2006.03.002

Dion, P. A., Daoud, H., and Rouleau, G. A. (2009). Genetics of motor neuron disorders: new insights into pathogenic mechanisms. *Nat. Rev. Genet.* 10, 769–782. doi: 10.1038/nrg2680

Doherty, G. J., and McMahon, H. T. (2009). Mechanisms of endocytosis. *Annu. Rev. Biochem.* 78, 857–902. doi: 10.1146/annurev.biochem.78.081307.110540

Druyan, S., de Oliveira, J. E., and Ashwell, C. M. (2008). Focused microarrays as a method to evaluate subtle changes in gene expression. *Poult. Sci.* 87, 2418–2429. doi: 10.3382/ps.2007-00513

Elmer, B. M., and McAllister, A. K. (2012). Major histocompatibility complex class I proteins in brain development and plasticity. *Trends Neurosci.* 35, 660–670. doi: 10.1016/j.tins.2012.08.001

Fei, E., Jia, N., Yan, M., Ying, Z., Sun, Q., Wang, H., et al. (2006). SUMO-1 modification increases human SOD1 stability and aggregation. *Biochem. Biophys. Res. Commun.* 347, 406–412. doi: 10.1016/j.bbrc.2006.06.092

Ferraiuolo, L., Heath, P. R., Holden, H., Kasher, P., Kirby, J., and Shaw, P. J. (2007). Microarray analysis of the cellular pathways involved in the adaptation to and progression of motor neuron injury in the SOD1 G93A mouse model of familial ALS. *J. Neurosci.* 27, 9201–9219. doi: 10.1523/JNEUROSCI.1470-07.2007

Ferraiuolo, L., Higginbottom, A., Heath, P. R., Barber, S., Greenald, D., Kirby, J., et al. (2011a). Dysregulation of astrocyte-motoneuron cross-talk in mutant superoxide dismutase 1-related amyotrophic lateral sclerosis. *Brain* 134, 2627–2641. doi: 10.1093/brain/awr193

Ferraiuolo, L., Kirby, J., Grierson, A. J., Sendtner, M., and Shaw, P. J. (2011b). Molecular pathways of motor neuron injury in amyotrophic lateral sclerosis. *Nat. Rev. Neurol.* 7, 616–630. doi: 10.1038/nrneurol.2011.152

Fischer, L. R., Culver, D. G., Tennant, P., Davis, A. A., Wang, M., Castellano-Sanchez, A., et al. (2004). Amyotrophic lateral sclerosis is a distal axonopathy: evidence in mice and man. *Exp. Neurol.* 185, 232–240. doi: 10.1016/j.expneurol.2003.10.004

Foran, E., Bogush, A., Goffredo, M., Roncaglia, P., Gustincich, S., Pasinelli, P., et al. (2011). Motor neuron impairment mediated by a sumoylated fragment of the glial glutamate transporter EAAT2. *Glia* 59, 1719–1731. doi: 10.1002/glia.21218

Garbuzova-Davis, S., Hernandez-Ontiveros, D. G., Rodrigues, M. C., Haller, E., Frisina-Deyo, A., Mirtyl, S., et al. (2012). Impaired blood-brain/spinal cord barrier in ALS patients. *Brain Res.* 1469, 114–128. doi: 10.1016/j.brainres.2012.05.056

Garbuzova-Davis, S., Rodrigues, M. C., Hernandez-Ontiveros, D. G., Louis, M. K., Willing, A. E., Borlongan, C. V., et al. (2011). Amyotrophic lateral sclerosis: a neurovascular disease. *Brain Res.* 1398, 113–125. doi: 10.1016/j.brainres.2011.04.049

Gentleman, R. C., Carey, V. J., Bates, D. M., Bolstad, B., Dettling, M., Dudoit, S., et al. (2004). Bioconductor: open software development for computational biology and bioinformatics. *Genome Biol.* 5:R80. doi: 10.1186/gb-2004-5-10-r80

Gerber, Y. N., Sabourin, J. C., Rabano, M., Vivanco, M., and Perrin, F. E. (2012). Early functional deficit and microglial disturbances in a mouse model of amyotrophic lateral sclerosis. *PLoS ONE* 7:e36000. doi: 10.1371/journal.pone.0036000

Gibb, S. L., Boston-Howes, W., Lavina, Z. S., Gustincich, S., Brown, R. H. Jr., Pasinelli, P., et al. (2007). A caspase-3-cleaved fragment of the glial glutamate transporter EAAT2 is sumoylated and targeted to promyelocytic leukemia nuclear bodies in mutant SOD1-linked amyotrophic lateral sclerosis. *J. Biol. Chem.* 282, 32480–32490. doi: 10.1074/jbc.M704314200

Gifondorwa, D. J., Jimenz-Moreno, R., Hayes, C. D., Rouhani, H., Robinson, M. B., Strupe, J. L., et al. (2012). Administration of recombinant heat shock protein 70 delays peripheral muscle denervation in the SOD1(G93A) mouse model of Amyotrophic Lateral Sclerosis. *Neurol. Res. Int.* 2012, 170426. doi: 10.1155/2012/170426

Gifondorwa, D. J., Robinson, M. B., Hayes, C. D., Taylor, A. R., Prevette, D. M., Oppenheim, R. W., et al. (2007). Exogenous delivery of heat shock protein 70 increases lifespan in a mouse model of amyotrophic lateral sclerosis. *J. Neurosci.* 27, 13173–13180. doi: 10.1523/JNEUROSCI.4057-07.2007

Graber, D. J., Hickey, W. F., and Harris, B. T. (2010). Progressive changes in microglia and macrophages in spinal cord and peripheral nerve in the transgenic rat model of amyotrophic lateral sclerosis. *J. Neuroinflammation* 7, 8. doi: 10.1186/1742-2094-7-8

Grammas, P., Martinez, J., and Miller, B. (2011). Cerebral microvascular endothelium and the pathogenesis of neurodegenerative diseases. *Expert Rev. Mol. Med.* 13, e19. doi: 10.1017/S1462399411001918

Guipponi, M., Li, Q. X., Hyde, L., Beissbarth, T., Smyth, G. K., Masters, C. L., et al. (2010). SAGE analysis of genes differentially expressed in presymptomatic TgSOD1G93A transgenic mice identified cellular processes involved in early stage of ALS pathology. *J. Mol. Neurosci.* 41, 172–182. doi: 10.1007/s12031-009-9317-1

Gupta, P. K., Prabhakar, S., Sharma, N. K., and Anand, A. (2012). Possible association between expression of chemokine receptor-2 (CCR2) and amyotrophic lateral sclerosis (ALS) patients of North India. *PLoS ONE* 7:e38382. doi: 10.1371/journal.pone.0038382

Gurney, M. E. (1994). Transgenic-mouse model of amyotrophic lateral sclerosis. *N. Engl. J. Med.* 331, 1721–1722. doi: 10.1056/NEJM199412223312516

Hall, E. D., Oostveen, J. A., and Gurney, M. E. (1998). Relationship of microglial and astrocytic activation to disease onset and progression in a transgenic model of familial ALS. *Glia* 23, 249–256. doi: 10.1002/(SICI)1098-1136(199807)23:3

Heath, P. R., and Shaw, P. J. (2002). Update on the glutamatergic neurotransmitter system and the role of excitotoxicity in amyotrophic lateral sclerosis. *Muscle Nerve* 26, 438–458. doi: 10.1002/mus.10186

Henkel, J. S., Beers, D. R., Siklos, L., and Appel, S. H. (2006). The chemokine MCP-1 and the dendritic and myeloid cells it attracts are increased in the mSOD1 mouse model of ALS. *Mol. Cell. Neurosci.* 31, 427–437. doi: 10.1016/j.mcn.2005.10.016

Henkel, J. S., Beers, D. R., Wen, S., Bowser, R., and Appel, S. H. (2009). Decreased mRNA expression of tight junction proteins in lumbar spinal cords of patients with ALS. *Neurology* 72, 1614–1616. doi: 10.1212/WNL.0b013e3181a41228

Jiang, M., Schuster, J. E., Fu, R., Siddique, T., and Heckman, C. J. (2009). Progressive changes in synaptic inputs to motoneurons in adult sacral spinal cord of a mouse model of amyotrophic lateral sclerosis. *J. Neurosci.* 29, 15031–15038. doi: 10.1523/JNEUROSCI.0574-09.2009

Jiang, Y. M., Yamamoto, M., Kobayashi, Y., Yoshihara, T., Liang, Y., Terao, S., et al. (2005). Gene expression profile of spinal motor neurons in sporadic amyotrophic lateral sclerosis. *Ann. Neurol.* 57, 236–251. doi: 10.1002/ana.20379

Kalathur, R. K., Hernandez-Prieto, M. A., and Futschik, M. E. (2012). Huntington's disease and its therapeutic target genes: a global functional profile based on the HD Research Crossroads database. *BMC Neurol.* 12:47. doi: 10.1186/1471-2377-12-47

Kawahara, Y., Ito, K., Sun, H., Ito, M., Kanazawa, I., and Kwak, S. (2004). Regulation of glutamate receptor RNA editing and ADAR mRNA expression in developing human normal and Down's syndrome brains. *Brain Res. Dev. Brain Res.* 148, 151–155. doi: 10.1016/j.devbrainres.2003.11.008

Kieran, D., Kalmar, B., Dick, J. R., Riddoch-Contreras, J., Burnstock, G., and Greensmith, L. (2004). Treatment with arimoclomol, a coinducer of heat shock proteins, delays disease progression in ALS mice. *Nat. Med.* 10, 402–405. doi: 10.1038/nm1021

Kiernan, M. C., Vucic, S., Cheah, B. C., Turner, M. R., Eisen, A., Hardiman, O., et al. (2011). Amyotrophic lateral sclerosis. *Lancet* 377, 942–955. doi: 10.1016/S0140-6736(10)61156-7

Kimura, T., and Griffin, D. E. (2000). The role of CD8(+) T cells and major histocompatibility complex class I expression in the central nervous system of mice infected with neurovirulent Sindbis virus. *J. Virol.* 74, 6117–6125. doi: 10.1128/JVI.74.13.6117-6125.2000

Kon, M., and Cuervo, A. M. (2010). Chaperone-mediated autophagy in health and disease. *FEBS Lett.* 584, 1399–1404. doi: 10.1016/j.febslet.2009.12.025

Koopman, W. J., Distelmaier, F., Smeitink, J. A., and Willems, P. H. (2013). OXPHOS mutations and neurodegeneration. *EMBO J.* 32, 9–29. doi: 10.1038/emboj.2012.300

Kuhle, J., Lindberg, R. L., Regeniter, A., Mehling, M., Steck, A. J., Kappos, L., et al. (2009). Increased levels of inflammatory chemokines in amyotrophic lateral sclerosis. *Eur. J. Neurol.* 16, 771–774. doi: 10.1111/j.1468-1331.2009.02560.x

Kwak, Y. D., Wang, B., Li, J. J., Wang, R., Deng, Q., Diao, S., et al. (2012). Upregulation of the E3 ligase NEDD4-1 by oxidative stress degrades IGF-1 receptor protein in neurodegeneration. *J. Neurosci.* 32, 10971–10981. doi: 10.1523/JNEUROSCI.1836-12.2012

Lemmens, R., Moore, M. J., Al-Chalabi, A., Brown, R. H. Jr., and Robberecht, W. (2010). RNA metabolism and the pathogenesis of motor neuron diseases. *Trends Neurosci.* 33, 249–258. doi: 10.1016/j.tins.2010.02.003

Lenzken, S. C., Romeo, V., Zolezzi, F., Cordero, F., Lamorte, G., Bonanno, D., et al. (2011). Mutant SOD1 and mitochondrial damage alter expression and splicing of genes controlling neuritogenesis in models of neurodegeneration. *Hum. Mutat.* 32, 168–182. doi: 10.1002/humu.21394

Le Roy, C., and Wrana, J. L. (2005). Clathrin- and non-clathrin-mediated endocytic regulation of cell signalling. *Nat. Rev. Mol. Cell Biol.* 6, 112–126. doi: 10.1038/nrm1571

Lin, J., Diamanduros, A., Chowdhury, S. A., Scelsa, S., Latov, N., and Sadiq, S. A. (2009). Specific electron transport chain abnormalities in amyotrophic lateral sclerosis. *J. Neurol.* 256, 774–782. doi: 10.1007/s00415-009-5015-8

Liu, J. X., Brannstrom, T., Andersen, P. M., and Pedrosa-Domellof, F. (2013). Distinct changes in synaptic protein composition at neuromuscular junctions of extraocular muscles versus limb muscles of ALS donors. *PLoS ONE* 8:e57473. doi: 10.1371/journal.pone.0057473

Luo, Y., Xue, H., Pardo, A. C., Mattson, M. P., Rao, M. S., and Maragakis, N. J. (2007). Impaired SDF1/CXCR4 signaling in glial progenitors derived from SOD1(G93A) mice. *J. Neurosci. Res.* 85, 2422–2432. doi: 10.1002/jnr.21398

Malaspina, A., and De Belleroche, J. (2004). Spinal cord molecular profiling provides a better understanding of amyotrophic lateral sclerosis pathogenesis. *Brain Res. Brain Res. Rev.* 45, 213–229. doi: 10.1016/j.brainresrev.2004.04.002

Manfredi, G., and Xu, Z. (2005). Mitochondrial dysfunction and its role in motor neuron degeneration in ALS. *Mitochondrion* 5, 77–87. doi: 10.1016/j.mito.2005.01.002

Manzano, R., Toivonen, J. M., Olivan, S., Calvo, A. C., Moreno-Igoa, M., Munoz, M. J., et al. (2011). Altered expression of myogenic regulatory factors in the mouse model of amyotrophic lateral sclerosis. *Neurodegener. Dis.* 8, 386–396. doi: 10.1159/000324159

Martin, L. J. (2010). Mitochondrial and cell death mechanisms in neurodegenerative diseases. *Pharmaceuticals (Basel)* 3, 839–915. doi: 10.3390/ph3040839

Martin, S., Wilkinson, K. A., Nishimune, A., and Henley, J. M. (2007). Emerging extranuclear roles of protein SUMOylation in neuronal function and dysfunction. *Nat. Rev. Neurosci.* 8, 948–959. doi: 10.1038/nrn2276

Martin, L. J. (2011). Mitochondrial pathobiology in ALS. *J Bioenerg Biomembr* 43, 569–579. doi: 10.1007/s10863-011-9395-y.

Massey, A. C., Zhang, C., and Cuervo, A. M. (2006). Chaperone-mediated autophagy in aging and disease. *Curr. Top. Dev. Biol.* 73, 205–235. doi: 10.1016/S0070-2153(05)73007-6

Massignan, T., Casoni, F., Basso, M., Stefanazzi, P., Biasini, E., Tortarolo, M., et al. (2007). Proteomic analysis of spinal cord of presymptomatic amyotrophic lateral sclerosis G93A SOD1 mouse. *Biochem. Biophys. Res. Commun.* 353, 719–725. doi: 10.1016/j.bbrc.2006.12.075

Matsumoto, A., Tateishi, Y., Onoyama, I., Okita, Y., Nakayama, K., and Nakayama, K. I. (2011). Fbxw7beta resides in the endoplasmic reticulum membrane and protects cells from oxidative stress. *Cancer Sci.* 102, 749–755. doi: 10.1111/j.1349-7006.2011.01851.x

McMahon, H. T., and Boucrot, E. (2011). Molecular mechanism and physiological functions of clathrin-mediated endocytosis. *Nat. Rev. Mol. Cell Biol.* 12, 517–533. doi: 10.1038/nrm3151

Miyazaki, K., Ohta, Y., Nagai, M., Morimoto, N., Kurata, T., Takehisa, Y., et al. (2011). Disruption of neurovascular unit prior to motor neuron degeneration in amyotrophic lateral sclerosis. *J. Neurosci. Res.* 89, 718–728. doi: 10.1002/jnr.22594

Morimoto, N., Nagai, M., Ohta, Y., Miyazaki, K., Kurata, T., Morimoto, M., et al. (2007). Increased autophagy in transgenic mice with a G93A mutant SOD1 gene. *Brain Res.* 1167, 112–117. doi: 10.1016/j.brainres.2007.06.045

Mougeot, J. L., Li, Z., Price, A. E., Wright, F. A., and Brooks, B. R. (2011). Microarray analysis of peripheral blood lymphocytes from ALS patients and the SAFE detection of the KEGG ALS pathway. *BMC Med. Genomics* 4:74. doi: 10.1186/1755-8794-4-74

Narai, H., Manabe, Y., Nagai, M., Nagano, I., Ohta, Y., Murakami, T., et al. (2009). Early detachment of neuromuscular junction proteins in ALS mice with SODG93A mutation. *Neurol. Int.* 1:e16. doi: 10.4081/ni.2009.e16

Nateri, A. S., Riera-Sans, L., Da Costa, C., and Behrens, A. (2004). The ubiquitin ligase SCFFbw7 antagonizes apoptotic JNK signaling. *Science* 303, 1374–1378. doi: 10.1126/science.1092880

Offen, D., Barhum, Y., Melamed, E., Embacher, N., Schindler, C., and Ransmayr, G. (2009). Spinal cord mRNA profile in patients with ALS: comparison with transgenic mice expressing the human SOD-1 mutant. *J. Mol. Neurosci.* 38, 85–93. doi: 10.1007/s12031-007-9004-z

Oliveira, A. L., Thams, S., Lidman, O., Piehl, F., Hokfelt, T., Karre, K., et al. (2004). A role for MHC class I molecules in synaptic plasticity and regeneration of neurons after axotomy. *Proc. Natl. Acad. Sci. U.S.A.* 101, 17843–17848. doi: 10.1073/pnas.0408154101

Olsen, M. K., Roberds, S. L., Ellerbrock, B. R., Fleck, T. J., McKinley, D. K., and Gurney, M. E. (2001). Disease mechanisms revealed by transcription profiling in SOD1-G93A transgenic mouse spinal cord. *Ann. Neurol.* 50, 730–740. doi: 10.1002/ana.1252

Otomo, A., Pan, L., and Hadano, S. (2012). Dysregulation of the autophagy-endolysosomal system in amyotrophic lateral sclerosis and related motor neuron diseases. *Neurol. Res. Int.* 2012, 498428. doi: 10.1155/2012/498428

Pedotti, P., 't Hoen, P. A., Vreugdenhil, E., Schenk, G. J., Vossen, R. H., Ariyurek, Y., et al. (2008). Can subtle changes in gene expression be consistently detected with different microarray platforms? *BMC Genomics* 9:124. doi: 10.1186/1471-2164-9-124

Perrin, F. E., Boisset, G., Docquier, M., Schaad, O., Descombes, P., and Kato, A. C. (2005). No widespread induction of cell death genes occurs in pure motoneurons in an amyotrophic lateral sclerosis mouse model. *Hum. Mol. Genet.* 14, 3309–3320. doi: 10.1093/hmg/ddi357

Perrin, F. E., Boisset, G., Lathuiliere, A., and Kato, A. C. (2006). Cell death pathways differ in several mouse models with motoneurone disease: analysis of pure motoneurone populations at a presymptomatic age. *J. Neurochem.* 98, 1959–1972. doi: 10.1111/j.1471-4159.2006.04024.x

Petri, S., Schmalbach, S., Grosskreutz, J., Krampfl, K., Grothe, C., Dengler, R., et al. (2005). The cellular mRNA expression of GABA and glutamate receptors in spinal motor neurons of SOD1 mice. *J. Neurol. Sci.* 238, 25–30. doi: 10.1016/j.jns.2005.06.005

Polymenidou, M., and Cleveland, D. W. (2011). The seeds of neurodegeneration: prion-like spreading in ALS. *Cell* 147, 498–508. doi: 10.1016/j.cell.2011.10.011

Prifti, E., Zucker, J. D., Clement, K., and Henegar, C. (2008). FunNet: an integrative tool for exploring transcriptional interactions. *Bioinformatics* 24, 2636–2638. doi: 10.1093/bioinformatics/btn492

Rentzos, M., Nikolaou, C., Rombos, A., Boufidou, F., Zoga, M., Dimitrakopoulos, A., et al. (2007). RANTES levels are elevated in serum and cerebrospinal fluid in patients with amyotrophic lateral sclerosis. *Amyotroph. Lateral Scler.* 8, 283–287. doi: 10.1080/17482960701419232

Richardson, K., Allen, S. P., Mortiboys, H., Grierson, A. J., Wharton, S. B., Ince, P. G., et al. (2013). The effect of SOD1 mutation on cellular bioenergetic profile and viability in response to oxidative stress and influence of mutation-type. *PLoS ONE* 8:e68256. doi: 10.1371/journal.pone.0068256

Rosen, D. R., Siddique, T., Patterson, D., Figlewicz, D. A., Sapp, P., Hentati, A., et al. (1993). Mutations in Cu/Zn superoxide dismutase gene are associated with familial amyotrophic lateral sclerosis. *Nature* 362, 59–62. doi: 10.1038/362059a0

Rothstein, J. D., Martin, L. J., and Kuncl, R. W. (1992). Decreased glutamate transport by the brain and spinal cord in amyotrophic lateral sclerosis. *N. Engl. J. Med.* 326, 1464–1468. doi: 10.1056/NEJM199205283262204

Rotshenker, S. (2009). The role of Galectin-3/MAC-2 in the activation of the innate-immune function of phagocytosis in microglia in injury and disease. *J. Mol. Neurosci.* 39, 99–103. doi: 10.1007/s12031-009-9186-7

Sanagi, T., Yuasa, S., Nakamura, Y., Suzuki, E., Aoki, M., Warita, H., et al. (2010). Appearance of phagocytic microglia adjacent to motoneurons in spinal cord tissue from a presymptomatic transgenic rat model of amyotrophic lateral sclerosis. *J. Neurosci. Res.* 88, 2736–2746. doi: 10.1002/jnr.22424

Sargsyan, S. A., Blackburn, D. J., Barber, S. C., Monk, P. N., and Shaw, P. J. (2009). Mutant SOD1 G93A microglia have an inflammatory phenotype and elevated production of MCP-1. *Neuroreport* 20, 1450–1455. doi: 10.1097/WNR.0b013e328331e8fa

Saris, C. G., Groen, E. J., Koekkoek, J. A., Veldink, J. H., and Van Den Berg, L. H. (2013a). Meta-analysis of gene expression profiling in amyotrophic lateral sclerosis: a comparison between transgenic mouse models and human patients. *Amyotroph. Lateral Scler. Frontotemporal Degener.* 14, 177–189. doi: 10.3109/21678421.2012.729842

Saris, C. G., Groen, E. J., Van Vught, P. W., Van Es, M. A., Blauw, H. M., Veldink, J. H., et al. (2013b). Gene expression profile of SOD1-G93A mouse spinal cord, blood and muscle. *Amyotroph. Lateral Scler. Frontotemporal Degener.* 14, 190–198. doi: 10.3109/21678421.2012.749914

Sasaki, S., Warita, H., Abe, K., Komori, T., and Iwata, M. (2001). EAAT1 and EAAT2 immunoreactivity in transgenic mice with a G93A mutant SOD1 gene. *Neuroreport* 12, 1359–1362. doi: 10.1097/00001756-200105250-00014

Schutz, B. (2005). Imbalanced excitatory to inhibitory synaptic input precedes motor neuron degeneration in an animal model of amyotrophic lateral sclerosis. *Neurobiol. Dis.* 20, 131–140. doi: 10.1016/j.nbd.2005.02.006

Scorisa, J. M., Duobles, T., Oliveira, G. P., Maximino, J. R., and Chadi, G. (2010). The review of the methods to obtain non-neuronal cells to study glial influence on Amyotrophic Lateral Sclerosis pathophysiology at molecular level *in vitro*. *Acta Cir. Bras.* 25, 281–289. doi: 10.1590/S0102-86502010000300011

Shideman, C. R., Hu, S., Peterson, P. K., and Thayer, S. A. (2006). CCL5 evokes calcium signals in microglia through a kinase-, phosphoinositide-, and nucleotide-dependent mechanism. *J. Neurosci. Res.* 83, 1471–1484. doi: 10.1002/jnr.20839

Singh, R. K., Cooper, T. A. (2012). Pre-mRNA splicing in disease and therapeutics. *Trends Mol. Med.* 18, 472–82. doi: 10.1016/j.molmed.2012.06.006

Smyth, G. K. (2005). "Limma: linear models for microarray data," in *Bioinformatics and Computational Biology Solutions using R and Bioconductor*, eds V. C. R.

Gentleman, S. Dudoit, R. Irizarry, and W. Huber (New York, NY: Springer), 397–420.

Sunico, C. R., Dominguez, G., Garcia-Verdugo, J. M., Osta, R., Montero, F., and Moreno-Lopez, B. (2011). Reduction in the motoneuron inhibitory/excitatory synaptic ratio in an early-symptomatic mouse model of amyotrophic lateral sclerosis. *Brain Pathol.* 21, 1–15. doi: 10.1111/j.1750-3639.2010.00417.x

Takeuchi, H., Kobayashi, Y., Yoshihara, T., Niwa, J., Doyu, M., Ohtsuka, K., et al. (2002). Hsp70 and Hsp40 improve neurite outgrowth and suppress intracytoplasmic aggregate formation in cultured neuronal cells expressing mutant SOD1. *Brain Res.* 949, 11–22. doi: 10.1016/S0006-8993(02)02568-4

Tateishi, T., Yamasaki, R., Tanaka, M., Matsushita, T., Kikuchi, H., Isobe, N., et al. (2010). CSF chemokine alterations related to the clinical course of amyotrophic lateral sclerosis. *J. Neuroimmunol.* 222, 76–81. doi: 10.1016/j.jneuroim.2010.03.004

Tateno, M., Sadakata, H., Tanaka, M., Itohara, S., Shin, R. M., Miura, M., et al. (2004). Calcium-permeable AMPA receptors promote misfolding of mutant SOD1 protein and development of amyotrophic lateral sclerosis in a transgenic mouse model. *Hum. Mol. Genet.* 13, 2183–2196. doi: 10.1093/hmg/ddh246

Tian, F., Morimoto, N., Liu, W., Ohta, Y., Deguchi, K., Miyazaki, K., et al. (2011). *In vivo* optical imaging of motor neuron autophagy in a mouse model of amyotrophic lateral sclerosis. *Autophagy* 7, 985–992. doi: 10.4161/auto.7.9.16012

Turner, B. J., and Talbot, K. (2008). Transgenics, toxicity and therapeutics in rodent models of mutant SOD1-mediated familial ALS. *Prog. Neurobiol.* 85, 94–134. doi: 10.1016/j.pneurobio.2008.01.001

Turner, M. R., Hardiman, O., Benatar, M., Brooks, B. R., Chio, A., De Carvalho, M., et al. (2013). Controversies and priorities in amyotrophic lateral sclerosis. *Lancet Neurol.* 12, 310–322. doi: 10.1016/S1474-4422(13)70036-X

Urushitani, M., Kurisu, J., Tateno, M., Hatakeyama, S., Nakayama, K., Kato, S., et al. (2004). CHIP promotes proteasomal degradation of familial ALS-linked mutant SOD1 by ubiquitinating Hsp/Hsc70. *J. Neurochem.* 90, 231–244. doi: 10.1111/j.1471-4159.2004.02486.x

Usuki, S., Kamitani, T., Matsuo, Y., and Yu, R. K. (2012). Pathobiochemical effect of acylated steryl-beta-glucoside on aggregation and cytotoxicity of alpha-synuclein. *Neurochem. Res.* 37, 1261–1266. doi: 10.1007/s11064-011-0662-4

Van Gelder, R. N., Von Zastrow, M. E., Yool, A., Dement, W. C., Barchas, J. D., and Eberwine, J. H. (1990). Amplified RNA synthesized from limited quantities of heterogeneous cDNA. *Proc. Natl. Acad. Sci. U.S.A.* 87, 1663–1667. doi: 10.1073/pnas.87.5.1663

Veugelers, B., Theys, P., Lammens, M., Van Hees, J., and Robberecht, W. (1996). Pathological findings in a patient with amyotrophic lateral sclerosis and multifocal motor neuropathy with conduction block. *J. Neurol. Sci.* 136, 64–70. doi: 10.1016/0022-510X(95)00295-D

Wang, L., Gutmann, D. H., and Roos, R. P. (2011a). Astrocyte loss of mutant SOD1 delays ALS disease onset and progression in G85R transgenic mice. *Hum. Mol. Genet.* 20, 286–293. doi: 10.1093/hmg/ddq463

Wang, R., Yang, B., and Zhang, D. (2011b). Activation of interferon signaling pathways in spinal cord astrocytes from an ALS mouse model. *Glia* 59, 946–958. doi: 10.1002/glia.21167

Weydt, P., Weiss, M. D., Moller, T., and Carter, G. T. (2002). Neuro-inflammation as a therapeutic target in amyotrophic lateral sclerosis. *Curr. Opin. Investig. Drugs* 3, 1720–1724. doi: 10.1016/0022-510X(95)00295-D

Wootz, H., Enjin, A., Wallen-Mackenzie, A., Lindholm, D., and Kullander, K. (2010). Reduced VGLUT2 expression increases motor neuron viability in Sod1(G93A) mice. *Neurobiol. Dis.* 37, 58–66. doi: 10.1016/j.nbd.2009.09.006

Xu, R., Wu, C., Zhang, X., Zhang, Q., Yang, Y., Yi, J., et al. (2011). Linking hypoxic and oxidative insults to cell death mechanisms in models of ALS. *Brain Res.* 1372, 133–144. doi: 10.1016/j.brainres.2010.11.056

Yamamoto, M., Tanaka, F., and Sobue, G. (2007). [Gene expression profile of spinal ventral horn in ALS]. *Brain Nerve* 59, 1129–1139.

Yamanaka, K., Chun, S. J., Boillee, S., Fujimori-Tonou, N., Yamashita, H., Gutmann, D. H., et al. (2008). Astrocytes as determinants of disease progression in inherited amyotrophic lateral sclerosis. *Nat. Neurosci.* 11, 251–253. doi: 10.1038/nn2047

Yoshihara, T., Ishigaki, S., Yamamoto, M., Liang, Y., Niwa, J., Takeuchi, H., et al. (2002). Differential expression of inflammation- and apoptosis-related genes in spinal cords of a mutant SOD1 transgenic mouse model of familial amyotrophic lateral sclerosis. *J. Neurochem.* 80, 158–167. doi: 10.1046/j.0022-3042.2001.00683.x

Yu, L., Guan, Y., Wu, X., Chen, Y., Liu, Z., Du, H., et al. (2013). Wnt signaling is altered by spinal cord neuronal dysfunction in amyotrophic lateral sclerosis transgenic mice. *Neurochem. Res.* 38, 1904–1913. doi: 10.1007/s11064-013-1096-y

Zhang, R., Gascon, R., Miller, R. G., Gelinas, D. F., Mass, J., Lancero, M., et al. (2006). MCP-1 chemokine receptor CCR2 is decreased on circulating monocytes in sporadic amyotrophic lateral sclerosis (sALS). *J. Neuroimmunol.* 179, 87–93. doi: 10.1016/j.jneuroim.2006.06.008

Zhao, P., Ignacio, S., Beattie, E. C., and Abood, M. E. (2008). Altered presymptomatic AMPA and cannabinoid receptor trafficking in motor neurons of ALS model mice: implications for excitotoxicity. *Eur. J. Neurosci.* 27, 572–579. doi: 10.1111/j.1460-9568.2008.06041.x

Zhong, Z., Deane, R., Ali, Z., Parisi, M., Shapovalov, Y., O'banion, M. K., et al. (2008). ALS-causing SOD1 mutants generate vascular changes prior to motor neuron degeneration. *Nat. Neurosci.* 11, 420–422. doi: 10.1038/nn2073

24

Resentment, hate, and hope in amyotrophic lateral sclerosis

C. Oster[1]* *and F. Pagnini*[2,3]

[1] The Healers Campaign, Haslett, MI, USA
[2] Department of Psychology, Catholic University of Milan, Milan, Italy
[3] Niguarda Ca' Granda Hospital, Milan, Italy

Edited by:
Gianluca Castelnuovo, Università Cattolica del Sacro Cuore, Italy

Reviewed by:
Paraskevi Theofilou, Sotiria Hospital for Thoracic Diseases, Greece
Julian B. Nesci, Austin Health, Australia

***Correspondence:**
C. Oster, The Healers Campaign, Haslett, MI 48840, USA.
e-mail: drcraigoster@comcast.net

Amyotrophic lateral sclerosis (ALS) is a fatal and progressive neurodegenerative disease. Despite much research having been conducted about psychological issues involved in living with ALS, anger, and resentment have yet to be investigated. Moreover, the construct of "hope" has received little attention, so far. An online survey was created to investigate hate, resentment, and hope issues in people with ALS, in relation to the willingness to adopt a strict nutrient-dense diet if it were shown to increase longevity. Results indicate that there is a high level of hope in the sample. People who have lived with ALS for more time expressed a higher level of hope to live 10 years or more. Those who are married were more likely to have hope of living 10 years or longer and more likely to have lower levels of hate against ALS. Dietary self-care choices appear to be related to hope issues. Resentment and hate tended to be higher in people who have had ALS for less time, and in women. Despite some methodological limitations, the results suggest that hope, hate, and resentment could be important issues to explore in future studies.

Keywords: anger, resentment, hope, amyotrophic lateral sclerosis, quality of life, caregivers, ALS, will to live

INTRODUCTION

Amyotrophic lateral sclerosis (ALS) is a fatal and progressive neurodegenerative disease, which affects motor neurons in the anterior horn of the spinal cord, the brainstem, and the motor cortex. It is a rare disease, with an incidence of 1.89 per 100,000/year in western countries (Worms, 2001). People with ALS experience a progressive muscle weakness, becoming relentlessly immobile, developing impaired speech, and respiration problems. In the late stages of the disease, progressing paralysis can result in a "locked-in" state in which only residual muscular movement is possible.

Despite the average life expectancy of about 3 years after symptom onset (Ilzecka et al., 2003), the progression of the disease is unpredictable, with 10% of patients with ALS living more than 10 years (Andrews, 2009). So far, research has not demonstrated that it is possible to stop the progression of the disease. Therefore, the improvement of patients' quality of life is often considered one of the primary goals of clinical management (Simmons, 2005; Pagnini, 2012).

Many psychological issues have been investigated in ALS, including psychological well-being, anxiety, and depression (Pagnini et al., 2012a), pain (Brettschneider et al., 2008), hopelessness (Plahuta et al., 2002), spiritual and existential well-being (Dal Bello-Haas et al., 2000). However, no study to our knowledge has investigated the topics of hate and resentment. Moreover, despite its clinical importance (Fanos et al., 2008), the issue of hope has received little empirical investigation. To date, no study has investigated the relationship among hate, resentment, and hope and their development through time.

Hate and resentment, as well as hope, are often reported as a psychological response toward a chronic and non-treatable illness. Clinical practice (Radunovic et al., 2007), as well as patients' perspectives (Melazzini, 2007), often report of anger reactions, expressed in various ways by the patient. Not surprisingly, a study by Palmieri et al. (2010) observed high levels of anger in the considered ALS population. The "relationship" established with the disease seems to change over time (De Groot et al., 2007), probably because of the advancement of the disease and/or a grief elaboration process. Clinical practice suggests that ALS is often the target of hate by the people who have it; resentment is another emotion expressed by the patients, as well as by their caregivers, but there are very few scientific data pertaining to those reactions.

The diagnosis of ALS may threaten hope, especially with the belief that there is nothing that can be done to change a patient's fate. However, many clinicians suggest that "hope" is a very important issue for the psychological well-being of patients and their caregivers (Centers, 2001). In the ALS scientific literature, the concept of "hope" is less investigated than the one of "hopelessness" (Plahuta et al., 2002). Hopelessness is related to depressive features, and with low levels of quality of life (Ganzini et al., 1999); moreover, hopelessness seems to predict the desire for assisted suicide (Ganzini et al., 2002).

Our rationale in this study was to investigate the prevalence and degree of hate and resentment in a sample of the ALS population, and to understand their relationships with time since diagnosis, hope, marital status, and other demographic characteristics. A further innovation of this research is the examination of these three variables in relationship to the willingness to extend one's longevity through nutritional self-care. This variable was included, because clinical considerations made by Oster (the manuscript's first author, who is an 18 years ALS survivor) suggest that some people with ALS would not be willing to adopt a healthier diet even if it were to be shown to extend life. We wanted to investigate the prevalence of this mindset in our study's subject population, and to discover whether the variables of hate, resentment, and hope were related to this attitude.

MATERIALS AND METHODS

An online questionnaire was created with a Google spreadsheet, as part of a larger study. The overall survey was composed by 65 items, with both opened-ended and closed-ended questions; in case of closed-ended questions, subjects could choose among different sentences. The time requested to complete the entire survey ranged between 10 and 20 min. The survey was created with Google Documents tool and was accessible by subjects through a dedicated template. All the items were generated *ex novo* (therefore no cut-off-points could be expected). There were no forced answers. For the purpose of this study, we only used a selected sub-sample of items.

People with ALS were invited with messages that were posted in ALS forums, facebook, and a newsletter, as well as with an announcement on "The Healers" website. The purpose of the survey was described before subjects were asked to complete the questionnaire, stating that results would be analyzed only for research purposes, and there was no possibility to link the published data to their true identity.

Together with demographical data, subjects were asked to provide answers about hate, resentment, and hope, with questions like "Do you believe that there will be a cure for ALS in your lifetime?" and "What statement best describes the level of resentment that you feel about living with ALS?" Multiple answers were possible.

The analyses, both descriptive and inferential, were, carried out with Excel and SPSS software, are mainly descriptive statistics and cross-tabs analysis, using the Pearson's chi-squared test.

RESULTS

A total of 83 subjects with ALS completed the survey. The sample's characteristics are reported in **Table 1**. Missing values were excluded.

The answers provided to the questions are presented in the **Figures 1–5**.

People who answered positively to the question about the hope to live more than 10 years had a lower frequency of resentment, χ^2 $(6, N = 82) = 11.14$, $p < 0.05$, and hate χ^2 $(6, N = 81) = 13.48$, $p < 0.05$, toward the illness.

The level of resentment of ALS reported by subjects is highly related to the level of resentment perceived in the caregiver, χ^2 $(6, N = 81) = 41.09$, $p < 0.001$, and the level of hate toward ALS, χ^2 $(6, N = 81) = 58.21$, $p < 0.001$. The caregiver's resentment perceived by the patient is also related to the level of hate expressed by the subject, χ^2 $(6, N = 80) = 21.19$, $p < 0.05$. It seems that there is a tendency for a positive correlation among these three variables.

Subjects who have the hope to live 10 or more years would be more willing to follow a strict diet if it would increase the life expectancy by 1 year χ^2 $(6, N = 75) = 21.93$, $p < 0.01$, but no differences were found about the willingness to take a new drug with uncomfortable side effects. Both the questions about "hope" presented no differences with regards to the demographic variables.

Women report higher level of resentment, with higher frequencies of moderate/strong resentment answers, in comparison with males χ^2 $(3, N = 81) = 6.44$, $p < 0.05$. There is a similar tendency, non-significant ($p < 0.1$), with women reporting a higher hate level. Splitting the sample into two groups, using the median of the time since diagnosis, subjects who have had the disease for less time present with higher level of resentment χ^2 $(3, N = 81) = 8.05$, $p < 0.05$, and hate χ^2 $(3, N = 82) = 9.89$, $p < 0.05$.

The subjects who report a higher level of caregiver's resentment indicate with greater frequency the answer "yes" to the question "Do you believe that there is a relation between your dietary habits and the losses that you have experienced subsequent to ALS?" χ^2 $(9, N = 78) = 20.32$, $p < 0.05$.

Regarding hope, people who do not believe that there will be a cure for ALS in their lifetime were more likely to believe that they will not live for 10 years, compared to those who have the hope that a cure will be found χ^2 $(1, N = 78) = 4.67$, $p < 0.05$. People who answered "yes" to both the hope questions ($N = 21$), compared to those who answered "no" ($N = 11$), had ALS for a longer time (but without statistical differences), were more likely to be married χ^2 $(5, N = 32) = 13.38$, $p < 0.05$ and reported a lower level of hate against ALS χ^2 $(4, N = 32) = 8.06$, $p < 0.05$.

Considering the resentment level expressed by the subjects, in comparison with the resentment level that the subjects reported to be experienced by the caregivers, about half of the subjects (51.2%) express an equal level of resentment, the 21.3% report higher level of resentment experienced by the patient, while the 27.5% indicate the contrary. No differences arose about demographics or hope levels reported (all Chi Squares without significant results).

DISCUSSION

The present study from an online survey completed by men and women with ALS and analyzed with cross-sectional analyses – aimed to investigate levels of hate, resentment, and hope, and the relationships among them. These variables were also examined in relationship to the willingness to extend longevity through a commitment to disciplined nutritional self-care. To our knowledge, this is one of the first attempts to investigate, with a survey methodology, the point of view of people with ALS about the hope for longevity and a cure, and the level of hate and resentment toward the illness. Furthermore, we are not aware of any study examining motivation regarding nutritional self-care, related to the will to live.

In our sample, most of the subjects (70%) hoped to be able to live more than 10 years. The hope for a cure was somewhat less present. A third of the people who reported hope of seeing a cure in their lifetime, and more than half of the sample who reported not believing that they will have the chance to see a cure. These two issues were correlated. Interestingly, people in a marriage were more likely to have hope of living 10 years or longer and more likely to have lower levels of hate against ALS.

To hate ALS involves hating having ALS and all of the potentially frustrating and otherwise emotionally challenging experiences that occur in the lives of people with ALS, as well as hating the

Table 1 | Sample characteristics ($N = 83$).

		Frequency	%
Months since diagnosis [*M*, (SD)]	44.12 (84.32)		
Sex	Female	41	50
	Male	41	50
Marital status	Now married	56	68.3
	Widowed	4	4.9
	Divorced	11	13.4
	Separated	3	3.7
	Never married	3	3.7
	other	5	6.1
Highest degree	Less than high school	1	1.2
	High school graduate	18	22.2
	Some college credit	15	18.5
	Associate degree (e.g., AA, AS)	5	6.2
	Bachelor's degree (e.g., BA, AB, BS)	23	28.4
	Master's degree (e.g., MA, MS, MEng, MEd, MSW, MBA)	12	14.8
	Professional degree (e.g., MD, DDS, DVM, LLB, JD)	4	4.9
	Doctorate degree (e.g., PhD, EdD)	2	2.5
	other	1	1.2
Work activity	Employed for wages	13	15.9
	Self-employed	4	4.9
	Unemployed	12	14.6
	Retired	39	47.6
	Unable to work	13	15.9
	Other	1	1.2
Race	Asian	1	1.2
	Black or African American	1	1.2
	White	76	92.7
	Hispanic	4	4.9
Country/province	USA	73	89
	South America	1	1.2
	Europe	5	6.1
	Australia	1	1.2
	Canada	1	1.2
	Mexico	1	1.2
Life environment	City	28	34.1
	Country/Rural	10	12.2
	Suburban	28	34.1
	Small town	15	18.3
	Other	1	1.2

way one's own physiology is performing. Perhaps, our finding regarding marriage and hope suggests that people in marriages may build a vision of hope together, and that the meaning of their shared marital commitment could be protective against what is involved in hating one's life with ALS. Research into this area could give clinicians greater understanding of strategies that could facilitate greater hope as well as less resentment and hate in people with ALS. It must be pointed out that some people with ALS may value hating and resenting ALS as the best strategy for them in terms of coping and life satisfaction, and we have much to learn from them about their experiences in living with ALS.

The majority of the sample indicated a strong or moderate resentment level; a similar indication was given subjects' perception of caregiver resentment level. About a third of the sample reported sporadic episodes of hate, while less than a fifth of the subjects indicated to always hate the disease. The current study suggests a prevalence of these distressing emotional experiences that is high enough to warrant investigation of the nature of these experiences and the meanings that they have for the people having them.

We postulate that there may be cognitive interpretations of experiences of living with ALS that may increase the likelihood of experiencing resentment and hatred. If so, then clinicians could

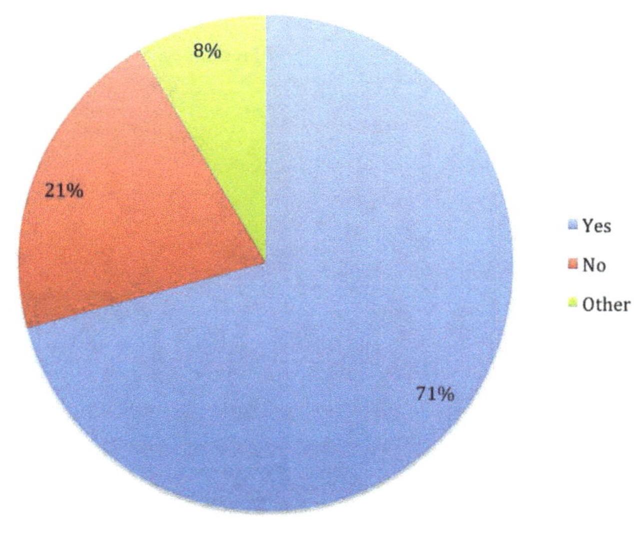

FIGURE 1 | Do you have hope that you could live 10 years or longer regardless of whether an effective pharmaceutical treatment were to be discovered? (*N* = 82).

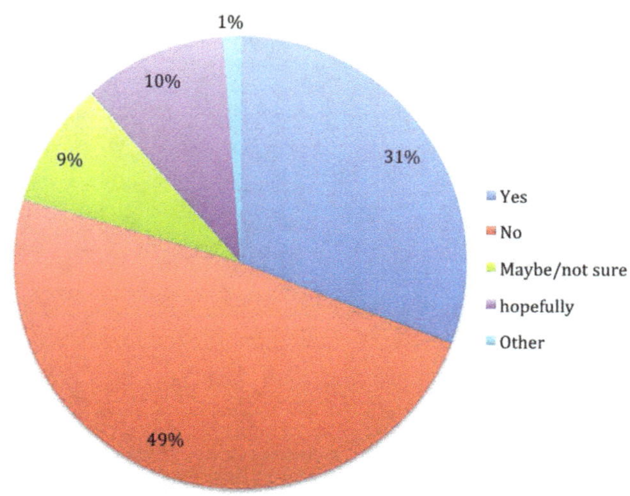

FIGURE 2 | Do you believe that there will be a cure for ALS in your lifetime? (*N* = 78).

work with ALS patients to learn to interpret events in ways that are less emotionally and physiologically distressing. This is what was personally observed by Oster, first author of this paper and an 18 year survivor of ALS, in his self-case study. Oster has experienced much more positive experiences of living with ALS through working with a psychoanalyst psychologist for over 12 years, and experiences less hate and resentment toward ALS. Oster states that he has learned to see the world differently, based to a large extent upon learning to interpret and understand living with ALS differently (unpublished data). There are no or very few studies about psychological interventions in ALS, as recently pointed noted (Pagnini et al., 2012b). However, psychological treatments with people with other chronic illnesses presented a high capacity to improve the well-being and to reduce the anger response, promoting acceptance (Telford et al., 2006).

Other researchers have evaluated that patient hopefulness is the result of an active style of coping, although their construct of hope was more comprehensive than our definition (Fanos et al., 2008). Furthermore, previous research has demonstrated that lower levels of well-being are associated with reduced longevity (Pagnini et al., 2012a); therefore, we believe that it would be worthwhile for additional research on the relationship between the variables of hate, resentment, and hope in relationship to well-being to help understand whether these variables factor into longevity with ALS.

The analyses of the relationships among resentment, hate, and hope provide interesting results. Subjects who reported hope of living 10 years or more reported less hate and resentment toward ALS. Further research is required to understand hope in relationship to hate and resentment, and to answer the following questions. Is hope in ALS protective regarding the experience of hating and resenting ALS? And/or, do tendencies to experience greater hate and resentment regarding losses, challenges, limitations, and frustrations lessen hope in people with ALS? Aside from the relationship of lower levels of hating ALS being associated with being married and having hope of surviving 10 years post-diagnosis, it is unclear from our findings what causes some people to always hate ALS and others to never hate it. Research is needed to understand the meanings and experiences of the people who always hate ALS and those who report to never hate ALS.

Levels of hate and resentment were correlated; moreover, subjects' estimation of the level of resentment in the caregiver was related to their own resentment level, without statistical differences between them. To our knowledge, this is a new finding, yet there is the issue that our research relied upon the perception that the person with ALS has of their caregiver. So, we do not know the extent to which this finding reflects actual symmetry between the person with ALS and their caregiver. Researchers have demonstrated symmetry between people with ALS and caregivers in regards to distress, but this has not been previously studied in regards to resentment (Rabkin et al., 2000).

There were differences in gender in the report of resentment and hate related to the illness. Women indicated higher level of resentment and a higher level of hate, with the latter emotion only expressing a tendency toward significance. The novelty of this data suggests caution in its interpretation, but a possible explanation is that women are more devastated by being robbed of their caregiving role as well as by being forced into being a recipient. Cultural norms may play a role in gender differences found. Cultural norms emphasize the physical appearance of the woman being linked to feeling valued, loved, included, but the perception of the body after the diagnosis of ALS may be related to discard, pity, and contempt. Furthermore, men may have a tendency to have been recipients of nurturing and caregiving from not only mothers but also wives, therefore adapting more easily to being put in the role of being taken care of. Further investigations and data are required regarding these cautious interpretations, as well as regarding whether or not some of women's greater resentment than men about ALS is related to some extent to greater distress with receiving the

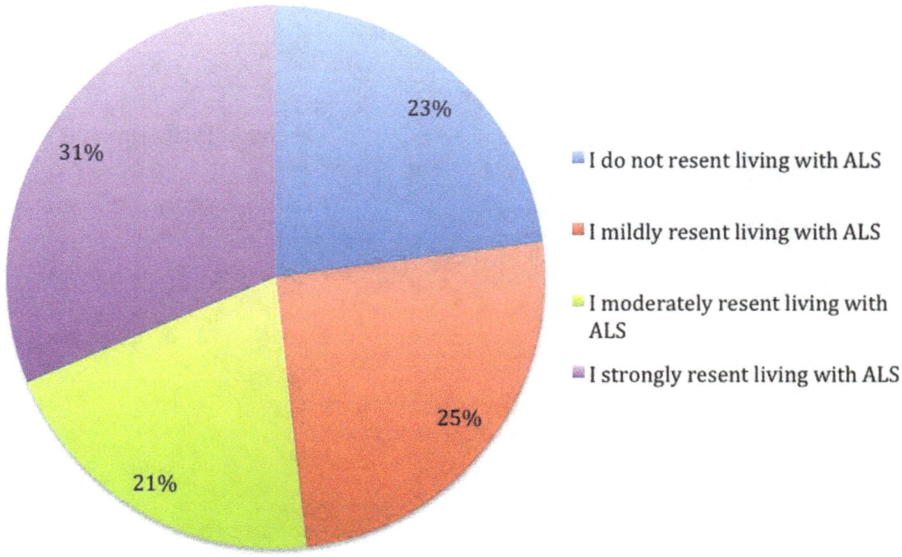

FIGURE 3 | What statement best describes the level of resentment that you feel about living with ALS? ($N = 83$).

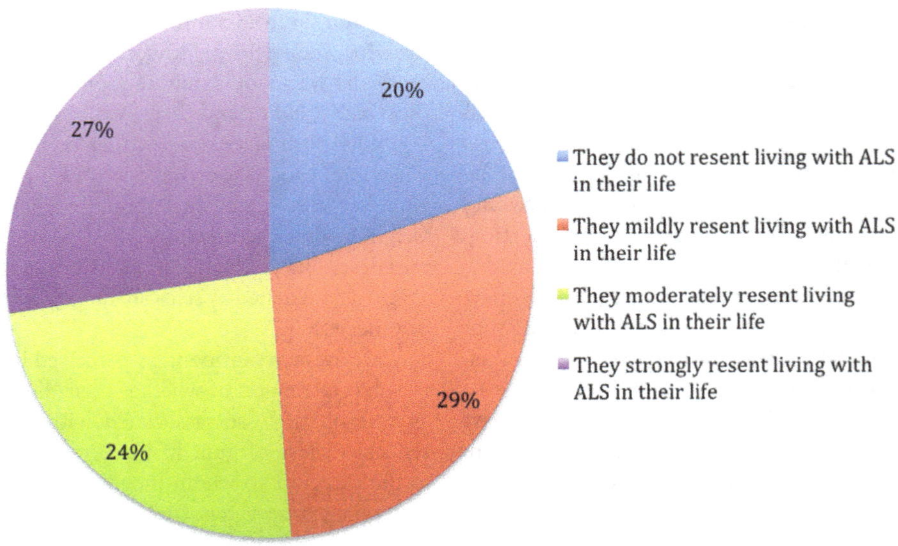

FIGURE 4 | What statement do you guess best describes the level of resentment that your primary caregiver feels about living with ALS in their life? ($N = 80$).

very personal assistance required with urination and bathing as a recipient of caregiving.

The time since diagnosis is another issue that discriminates hate and resentment levels, as well as reported hope. In our sample, subjects who have had ALS for a longer time reported higher levels of hope as well as lower levels of both hate and resentment. A possible explanation to these findings may be related to the relationship established with the illness and a grief elaboration process. Living with the illness could promote its acceptance; therefore, the amount of time spent with ALS may play a positive role in diminishing hate and resentment toward the illness. Moreover, the reason why people who survive ALS longer have more hope of living longer could be related to the course of the illness being less quick than initially perceived, resulting in less hate and resentment toward ALS.

In the light of our findings, and because of the quality of life issues involved, we suggest that clinicians attempt to understand the meanings of patients' hate and resentment toward ALS and not take it at face value. Although, it appears that the passage of time may in many cases increase hope and decrease both hate and

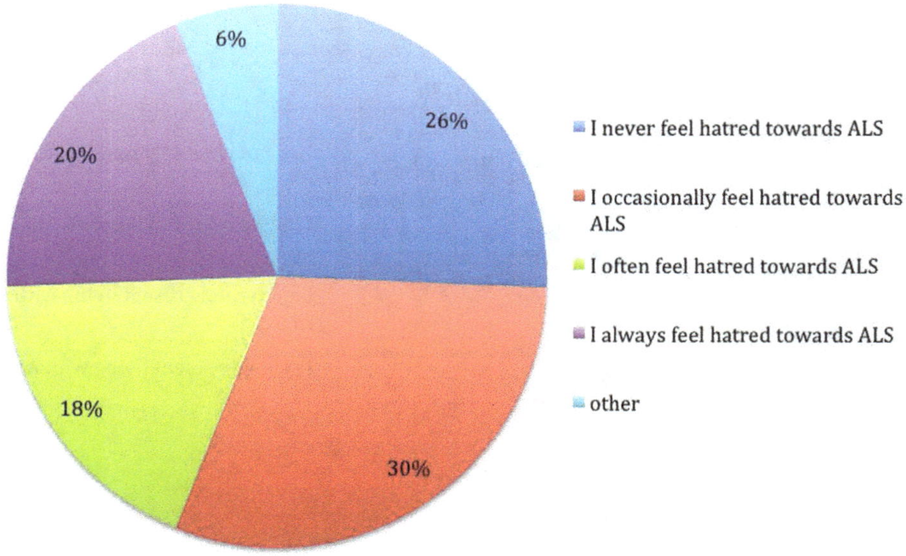

FIGURE 5 | What statement most accurately describes your feelings in the last 6 months regarding "hating" ALS? (*N* = 82).

resentment, it is possible that some people could get stuck in the grieving process because of the immensity of the losses that may occur with ALS.

The investigation of hope provided interesting results about the motivation toward following medical indications. The subjects who have the hope to live more than 10 years or more reported, as a group, more willingness to follow a strict nutrient-dense diet if scientific research indicated that such a diet increased life expectancy by 1 year, but declared that they would not agree to consume drugs with uncomfortable side effects, even if these would increase life expectancy by 1 year. It seems likely that people who already have the hope to maintain a positive level of quality of life may be more interested in maintaining it, as compared to worsening their quality of life to gain 1 year of survival.

It is noteworthy that some subjects, whether or not they have the hope of 10 years survival, would be willing to sacrifice 1 year of life rather than eating a nutrient-dense diet if it were demonstrated to be healthier for ALS. 18% (14 subjects) of the population in our study would be willing to refrain from a healthier diet, instead of extending their lives by 1 year. Slightly less than 5% (four subjects) of the population in our study would be willing to refrain from a healthier diet, instead of extending their lives by two or more years. To our knowledge, this is the first time that people with ALS have reported and been documented to be willing to sacrifice months off of their lives in order to eat whatever they desire. One subject in our study, whose response was categorized as "other" stated that they would only follow a life extending diet if it tasted good. Others reported that it would depend upon the quality of life that they would have, if they were to practice the hypothetical diet.

Additional research is required to discover what the meanings are for the people with ALS who would cut their lives short, rather than choose to focus on their longevity through life style changes. It appears that there is a cost-benefit analysis going on in terms of time, given that over three times as many subjects (14 of them) would refrain from a nutrient-dense diet that would extend their lives for a single year, as compared to the subjects (only four of them) who would refrain from consuming a nutrient-dense diet that would extend their lives by two or more years. Research is needed to understand whether or not actual self-care dietary behavioral choices are predictive of longevity in a way other than what has been established about people with ALS who maintain weight having a greater longevity (Paganoni et al., 2011). Another area deserving research is whether or not hope in ALS is related to longevity, mediated by self-care dietary behavioral choices, dietary, or otherwise.

Caregivers' resentment, as perceived by the subjects, is related to subjects' reports of whether their dietary habits have changed as a result of losses associated with the disease. Perhaps this reflects a sense of guilt in the person with ALS, in relationship to the caregiver to whom they may feel burdensome. Some previous papers have reported on a sense of feeling guilty toward the caregiver as one of the most distressing issues for a person with ALS (Bolmsjo, 2001). It seems possible that if a subject indicates higher caregiver resentment, that the reported perception of caregiver's resentment could be to some extent a projection of an inner sense of guilt. Another possibility is that the person may accurately perceive the high resentment of the caregiver, and therefore experience some guilt that leads to his/her having a lower enjoyment of life, including dietary habits. Clinically addressing and attenuating caregivers' resentment could possibly reduce the ALS diagnosed persons' resentment level, to the extent that part of the latter's resentment of ALS is related to being dependent upon a caregiver with high resentment. Previous research has demonstrated that caregiver depression is related to the depression experienced by the patient, and therefore, addressing caregiver depression may also reduce patient distress (Pagnini et al., 2010, 2012a).

This study presents some limitations. The use of non-validated instruments, such as the survey questions that we have created, may reduce the validity of the results. Further studies with validated questionnaires about anger, hate, and resentment are warranted. The cross-sectional design does not allow any causal inferences between variables, even if these can be discussed in the interpretation. Moreover, the sample size was small and it is possible that some correlations would be underestimated. Finally, the choice of an Internet-based survey may limit the external validity of the study to people with ALS who have access to Internet, and who can easily communicate with a keyboard, augmentative communication, or with personal assistance. The self-selection of the sample may further reduce the generalizability of results, and there was no premorbid attitudinal assessment to compare to the current attitudes. The only inclusion criteria was a self-reported diagnosis of ALS, and we had no chance to verify this information. However, subjects did not receive any compensation, therefore we consider the chance of subjects' participation without ALS not probable. Moreover, there is a balance between male and females in our sample, but it seems that ALS is lightly more prevalent in males, suggesting that the sample could be non-completely representative. Therefore, further studies with representative samples, longitudinal and experimental designs are required to confirm and deepen the findings presented in this paper.

CONCLUSION

The present study is a first attempt to investigate hate, resentment, and hope in ALS, in relationship to each other and in relationship to the willingness to follow a strict nutrient-dense diet, if it were shown to increase longevity. We conducted an online survey, where people with ALS were directly invited to provide answers. Results indicate that there is a massive presence of hope in our sample, with heterogeneous levels of hate and resentment; the three constructs were interrelated. Subjects with hope of living 10 years or more were more likely to report a willingness to make dietary lifestyle changes if such changes were demonstrated to increase longevity. Resentment and hate tended to be higher in people who have had ALS for less time, and in women. People who have lived with ALS for more time expressed a higher level of hope to live 10 years or more.

The main findings of this research indicate that hate, resentment, and hope could be important issues to investigate in future ALS studies. Their roles in the acceptance process of the illness, and how hate and resentment feelings as well as hopelessness may be clinically treated, are important topics to be explored by ALS researchers and clinicians. In particular, the development of specific psychological interventions, or research about existing psychological treatments applied to people with ALS, seems important to improve patients' and caregivers' quality of life (Pagnini et al., 2012b).

REFERENCES

Andrews, J. (2009). Amyotrophic lat- eral sclerosis: clinical management and research update. *Curr. Neurol. Neurosci. Rep.* 9, 59–68.

Bolmsjo, I. (2001). Existential issues in palliative care: interviews of patients with amyotrophic lateral sclerosis. *J. Palliat. Med.* 4, 499–505.

Brettschneider, J., Kurent, J., Ludolph, A., and Mitchell, J. D. (2008). Drug therapy for pain in amyotrophic lat- eral sclerosis or motor neuron dis- ease. *Cochrane Database Syst. Rev.* CD005226.

Centers, L. C. (2001). Beyond denial and despair: ALS and our heroic potential for hope. *J. Palliat. Care* 17, 259–264.

Dal Bello-Haas, V., Andrews-Hinders, D., Bocian, J., Mascha, E., Wheeler, T., and Mitsumoto, H. (2000). Spir- itual well-being of the individual with amyotrophic lateral sclerosis. *Amyotroph. Lateral Scler.* 1, 337–341.

De Groot, I. J., Post, M. W., van Heuveln, T., Van den Berg, L. H., and Lindeman, E. (2007). Cross- sectional and longitudinal correla- tions between disease progression and different health-related qual- ity of life domains in persons with amyotrophic lateral sclerosis. *Amy- otroph. Lateral Scler.* 8, 356–361.

Fanos, J. H., Gelinas, D. F., Foster, R. S., Postone, N., and Miller, R. G. (2008). Hope in palliative care: from narcissism to self-transcendence in amyotrophic lateral sclerosis. *J. Pal- liat. Med.* 11, 470–475.

Ganzini, L., Johnston, W. S., and Hoff- man, W. F. (1999). Correlates of suf- fering in amyotrophic lateral sclero- sis. *Neurology* 52, 1434–1440.

Ganzini, L., Silveira, M. J., and John-ston, W. S. (2002). Predictors and correlates of interest in assisted sui- cide in the final month of life among ALS patients in Oregon and Wash- ington. *J. Pain Symptom. Manage.* 24, 312–317.

Ilzecka, J., Stelmasiak, Z., and Balicka, G. (2003). Respiratory function in amyotrophic lateral sclerosis. *Neu- rol. Sci.* 24, 288–289.

Melazzini, M. (2007). Amyotrophic lat- eral sclerosis viewed from a patient's perspective. *Monaldi Arch. Chest Dis.* 67, 4–5.

Paganoni, S., Deng, J., Jaffa, M., Cud- kowicz, M. E., and Wills, A. M. (2011). Body mass index, not dys- lipidemia, is an independent predic- tor of survival in amyotrophic lateral sclerosis. *Muscle Nerve* 44, 20–24.

Pagnini, F. (2012). Psychological wellbeing and quality of life in amyotrophic lateral sclero- sis: a review. *Int. J. Psychol.* doi:10.1080/00207594.2012.691977

Pagnini, F., Lunetta, C., Banfi, P., Rossi, G., Gorni, K., Castelnuovo, G., et al. (2012a). Anxiety and depression in patients with amyotrophic lateral sclerosis and their caregivers. *Curr. Psychol.* 31, 79–87.

Pagnini, F., Simmons, Z., Corbo, M., and Molinari, E. (2012b). Amy- otrophic lateral sclerosis: time for research on psychological interven- tion? *Amyotroph. Lateral Scler.* 13, 416–417.

Pagnini, F., Rossi, G., Lunetta, C., Banfi, P., Castelnuovo, G., Corbo, M., et al. (2010). Burden, depres- sion, and anxiety in caregivers of people with amyotrophic lateral sclerosis. *Psychol. Health Med.* 15, 685–693.

Palmieri, A., Soraru, G., Albertini, E., Semenza, C., Vottero-Ris, F., D'Ascenzo, C., et al. (2010). Psy- chopathological features and suici- dal ideation in amyotrophic lateral sclerosis patients. *Neurol. Sci.* 31, 735–740.

Plahuta, J. M., McCulloch, B. J., Kasarskis, E. J., Ross, M. A., Wal- ter, R. A., and McDonald, E. R. (2002). Amyotrophic lateral sclero- sis and hopelessness: psychosocial factors. *Soc. Sci. Med.* 55, 2131–2140.

Rabkin, J. G., Wagner, G. J., and Del Bene, M. (2000). Resilience and distress among amyotrophic lateral sclerosis patients and caregivers. *Psy- chosom. Med.* 62, 271–279.

Radunovic, A., Mitsumoto, H., and Leigh, P. N. (2007). Clinical care of patients with amyotrophic lateral sclerosis. *Lancet Neurol.* 6, 913–925.

Simmons, Z. (2005). Management strategies for patients with amy- otrophic lateral sclerosis from diagnosis through death. *Neurologist* 11, 257–270.

Telford, K., Kralik, D., and Koch, T. (2006). Acceptance and denial: implications for people adapting to chronic illness: literature review. *J. Adv. Nurs.* 55, 457–464.

Worms, P. M. (2001). The epidemiology of motor neuron diseases: a review of recent studies. *J. Neurol. Sci.* 191, 3–9.

Permissions

All chapters in this book were first published in CMMMNDALS, by Frontiers; hereby published with permission under the Creative Commons Attribution License or equivalent. Every chapter published in this book has been scrutinized by our experts. Their significance has been extensively debated. The topics covered herein carry significant findings which will fuel the growth of the discipline. They may even be implemented as practical applications or may be referred to as a beginning point for another development.

The contributors of this book come from diverse backgrounds, making this book a truly international effort. This book will bring forth new frontiers with its revolutionizing research information and detailed analysis of the nascent developments around the world.

We would like to thank all the contributing authors for lending their expertise to make the book truly unique. They have played a crucial role in the development of this book. Without their invaluable contributions this book wouldn't have been possible. They have made vital efforts to compile up to date information on the varied aspects of this subject to make this book a valuable addition to the collection of many professionals and students.

This book was conceptualized with the vision of imparting up-to-date information and advanced data in this field. To ensure the same, a matchless editorial board was set up. Every individual on the board went through rigorous rounds of assessment to prove their worth. After which they invested a large part of their time researching and compiling the most relevant data for our readers.

The editorial board has been involved in producing this book since its inception. They have spent rigorous hours researching and exploring the diverse topics which have resulted in the successful publishing of this book. They have passed on their knowledge of decades through this book. To expedite this challenging task, the publisher supported the team at every step. A small team of assistant editors was also appointed to further simplify the editing procedure and attain best results for the readers.

Apart from the editorial board, the designing team has also invested a significant amount of their time in understanding the subject and creating the most relevant covers. They scrutinized every image to scout for the most suitable representation of the subject and create an appropriate cover for the book.

The publishing team has been an ardent support to the editorial, designing and production team. Their endless efforts to recruit the best for this project, has resulted in the accomplishment of this book. They are a veteran in the field of academics and their pool of knowledge is as vast as their experience in printing. Their expertise and guidance has proved useful at every step. Their uncompromising quality standards have made this book an exceptional effort. Their encouragement from time to time has been an inspiration for everyone.

The publisher and the editorial board hope that this book will prove to be a valuable piece of knowledge for researchers, students, practitioners and scholars across the globe.

List of Contributors

Valeria Crippa, Mariarita Galbiati, Paola Rusmini, Elisa Giorgetti, Riccardo Cristofani and Angelo Poletti
Sezione di Biomedicina e Endocrinologia, Dipartimento di Scienze Farmacologiche e Biomolecolari, Centro di Eccellenza sulle Malattie Neurodegenerative, Università degli Studi di Milano, Milano, Italy
Centro Inter Universitario sulle Malattie Neurodegenerative, Università degli Studi di Firenze, Milano, Genova e Roma Tor Vergata, Italy

Alessandra Boncoraglio
Sezione di Biomedicina e Endocrinologia, Dipartimento di Scienze Farmacologiche e Biomolecolari, Centro di Eccellenza sulle Malattie Neurodegenerative, Università degli Studi di Milano, Milano, Italy
Centro Inter Universitario sulle Malattie Neurodegenerative, Università degli Studi di Firenze, Milano, Genova e Roma Tor Vergata, Italy
Department of Cell Biology, University Medical Center of Groningen, Groningen, Netherlands

Tanya Aggarwal
Department of Neuroscience and Brain Technologies, Istituto Italiano di Tecnologia, Genova, Italy

Serena Carra
Department of Cell Biology, University Medical Center of Groningen, Groningen, Netherlands
Sezione di Fisiologia e Neuroscienze, Dipartimento di Scienze Biomediche, Metaboliche e Neuroscienze, Università degli Studi di Modena e Reggio Emilia, Modena, Italy

Maria Pennuto
Department of Neuroscience and Brain Technologies, Istituto Italiano di Tecnologia, Genova, Italy
Dulbecco Telethon Institute Laboratory of Neurodegenerative Diseases, Centre for Integrative Biology (CIBIO), University of Trento, Italy

Melissa Bowerman, Frédérique Scamps and Cédric Raoul
The Neuroscience Institute of Montpellier, INM, INSERM UMR1051, Saint Eloi Hospital, Montpellier, France

Thierry Vincent
The Neuroscience Institute of Montpellier, INM, INSERM UMR1051, Saint Eloi Hospital, Montpellier, France
Department of Immunology, Saint Eloi Hospital, Montpellier, France

Florence E. Perrin
The Neuroscience Institute of Montpellier, INM, INSERM UMR1051, Saint Eloi Hospital, Montpellier, France
Integrative Biology of Neuroregeneration, Faculty of Science, University of Montpellier 2, Montpellier, France

William Camu
The Neuroscience Institute of Montpellier, INM, INSERM UMR1051, Saint Eloi Hospital, Montpellier, France
Department of Neurology, ALS Reference Center, Gui-de-Chauliac Hospital, Montpellier, France

Laura Jelsone-Swain
Department of Radiology, University of Michigan, Ann Arbor, MI, USA

Carol Persad, Kristen L. Votruba and Sara L. Weisenbach
Department of Psychiatry, University of Michigan, Ann Arbor, MI, USA

Timothy Johnson
Department of Biostatistics, University of Michigan, Ann Arbor, MI, USA

Kirsten L. Gruis
Department of Neurology, The State University of New York Upstate Medical University, Syracuse, NY, USA

Robert C. Welsh
Department of Radiology, University of Michigan, Ann Arbor, MI, USA
Department of Psychiatry, University of Michigan, Ann Arbor, MI, USA

Yannick N. Gerber
Institute for Neurosciences of Montpellier (INM), INSERM U 1051, Montpellier, France
"Integrative Biology of Neurodegeneration," IKERBASQUE Basque Foundation for Science, Neuroscience Department, University of the Basque Country, Bilbao, Spain

Alain Privat
Institute for Neurosciences of Montpellier (INM), INSERM U 1051, Montpellier, France

Florence E. Perrin
Institute for Neurosciences of Montpellier (INM), INSERM U 1051, Montpellier, France
"Integrative Biology of Neurodegeneration," IKERBASQUE Basque Foundation for Science, Neuroscience Department, University of the Basque Country, Bilbao, Spain
"Integrative Biology of Neuroregeneration," Faculty of Science, University of Montpellier 2, Montpellier, France

Fabiola Rojas, Nicole Cortes, Sebastian Abarzua, Agnieszka Dyrda and Brigitte van Zunder
Faculty of Biological Sciences and Faculty of Medicine, Center for Biomedical Research, Universidad Andres Bello, Santiago, Chile

Paul R. Heath, Janine Kirby and Pamela J. Shaw
Sheffield Institute for Translational Neuroscience, University of Sheffield, Sheffield, UK

Kim A. Staats
KU Leuven Laboratory of Neurobiology and Leuven Research Institute for Neuroscience and Disease (LIND), Leuven, Belgium
VIB Vesalius Research Center, KU Leuven, Leuven, Belgium
VIB Autoimmune Genetics Laboratory, KU Leuven, Leuven, Belgium
Department of Microbiology and Immunology, University of Leuven, Leuven, Belgium

Susann Schönefeldt, Marike Van Rillaer and Adrian Liston
VIB Autoimmune Genetics Laboratory, KU Leuven, Leuven, Belgium
Department of Microbiology and Immunology, University of Leuven, Leuven, Belgium

Annelies Van Hoecke and Ludo Van Den Bosch
KU Leuven Laboratory of Neurobiology and Leuven Research Institute for Neuroscience and Disease (LIND), Leuven, Belgium
VIB Vesalius Research Center, KU Leuven, Leuven, Belgium

Philip Van Damme and Wim Robberecht
KU Leuven Laboratory of Neurobiology and Leuven Research Institute for Neuroscience and Disease (LIND), Leuven, Belgium
VIB Vesalius Research Center, KU Leuven, Leuven, Belgium
Neurology, University Hospitals Leuven, Leuven, Belgium

Rafael Lazo-Gómez, Uri N. Ramírez-Jarquín, Luis B. Tovar-y-Romo and Ricardo Tapia
División de Neurociencias, Instituto de Fisiología Celular, Universidad Nacional Autónoma de México, D. F., México

Ruben G. L. Real
Department of Psychology I, Institute of Psychology, University of Würzburg, Würzburg, Germany

Thorsten Dickhaus
Weierstrass Institute for Applied Analysis and Stochastics, Research Group "Stochastic Algorithms and Nonparametric Statistics", Berlin, Germany

Albert Ludolph
Department of Neurology, University of Ulm, Ulm, Germany

Martin Hautzinger
Department of Clinical Psychology and Psychotherapy, University of Tübingen, Tübingen, Germany

Andrea Kübler
Department of Psychology I, Institute of Psychology, University of Würzburg, Würzburg, Germany
Institute for Medical Psychology and Behavioural Neurobiology, University of Tübingen, Tübingen, Germany

Yoshiaki Furukawa
Laboratory for Mechanistic Chemistry of Biomolecules, Department of Chemistry, Keio University, Yokohama, Japan

Jerònia Lladó, Laia Tolosa and Gabriel Olmos
Grup de Neurobiologia Celular, Departament de Biologia, Universitat de les Illes Balears, Palma de Mallorca, Spain
Institut Universitari d'Investigacions en Ciències de la Salut (IUNICS), Universitat de les Illes Balears, Palma de Mallorca, Spain

Mariko Ogawa and Yoshiaki Furukawa
Laboratory for Mechanistic Chemistry of Biomolecules, Department of Chemistry, Keio University, Yokohama, Japan

Jesús S. Mora and Teresa Salas
ALS Unit, Department of Neurology, Hospital Carlos III, Madrid, Spain

María L. Fajardo
Department of Epidemiology, Consejería de Salud de Andalucía, Huelva, Spain

Lourdes Iváñez
Department of Epidemiology, Consejería de Salud de Andalucía, Sevilla, Spain

Francisco Rodríguez-Santos
Department of Clinical Psychology, School of Psychology, Universidad Autónoma, Madrid, Spain

Svitlana Garbuzova-Davis
Department of Neurosurgery and Brain Repair, Center of Excellence for Aging and Brain Repair, Morsani College of Medicine, University of South Florida, Tampa, FL, USA
Department of Molecular Pharmacology and Physiology, Morsani College of Medicine, University of South Florida, Tampa, FL, USA
Department of Pathology and Cell Biology, Morsani College of Medicine, University of South Florida, Tampa, FL, USA

Paul R. Sanberg
Department of Neurosurgery and Brain Repair, Center of Excellence for Aging and Brain Repair, Morsani College of Medicine, University of South Florida, Tampa, FL, USA
Department of Molecular Pharmacology and Physiology, Morsani College of Medicine, University of South Florida, Tampa, FL, USA
Department of Pathology and Cell Biology, Morsani College of Medicine, University of South Florida, Tampa, FL, USA
Department of Psychiatry, Morsani College of Medicine, University of South Florida, Tampa, FL, USA

Luis B. Tovar-y-Romo, Uri Nimrod Ramírez-Jarquín, Rafael Lazo-Gómez and Ricardo Tapia
División de Neurociencias, Instituto de Fisiología Celular, Universidad Nacional Autónoma de México, Mexico City, Mexico

Margaret Wong
Department of Pathology, Division of Neuropathology, Johns Hopkins University School of Medicine, Baltimore, MD, USA

Barry Gertz and Barry A. Chestnut
Department of Pathology, Division of Neuropathology, Johns Hopkins University School of Medicine, Baltimore, MD, USA
Department of Pathology, Pathobiology Graduate Program, Johns Hopkins University School of Medicine, Baltimore, MD, USA

Lee J. Martin
Department of Pathology, Division of Neuropathology, Johns Hopkins University School of Medicine, Baltimore, MD, USA
Department of Pathology, Pathobiology Graduate Program, Johns Hopkins University School of Medicine, Baltimore, MD, USA
Department of Neuroscience, Johns Hopkins University School of Medicine, Baltimore, MD, USA

Arianna Palmieri, Johann Roland Kleinbub, Vincenzo Calvo, Irene Messina and Marco Sambin
Department of Philosophy, Sociology, Pedagogy and Applied Psychology, University of Padova, Padova, Italy

Gianni Sorarù and Irene Grasso
Department of Neurosciences, University of Padova, Padova, Italy

Laura Mòdol, Renzo Mancuso, Albert Alé, Isaac Francos-Quijorna and Xavier Navarro
Department of Cell Biology, Physiology, and Immunology, Centro de Investigación Biomédica en Red sobre Enfermedades Neurodegenerativas, Institute of Neurosciences, Universitat Autònoma de Barcelona, Bellaterra, Spain

Emiliano Trias, Pablo Díaz-Amarilla, Silvia Olivera-Bravo and Eugenia Isasi
Instituto de Investigaciones Biológicas Clemente Estable, Montevideo, Uruguay

Derek A. Drechsel, Nathan Lopez and C. Samuel Bradford
Department of Biochemistry and Biophysics, Oregon State University, Corvallis, OR, USA
Environmental Health Sciences Center, Oregon State University, Corvallis, OR, USA

Kyle E. Ireton
Department of Biochemistry and Biophysics, Oregon State University, Corvallis, OR, USA
Environmental Health Sciences Center, Oregon State University, Corvallis, OR, USA
Institut Pasteur de Montevideo, Montevideo, Uruguay

Joseph S. Beckman
Department of Biochemistry and Biophysics, Oregon State University, Corvallis, OR, USA
Environmental Health Sciences Center, Oregon State University, Corvallis, OR, USA
Linus Pauling Institute, Oregon State University, Corvallis, OR, USA

Luis Barbeito
Institut Pasteur de Montevideo, Montevideo, Uruguay
Florent Schmitt, Ghulam Hussain, Luc Dupuis, Jean-Philippe Loeffler and Alexandre Henriques
Mécanismes Centraux et Périphériques de la Neurodégénerescence, INSERM U1118, Strasbourg, France
UMRS1118, Fédération de Médecine Translationnelle de Strasbourg, Université de Strasbourg, France

Ralf Stutzki and Stella Reiter-Theil
Clinical Ethics Support and Accompanying Research, University Hospital Basel/Psychiatric University Hospitals Basel, Institut für Bio- und Medizin Ethik, University of Basel, Basel, Switzerland

Ursula Schneider and Markus Weber
Muskelzentrum/ALS Clinic, Kantonsspital St. Gallen, St. Gallen, Switzerland

Melissa S. Rotunno and Daryl A. Bosco
Department of Neurology, University of Massachusetts Medical Center, Worcester, MA, USA

Gabriela P. de Oliveira, Chrystian J. Alves and Gerson Chadi
Department of Neurology, Neuroregeneration Center, University of São Paulo School of Medicine, São Paulo, Brazil

C. Oster
The Healers Campaign, Haslett, MI, USA

F. Pagnini
Department of Psychology, Catholic University of Milan, Milan, Italy
Niguarda Ca' Granda Hospital, Milan, Italy

Index

www.ingramcontent.com/pod-product-compliance
Lightning Source LLC
LaVergne TN
LVHW060537210926
848485LV00005B/1216
* 9 7 8 1 6 3 9 8 7 0 4 4 8 *